HANDBOOK OF PLASTIC SURGERY

Edited by

Steven E. Greer, M.D.
New York, New York, U.S.A.

Prosper Benhaim, M.D.
David Geffen School of Medicine at UCLA
Los Angeles, California, U.S.A.

H. Peter Lorenz, M.D.
Stanford University School of Medicine
Stanford, California, U.S.A.

James Chang, M.D.
Stanford University School of Medicine
Stanford, California, U.S.A.

Marc H. Hedrick, M.D.
David Geffen School of Medicine at UCLA
Los Angeles, California, U.S.A.

MARCEL DEKKER

MARCEL DEKKER NEW YORK

Library of Congress Cataloging-in-Publication Data
A catalog record for this book is available from the Library of Congress.

ISBN: 0-8247-4296-6

This book is printed on acid-free paper.

Headquarters
Marcel Dekker
270 Madison Avenue, New York, NY 10016, U.S.A.
tel: 212-696-9000; fax: 212-685-4540

Distribution and Customer Service
Marcel Dekker
Cimarron Road, Monticello, New York 12701, U.S.A.
tel: 800-228-1160; fax: 845-796-1772

World Wide Web
http://www.dekker.com

Current printing (last digit):

10 9 8 7 6 5 4 3 2 1

PRINTED IN THE UNITED STATES OF AMERICA

Preface

The idea for the *Handbook of Plastic Surgery* came to me during my second year in general surgery training at New York University when I was on the plastic surgery service. I had read an excellent single volume hardback reference book on plastic surgery, but still wanted a more "high-yield" portable handbook to carry with me. A year later, while doing my first year of full-time research at the Institute of Reconstructive Plastic Surgery at NYU, I sought out a publishing partner and began the task of editing and writing portions of a comprehensive handbook with the assistance of co-editors/authors who have distinguished themselves in academic plastic surgery. I am most grateful to the select few who had the foresight and confidence in us to support this project. It was a pleasure working with all the authors of this book.

I wanted the book to be an edited project with recognized luminaries of each field contributing. At the same time, I also realized that surgical residents are highly educated and underutilized resources who could provide much of the content of the chapters in a timely manner. When paired with their respective attending surgeons, the resident/attending chapters could provide a quality of work not otherwise possible for such a handbook and would incorporate both resident and attending perspectives alike in order to maximize the educational content of this book. This concept was key to the project.

Being an edited book with numerous authors, the reader will note slightly different styles among the chapters, and that is intentional. It certainly would not have been appropriate for us to instruct senior, highly respected plastic surgeons with international reputations to alter their style to meet some arbitrary rigid style constraints.

The goal of the *Handbook* was to be comprehensive enough to serve as one of several study resources for both the written and oral board examinations in plastic surgery that would complement other established resources as an easy-to-use, practical, and high-yield alternative. Even established plastic surgeons studying for a recertification board examination will find a wide breadth of information presented in a pragmatic approach useful for review in an efficient, yet detailed, format. Unlike many formal textbooks, the outline nature of the book is also designed to be a quick-read for fellows, residents, and medical students on call or preparing for patient rounds.

Although a tall task, our desire was to find a niche of utility that spans the gamut from medical student to practicing plastic surgeon. We also wanted the Handbook to be useful to several specialties. Plastic surgery, otolaryngology, dermatology, and emergency medicine all have overlapping areas of practice covered in this *Handbook*, as do orthopedic surgery and plastic surgery with the hand and microsurgery sections.

The *Handbook of Plastic Surgery* is modeled after a few successful handbooks in medicine. The bullet point outline of the book is inspired by the high yield format of the *Washington Manual* of internal medicine and the *Mont Reid Surgical Handbook* of general surgery. The ten major sections are organized like many other plastic surgery texts, but with some exceptions. The Patient Management section includes chapters that I found lacking in other sources. The Pediatric Plastic Surgery section has many topics usually found under Head and Neck sections. Likewise, we felt that Breast and Microsurgery deserved to be separate sections.

Many people graciously contributed their time to this project. Dr. Benhaim deserves special recognition for the hundreds of hours of work that he put into this book editing all of the chapters within his section and the other sections. His assistance in coordinating with the other attendings was crucial toward maintaining the momentum of the book. I am also grateful to our publisher, Marcel Dekker, for seeing this project to its completion.

Steven E. Greer, M.D.
Editor-in-Chief

Contents

Part IV Head and Neck

Part V Pediatric Plastic Surgery

Part VI Microsurgery

Part VII Hand Surgery

1

Bleeding, Blood Products, and Hemostasis

Loren J. Borud, M.D.
Beth Israel Deaconess Medical Center, Boston, Massachusetts, U.S.A.

I. BLEEDING AND PLASTIC SURGERY

A. Basic Tenets

1. Blood loss is of fundamental concern in all surgical patients. Major bleeding can be life threatening, especially in pediatric patients undergoing substantial reconstructive procedures.
2. In facial aesthetic surgery, hematoma is the most frequent major complication, occurring in 1–3% of patients, with about twice that incidence in males.
3. Even in procedures as straightforward as skin grafting, hematomas interfere with neovascularization and are the number one cause of skin graft failure.
4. By adhering to the following basic surgical principles, most abnormal surgical bleeding can be avoided.

B. Adequate Preoperative Evaluation

1. A careful medical and family history can alert the plastic surgeon to most systemic coagulopathies.
2. High-risk patients or any patient undergoing a major reconstructive procedure should have a basic laboratory evaluation consisting of hematocrit, prothrombin time (PT), and activated partial thromboplastin time (aPTT).
3. Patients on warfarin, heparin, or aspirin should be questioned closely about the indication and duration of anticoagulant therapy.
4. Often, consultation with medical colleagues or hematologists is required.

C. Avoidance of Antiplatelet Medication

1. Patients are often unaware that aspirin, nonsteroidal anti-inflammatory medications, and many other nonprescription medications can interfere with normal clotting mechanisms.
2. "Herbal medications" such as ginger, ginkgo biloba, ginseng, and grapeseed extract have been shown to reduce platelet aggregation and should be discontinued before surgery.

D. Autologous Donation

1. Although not frequently indicated in plastic surgical procedures, patients undergoing ablative and/or reconstructive procedures associated with significant blood loss should be counseled about the possibility of autologous donation. Depending on the blood bank protocol, donation begins 2–4 weeks before surgery, sometimes in small-volume donations every 3 days.
2. In special cases, recombinant erythropoietin can be used to restore blood cell mass before surgery.

3. Autologous blood should not be transfused into the patient unless the blood is truly needed. Case reports of multisystem organ failure and death from autologous blood transfusions (possibly due to laboratory contamination) have been reported.

E. Meticulous Surgical Technique and Drainage

1. There is no substitute for meticulous hemostasis with cautery and suture ligation of larger vessels.
2. Placement of drains never prevents a hematoma, but they sometimes alert the clinician to ongoing postoperative blood loss.

F. Perioperative Management

1. Even a single Valsalva maneuver during traumatic extubation can result in a hematoma following soft tissue procedures, especially facialplasty and blepharoplasty.
2. Wide blood pressure fluctuations should be avoided with antihypertensive agents, sedation, and appropriate analgesics.

G. Dressings

1. For many plastic surgical procedures, dressings play a significant role in preventing hematomas.
2. Bolstered dressings and pressure dressings are used in most skin graft procedures.
3. Compression dressing are used by some plastic surgeons following abdominoplasty, facialplasty, and other subcutaneous procedures, but their use for these indications is not proven scientifically.

II. HEMOSTASIS

A detailed description of the complex mechanism of hemostasis is beyond the scope of this text. Briefly, the first events following injury are platelet degranulation, vasoconstriction, and formation of a platelet plug. Bleeding time is a measure of this process.

A. The Clotting Cascade

The currently accepted understanding of the clotting cascade is seen in Fig. 1.

B. PT and aPTT

Elevations in PT occur due to lack of the vitamin K–dependent factors (II, VII, IX, and X). Elevations in aPTT occur due to either a deficiency in the intrinsic pathway (high molecular weight kininogen, prekallikrein, XII, XI, IX, and VIII) or a deficiency in the common pathway (fibrinogen, II, V, and X).

III. HEREDITARY COAGULOPATHIES

The most commonly encountered hereditary coagulopathies (in patients or in examinations) are listed here.

A. Hemophilia A

1. X-linked deficiency of factor VIII.
2. The most common "hemophilia," with an incidence of 1/10,000 males.
3. Characterized by elevated PTT, normal PT and bleeding time (BT), and decreased VIII: C (i.e., functional factor VIII).
4. Recombinant factor VIII is now generally available for treatment.

B. Hemophilia B

1. Another X-linked disorder.
2. Also known as Christmas disease.
3. Accounts for only about 15% of all hemophilia.
4. Characterized by increased PTT, normal PT, BT, and decreased factor IX levels.
5. Recombinant factor IX is generally available.

C. Factor XI Deficiency

1. Also known as Rosenthal's syndrome.
2. Again, characterized by isolated PTT elevation.
3. Only described in descendents of Ashkenazi Jews, this disorder is frequently subclinical and not always known to adult patients undergoing surgery.
4. Recombinant factor XI is not available at this time in the United States.
5. Fresh-frozen plasma is used in high-risk patients.

D. Von Willebrand's Disease

1. The most common hereditary coagulopathy, this disease affects men and women equally, with an incidence of 1/800.

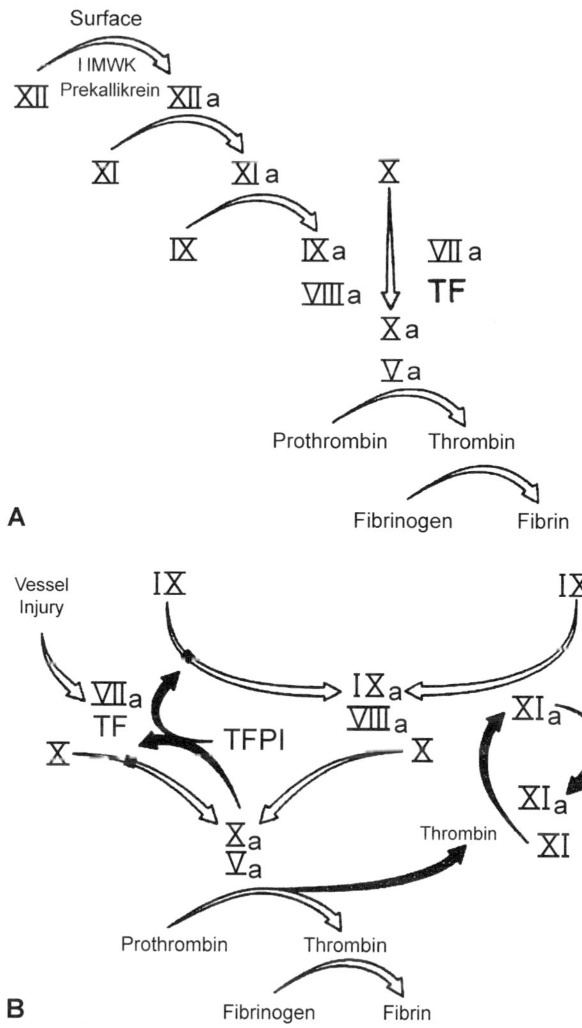

Figure 1 (A) Classic coagulation cascade and (B) revised model. (From Gailani D; Broze GJ. Factor XI activation by thrombin and factor XIa. *Semin. Thromb. Haemost* 19:396, 1993.)

2. Generally, this coagulopathy is characterized by elevated PTT with normal PT but an abnormal bleeding time.
3. Treatment is with cryoprecipitate or DDAVP.

IV. TRANSFUSION RISKS

Transfusion risks are rapidly changing due to improved screening methods.

A. Systemic Reactions

1. "Transfusion reactions" consisting of mild fever and urticaria are as common as 1–2%.
2. Anaphylaxis incidence is 1/150,000.
3. Serious hemolytic reactions incidence is 1/6000.

B. Infectious Complications

U.S. government figures for infections per unit transfusion are:

1. Hepatitis B: 1/63,000
2. Hepatitis C: 1/4100
3. Hepatitis non-ABC: 1/5,900
4. HIV: 1/450,000

V. OCCUPATIONAL RISKS OF BLOOD PRODUCT EXPOSURE

Risks to the health care provider during surgical procedures depend on the specialty. Orthopedic and gynecologic procedures are more prone to such exposure than plastic surgery. Nonetheless, incidents and occupational exposure are extremely disconcerting to the health care provider. In some reports, blood exposure to at least one operating room staff member or surgeon occurs as frequently as 17–33%.

A. Avoiding Needlesticks

It may be of some solace to the surgeon that hollow point needles, which contain a column of blood, are much more dangerous than suture needles. Adherence to the following principles can reduce incidence of occupational exposure for surgeons:

1. Universal precautions—assume every patient has a bloodborne infectious disease.
2. Use of barriers—eye protection, double gloving, sleeve protectors. In double gloving, it has been shown that the outer glove "wipes off" much of the blood on a suture needle, decreasing the inoculum to the surgeon in the event of needle stick.
3. Sharps precautions—especially in high-risk cases, sharps should not be passed from hand to hand, but by way of a water basin or separate Mayo stand.

B. Management of Needlesticks

1. The injured surgeon or staff should immediately scrub out and wash the area vigorously with Betadine.
2. Unless immediate patient safety is endangered, the injured individual should proceed immediately to employee health or the emergency room.
3. It is thought by most infectious disease specialists that triple HIV prophylaxis therapy (retrovir, epivir, and crixivan) is most efficacious when started within hours of the needlestick.
4. Both the patient and the injured worker are tested for HIV and hepatitis. In cases of the HIV-positive patient, triple therapy should be continued for several weeks, with intermittent serological examination as dictated by the local protocol.

VI. THE JEHOVAH'S WITNESS PATIENT

The Jehovah's Witness patient is religiously opposed to transfusion of blood products. An informed consent discussion should take place with appropriate documentation in the medical record. The specific views of the individual patient should be carefully documented. Some such patients are willing to accept autologous blood, autotransfusion blood (i.e., cell saver blood), DDAVP, or erythropoietin therapy.

2

Postoperative Care and Flap Monitoring

Thomas A. Davenport, M.D.*

Memorial Sloan-Kettering Cancer Center, New York, New York, U.S.A.

Joseph J. Disa, M.D.

Memorial Sloan-Kettering Cancer Center and Cornell University College of Medicine, New York, New York, U.S.A.

I. INTRODUCTION

The postoperative care principles for plastic surgery patients are the same as for any other surgical patient. As is the case with other specialties, there are specific instances where plastic surgery patients require more specific attention in order to prevent or detect postoperative problems.

II. FLUID STATUS

A. In terms of fluid status, plastic surgery patients can be approached with the same parameters as other surgical patients. Patients should be monitored and fluid administered to ensure adequate volume status.

B. **Monitor fluid status** using urine output, daily weights, heart rate, and with invasive monitoring (central venous pressure catheter, Swan-Ganz catheter, arterial lines) and renal function tests when necessary.

C. **Give standard intravenous fluid** such as lactated Ringer's or normal saline for 24 hours, then 5% dextrose in 1/2 normal saline afterward for the noncomplicated patient.

D. **Carefully monitor free flap patients for hypovolemia** to avoid hypotension and loss of perfusion pressure to the flap. *Pressors should be used only when absolutely necessary.* Pressors should not be used to treat most episodes of hypotension, since pressors may affect flap perfusion significantly.

III. MONITORING VITAL SIGNS

A. Heart Rate

1. Causes of tachycardia include pain, hypovolemia, arrhythmia, and anemia secondary to blood loss.
2. Causes of bradycardia include arrhythmia (heart block) and use of beta blockers.

B. Blood Pressure

1. Hypertension can result in hemorrhage and hematoma.
2. Hypotension should be monitored carefully in flap surgery to prevent flap ischemia.

C. Temperature

1. Fever may herald infection.

* *Current affiliation*: Long Island Plastic Surgery, Garden City, New York, U.S.A.

IV. RESPIRATORY CARE AND AIRWAYS

A. **Atelectasis** is the most common cause of early postoperative fevers and may progress to pneumonia. The use of inspiratory spirometry and ambulation help reduce atelectasis.

B. **Adequate pain control**, particularly in trunk surgery, will reduce chest wall splinting and subsequent atelectasis.

C. **Airways** in head and neck surgical patients after extubation should be monitored. Head of bed elevation, steroids, and careful monitoring of fluid status may help to prevent airway edema. Elective tracheostomy may be required.

V. DIET

Diet should be individualized by type and location of procedure and preoperative alimentary status.

VI. DRAINS

Drains may help prevent seroma formation, eliminate dead space, promote adherence of flaps, and monitor postoperative bleeding. They should be placed in a dependent position in and away from vessels or anastomoses.

A. **Closed-suction systems** include Jackson-Pratt, Reliavac, and Hemovac systems. These drains create different amounts of suction pressure and should be chosen accordingly. Blake drains have a continuous side port system instead of side holes in the drain portion.

B. **Passive systems** have no suction chamber system, and the fluid drains directly into an overlying dressing through a Penrose drain.

VII. PERIOPERATIVE ANTIBIOTICS

A. **Gram-positive coverage** may be used unless infection is already present or there is suspicion of Gram-negative or other infection.

B. **Postoperative antibiotics** may be used, depending on the surgical procedure and circumstance.

VIII. NAUSEA

A. **Postoperative nausea** is a common complication of general anesthesia.

B. **Postoperative emesis** can cause hematoma, especially in facial cosmetic surgery patients, and should be treated promptly.

C. **Common antiemetics** include prochlorperazine, ondansetron, droperidol, and benzodiazepines.

D. **Nasogastric tube drainage** should be used in esophageal and head and neck reconstruction patients for gastric decompression.

IX. PAIN

A. **Infection or hematoma** can cause an increase in postoperative pain.

B. **Wound inspection** should be prompt and dressings should be removed for pain out of proportion to what is expected from a specific surgical procedure.

C. **Long-acting local anesthetics** can also be used at the end of the procedure to help in postoperative pain control.

D. **Respiratory depression** can result from an overdose of narcotic pain medication.

X. SPECIAL SUBJECTS

A. Craniofacial Surgery

1. **Conduct neurologic exams** and **monitor drain output** regularly.
2. **Monitor vision**, if possible, to detect optic nerve compression or damage.
3. **Monitor dental occlusion** in patients with intermaxillary fixation.
4. **Monitor respiratory status** for possible air embolus.
5. **Monitor wounds** for cerebrospinal fluid (CSF) leak.
6. **Head of bed elevation** helps to reduce edema and headache.
7. **Mouth care** with irrigation and Peridex.
8. **Wire cutters** should be kept at the bedside for intermaxillary fixation patients to allow emergent release of the intermaxillary fixation in cases of postoperative emesis or airway compromise.
9. **Steroids** can be used in specific cases to reduce postoperative edema.

B. Cleft Lip/Palate Surgery

1. **Monitor airway** for edema postoperatively.
2. **Monitor wound** for oral bleeding and possible aspiration of blood.

3. **Monitor fluid status** postoperatively, as patients have a tendency to reject oral hydration.
4. **Monitor wounds** in cleft lip and lip adhesion patients for dehiscence.
5. **Splint arms** postoperatively in young children to prevent disruption of the operative site incisions.
6. **Tongue sutures** may be used to facilitate airway management in cases of airway obstruction.

C. Hand Surgery

1. **Splints/casts** should secure hand and arm in position of safety, position of function, or other position that is most appropriate for the specific procedure performed.
2. **Monitor swelling** of hand/arm. Keep hand elevated, when possible, to reduce swelling.
3. **Hand dressings** should be loose enough to avoid restriction of venous or lymphatic return.
4. **Hand wounds** should be monitored for hematoma, cellulitis, and lymphangitis.

D. Cosmetic Surgery

1. **Compression garments** are used after suction lipectomy and facelifts by some surgeons to minimize postoperative bleeding and tissue edema.
2. **Cool compresses** help reduce swelling in facial cosmetic surgery patients.
3. **Head of bed elevation** helps to reduce swelling in facial surgery patients.
4. **Drains** may help minimize or possibly prevent hematoma or seroma formation.
5. **Nasal splints** help to protect positioning in rhinoplasty patients.
6. **Vision monitoring** is important in periocular surgery patients.

E. Breast Surgery

1. **Limited dressings** make early wound monitoring for hematoma easier.
2. **Drains** may help to reduce hematoma or seroma formation.
3. **Postsurgical bras** may make patients more comfortable and dressings easier to change.

XI. SKIN GRAFTS

A. **Bolster or wrap dressings** should be removed for drainage or odor.

B. **Splints or casts** should be used in areas of skin movement to immobilize the graft bed.

C. **Elevation** is important in grafts to the extremities to reduce edema below the graft.

D. **Donor sites** should be monitored for cellulitis.

XII. SURGICAL FLAPS

A. **Careful monitoring** for vascular compromise is mandatory.

B. **Maintaining the position of flaps** using splints or cushions is important in the early postoperative period.

C. **Drains** help to reduce fluid collections that may compromise the flap perfusion.

D. **Dressings** should be minimal to make flap monitoring easier.

E. **Anticoagulation therapy** may be used postoperatively in free-flap patients.

XIII. FREE-FLAP MONITORING

The refinement of microvascular techniques has brought the failure rate of free tissue transfers to only a few percent. Inherent in optimizing flap survival rate is the early identification of vascular compromise. In order to avoid flap ischemia and the "no-reflow" phenomenon, it is important that vascular compromise be detected early. Several systems of flap monitoring have been devised with different institutional preferences.

A. **Clinical observation (*the gold standard*)**: flap color, blanch test (capillary refill), flap bleeding.

B. **Pulse oximetry** is useful with finger or extremity replantations. Loss of pulsatile flow indicates arterial compromise. Oxygen saturation less than 85% indicates venous compromise.

C. **Temperature** is used with flaps containing a skin paddle or with extremity replants. The flap temperature is compared with local skin temperature as a control. A temperature difference of 3°C or absolute temperature of less than 30°C is suggestive of flap compromise.

D. **Conventional Doppler**: An 8 MHz hand-held Doppler probe is used to perform periodic detection of venous and arterial Doppler signals. It can be difficult to determine a proper signal with other vessels in close proximity. The venous signal can be checked via augmentation with flap compression.

E. **Implantable Doppler** involves 20 MHz probes with an implantable cuff that can be disconnected from the monitor and remains in the patient. It is very useful in buried flaps such as jejunal flaps or vascularized bone transfers.

F. A **laser Doppler** monitor uses a measurement of reflected laser light from a helium neon laser and can be used on the cutaneous surface of a flap or internally with an implantable probe. This technique measures the average velocity of red blood cells moving in capillaries below the probe and the amount of blood in the tissue, as determined by the total intensity of the reflected light.

G. Several other methods of free flap monitoring have been shown to be effective, including transcutaneous oxygen saturation, tissue pH, photoplethysmography, electrical impedance plethysmography, and implantable thermocouplers.

H. **Signs of free-flap compromise** include:

- **Color changes** such as pale or blue appearance or loss of capillary refill
- **Loss of Doppler signal**, either venous or arterial
- **Flap swelling** may indicate venous thrombosis
- **Decrease in flap temperature** compared to control skin temperature
- **Loss of pulse oximetry signal** or oxygen saturation

3

Cardiopulmonary Complications in Plastic Surgery

Arthur W. Perry, M.D.
The University of Medicine and Dentistry of New Jersey—Robert Wood Johnson Medical School, Piscataway, New Jersey and The University of Pennsylvania School of Medicine, Philadelphia, Pennsylvania, U.S.A.

Steven E. Greer, M.D.
New York, New York, U.S.A.

Charles A. Bush, M.D.
The Ohio State University College of Medicine, Columbus, Ohio, U.S.A.

I. INTRODUCTION

A. The majority of serious or fatal complications in plastic surgery involve the cardiopulmonary system. The most common is *pulmonary embolism*. Others are unique to plastic surgery, such as *lidocaine toxicity*.

B. Given that almost any minor complication is unacceptable in elective cosmetic surgery, serious or fatal outcomes are even more tragic. Many of these complications can easily occur in the office surgery suite setting where prompt medical support is not available. It is therefore imperative that the plastic surgeon be an expert at diagnosing and treating cardiopulmonary complications.

C. For the medical student and junior resident, a review of the pertinent cardiovascular history, a physical examination, and a basic electrocardiograph interpretation is warranted. (See Appendix B.)

II. LIDOCAINE TOXICITY

A. Lidocaine is an amide local anesthetic that works by interfering with neuronal action potentials. Its most profound toxic effects are on the central nervous system (CNS) and cardiac conduction systems.

B. The action of lidocaine is virtually instantaneous.

C. Lidocaine is effective in concentrations as low as 0.025%.

D. Contraindications to lidocaine include:

- Heart block.
- Congestive heart failure.
- Certain arrhythmias.
- Decreased liver function—as an amide, lidocaine is metabolized in the liver, producing monoethylglycine xylidide and glycine xylidide. These both have overlapping toxicity with lidocaine. The ester **procaine** is a better choice when liver function is impaired.
- Decreased renal function—75% of lidocaine metabolites are excreted into the urine. Lidocaine metabolite levels will rise if excretion is altered.

E. Pharmacokinetics

Toxicity is dependent on the proportion of free versus protein-bound lidocaine. Most is bound to **alpha-1 acid glycoprotein**. Cancer, trauma, myocardial infarction, smoking, uremia, oral contraceptives affect the levels.

A multitude of drugs interact with lidocaine:

- Beta blockers
- Tricyclic antidepressants
- Various diet pills
- Cimetidine

Physiologic conditions influencing lidocaine metabolism include:

- Hypokalemia and hyperkalemia
- Hyphosphatemia
- Hypoalbuminemia

F. Dose Limits

Conventional Subcutaneous Administration

- The generally accepted upper limit of lidocaine use is **4–5 mg/kg**; the upper limit increases to **7 mg/kg** when lidocaine is mixed with epinephrine.
- This usage is based on injection into highly vascular tissues such as muscle.
- The epinephrine causes vasoconstriction and flattens the distribution curve of the lidocaine so that it is absorbed systemically over a period of time that is 50% longer than without epinephrine.

Highly Diluted Method (Tumescent/Wet/Superwet Techniques)

- When lidocaine is administered **into fat** in concentrations of less than 0.1%, along with very diluted epinephrine (1:1,000,000), it is apparent that much larger amounts can be used.
- This technique has been shown to alter the pharmacokinetics dramatically. Lidocaine is absorbed over as long as 24 hours, with peak levels occurring at 10–12 hours postop.
- The actual amount that can be used is debatable. Lidocaine doses of 22 mg/kg have been shown to result in nontoxic blood levels. Some have used significantly higher doses.

Symptoms

- With serum lidocaine levels of 1.5 μg/mL, symptoms of restlessness, drowsiness, dizziness, euphoria, and paresthesias may occur. These can be masked by the use of other drugs such as narcotics and benzodiazepines.
- At higher levels, confusion, agitation, visual disturbances, and vertigo occur, followed by nausea and muscle tremors. Seizures, psychosis, and respiratory depression follow.
- Above 8 μg/mL, coma and cardiovascular and respiratory collapse occur.

ECG Signs (See Appendix)

- Lidocaine blocks cardiac sodium channels.
- Sinus arrest and, rarely, complete heart block can occur.

Treatment

- The best treatment is prevention. Short of that, at the first sign of toxicity, the patient should have intravenous access established and should be transferred to the hospital. Because of the long half-life of lidocaine and the altered volume status in patients who have undergone liposuction, there is no role for observation in the office or at home. Patients showing signs of lidocaine toxicity should be admitted to the intensive care unit and have plasma lidocaine levels repeatedly monitored.
- Treatment of symptomatic arrhythmias with appropriate drugs, as indicated by Advanced Cardiac Life Support algorithms, is indicated.
- Consideration of hemodialysis should be given in severe cases.

Misuse of Lidocaine

- There is no advantage to using large doses of lidocaine when a surgical procedure is performed under general or epidural anesthesia.
- Most plastic surgeons who usually perform liposuction under general or epidural anesthesia and administer tumescent lidocaine should consider not using lidocaine or using lower doses.

General Precautions with Lidocaine Use

- Lidocaine toxicity is a rising complication of liposuction procedures.
- Large-volume lidocaine administration can be painful.
- Large-volume lidocaine use is very dependent on the cardiovascular and renal systems working in perfect unison.
- When intravascular volume depletion occurs, such as with postoperative nausea, dangerously high lidocaine levels can result.
- When lidocaine is used as the sole means of anesthesia, consider performing smaller procedures to limit the total dose of lidocaine. If large volumes of lidocaine are used, patients should be monitored overnight, with careful attention to volume, neurologic status, and cardiac status.

III. EPINEPHRINE

Epinephrine is extremely useful in plastic surgery. The vasoconstriction produced by epinephrine dramatically decreases blood loss, with low risk for rebound bleeding. As an adrenergic agent acting through a second messenger system, its onset is delayed approximately 7–8 minutes.

A. Relative Contraindications

1. Hypertension
2. Stenotic heart valve disease
3. Coronary artery disease
4. Peripheral vascular disease
5. Hyperthyroidism
6. Psychosis
7. Ventricular arrhythmias
8. Distal appendages supplied by end-arteries, such as fingers or penis, due to the risk of infarction

B. Dose Limits

1. Unlike lidocaine, there is no well-described limitation to epinephrine dosing. Using data from pheochromocytoma studies, a serum level of 133 μg/mL has been considered the upper limit of normal.
2. Peak serum levels are achieved approximately within 30 minutes following injection.
3. Injected submucosally, the safe limit is considered to be **6.7 μg/kg**. Conventional subcutaneous limits are not known, but physiologic parameters are readily measurable (pulse, blood pressure).
4. Highly diluted method—Burk showed that doses up to 10 mg are safe when diluted as 1 mg of 1:1000 solution in 1 L of saline. Peak epinephrine levels occur 3 hours after administration of this subcutaneous dilute solution.

C. Symptoms of Epinephrine Excess

1. Tachycardia, hypertension, arrhythmia, psychosis, flushing, sweating, and palpitations.
2. **ECG signs** (see Appendix B)—epinephrine decreases the amplitude of the T wave. In higher doses, the T wave may become biphasic and there can be ST changes. These changes are attributed to myocardial ischemia. Sinus tachycardia, PVCs, ventricular tachycardia, ventricular fibrillation, and ST segment changes of myocardial injury may also occur.
3. **Treatment**
   - Immediate intravenous access is established while preparations for transfer to a hospital are being made.
   - **Beta-blockers** or the cautious use of **phentolamine (alpha-blocker)** may be useful in reversing the adrenergic stimulation. Phentolamine must be used with caution in patients with coronary artery disease.
   - Phentolamine can be injected locally to prevent necrosis after inadvertent injection of epinephrine into digits.

IV. PHENOL TOXICITY

A. Baker and Gordon popularized the phenol chemical peel in the 1960s. Although now less popular than other forms of chemical peel and laser resurfacing, there is still a place for phenol peeling, and it is again rising in popularity.

B. Phenol is metabolized by the liver and excreted in the urine.

C. Phenol is a myocardial irritant and depressant and can cause fatal arrhythmias.

D. Respiratory depression, nephrotoxicity, and hepatic injury may also occur.

E. The amount of phenol absorbed through the intact skin is variable and dependent on pattern of use.

F. Experience has shown that cardiac arrhythmias are rare if the peel is performed in segments.

G. Continuous EKG monitoring must be performed.

V. PULMONARY EDEMA AND CONGESTIVE HEART FAILURE

A. Large-volume liposuction using subcutaneous infiltration may result in the administration of large amounts of fluid. Superwet techniques involve injection of 1 mL of fluid for every 1 mL of fat to be suctioned. Tumescent techniques give 2 mL of fluid for every 1 mL of fat suctioned. With the concomitant "third spacing" that occurs during and after liposuction and the administration of fluid by "clysis," intravenous fluid management may be complicated.

B. For the average healthy person, volume deficit from dehydration and insensible loss prior to surgery is made up by the anesthesiologist prior to induction, and then **a total of twice the volume of total fluid suctioned (fat and water) should be administered**. This is a combination of fluid by clysis and intravenously. Therefore, intravenous fluids are often unnecessary. Lactated Ringer's solution is preferred when necessary.

C. Pulmonary edema may result from excessive volume administration or from preexisting or new-onset heart or renal failure.

D. Patients should be adequately screened prior to surgery. A cardiac preoperative evaluation should be done on any patient who has used **Phentermine-fenfluramine (Phen-fen)**.

E. Placement of a Foley catheter should be strongly considered to facilitate monitoring of fluid status.

VI. PULMONARY EMBOLISM AND DEEP VENOUS THROMBOSIS (DVT)

The most common cause of death following liposuction is pulmonary emboli. Certain risk factors can increase the chance of these events. **Virchow's triad** of stasis, trauma, and a hypercoagulable state are still valid. Stasis is inherent in all surgery, and surgery is clearly considered a form of trauma from a physiologic perspective. Gentle surgery and adequate hydration mitigate against these risk factors.

A. **Oral contraceptives** increase the chance of a DVT from 2 to 12 times. This risk increases if >50 μg of estrogen is used. It is probably safest if these drugs are stopped 4 weeks prior to surgery and not started until 2 weeks postop.

B. Some form of DVT prophylaxis should be used in every case. Either **miniheparin** (5000 U subcutaneous, 2 h preop) or **pneumatic compression stockings** should be used. Having the patient walk just prior to surgery and early after surgery also makes a difference.

C. Postop preventive care—assure that the foot of the bed is elevated. Two to three inches of books placed under the foot of the bed will help venous drainage.

D. **Symptoms of DVT**

- Hot, tender calf (often unreliable)
- Fever
- Unilateral or bilateral inappropriate swelling
- Homan's sign—considered present if pain in the calf containing a DVT is elicited with dorsiflexion of the ankle

E. **Symptoms of pulmonary embolism**

- Pleuritic chest pain
- Nervousness

F. **ECG changes** (see Appendix B) include sinus tachycardia, right bundle branch block (incomplete or complete), signs of right ventricle ischemia (Q waves in leads 2, 3, and AVF; appearance of S wave in leads 1 and V6).

G. **Diagnostic work-up**

- Physical examination
- Duplex Doppler studies—low threshold for examination
- Venogram
- V/Q scan

VII. FAT EMBOLISM

It is important to distinguish fat emboli from thrombopulmonary emboli, as the treatments are different.

While most common following trauma and orthopedic surgery, this complication is rather rare in liposuction procedures. Fat theoretically can be liberated from tissue and sent streaming along blood vessels, stopping in end organs such as the lungs. Fat that lodges in the lungs releases free fatty acids, leading to adult respiratory distress syndrome (ARDS).

Signs and symptoms—hypoxia, tachypnea, fever, tachycardia.

ECG signs—tachycardia.

Other diagnostic studies—plain chest films display diagnostic diffuse patchy infiltrates within 24 hours. In contrast to thromboembolism, pulmonary scans are unreliable.

Treatment—oxygen, positive end-expiratory pressure (PEEP), and corticosteroids. Unlike pulmonary embolism, Dextran and heparin are contraindicated.

VIII. HERBAL MEDICINE DRUG INTERACTIONS

St. John's wort—contains a mild MAO inhibitor and may intensify some anesthetics.

Yohimbe—also displays MAO inhibitor effects and may increase the potency of anesthetics.

Gingko biloba—a powerful anticoagulant.

Ginger, garlic, cayennne, bilberry—antiplatelet activity.

Ginseng—associated with hypertension.

Melatonin—increases anesthesia potency.

Echinacea—affects liver function and drug metabolism.

A multitude of "understudied drugs" are currently in common use. Each drug should be investigated and considered for discontinuation prior to surgery.

4

Flap Loss, Infections, and Other Complications

Kaveh Alizadeh, M.D.*
Memorial Sloan-Kettering Cancer Center, New York, New York, U.S.A.

Joseph J. Disa, M.D.
Memorial Sloan-Kettering Cancer Center and Cornell University Medical College, New York, New York, U.S.A.

The fate of any flap surgery is dependent on the technical execution of the procedure by the surgeon and an early recognition of potential complications with prompt intervention to salvage the flap. It is important to know that prevention of any surgical complication begins in the preoperative phase.

I. PREOPERATIVE ASSESSMENT

A. Patient Selection

1. **Advanced age** is not a factor in the outcome of flaps once the preexisting medical conditions are well controlled.
2. **Systemic disease**, including diabetes, cardiovascular, renal, and pulmonary conditions, can increase the risk of anesthetic complications, but by themselves they do not constitute a contraindication to flap surgery.
3. **History of tobacco smoking** is not a contraindication to flap surgery; however, there is an increased incidence of donor-site wound complications. There is no association with flap loss with free tissue transfer, but pedicle flaps may be less reliable (e.g., TRAM flaps).

* *Current affiliation*: Long Island Plastic Surgery, Garden City, New York, U.S.A.

B. Zone of Injury

1. **Posttraumatic wounds**, especially after a crush injury, may cause damage to local recipient vessels and may make them unsuitable for anastomoses. This is frequently encountered in lower extremity trauma where a large soft tissue defect necessitates a free flap. Ideally, the vascular anastomosis should be performed outside the zone of injury.
2. **Previous irradiation** can lead to blood vessel fibrosis and thickness. Surgical manipulation of these vessels can lead to intramural wall dissection and formation of red and white thrombi. Unless the donor vessels are limited, most surgeons would prefer to carry out the anastomosis outside the radiation field.

C. Golden Rules

1. **Adequately debride** the recipient wound of all devitalized tissue.
2. **Properly design** a donor flap that has adequate vessel length, thus avoiding vein grafts whenever possible.
3. Choose the site of anastomosis **outside the zone of injury** whenever possible.

II. INTRAOPERATIVE FACTORS

A. **Anastomotic technique**, regardless of all the other variables, is the single most important factor in the ultimate patency of the vessel and requires precise, nontraumatic, and timely approximation of the vessels and/or nerves.

B. **Vessel size** has been shown to be directly proportional to flap success rate, especially once the size diminishes to 1 mm in diameter.

C. **Twisting and kinking** of the pedicle should be avoided at all costs. This is accomplished by marking the side of the vessel with a pen marker, carrying out the anastomosis under minimal tension, and checking the position of the vessels prior to the final flap inset.

D. **Vasospasm** is minimized with the aid of pharmacologic agents such as lidocaine and papaverine and meticulous surgical technique during flap harvest and microanastomosis.

E. **External compression** can lead to thrombosis. It may be the result of a tight dressing, perivascular hematoma, or a narrow tunnel for the pedicle.

III. POSTOPERATIVE MANAGEMENT

A. **The setting** of postoperative management begins in the postanesthesia care unit (PACU), where the flap can be observed and monitored at least every hour. Pedicled flaps may be observed on the floor, while free flaps require hourly monitoring for at least the first 48 hours.

B. **Aggressive management** means avoidance of scenarios that ultimately lead to vascular spasm and thrombosis:

- **Hypovolemia:** maintain adequate volume
- **Hypotension:** maintain blood pressure (at a level that ensures appropriate perfusion pressure)
- **Hypothermia:** maintain temperature above 36°C
- **Hypoxia:** maintain oxygen saturation above 93%
- **Anxiety and pain** may be controlled with narcotics and sedatives
- **Flap monitoring** involves clinical observation with the aid of Doppler monitoring and temperature probes (see Chapter 3)

IV. COMPLICATIONS

The most common complications in flap surgery are outlined below.

A. **Hematomas** are usually noted within the first 48 h after surgery. Hematomas can occur at the donor or recipient sites. An untreated hematoma can lead to flap compromise due to extrinsic compression of the flap or vascular pedicle. Once diagnosed, the only management would be emergent exploration and evacuation of the hematoma with careful inspection of the vascular pedicle to ascertain its patency.

B. **Infection** in the vicinity of the pedicle can lead to thrombosis. They usually occur on postoperative days 3–14. Management includes early operative intervention, adequate debridement of infected tissues, and treatment with topical and systemic antibiotics. High infection rates have been reported in traumatic wounds that undergo delayed reconstruction (5–90 days after injury).

C. **Venous congestion** of the flap may occur early or may be a late presentation of a failing flap. The presenting signs include:

- **Red flap** with rapid refill
- **Dark blood** oozing from a percutaneous needle stick
- **Bluish discoloration** evolving over the surface of the flap as time progresses
- **Pronounced swelling**, often due to poor venous outflow

D. **Primary arterial thrombosis** of the vessels is usually encountered in the immediate (1–48 h) postoperative period and is due to formation of a clot at the site of the anastomosis. Early signs include:

- **Increased discrepancy between the flap and control tissue temperatures**. A difference of greater than 3°C is considered significant.
- **Sluggish capillary refill** consistent with arterial insufficiency.
- **Whitish discoloration** of the flap over time.
- **Loss of tissue turgor**.
- **Diminished or absent Doppler signals** are harbingers of impending flap failure.

E. **Secondary thrombosis** occurs away from the anastomotic site downstream in the microcirculation and presents with a slow, progressive loss of the flap. This should not be confused with the **no-reflow phenomenon**, noted in tissues with prolonged ischemia that fail to reperfuse despite reconstitution of their blood supply. Early signs of secondary thrombosis occur about 5–6 days after surgery and include:

- "Delayed" skin graft take over the muscle flap
- Progressive eschar formation along the edges of the flap though good bleeding is noted by pricking the center of the flap near the pedicle.

F. **Total flap failure** despite multiple operative interventions may require a second flap once the physiological and psychological needs of the patient have been addressed. A review of the literature reveals the following data:

- Total flap loss: 1–4%
- Flap salvage rate: 57–75%

V. MANAGEMENT

A. **Emergent reexploration** of the flap is the only way to assess and salvage a failing flap. Once back in the operating room, the surgeon needs to provide adequate exposure of the vascular pedicle and carefully run the checklist of all the factors listed in this chapter that could cause the thrombosis. Once the cause is established, the appropriate treatment can be carried out.

B. There are no definite indications for anticoagulation or antifibrinolytic therapy when mechanical or vascular factors are optimal—i.e., elective free flap surgery. However, these modalities are helpful when the microsurgeon is faced with a failing or failed flap that requires reoperation.

C. **Leech therapy** is the only modality that is uniformly accepted to be effective for salvage in venous insufficiency, especially when the number and size of veins available are inadequate (e.g., ear or digital replantation). The medicinal leech ***Hirudo medicinalis*** has three sharp jaws that create an Y-shaped wound into which it secretes **hirudin**, a polypeptide anticoagulant. Leeches contain ***Aeromonas hydrophila*** as a predominant enteric organism, which can cause flap or systemic infection. All patients undergoing leech therapy must be covered with third-generation cephalosporin, ciprofloxicin, or trimethoprin-sulfamethaxasole as prophylaxis against infection with ***Aeromonas hydrophila***.

5

Wound Healing

Ziv Peled, M.D.
University of Connecticut School of Medicine, Farmington, Connecticut, U.S.A.
Robert D. Galiano, M.D.
New York University School of Medicine, New York, New York, U.S.A.
Michael T. Longaker, M.D.
Stanford University School of Medicine, Stanford, California, U.S.A.

I. INTRODUCTION

A. Wound healing is a complex biologic response that ultimately results in a mature scar.

B. Several phases define healing, namely, inflammation, epithelialization, extracellular matrix synthesis and remodeling, and wound contraction. Although in the past these were considered distinct stages, a more accurate conceptualization of tissue repair recognizes that these are overlapping and present in some degree throughout most of the course of a healing wound.

C. These processes require the coordinated integration of a variety of cellular activities, including phagocytosis, chemotaxis, mitogenesis, neovascularization, and the synthesis and degradation of collagen and other matrix molecules.

D. This complex response to cutaneous injury eventually leads to the formation of a scar. This is in contrast to the regenerative repair seen in early gestation fetal skin repair.

II. TYPES OF WOUND HEALING

There are four general types of wound healing: primary, delayed primary, secondary, and the healing that occurs in partial-thickness wounds.

A. Primary Healing

Wounds are closed by reapproximation using suture or by some other mechanical means within hours of their creation.

B. Delayed Primary Healing

1. To allow normal host defenses to debride the area, contaminated or poorly delineated wounds are left open and unopposed to prevent infection.
2. By day 3 postinjury, local inflammatory cell recruitment into the wound has occurred to destroy contaminating bacteria. Furthermore, granulation tissue composed of inflammatory cells, extracellular matrix, and new capillaries begins to form.
3. Following a delay of several days, the wound edges are surgically approximated. Collagen metabolism is undisturbed and tensile strength develops as if closure had been immediate.

C. Secondary Healing

1. An open full-thickness wound is allowed to close by both wound contraction and epithelialization.

2. The circumference of the wound contracts by yet incompletely understood mechanisms. However, myofibroblasts are thought to play a pivotal role. Hypothesized to be derived from fibroblasts, myofibroblasts contain a well-defined actin microfilament system. These cells appear in the wound on approximately the third day after wounding and disappear as contraction is completed.
3. Current evidence suggests a direct correlation between the number of myofibroblasts and the extent of wound contraction.

D. Healing of Partial-Thickness Wounds

1. In this type of wound, only the epithelium and the superficial portion of the dermis is injured. Epithelial cells that remain within the dermal appendages, hair follicles, and sebaceous glands proliferate to close the wound.
2. Thus, epithelialization is the main process by which the exposed dermis is covered in partial thickness wounds, with minimal collagen deposition and wound contraction.

III. PHASES OF WOUND HEALING

A. Introduction

Wound repair involves the regulation of a defined sequential cascade of overlapping processes and the coordinated completion of a variety of cellular activities, including phagocytosis, chemotaxis, mitogenesis, and the synthesis of extracellular matrix components. In order for successful healing to occur, these activities must occur in a carefully regulated and reproducible fashion that correlates with the appearance of different cell types present in the wound. Each phase of this complex response to injury is discussed below.

B. Tissue Injury

1. Injury initiates a regulated sequence of events, including coagulation, inflammation, cell replication, angiogenesis, epithelialization, and matrix synthesis and turnover.
2. Vascular injury leads to rapid constriction of affected vessels and activation of the coagulation cascade in order to limit blood loss.
3. Inflammatory cells release vasoactive amines and other mediators, which contribute to vessel permeability and the leak of plasma and proteins into the wound and permit effector cells to enter the environment.

C. Coagulation

1. **Platelets**. Hemostasis, achieved by trapping platelets in the clot, eventually leads to coagulation. These trapped platelets are also essential for the normal inflammatory response by releasing vasoactive amines. These include serotonin, from dense bodies, and cytokines, including platelet-derived growth factor (PDGF), transforming growth factor-beta (TGF-β), epidermal growth factor (EGF), and platelet factor IV, from their α granules. The released serotonin increases microvascular permeability, while the growth factors initiate the wound-healing cascade by attracting and activating macrophages, fibroblasts, and endothelial cells, and by stimulating granulation tissue formation.
2. **Fibrin** is the end product of both the intrinsic and extrinsic coagulation pathways. Derived from factor I, also known as fibrinogen, fibrin is essential to early wound healing because it provides the matrix foundation into which cells can migrate. In addition, fibrin can also serve as a reservoir for peptide growth factors. This infrastructure consists of fibronectin and traps platelets, bloodborne cells, and plasma proteins. Removal of the fibrin provisional matrix is known to impede wound repair.

D. Early Inflammation

1. **Complement**. The inflammatory phase of wound healing is characterized by the activation of complement and the initiation of the classical molecular cascade, which leads to infiltration of polymorphonuclear cells (PMNs) into the wound milieu within 24–48 h.
2. **PMNs**. A number of chemical messengers released from the damaged tissue, platelets, and bacteria attract PMNs into the wound site. These biochemical agents include complement components such as C5a, formylmethionyl peptide products from bacteria, and TGF-β. Upon entering the wound environment, PMNs begin to adhere to the endothelial cells in the adjacent blood vessels by a process called margination. Thereafter, they begin to actively move through

the vessel wall, a process known as diapedesis. The major function of PMNs is to remove bacteria and foreign debris from the wound. However, depletion of these cells is not thought to significantly alter healing in normal wounds.

3. **Epithelialization** results in the formation of a barrier between the internal and external environments. Within hours of the injury, migration of epithelial cells across the wound (i.e., reepithelialization) begins. The cells at the leading edge begin to lose their basement membrane adhesion, flatten, send out cytoplasmic projections, secrete proteases, and phagocytize a path for the impending keratinocyte migration. One to 2 days after injury, epithelial cells at the wound edges begin to proliferate behind the migrating epithelium.
    - Full-thickness wounds—the edge of the wound is the sole source of the migrating epithelium. As a result, these types of wounds heal more slowly and with more inflammation; these delays are thought to result in a greater propensity for hypertrophic scar formation.
    - Partial-thickness wounds—these include skin graft donor sites, which epithelialize more rapidly in a moist environment. The rate of epithelialization is slowed by dry eschars (scabs). In addition, as in all open wounds, as long as the dermis is not completely destroyed, epithelialization can occur through the migration of epithelial cells from the remaining dermal appendages, sweat glands, and hair follicles. An example of this type of healing is a second-degree burn or partial-thickness skin graft donor site.
    - Growth factors—these are potent stimulators of epithelial mitogenesis and chemotaxis. Key players include EGF, basic fibroblast growth factor (bFGF), and keratinocyte growth factor (KGF).

E. Late Inflammation

1. **Macrophages** are the key regulatory cells present in the healing wound. When depleted of circulating monocytes and tissue macrophages, wounds in experimental animal models have been shown to heal with poor debridement, delayed fibroblast proliferation, inadequate angiogenesis, and poor fibrosis. Upon entering a wound through a blood vessel wall, monocytes differentiate into wound macrophages that act as phagocytic cells. By 48–72 h postwounding, macrophages are the predominant cell type within the wound. In addition, macrophages are the primary producers of growth factors responsible for both the production and accumulation of the extracellular matrix (ECM) by fibroblasts and proliferation of smooth muscle and endothelial cells resulting in angiogenesis. Chemoattractants for macrophages include complement, clotting components, immunoglobulin G (IgG) fragments, collagen and elastin breakdown products, and cytokines, such as leukotriene B_4, platelet factor IV, PDGF, and TGF-β.
2. **Lymphocytes**. Attracted by interleukin-1 (IL-1), IgG, and complement products, lymphocytes are the last cells to enter the wound during the inflammatory phase (>72 h after wounding). Although the role of lymphocytes in wound healing has not been clearly defined, IL-1 is believed to have a role in the regulation of collagenase, implicating lymphocyte involvement in collagen and ECM remodeling.

F. Proliferation

1. **Fibroblasts**. By day 7, fibroblasts are the predominant cell type in the wound. Stimulated by cytokines, they migrate through the ECM into the wound. Between 5 and 7 days postwounding, fibroblasts begin to synthesize collagen, which increases in a linear fashion for 2–3 weeks.
2. **Collagens** are the most abundant ECM in the human body. To date, at least 19 different types of collagen have been discovered.
    - Collagen types include (a) type I collagen, the major structural component of bones, skin, and tendons; (b) type II collagen, found predominantly in cartilage; (c) type III collagen, found in association with type I collagen in varying ratios, depending on the type of tissue; (d) type IV collagen, found in the basement membrane; and (e) type V collagen, found in the cornea.
    - Upon injury, the exposed collagen elicits the chemotactic response of the wound-healing cells and promotes platelet aggregation. Eventually, the migrating fibroblasts synthesize and secrete types I and

III collagen to form the foundation of the wound extracellular matrix.

- Collagen metabolism begins with the synthesis of the procollagen α chains on membrane-bound ribosomes. Chromosomes 17 and 7 encode the $\alpha 1$ and $\alpha 2$ chains of type I collagen, respectively. Type I collagen consists of two $\alpha 1$ and one $\alpha 2$ chains. Through hydroxylation of proline and lysine amino acids, the α chains then interact to form a triple helical molecule, which is important for thermal stability. In addition, without the triple helix the collagen cannot be exported from the cell. Within the cell, cross-linking between the chains by means of disulfide bonds also occurs. Procollagen is then packaged into secretory vesicles that move to the cell surface. At the cell membrane, procollagen is cleaved into collagen by procollagen peptidase, and subsequently the collagen is released extracellularly into the wound. The importance of collagen in wound healing is dramatically exemplified by scurvitic wounds, which heal poorly.

3. **Angiogenesis**. Ongoing throughout the previously mentioned phases, angiogenesis describes the process of forming new blood vessels.

   - Platelets. Upon entering the wound, platelets release numerous cytokines, including TGF-β and PDGF, that promote angiogenesis by attracting macrophages and PMNs.
   - Macrophages, in turn, release a number of angiogenic substances including vascular endothelial growth factor (VEGF), tumor necrosis factor-alpha (TNF-α), and bFGF.

G. Remodeling

By approximately 21 days, equilibration of collagen synthesis and breakdown is reached. More specifically, a steady state of collagen synthesis and breakdown is achieved as the ECM is continually remodeled. The increase in tensile strength of a skin wound plateaus at around 6–7 weeks.

1. **Matrix metalloproteinases (MMPs)** are produced by fibroblasts, granulocytes, and macrophages. TGF-β is thought to decrease the activity of matrix metalloproteinases, while the activity of their inhibitors, tissue inhibitors of matrix metalloproteinases (TIMPs), are increased. Thus, TGF-β promotes matrix accumulation.
2. **Fibronectin** is a matrix molecule found in the tissue stroma and the basal lamina that acts as a scaffold for collagen deposition. Produced by fibroblasts, epithelial cells, and macrophages, fibronectin is involved in wound contraction, cell–cell and cell–matrix interaction, cell migration, collagen matrix deposition, and epithelialization. Fibronectin has the ability to bind a wide variety of molecules involved in wound healing, including collagen types I and IV, actin, fibrin, hyaluronic acid, dermatan and heparan sulfates, fibronectin itself, and fibroblast surface receptors. Among the first proteins laid down in a fresh wound, the main function of fibronectin is to promote cell–cell and cell–matrix interactions, cross-linking to fibrin clot and facilitating fibroblast attachment. As the wound matures, fibronectin decreases and type I collagen replaces type III collagen.
3. **Stroma (ground substance)** is another vital component of the wound architecture, consisting of proteoglycans and glycosaminoglycans (GAGs). Although proteoglycans are known to create a charged, hydrated environment that facilitates cell mobility and provides viscoelastic properties of normal connective tissues, their role in wound healing remains unclear. However, proteoglycans are covalently linked to a special type of polysaccharide that may be important to wound matrix, namely, GAGs. There are four known types of GAGs involved in wound healing: chondroitin sulfate, heparan sulfate, keratan sulfate, and hyaluronic acid (HA). Unlike other GAGs, HA is a repeating sequence of nonsulfated disaccharides without a protein core and appears earlier in the wound than the other GAGs, all of which are sulfated and have protein cores. These proteoglycans have been shown to bind and in some cases present extracellular growth factors to their cell surface receptors.

IV. GROWTH FACTORS IN WOUND HEALING

Growth factors (GFs) are proteins that affect a myriad of cellular processes, including migration, proliferation, differentiation, and ECM production. In addition, they are responsible for modulating the inflammatory response. Weighing between 4,000 and 60,000 daltons, GFs exert their effects via membrane receptors, which in turn initiate a cascade of intracellular activity, and through endocrine, paracrine, autocrine, and intracrine mechanisms. Endocrine GFs are produced by a specific cell type and, thereafter, transported via the bloodstream to act on a cell at a distant site. Paracrine GFs are produced by a specific cell type and act on an adjacent cell. Autocrine GFs exert their effects on the same cell that produced them. Finally, intracrine GFs act within the cell that produced them. The majority of the GFs involved in the wound-healing process act via the paracrine or autocrine mechanisms. GFs were initially named for their first known actions or the first cells known to produce them. With further study, scientists have discovered that many different cell types may produce any one GF, and virtually all GFs are known to have more than one function. Thus, the names of various GFs can often be misleading. The following is a brief discussion of some of the more common GFs known to be involved in the adult wound-healing process. To date, although many GFs have begun clinical trials, only one, PDGF, has received FDA approval for the treatment of chronic wounds.

KGF and VEGF will likely be approved soon.

A. Epidermal Growth Factor (EGF)

EGF is a 53-amino-acid polypeptide that is released from platelets during platelet degranulation. EGF is mitogenic and chemotactic for several cell types, including epithelial cells, endothelial cells, and fibroblasts, all of which have receptors for this molecule. In addition, EGF stimulates angiogenesis and collagenase activity at the wound site.

B. Fibroblast Growth Factor (FGF)

FGFs are a large family of GFs. FGF-2, in particular, is a well-established angiogenic factor and mitogen for fibroblasts. FGF-2 is produced primarily by macrophages and endothelial cells. FGF-2 also stimulates collagen and ECM synthesis and promotes wound contraction and epithelialization.

C. Keratinocyte Growth Factor (KGF)

KGF, also known as FGF-7, is a protein produced by fibroblasts early in the course of tissue repair. Epithelial cells, such as keratinocytes, are the only known cells with receptors for KGF. As such, this molecule is believed to play an important role in mesenchymal-epithelial signaling and reepithelialization during wound healing.

D. Platelet-Derived Growth Factor (PDGF)

PDGF is a 30–32 kDA glycoprotein made up of two subunits called A and B. These two subunits form a heterodimer that is produced primarily by platelets and stored in the α granules. Other cells such as macrophages and epidermal cells release similar PDGF-like substances. PDGF is known to modulate numerous functions such as fibroblast and smooth muscle cell proliferation/chemoattraction, activation/chemoattraction of macrophages, and stimulation of neutrophils. It is also thought that PDGF participates in the process of neovascularization, but this function may be secondary to its effects on the other cells involved in the wound-healing process.

E. Transforming Growth Factor-β (TGF-β)

TGF-β exists as a homodimer with a molecular weight of 25,000 kDA and has been isolated from nearly all types of tissues. TGF-β is one of the most well-studied growth factors. Consisting of three different isoforms (β1, β2, β3) in humans, TGF-β is chemotactic for macrophages and fibroblasts and is involved in extracellular matrix synthesis and remodeling. Produced initially by platelets (and stored within the α granules) and macrophages, TGF-β acts via the autocrine mechanism on monocytes to stimulate the secretion of other growth factors such as FGF, PDGF, TNF-α, and IL-1. Furthermore, TGF-β is perhaps the most potent stimulator of collagen and extracellular matrix synthesis and has, therefore, been implicated in scar formation. Several experimental studies have successfully employed strategies to attenuate the effects of TGF-β (i.e., antibodies to TGF-β1 and TGF-β2) and have demonstrated reduced scar formation as a result. Not all members of the TGF-β family have detrimental effects. Actually, TGF-β1 has been shown, like vitamin A, to reverse the inhibition of wound healing caused by glucocorticoids in an animal incisional model. Also, recent studies suggest that TGF-β3 may have antiscarring activity, in contrast to TGF-β1 and TGF-β2. This is, however, controversial.

F. Transforming Growth Factor-α (TGF-α)

TGF-α is a molecule that is produced by macrophages, platelets, keratinocytes, and other epidermal cells. Similar to EGF, it binds the EGF receptor and acts in an autocrine manner to exert its effects. It is chemotactic and mitogenic for epithelial, endothelial, and mesenchymal cells. TGF-α may also be mitogenic for fibroblasts in vivo.

G. Interleukin-1 (IL-1)

Initially described as a mitogen for lymphocytes, IL-1 is produced by macrophages and neutrophils and is now known to be chemotactic for epithelial cells, monocytes, neutrophils, as well as lymphocytes. IL-1 is thought to play an important role in the processes of wound repair and remodeling, based on its mitogenic effects on fibroblasts and its ability to synthesize collagen, to promote collagenase and to promote hyaluronidase activity.

H. Tumor Necrosis Factor-α (TNF-α)

TNF-α is a 157-amino-acid molecule produced by macrophages and neutrophils. Its primary functions are to stimulate fibroblast proliferation and to promote collagen and collagenase synthesis.

I. Vascular Endothelial Growth Factor (VEGF)

A family of at least three different isomers (VEGF-A, -B, and -C), the VEGFs act on defined tyrosine kinase receptors on endothelial cells and are extremely important in angiogenesis. They have been used in ischemic flap models to stimulate neovascularization and in tissue engineering research to improve tissue vascularity.

J. Insulin-like Growth Factors (IGF)

IGF-I is the main member of this family involved in wound healing. It is released by many cells involved in wound healing, including fibroblasts and macrophages. Its actions are modulated by so-called IGF-binding proteins found in the extracellular matrix. They are potent anabolic agents that have also been demonstrated to enhance cell migration and proliferation.

V. CHRONIC WOUNDS

Chronic wounds are one of the most costly medical problems encountered in the United States. Among the most common types of chronic wounds are pressure ulcers, venous stasis ulcers, and diabetic foot ulcers. In 1997, 6.5 million people in the United States suffered from one of these chronic conditions. The estimated annual cost of treating these wounds was in excess of $3.3 billion dollars and continues to rise. The key to wound healing is the balance between tissue formation and tissue degradation. In successful wound healing, the timing and character of ECM deposition and turnover as well as protein synthesis and proteolysis is well synchronized and specific. In chronic wounds, the normal sequence of repair or the imbalance between tissue production and turnover is disrupted, resulting in either delayed or absent repair. The microenvironment created by chronic wounds is often hostile to the repair process, being deficient in some growth factors. In support of this, wound fluid derived from acute wounds has been shown to stimulate proliferation of fibroblasts and keratinocytes, whereas wound fluid derived from chronic wounds decreases proliferation of these same cell types. In addition, most chronic wounds also are characterized by varying degrees of infection, host malnutrition or a catabolic state, and local tissue hypoxia.

A. Matrix Metalloproteinases (MMPs)

MMPs are a family of zinc-dependent endopeptidases that include gelatinases, collagenases, and stromelysins. During wound healing, MMPs modulate much of the ECM turnover. Thus, an imbalance between matrix deposition and degradation in favor of tissue turnover has been postulated as one possible mechanism for the delayed healing seen in chronic wounds. MMP-2 and MMP-9 have been described in chronic wound fluid but are noticeably absent from acute wound fluid. In addition, tissue inhibitor of MMP (TIMP-1) has been found to be decreased in chronic wounds, while active gelatinases have been found in increased amounts when compared with acute wounds.

B. Cytokine Function

Even if certain growth factors are present in chronic wound fluid, they may not function normally. Recent data about chronic wound fluid suggest that peptide growth factors may not function optimally due to the presence of excess proteolysis; this may be due to bacterial enzymes in contaminated wounds that degrade peptides, including growth factors.

C. Hypoxia

While tissue hypoxia is present in *all* wounds to some degree or another, the persistent lack of oxygen and nutrients to a wound will serve as a major impediment to successful healing. For example, it has been shown experimentally that cells exposed to a hypoxic environment respond by proliferating, by migrating more rapidly, and by synthesizing growth factors such as VEGF. In this way, the cells are directing their own repair and recruiting endothelial cells to reverse their hypoxic environment. However, cells exposed to chronic, long-standing hypoxia (as seen in most chronic wounds) stop proliferating and may even enter apoptosis. It is axiomatic in surgery that a wound needs a reliable blood supply to heal; as clinicians, this is one of the variables that plastic surgeons can affect. By decreasing local tissue edema (which increases the diffusion distance of oxygen and nutrients from capillaries to wound cells) and enhancing local blood flow (which may mean something as simple as warming the patient or as drastic as a free flap or bypass to restore vascular flow), the delivery of oxygen to a healing wound should be a goal to be reached when dealing with any recalcitrant wound.

VI. FETAL WOUND HEALING

Over the past decade, our experience with fetal surgery has led to some remarkable advances in the treatment of previously fatal conditions. Observations from these procedures indicate that the human fetus is capable of healing without a scar. This discovery has led to intense research, with the ultimate goal of repairing adult wounds without scars. The fundamental question in elucidating this phenomenon is: Are the differences between scarless fetal wound repair and scarring adult-type wound repair a function of the fetal environment (extrinsic differences) or are they a unique function of the fetal cells themselves (intrinsic differences)?

A. Extrinsic Differences

1. **Amniotic fluid**—The fetus is continuously bathed in warm amniotic fluid that is rich in GFs and ECM components such as hyaluronic acid (HA) and fibronectin.
2. **Sterility**—The amniotic fluid and entire fetal environment are sterile.

B. Intrinsic Differences

1. **Hypoxemia**—The fetus is profoundly hypoxemic compared with the adult. Although high tissue oxygenation is necessary for wound healing in the adult, the relative hypoxemia in fetal tissues may promote greater production of certain growth factors and for matrix molecules, resulting in a reduction or elimination of scar formation.
2. **Immune response**—Major differences between fetal and adult acute inflammatory responses include the degree of the response, the character of the response, and the function of inflammatory cells, once recruited into the wound. Histologically, there are few granulocytes in fetal wounds. For example, it has been noted that fetal lamb wounds showed less acute inflammatory response with a large number of macrophages, while having relatively few neutrophils. This is in contrast to a large number of neutrophils acutely seen in adult wounds. Furthermore, the amounts and types of cytokines and GFs produced by the various inflammatory cells during fetal wound healing may differ markedly from those seen during adult wound repair. These differences would certainly influence the phenotypic outcome of the wound repair mechanism.
3. **ECM**—The ECM of fetal wounds is rich in HA, an important structural and functional component of the wound matrix whenever rapid tissue proliferation occurs. Although present early in both fetal and adult wound healing, HA deposition is sustained in fetal wound matrix, which may provide the local environment that promotes regeneration rather than scar formation. In the adult, subsequent to the initial deposition of HA, hyaluronidase is produced to degrade the HA, and the wound matrix is replaced by collagen. As alluded to, this process of early HA degradation may not occur in the fetus. In addition, there is an enhanced production of fibronectin and deposition of highly organized collagen architecture in the dermis of fetal cutaneous wounds.

C. Growth Factors

The exact role of GFs in scarless fetal wound healing remains unknown. Nevertheless, given the prominent role that GFs play in overall fetal development, it is highly suggestive that these cytokines may also play an important role in scarless fetal wound healing.

6

Suture Materials

Steven E. Greer, M.D.
New York, New York, U.S.A.

I. INTRODUCTION

A. Suture materials can be categorized in a number of ways, based on the following different characteristics:

- Absorbable vs. nonabsorbable
- Braided vs. monofilament
- Synthetic vs. biological
- Suture size
- Needle shape (straight; 1/4, 3/8, 1/2, or 5/8 circle; customized shapes)
- Needle size
- Needle point (cutting vs. tapered)
- Single vs. double needle (single-ended vs. double-ended)

B. The ideal suture is easily handled by the surgeon, easy to tie, and retains strength for the required period of time.

II. TENSILE STRENGTH RETENTION

A. Since different tissue types and wound closures require different durations of suture strength, suture materials with various absorption rates and tensile strengths have been engineered.

B. Nonabsorbable sutures permanently retain their tensile strength, although not all nonabsorbable sutures are completely "permanent."

III. TISSUE REACTION

A. Some suture materials evoke more of an inflammatory tissue reaction than do others.

B. The biological materials, such as silk or collagen (gut), are more reactive than synthetic types.

C. Braided sutures possibly induce more scarring when placed superficially and have a greater risk for wound infection by harboring organisms within the interstices of the braids.

IV. HANDLING ABILITY

A. "Memory" describes the tendency of suture to retain its straight shape and to spring back and resist tight curves (i.e., as in knots). Memory reduces the handling ability of sutures.

B. Braided suture has less memory and is easier to tie and work with, but has the disadvantage of evoking a greater inflammatory tissue reaction.

V. SUTURE SIZE

A. Suture size is quantified by the 0-gauge system. The more 0s a suture has, the smaller is its diameter. 1-0 is the largest, followed by 2-0 or 00, 3-0 or 000, etc.

B. The opposite is true for sutures described by whole numbers: number 2 suture is larger than number 1 suture, which is larger than 0 suture.

C. The smallest possible suture that provides the desired tensile strength appropriate for a specific tissue type should be used.

D. Large monofilament and small suture of any type are more difficult to handle.

E. Wetting the surgeon's gloves facilitates small-gauge suture handling.

Absorbable monofilament sutures are as follows:

Suture material	Brand names	Tensile strength retention	Frequent uses
Surgical gut, plain or chromic (beef or sheep collagen)		Varies by individual, but usually retains almost 0% tensile strength by 2 weeks	General soft tissue approximation; good for certain pediatric wounds to avoid a second distressful removal procedure
Poliglecaprone	MONOCRYL	50% tensile strength remains at 1 week	General soft tissue approximation; designed as a synthetic replacement of gut
Polydioxanone	PDS II, BIOSYN, MAXON	50% tensile strength remains at 4 weeks; completely absorbed within 210 days; slight differences occur among brands	Long-term strength in general soft tissue approximation; designed to be an absorbable alternative to nonabsorbable monofilament sutures

Absorbable braided sutures are as follows:

Suture material	Brand names	Tensile strength retention	Frequent uses
Polyglactin 910 (synthetic polyester composed of glycolide and lactide)	Coated VICRYL, VICRYL Rapide, POLYSORB	75% tensile strength remains at 2 weeks, completely absorbed in 70 days; slight differences occur among brands; VICRYL Rapide loses tensile strength slightly faster than coated VICRYL	Short-term wound support and closure of dead space in subcutaneous soft tissue layers; ligation
Polyglycolic acid (homopolymer)	DEXON	Similar to polyglactin 910; complete absorption within 60–90 days	Closure of dead space in subcutaneous soft tissue layers
90/10 Caprilactone/Glycolide	PANACRYL	60% tensile strength at 6 months	Designed to be a long-term absorbable suture to replace some roles of nonabsorbable suture such as polypropylene (fascia closure, orthopedic applications)

Nonabsorbable monofilament sutures are as follows:

Suture material	Brand names	Tensile strength retention	Frequent uses
Nylon (in black or clear)	ETHILON, NUROLON, MONOSOF	Virtually permanent tensile strength retention	General soft tissue approximation
Polypropylene	PROLENE, SURGIPRO	No loss of tensile strength	Superficial skin closure for less scarring than braided or gut sutures, abdominal fascia closure, other general subcutaneous tissue approximations
Expanded polytetra-fluoroethylene	Gore-Tex	Virtually permanent tensile strength retention	Vascular surgery anastomosis of tissue to synthetic grafts
Stainless steel		Virtually permanent tensile strength retention	Bone and ligament repairs; sternotomy closure; dangerous to work with due to the high risk of puncture wounds to the surgeon

VI. SURGICAL NEEDLE ANATOMY

A. Swage (Suture Attachment End)

1. Most needles are crimped around the suture, while some have an eye for threading the suture through. Special rhinoplasty needles have the swage in the middle of the body.

Nonabsorbable braided sutures are as follows:

Suture material	Brand names	Tensile strength retention	Frequent uses
Silk	Perma-Hand	Very slow absorption and loss of tensile strength; becomes encapsulated	Vessel ligation
Nylon	BRALON	Virtually permanent tensile strength retention	
Polyester fiber (in green or white)	MERSILENE, SURGIDAC	Virtually permanent tensile strength retention	General soft tissue approximation
Extra polyester fiber	ETHIBOND	Virtually permanent tensile strength retention	Cardiac valve replacement surgery

2. The swage can be designed to pull off from the suture (pop-off) or to be cut away.
3. A swage and overall needle diameter equal to or smaller than the suture reduces leaking in a vessel anastomosis.

B. Body

1. The body can be straight or curved.
2. The curve can be from 1/4 to 5/8 of a circle in circumference.
3. A 3/8 curve is often used for microsurgery and skin closure, and 5/8 for confined spaces such as the pelvis and rectum.

C. Point

1. The point can be **cutting** (sharp edge toward the inner concave curvature), **reverse cutting** (sharp edge toward the outer convex curvature), **tapered** (round tapering to a point), or **blunt**.
2. A cutting point provides good cosmetic results in skin and is effective for penetrating tissues with high resistance (e.g., dermis, tendons, and sternum).
3. A reverse cutting needle reduces the tendency of the knot to tear through tissue (fascia, ligament, tendon, and eye).
4. A taper needle is best for anastomoses (biliary, vessel, nerve) and for minimizing leaks.
5. Blunt-tip needles are usually reserved for friable tissue and are sometimes selected by surgeons for increased safety when operating on patients with communicable diseases.

VII. MICROSURGERY SUTURES AND NEEDLES

A. Microsurgical vessel anastomoses and nerve repairs require specialized instruments and sutures that are small enough to be used on structures as small as 1 mm in diameter.

B. The majority of microsurgical sutures are nonabsorbable, nonbraided nylon. At the small sizes used, handling and memory are not significant issues.

C. Most free flap arterial/venous anastomoses (vessel diameter usually 2–4 mm) and peripheral nerve repairs can be performed with 9-0 nylon sutures. Smaller digital arteries and veins, as in digital replantation, are more appropriately anastomosed with 10-0 sutures.

D. Suture diameters for microsurgery sutures are 25 μm for 10-0 sutures and 35 μm for 9-0 sutures.

E. Most microsurgery needles are 75, 100, or 130 μm in size. Careful matching of needle size and suture diameter must be performed in order to prevent a needle that is too big for a given suture, which may result in leaking at an anastomosis.

F. A tapered 3/8-circle needle is the most frequently used needle in microsurgical applications. Urologists will often use a cutting, large-diameter needle for microsurgical repair of a thick-walled vas deferens.

VIII. OTHER WOUND CLOSURE MATERIALS

A. **Surgical staples**

- Stainless steel staples were developed primarily as a faster wound closure method. They cause more scarring than subcuticular suture but are acceptable in plastic surgery for certain situations.

- In the scalp, staples are preferred, as they are less traumatic to the hair follicle and easier to remove than sutures.
- The surgeon's preference and experience determines their use on other areas.

B. **Adhesive Strips**, also known as steristrips or butterfly bandages, are designed for the tension loads of coapted wound edges. They are usually used to augment subcuticular sutures, but can be used in lieu of sutures for very small low-tension lacerations.

C. **Fibrin Sealant**. Recently approved for clinical use, fibrin sealant provides a biological hemostatic barrier to wounds not amenable to suture hemostasis, such as in the liver or spleen.

D. **The skin adhesive** 2-octyl cyanoacrylate (Dermabond®) has been approved for sutureless skin closure of small lacerations.

IX. FUTURE WOUND CLOSURE ADVANCES

A. **Growth factor–impregnated suture**—Animal studies have shown beneficial effects of the slow release of growth factors impregnated in absorbable suture into the wound. Tendon and ligament healing may be expedited.

B. **Anastomotic clips**—Various vascular surgery and microsurgery anastomotic ring clips have been developed to replace the more time-consuming suture methods.

C. **More practical fibrin sealant**—The current fibrin sealant systems require refrigeration of the component ingredients and mixing just prior to use, making them impractical for battlefield wounds or bedside procedures. Work is underway to make the ingredients stable at room temperature.

7

Clinical Wound Care

Steven E. Greer, M.D.
New York, New York, U.S.A.

The majority of wounds should show clinically apparent signs of healing within 2–4 weeks if no underlying problems exist. Most factors causing delayed healing can be eliminated with once-a-day hands-on care of the patient by the surgeon. Chronic wounds are often neglected under a dressing by nurses and surgeons, and this problem needs to be recognized. Wound debridement is essential to good outcomes.

I. SYSTEMIC FACTORS ASSOCIATED WITH DELAYED WOUND HEALING

The surgeon must be aware of the factors that can impair healing before implementing a proper prevention and treatment plan.

A. **Diabetes**—See Chapters 91 and 92

B. **Malnutrition**—25–50% of all acute care patients are malnourished. Poor caloric intake can cause malnutrition, and it can also occur with normal caloric intake if the patient is cachectic. **Cachexia** results from malabsorption or increased metabolism secondary to a systemic illness. There is no distinct cut-off point of any single parameter that defines malnutrition. Current guidelines indicate that malnutrition is likely present if **serum albumin is < 3.5 mg/dL, total lymphocytes (TLC) are < 1800/mm^3, or body weight has decreased >15%**. Increased dietary protein has been associated with improved wound healing.

- Specific nutrient deficiencies have been identified. These include: **arginine** (T-lymphocyte function), **linoleic acid** (precursor for prostanoids and inflammation), **cystine** (collagen formation), **glutamine, vitamin A** (retinal, retinol, retinoic acid, epithelial tissue maintenance), **vitamin E, vitamin C** (collagen synthesis), **ferrous iron** (hydroxylation of lysine and proline), **calcium** (cleavage of procollagen), **cuprous ion** (lysine metabolism), and **zinc (cell replication).**
- Trace elements should be supplemented, as should vitamin B6 in alcoholics and vitamin A with steroid use. Vitamin C stores are quickly depleted, and most severely ill patients will benefit from daily supplements. Unlike vitamin C, the human body has a 4-year store of vitamin E. Despite its popularity, there is no evidence that topical or systemic supplementation of vitamin E improves wound healing or scar formation.

C. **Marked obesity**—A well-known risk factor for wound complications of dehiscence, infection, and delayed healing.

D. **Age**—Some studies have shown that wounds heal less effectively with increasing age.

E. **Tobacco**—Nicotine constricts vessels and carbon monoxide decreases oxygen delivery. These short-term effects last for several hours. Respiratory tract changes persist for weeks. Peripheral vascular disease is usually a permanent effect.

F. **Corticosteroids**—Vitamin A can partially counteract the effects of steroids.

G. **Immunosuppression**—Congenital disorders, steroids, malnutrition, diabetes, and malignancies result in immunosuppression. AIDS slightly impairs healing.

H. **Genetic disorders**—Ehlers-Danlos and Marfan's syndromes have various deficiencies in collagen synthesis. Many other genetic disorders are known to have an effect on wound healing.

I. **Chemotherapy**—The evidence is contradictory. Chemotherapy, particularly adriamycin and 5-FU, might slightly impair healing. A several-week postoperative delay, when possible, is recommended.

J. **Renal or liver failure**—Some evidence suggests a slight impairing effect, but comorbidities such as diabetes confuse interpretation of the studies.

K. **Massive or metastatic cancer**—Directly impairs healing in addition to the effects of chemotherapy or radiation therapy. Smaller localized tumors are not thought to significantly impair healing.

II. LOCAL FACTORS CAUSING DELAYED WOUND HEALING

A. **Necrotic tissue** is probably the single most detrimental factor to wound healing, and also the factor that surgeons are most equipped to correct.

B. Wound contamination is ubiquitous and simply refers to colonized organisms on the surface. **Wound infection** denotes a deeper penetration of the wound by bacteria that induce an inflammatory response. Foul smell indicates anaerobes. The overall bioburden is greater in undermined or necrotic wounds. Bacterial loads greater than 10^5 bacteria per gram of tissue or greater impair healing.

C. Diagnoses are primarily made from clinical signs such as erythema, pain, odor, and drainage. Wound **swab cultures** are unreliable and should rarely be used. **Quantitative** biopsy cultures are the gold standard, but cost limitations prevent their routine use in most medical centers. Multiple needle-stick aspiration of a wound is a slightly less specific test compared to the tissue biopsy gold standard. Culture of pus or necrotic tissue is seldom reliable, as it will infrequently represent the same organisms infecting the viable tissue. **β-Hemolytic streptococci** are particularly detrimental to healing.

D. Systemic antibiotics are of limited use in wound infection treatment unless administered within 4 h of wounding. Adequate tissue levels are usually not achieved. Topical antibacterial such as silver sulfadiazine (Silvadene®), mafenide acetate (Sulfamylon®), and gentamycin reach adequate tissue levels but are also injurious to tissue cells. **Mafenide 5% solution** appears to be able to fight infection without causing tissue damage.

E. **Osteomyelitis**. Diabetic wounds that can be probed down to bone have a 90% chance of having osteomyelitis. Sensitive physical exam signs are crepitance or a spongy bone consistency. The presence of osteomyelitis in pressure ulcers is less certain and may warrant radiological workup. MRI and nuclear medicine scans can be useful for ruling out (false-positive rates are too high to reliably rule in) osteomyelitis and therefore reducing the length of antibiotic therapy.

F. **Arterial ischemia or venous insufficiency** (see Chapters 91 and 92).

G. **Edema** decreases oxygen diffusion to cells. Edema is a very potent inhibitor to healing, particularly in the lower extremity. Elevation of the wound and/or compression garments should be emphasized.

H. **Radiation exposure** (see Chapter 26)

I. **Foreign bodies**

J. **Tension**

K. **Pressure and shear forces** (see Chapter 95)

L. **Dry environment** inhibits epithelialization and healing.

M. **Urinary or fecal incontinence** may contaminate the wound and impair healing. In addition, these are important risk factors to the development of skin ulcers.

III. TISSUE-SPECIFIC CONSIDERATIONS

A. **Tendon**—Scarring and adhesions of the tendon sheaths often produce functional deficits, particularly in hand surgery. The blood supply from the **vincula** is important to keep intact in order to reduce adhesions. However, most tendon nutrient is delivered by synovial diffusion. Early passive motion helps reduce adhesion as well. Growth factors, proline analogues, and electrical stimulation may promote tendon healing.

B. **Bone**—Healing of externally reduced fractures initiates in the fracture hematoma, which develops into a **soft callus** with osteoprogenitor cells. Endochondral ossification then ensues in long bones. Healing of internally reduced fractures proceeds without a callus in a direct bone-to-bone healing. The fracture site becomes transiently ischemic from the severed local blood supply and promotes the healing transformation. Vascularized bone grafts heal from **osteogenesis** by creating bone from the surviving osteoblasts in the graft. Nonvascular bone grafts mostly heal by **osteoconduction** whereby the dead cells and the ossified matrix serve as a scaffold for surrounding cells to migrate and deposit new bone. **Ostoeinduction** is the transformation of surrounding undifferentiated cells, such as dura mater or periosteum, into osteoblasts and bone. Osteomyelitis must be debrided and eliminated before surrounding soft tissue can heal.

C. **Cartilage—Chondrocytes** produce **chondroitin sulfate** and collagen at a low metabolic rate. The inflammatory healing sequence is difficult to initiate in damaged cartilage, and defects often are permanent. In contrast to osteocytes, chondrocytes have little reparative ability and heal with fibrous scar.

D. **Nerve—Wallerian degeneration** occurs in the axonal dendrite of a peripheral nerve distal to the site of injury. **Schwann cells** repair the myelin sheath and allow axons to migrate across the damaged region.

E. **Skin**—Scar, keloid, hypertrophic scarring (see Chapters 5 and 14).

IV. CHRONIC WOUNDS

Chronic wounds are wounds that have failed to proceed in an orderly and timely process to produce anatomic and functional integrity. Some have set arbitrary time limits to define chronic wounds, but a strict definition does not exist.

A. There are approximately 3–5 million chronic wounds in the United States at any time. In the early 1990s, pressure ulcers alone were a $1.3 billion problem. Approximately 2 million diabetics have chronic wounds leading to many of the 60,000 amputations performed each year in the United States.

B. **Diabetic ulcers** (see Chapters 91 and 92)

C. **Venous ulcers** (see Chapters 91 and 92)

D. **Pressure ulcers** (see Chapter 95)

E. **Irradiated wounds** (see Chapter 26)

V. DEBRIDEMENT

A. The only accepted method is **sharp debridement**. However, sharp debridement performed at the bedside is often inadequate due to bleeding and incomplete anesthesia, making the operating room the appropriate place for this procedure. Unfortunately, many surgeons classify patients with chronic wounds as poor surgical candidates, and many physicians and nurses do not have privileges to perform sharp debridement.

B. An entire industry focusing on alternatives to sharp debridement has developed. Few of these modalities currently have controlled data showing efficacy, much less superiority to sharp debridement. Enzymatic debridement simultaneously also allows for rapid bacterial proliferation, offsetting the small benefits of debridement.

C. Scalpel and scissors should remove necrotic tissue. Wounds with "soupy" exudate can be debrided by a **curette** or a scrub brush.

D. The anatomy of the sacrum, trochanter, and foot needs to be appreciated to delineate necrotic tissue from normal ligaments and tendons. Healthy ligament and tendon does not always briskly bleed, and adjacent structures such as the rectum or major arteries can be penetrated with aggressive debridement.

E. **Fluorescein** and subatmospheric pressure dressing therapy can help to contrast living and necrotic tissue and facilitate the debridement.

VI. PASSIVE DRESSINGS

A. Passive dressings have been approved by the FDA for safety, but their efficacy has not been proven to be better than simple gauze dressings.

B. Some dressings do have advantages of less frequent dressing changes due to greater absorption of exudate, maintenance of beneficial moist environment, etc., but the translational effects on improved wound healing have not been proved.

C. The surgical primary closure wound requires a dry dressing for 24 h.

D. Abrasions or skin graft donor sites require a semi-occlusive dressing to maintain a moist environment optimal for epithelialization.

E. Full-thickness wounds with drainage benefit from absorbent dressings.

F. Adhesive skin sealants have been approved for use and are a promising alternative to sutures and dry gauze for primary closure of simple lacerations/incisions.

VII. SPECIAL ADJUVANT WOUND THERAPIES

A. Electrical Stimulation (ES)

1. Several varieties of electrical stimulation (ES) have been used for wound healing. This is one of the best-studied adjuvant therapies and has considerable randomized controlled data supporting it.
2. The electric current is usually delivered via an electrode within saline gauze in the wound. It can be delivered in **low-intensity direct current (LIDC), high-voltage pulsed current (HVPC), alternating current (AC), or pulsed electromagnetic energy**. HVPC has the most impressive supporting data from in vitro, animal, and human studies.
3. There are several postulates on the mechanisms for the effectiveness. Normal skin has an electrical potential between the surface and

Dressing types	Examples	Composition	Major indications
Skin sealant	Dermabond	2-octyl cyanoacrylate	Primary closure of acute clean lacerations
Plain gauze		Dry or can be combined with saline	Numerous indications
Antiseptic-soaked gauze		Dakins, hydrogen peroxide, or povidone	Avoid on almost all wounds with the possible exception of exposed heart in a contaminated field
Nonadhering dressings	Adaptic (oil), Xeroform (bismuth), petrolatum gauze	Oil, petrolatum, 3% bismuth (for odor reduction only)	Skin graft donor and recipient sites, abrasions
Films	Op-site, Tegaderm	Usually polyurethane	Abrasions, skin graft donor sites, as a component of SPD
Hydrocolloids	Duoderm, Intracite, Ultec	Various colloidal particles in an adhesive mass	Skin graft donor sites, pressure ulcers, stomal sites
Hydrogels	Vigilon, Elastogel	90% water with various polymers	Abrasions or pressure ulcers
Foams	Allevyn, Lyofoam	Polyurethane or polyvinyl	Draining wounds
Calcium alginate	Sorbsan, Kaltostat	Calcium alginate polysaccharide	Wound volume measurement, dental impressions, draining wounds

subcutaneous layers. Acute injury allows a flow of current. ES creates a similar current that may be lacking in nonhealing wounds. Cells migrate along a current in a **galvanotaxic** manner. ES is galvanotaxic for beneficial inflammatory cells.

4. ES also has a direct stimulatory effect on fibroblasts, increases blood flow, and is bacteriostatic and bacteriocidal to some organisms.

B. Hyperbaric Oxygen

1. Most modern hyperbaric oxygen (HBO) chambers for wound healing allow a single patient to lie down within the chamber. The patient breathes 100% oxygen while the chamber pressure is usually compressed to 2.5 atmospheres of pressure for 90 minutes.
2. Pressures and duration of therapy differ.
3. Under these conditions, the partial pressure of oxygen dissolved in the plasma alone, not counting the hemoglobin, is adequate for the resting demands of most tissues.
4. The strongest data demonstrating the effectiveness of HBO are from studies on osteoradionecrosis. Other data are conflicting and not randomized or controlled. Moreover, it is not known whether 100% oxygen at ambient pressures is any less effective.

C. Subatmospheric Pressure Dressing (SPD)

1. Russian surgeons in the 1960s were among the first to use subatmospheric pressure dressing (SPD), followed by the Germans and Japanese. A commercially successful version was developed by American plastic surgeons in the early 1990s.
2. The general schematic for SPD involves some variety of a porous screen over the wound, whether it be gauze or sponge, which is hermetically sealed by a film dressing. An exiting tube is connected to a suction source to create a vacuum over the wound, optimally at 125 mmHg pressure below ambient.
3. SPD increases blood flow, decreases edema, decreases bacterial load, and promotes granulation tissue production. Controlled studies are underway, and empiric results on virtually any wound have been promising.
4. SPD can also be used as a very effective skin graft bolster. The dressing needs to be changed no more than twice per week.
5. The only absolute contraindication is a wound that has not been debrided of solid necrotic tissue.
6. Importantly, anticoagulated patients can hemorrhage due to SPD therapy.

D. Topical Growth Factors

1. Early clinical trials were disappointing. Later trials on uninfected wounds have had better results.
2. Multiple different growth factors applied sequentially may be more effective than a single growth factor.
3. A PDGF cream is currently marketed for diabetic foot wounds (see Chapter 5).

E. Bilayered Tissue Engineered Skin (APLIGRAF®; Generic Name: Graftskin)

1. All cells are derived from discarded neonatal foreskin. The epidermis is allogenic living cultured human keratinocytes, and the dermal layer consists of allogenic fibroblasts in a bovine collagen matrix.
2. Graftskin provides structural protection to the wound, and the cells provide cytokines and growth factors that may promote healing. The originally applied graftskin often melts away and is replaced by the patient's own healing tissue.
3. Studies have shown success with expediting the healing of venous ulcers.

F. AlloDerm®

1. AlloDerm is made from cadaver skin by completely removing the epidermis and the antigenic cellular components of the dermis (fibroblasts, etc.), leaving the collagen and matrix structural components of the dermis.
2. This acellular structure can be used as a supporting structure below ultrathin skin grafts, increasing durability.

VIII. APPROACH TO THE ACUTE WOUND

A. History

It is important to assess for the risk factors discussed in Sec. I. This step is often overlooked.

B. Physical Examination

Examine the wound for small foreign bodies, exposed bone, erythema, or skin blisters indicating an abscess, cellulitis, pain, degree of undermining, and necrotic tissue. Crepitance and expanding erythema can indicate myonecrosis or necrotizing fasciitis.

C. Treatment

1. Use the American College of Surgeons Committee on Trauma recommendation for tetanus immunization
2. **Irrigate and debride the wound**—Do not assume that this has been performed. This often requires an operating room to perform adequate debridement, particularly if an open fracture is present. High-pressure **pulsatile jet lavages** can be more effective than low-pressure systems.
3. **Abrasions** need to be carefully scrubbed and cleaned of fine debris to prevent traumatic tattoos (see Chapter 27).
4. **Contusions** should be evacuated of any hematoma. Posttraumatic cooling reduces inflammation After 24–48 h, heating assists in mobilization of hematoma.
5. **Avulsion**—Assess for viability. Rarely throw away tissue. Complete avulsions can be salvaged for skin grafts if the tissue is defatted (see Chapter 68). Larger avulsions of scalp and limbs might be salvaged by microsurgery (see Chapter 27).
6. **Primary closure**—Wounds should be closed with monofilament sutures and buried sutures to relieve tension. For contaminated wounds, antibiotic therapy may be effective if adequate blood levels can be achieved within 4 h of wounding. A minimal amount of sutures should be used to reduce foreign body effects. The wounds should be evaluated closely every 24 h for signs of infection with a low threshold for reopening the wound.
7. **Bites and puncture wounds** (see Chapter 15)
8. **Delayed primary closure**—The majority of contaminated wounds, including blast explosive war wounds according to recent studies, can be closed by immediate primary closure after receiving adequate debridement and pulsatile jet lavage irrigation. Human mouth wounds to the hand (from a bite or punch) are infamous exceptions. For these and other wounds unable to be closed immediately, delayed primary closure should be performed after approximately 3–7 days.
9. **Malnutrition assessment** (if the patient is admitted). Correct other risk factors discussed above as well (see Chapter 95).
10. **Special adjuvant therapies** (see above)

IX. SPECIFIC CONSIDERATIONS IN THE APPROACH TO THE CHRONIC WOUND

A. The approach to the chronic wound is generally the same as with any other wound, except that the wound assessment emphasizes the risk factors that could be responsible for the healing impairment.

B. In the acute-care setting, a wound that may have been present for years is only seen by the acute-care staff for a few days or weeks, and the big picture is often missed.

C. Proper nutrition and infection control cannot be overemphasized. Inadequate debridement, a harbinger of infection and inhibitor of epithelialization, is a common contributing factor of a chronic wound.

D. Obtaining proper pressure relief and incontinence control are very challenging multidisciplinary problems. To address these difficult issues that are often beyond the scope of the acute-care setting, the new paradigm of the wound healing center was created.

8

Angiosomes

G. Ian Taylor, M.D., F.R.C.S., F.R.A.C.S., and Andrew Ives, M.D.
Royal Melbourne Hospital, Melbourne, Australia

I. INTRODUCTION

A. Each angiosome is a three-dimensional anatomical territory of tissue supplied by a source artery and its accompanying vein(s) that span between the skin and bone (Fig. 1). They are linked together like a jigsaw by either reduced caliber (choke) vessels or vessels of the same caliber (true anastomoses).

B. A knowledge of the anatomy of the cutaneous arteries and veins is fundamental to the design of skin flaps and incisions.

C. Cutaneous arteries arise directly or indirectly from underlying source arteries. Arteries then follow the connective tissue framework of the deep tissues, between or within muscles. They then pierce the deep fascia, usually at fixed skin sites. From the deep fascia they course on its superficial surface for a variable distance, supplying it and the undersurface of the fat (Fig. 2).

D. They then travel through the fat to the subdermal plexus. In the subcutaneous plane, the cutaneous arteries and veins often travel with the cutaneous nerves.

E. Density, size, and direction of the cutaneous perforators varies from region to region of the body. The vessels are largest and longest where the skin is mobile and shorter and more dense in the fixed skin area regions.

F. Connections between adjacent arteries are either by true anastomoses, without change in caliber, or by reduced caliber choke vessels (Fig. 3).

G. The choke vessels that link adjacent arteries are like resistors in an electrical circuit. When a flap is raised, they provide initial resistance to the flow of blood to the tip of the flap from the base. When a skin flap is delayed, these vessels open up and dilate to enhance the circulation to the flap. This is due to hyperplasia and hypertrophy of the elements in the vessel wall as well as muscle relaxation.

H. Veins also form a three-dimensional plexus. Valvular veins directing blood in particular directions are connected by avalvular channels, which allow bidirectional flow between venous territories. Usually cutaneous veins partner arteries. Veins collect into horizontal channels of large-caliber vessels that are often related to cutaneous nerves and a longitudinal system of chain-linked arteries, or alternatively collect in a centripetal fashion into a common channel that passes vertically down with the cutaneous arteries to pierce the deep fascia. The veins then accompany the direct and indirect arteries, eventually draining into the venae comitantes of the source arteries in the deep tissue (Fig. 4). The venous territories match their arterial counterparts in the skin and deep tissue, especially the muscles.

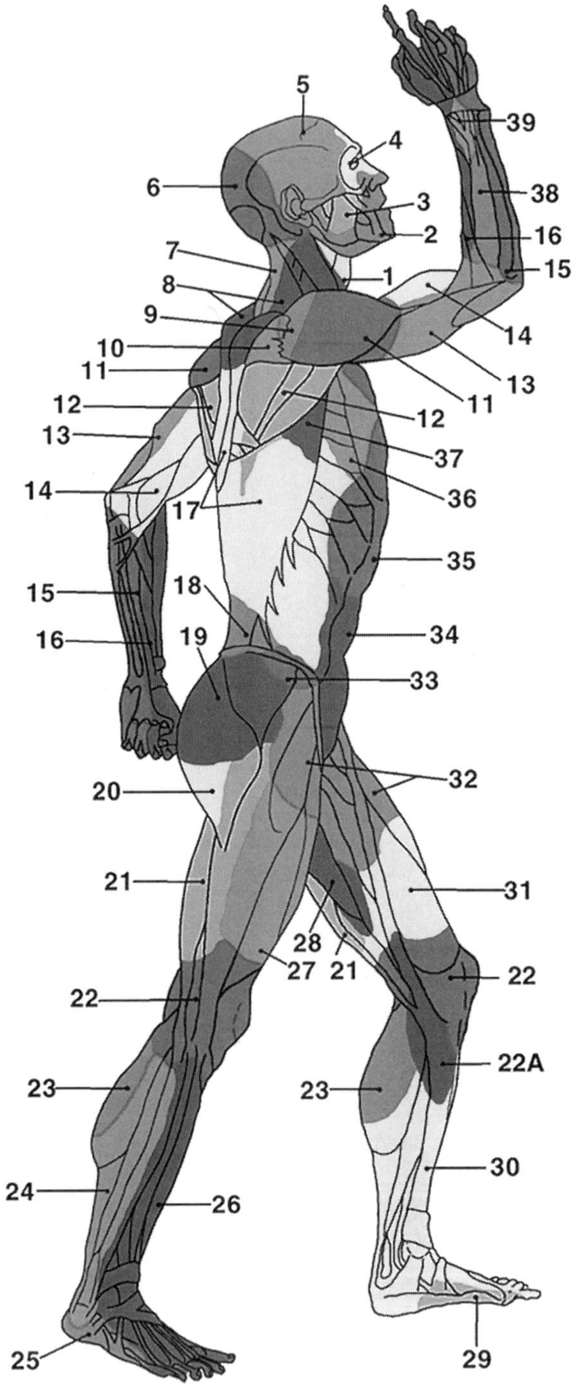

Figure 1 The angiosomes of the body: (1) thyroid; (2) facial; (3) buccal; (4) ophthalmic; (5) superficial temporal; (6) occipital; (7) deep cervical; (8) transverse cervical; (9) acromiothoracic; (10) suprascapular; (11) posterior circumflex scapular; (12) dorsal scapular; (13) profunda brachii; (14) brachial; (15) ulnar; (16) radial; (17) posterior intercostals; (18) lumbar; (19) superior gluteal; (20) inferior gluteal; (21) profunda femoris; (22) popliteal; (22A) descending geniculate; (23) sural; (24) peroneal; (25) lateral plantar; (26) anterior tibial; (27) lateral femoral circumflex; (28) adductor (profunda); (29) medial plantar; (30) posterior tibial; (31) superficial femoral; (32) common femoral; (33) deep circumflex iliac; (34) deep inferior epigastric; (35) internal thoracic; (36) lateral thoracic; (37) thoraco-dorsal; (38) posterior interosseous; (39) anterior interosseous. (From Taylor GI; Palmer JH. The angiosomes of the body. *Brit. J. Plast. Surg.* 40:113–141, 1987.)

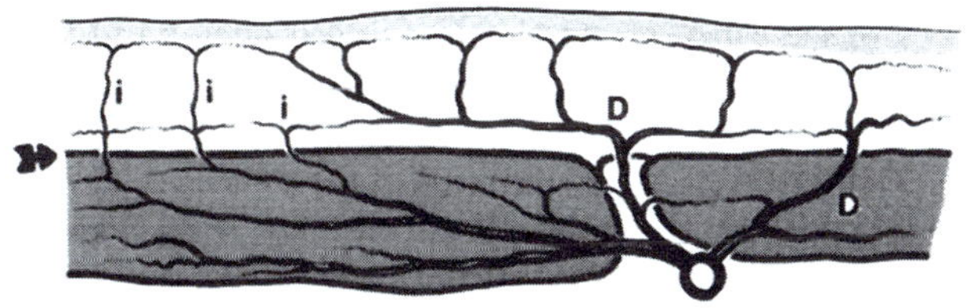

Figure 2 Schematic diagram of the direct (D) and indirect (i) cutaneous perforators of a source artery and their relationship to the deep fascia (arrow), the intermuscular septa, and the underlying muscle (shaded). (From Taylor GI; Palmer JH: The angiosomes of the body. *Brit. J. Plast. Surg.* 40:113–141, 1987.)

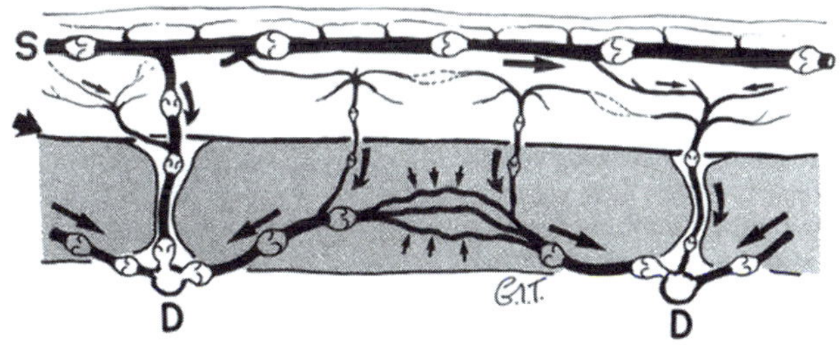

Figure 4 Composite diagram of the integument and underlying muscle (shaded) illustrating the superficial (S) and deep (D) venous systems with their interconnections. A large vena communicans connects these systems, and the alternative pathways of four venae comitantes are shown. Note the choke system of veins within the muscle (small arrows) and the diverging direction of flow of the muscular veins as determined by the orientation of their valves. (From Taylor GI; Caddy C; Watterson PA; Crock JG: The venous territories (venosomes) of the human body: experimental study and clinical implications. *Plast. Reconstr. Surg.* 86:185, 1990.)

II. ANGIOSOME CONCEPTS

A. Vessels Follow the Connective Tissue Framework of the Body

1. Major arteries are closely related to the axial skeleton. Their branches follow the intermuscular connective tissues where they divide to supply deeper structures. Cutaneous perforators arise from the source artery or one of its muscle branches either before or after it has entered the muscle. The cutaneous perforators then follow intermuscular or intramuscular connective tissue to pierce the deep fascia. After emerging from the deep fascia, the cutaneous vessels follow the connective tissue framework of the superficial fascia to reach the dermis.

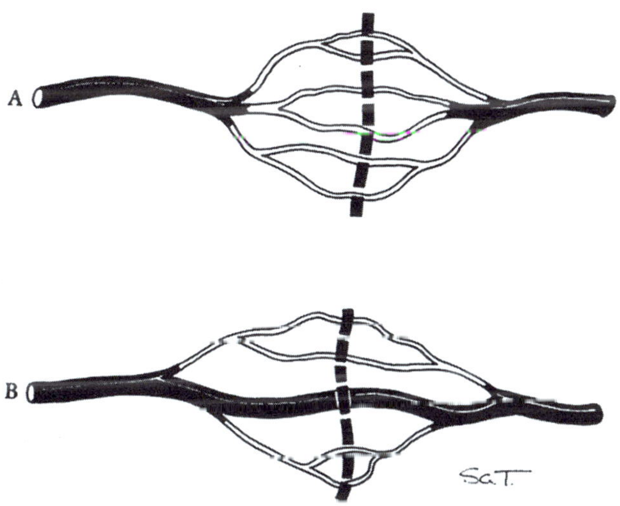

Figure 3 Schematic representation of choke anastomoses (A) and true anastomoses (B) between adjacent vascular territories. (From Taylor GI; Minabe T: The angiosomes of the mammals and other vertebrates. *Plast. Reconstr. Surg.* 89:181, 1992.)

2. In regions where the connective tissue is loose, the vessels travel within the connective tissue, allowing the arteries to pulsate and the veins dilate. In regions where the connective tissue forms tight fibrous sheets, such as the deep fascia, the vessels run beside or on the fascia, not within.
3. Applications—in flaps where the skin is relatively fixed to the deep fascia (scalp and limbs), fasciocutaneous flaps should include the deep fascia to protect the vessels. In flaps raised where the skin and subcutaneous tissue are mobile over the deep fascia, the deep fascia can be left since the vessels have already left this plane (e.g., in the anterior chest wall and the iliac fossae).

B. Vessels Radiate from Fixed to Mobile Areas

1. Vessels emerge from deep fascia to the skin where it is fixed or tethered. They then travel for a variable distance depending on the mobility of the skin.
2. Applications—long flaps should be based where the skin is fixed with their axis orientated along the lines of maximum skin mobility. Examples include the groin flap, the deltopectoral flap, and

various scalp flaps. The Doppler probe can be used to define the point of exit of these perforators from the deep fascia.

C. Vessels Hitchhike with Nerves

1. Cutaneous nerves are accompanied by longitudinal arteries and veins that are often the dominant supply to the region.
2. Applications—this relationship allows designing of long neurovascular flaps with the potential for sensation at the repair site.

D. Vessel Size and Orientation Are a Product of Tissue Growth and Differentiation

A fixed number of vessels supply the embryo, which are subsequently modified by growth and development of the fetus, child, and adult; for example, the scalp vessels "stretched" by the developing brain in the fetus and the breast in the pubertal female.

E. Vessels Obey "The Law of Equilibrium"

Debreuil-Chambardel stated that "the anatomical territories of adjacent arteries bear an inverse relationship to each other, yet combine to supply the same region." If one vessel is small, its partner is large to compensate, and vice versa.

F. Vessels Have a Relatively Constant Destination but May Have Variable Origins

1. This is typical of vessels that emanate from the groin to supply the skin of the lower abdomen and upper thigh. These vessels may arise directly from the femoral artery or one of its branches.
2. Application—variability may not be important in the raising of a pedicle flap, but it certainly is when the flap is being raised for microvascular transfer.

G. Vessels Form a Continuous Unbroken Network

1. Adjacent cutaneous arteries are linked together, especially in the subdermal plexus, by reduced-caliber "choke" anastomotic arteries and arterioles to form a continuous three-dimensional network in the integument. Hence, the same area of skin and subcutaneous tissue can be raised as a cutaneous, fasciocutaneous, septocutaneous, or musculocutaneous flap. Regardless of the flap design, the vessels that enter the flap at its base connect into the same vascular network.
2. Applications—one adjacent anatomical vascular territory can be captured with safety on the cutaneous artery at the base of the flap, and necrosis usually occurs at the next choke anastomosis in the arterial network or the one beyond. Flap survival can be extended by strategic division of vascular pedicles along the axis of the proposed flap.

III. EXAMPLES OF REGIONAL ANATOMY

A. Angiosomes of the Forearm (Fig. 5)

1. Skin—The perforators arise from the source arteries or from their muscular branches. They follow the intermuscular septa distally, but proximally often pierce the muscle bellies, where these are fixed either to bone or intermuscular septa. They become more numerous, but smaller distally, with the maximum number seen in the palm where the skin is most fixed.

Figure 5 Sites and relative size of the cutaneous perforators in (A) and (B) and the supply to the deep tissues shown schematically in (C) with the angiosome territories shaded. Note that the main link between angiosomes occurs within tissues, especially the muscles. BR = brachioradialis; PT = pronator teres; PL = palmaris longus; FCU = flexor carpi ulnaris; FDS = flexor digitorum superficialis; FDP = flexor digitorum profundus; FPL = flexor pollicis longus; FPB = flexor pollicis brevis; FDM = flexor digiti minimi; APB = abductor pollicis brevis; ADM = abductor digiti minimi; BR = brachioradialis; ECRL = extensor carpi radialis longus; ECRB = extensor carpi radialis brevis; EDM = extensor digiti minimi; EPL = extensor pollicis longus; EPB = extensor pollicis brevis; ECU = extensor carpi ulnaris; APL = abductor pollicis longus; ANC = anconeus. (From Inoue Y; Taylor GI: The angiosomes of the forearm: anatomic study and clinical applications. *Plast. Reconst. Surg.* 98:195, 1996.)

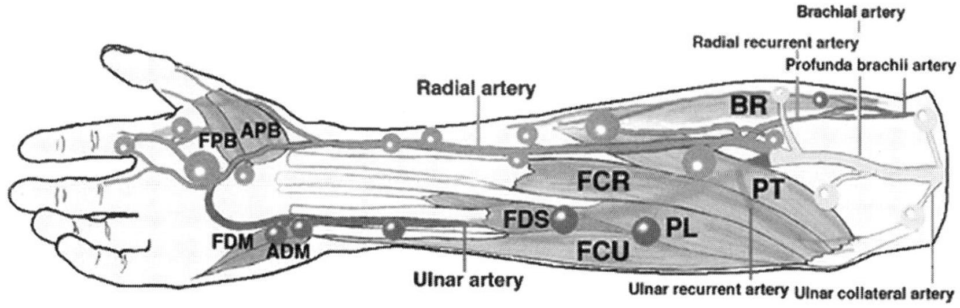
Brachial artery
Radial recurrent artery
Profunda brachii artery
Radial artery
BR
FPB
APB
FCR
PT
FDS
PL
FCU
FDM
ADM
Ulnar artery
Ulnar recurrent artery
Ulnar collateral artery

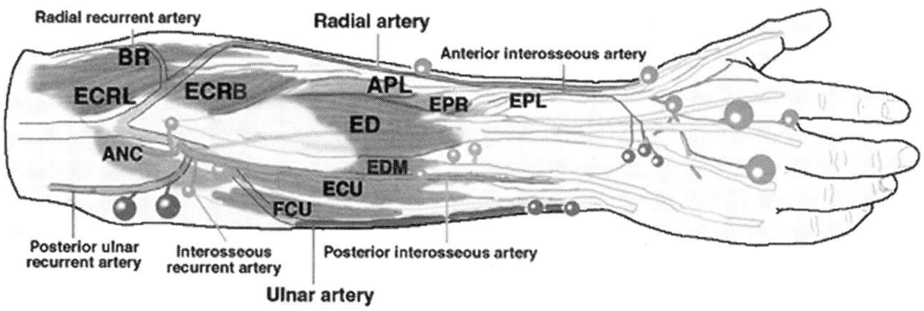
Radial recurrent artery
Radial artery
Anterior interosseous artery
BR
ECRL
ECRB
APL
EPB
EPL
ED
ANC
EDM
ECU
FCU
Posterior ulnar recurrent artery
Interosseous recurrent artery
Posterior interosseous artery
Ulnar artery

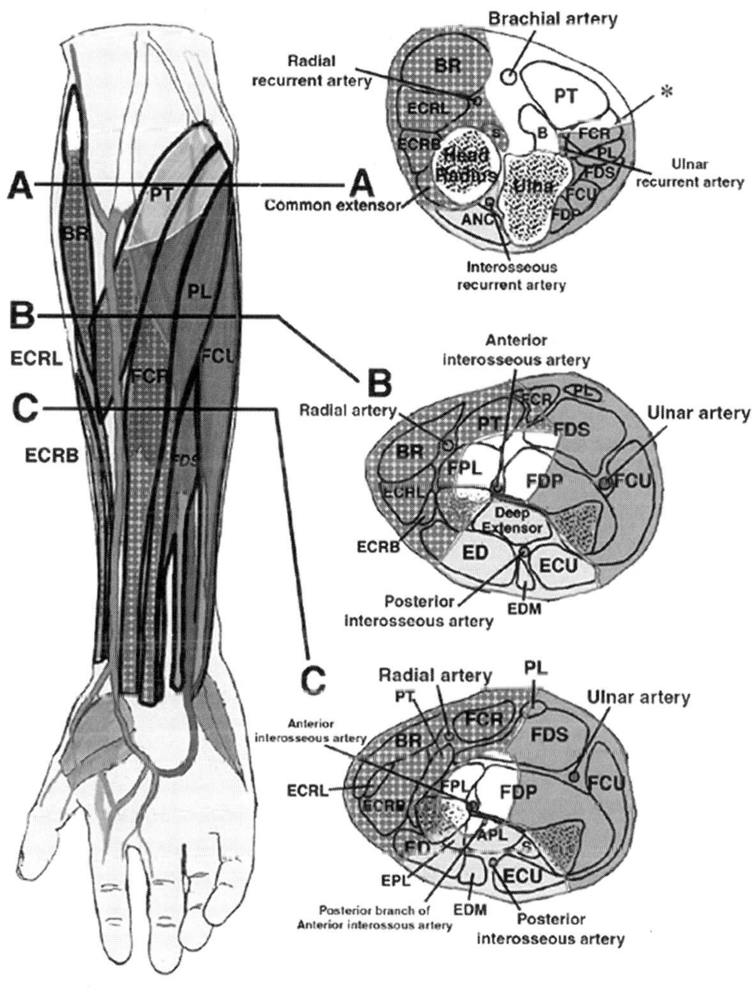
A
A
PT
BR
PL
B
B
ECRL
FCU
FCR
C
C
ECRB
FDS
Brachial artery
Radial recurrent artery
BR
PT
*
ECRL
ECRB
B
FCR
PL
FDS
Head Radius
Ulna
FCU
FDP
Ulnar recurrent artery
Common extensor
ANC
Interosseous recurrent artery
Anterior interosseous artery
Radial artery
Ulnar artery
FCR
PL
PT
FDS
BR
FPL
FDP
FCU
ECRL
Deep Extensor
ECRB
ED
ECU
Posterior interosseous artery
EDM
Radial artery
PL
PT
Ulnar artery
Anterior interosseous artery
BR
FCR
FDS
FCU
ECRL
ECRB
FPL
FDP
APL
ED
EPL
ECU
Posterior branch of Anterior interosseous artery
EDM
Posterior interosseous artery

2. Muscles—These are supplied by vascular pedicles from each angiosome territory that they span. They may be grouped as follows:

One territory	Two territories	Three territories	Four territories
Anconeus	Palmaris longus	Flexor digitorum superficialis	Pronator teres
Extensor carpi radialis longus	Flexor digitorum profundus	Flexor carpi radialis	
Flexor carpi ulnaris	Flexor pollicis longus	Pronator quadratus	
Extensor carpi radialis brevis	Brachioradialis		
Extensor digiti minimi	Extensor digitorum communis		
Extensor carpi ulnaris	Supinator		
	Abductor pollicis longus		
	Extensor pollicis brevis		
	Extensor pollicis longus		
	Extensor indicis proprius		

3. Clinical Implications
   - Volkmann's ischemic contracture: since flexor digitorum profundus (FDP) and flexor carpi ulnaris (FCU) lie the farthest from potential anastomotic pathways, these are most susceptible to ischemia and thus the first muscles to be affected by increases in compartment pressure (as identified by Tsuge).
   - Multiple muscle bellies cross the elbow joint in which intramuscular anastomoses exist between territories, thus creating potential bypasses for sudden blockages of the brachial artery at the elbow.
   - Flaps designed on the forearm can utilize all the tissues supplied by the one angiosome (e.g., the osseomusculocutaneous radial forearm flap) or can be extended to include the adjacent angiosome in each tissue layer. It is because of this link between angiosomes that occur mainly within the integument and muscles that necrosis of the remaining tissues at the donor site is uncommon when harvesting flaps based on either the radial, ulnar, or interosseous vessels.

B. Angiosomes of the Leg (Fig. 6)

In the lower leg, the source arteries and their venae comitantes travel adjacent to, but not within, the rigid fascial envelopes of the leg, being invested in loose connective tissue. They supply the following:

1. Skin—Cutaneous vessels arise from source arteries or their muscle branches that pierce deep fascia in longitudinal rows in the vicinity of the intermuscular septa, or beside tendons, and supply structures that they pass.
2. Muscles—They are supplied by vascular pedicles from each angiosome territory they span. They may be grouped as follows:

One territory	Two territories	Three territories
Tibialis anterior	Peroneous longus	Gastrocnemius
Extensor digitorum longus	Peroneus brevis	Soleus
Extensor hallucis longus	Flexor digitorum longus	Popliteus
Peroneus tertius	Flexor hallucis longus	Tibialis posterior

3. Clinical Implications
   - Since the anterior compartment muscles are supplied exclusively by the anterior tibial artery and confined in a compartment with rigid walls across which vascular connections are few, these muscles are at greatest risk of ischemia and may result in the painful condition of shin splints.
   - Intramuscular anastomoses form the main link between angiosomes. However, few muscle bellies extend across the knee joint (unlike at the elbow), with the main vascular connections being extramuscular through the geniculate vessels. Tenuous intramuscular links occur only through the popliteus and gastrocnemius muscles. This explains why sudden obstruction

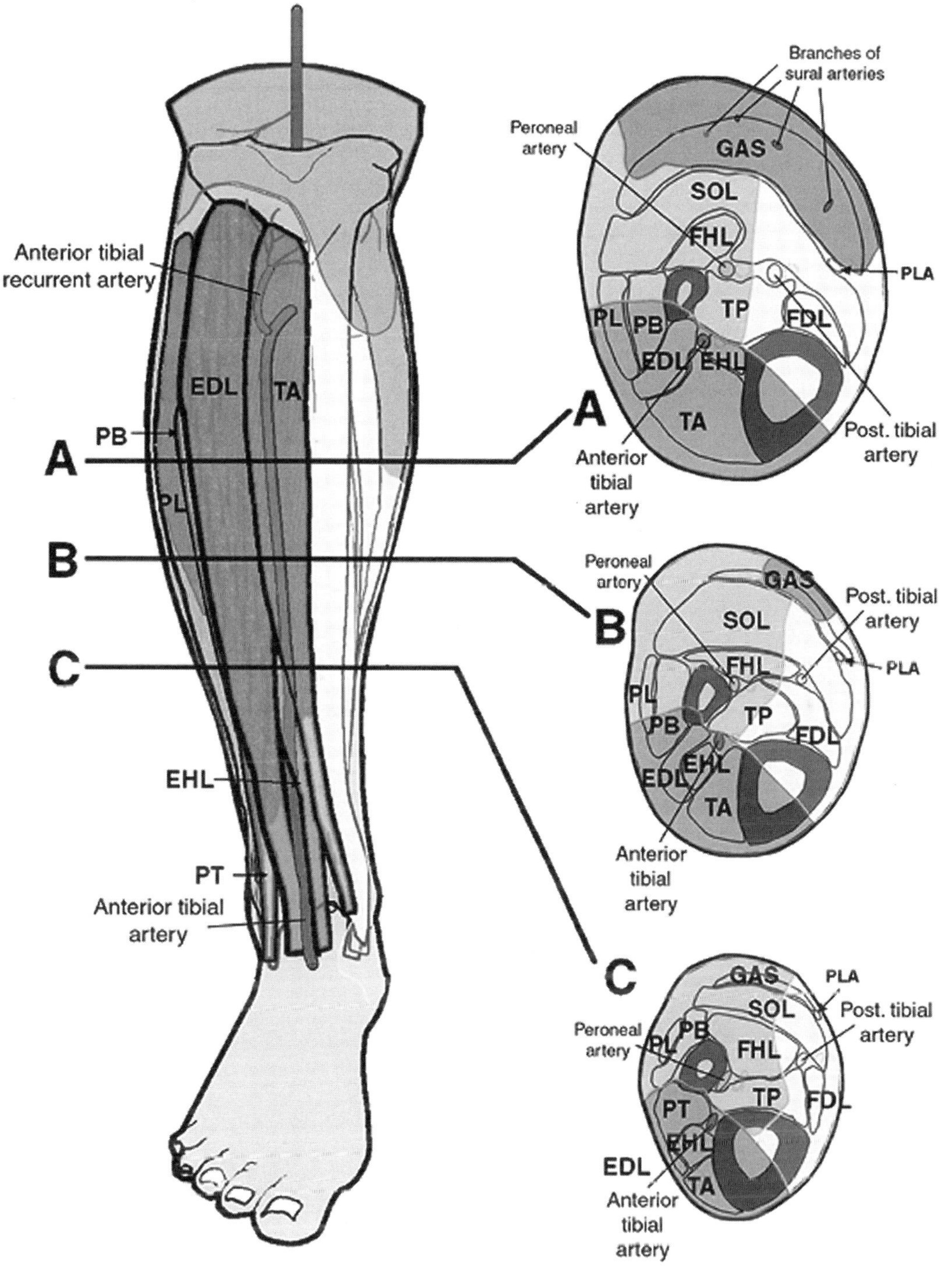

Figure 6 The site and relative size of the cutaneous perforators in (A) and (B) and the supply to the deep tissues shown schematically in (C) with the angiosome territories shaded. EDL = extensor digitorum longus; EHL = extensor hallucis longus; TA = tibialis anterior; PB = peroneus brevis; PL = peroneus longus; PT = peroneus tertius; GAS = gastrocnemius; SOL = soleus; FHL = flexor hallucis longus; FDL = flexor digitorum longus; PLA = plantaris; TP = tibialis posterior. (From Taylor GI; Pan W-R: The angiosomes of the leg: anatomic study and clinical implications. *Plast. Reconstr. Surg.* 102:599, 1998.)

of the popliteal artery has significant effects on the blood supply of the lower leg.

- In the lower leg, both soleus and tibialis posterior contain three territories and therefore form potential links among the three source vessels of the lower leg.
- The subcutaneous periosteal surface of the tibia contains anastomoses between the posterior and the anterior tibial arteries. Most pretibial lacerations occur superficial to the periosteum and shear off the cutaneous arteries, which emerge from this plexus, thus explaining the high incidence of traumatic flap necrosis.

C. Angiosomes of the Head and Neck (Fig. 7)

1. Skin and Superficial Musculoaponeurotic System (SMAS)

- Vessels follow the connective tissue framework. Main skin perforators pierce the deep fascia from fixed skin sites, especially around the base of the skull, the orbits, the nostrils, over the parotid gland, along the skin crease lines of the face, and beside the muscles in the neck. They then radiate into mobile skin areas and are intimately associated with the SMAS layer in the face, the platysma in the neck, and the galea in the scalp.
- Vascular arcades occur between the internal and external carotid arteries. Major veins often run a different course to the main arteries.
- In the neck, vessels are more sparse but emerge in regions of fixed skin, especially over the anterior border of trapezius, posterior and anterior border of sternocleidomastoid, and along the hyoid bone, clavicle, and sternum.

2. External Ear

The external ear is supplied by two angiosome territories, the superficial temporal and the posterior auricular.

3. Muscles

Once again, muscles may be grouped according to the number of angiosome territories they span and from which they receive a vascular supply. These muscles are subgrouped into regions. Together they form an important vascular connection via their intramuscular anastomoses, between branches of the internal carotid, external carotid, and subclavian vessels.

a. Muscles of Facial Expression—lying within the SMAS, these muscles contain within themselves major branches of the occipital, ophthalmic, superficial temporal, facial, superior and inferior thyroid arteries. The platysma forms a vascular link between external carotid and subclavian arteries via branches of the superior thyroid or submental branch of the facial artery above, and the transverse cervical and inferior thyroid arteries below.

b. Ocular Muscles—all lie within the territory of the ophthalmic artery

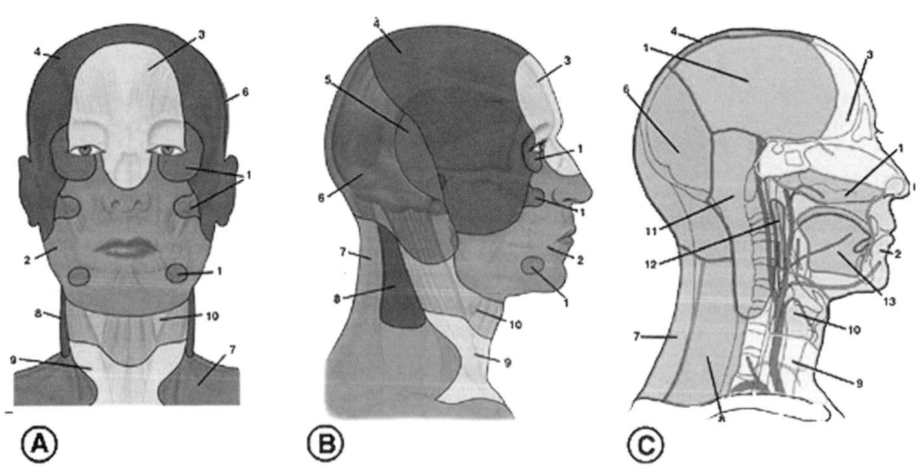

Figure 7 The angiosomes of the head and neck shown in anteroposterior (A), lateral (B), and sagittal (C) views: (1) internal maxillary; (2) facial; (3) ophthalmic; (4) superficial temporal; (5) posterior auricular; (6) occipital; (7) transverse cervical; (8) deep cervical; (9) inferior thyroid; (10) superior thyroid; (11) vertebral; (12) ascending pharyngeal; (13) lingual.

c. Muscles of Mastication

One territory	Two territories
Lateral pterygoid Medial pterygoid	Buccinator Temporalis Masseter

d. Posterior Neck Muscles

One territory	Two territories	Three territories
Obliquus capitis superior	Levator scapulae Rectus capitis posterior major Rectus capitus posterior minor	Splenius capitis Splenius cervicis Semispinalis capitis Semispinalis cervicis Obliquus capitis inferior Longissimus cervicis

Four territories	Five territories
Trapezius[a]	Trapezius[a] Longissimus capitis

[a] Note: Variation in number of angiosomes of trapezius due to variability in dorsal scapular artery origin.

e. Lateral Neck Muscles

Two territories	Four territories
Scalene anterior Scalene medius Scalene posterior	Sternomastoid

f Anterior Neck Muscles

One territory	Two territories	Three territories
Thyrohyoid	Sternohyoid Sternothyroid Longus cervicis Longus capitis	Digastric Omohyoid

4. Aerodigestive Tract

a. Nose

Two territories	Three territories
External nose	Internal nose

b. Tongue and Floor of Mouth

Extrinsic

One territory	Two territories
Geniohyoid Styloglossus Genioglossus Hyoglossus	Mylohyoid Stylopharngeus

Intrinsic

Two territories
Palate, pharynx, esophagus, and trachea

Five territories exist from hard palate to upper esophagus. There is a paucity of vessels in the midline.

5. The Glands

One territory	Two territories
Parotid Submandibular Sublingual	Thyroid

6. Clinical Implications

a. Vascular malformations of the head and neck seem to coincide with the choke anastomotic zones linking adjacent territories. Hence, the malformations are fed by two feeding vessels or more.

b. The rich anastomotic network within the SMAS layer and its prolongation onto the scalp as the galea accounts for the large number of flaps that can be raised in this area compared to the more fixed skin of other regions of the body.

c. The transverse forehead flap of McGregor often produces problems, especially at the tip of the flap as it tries to capture three territories in succession, unlike the scalping flap of Converse that captures two territories.

d. The buccinator flap can be safely raised on either of its pedicles along with overlying mucosa.

e. The sternocleidomastoid flap is very unpredictable when based superiorly with the skin paddle at its tip, since the flap extends over three or four territories, each linked by choke anastomoses.

9

Tissue Expansion

Nolan Karp, M.D.
New York University Medical Center, New York, New York, U.S.A.
Steven E. Greer, M.D.
New York, New York, U.S.A.

Since its description in 1957 for use in ear reconstruction, tissue expansion has become a powerful tool for the plastic surgeon. It involves the process of applying gradual force to overlying skin or myocutaneous segments in an effort to expand the overlying tissue, creating a larger surface area. The force is applied by underlying expandable preformed prosthetic envelopes.

I. TISSUE EXPANDERS

A. Expanders are silicone prosthetic envelopes that have self-sealing injection ports. The ports can be internal or external and either incorporated or separate from the expander envelope.

B. Fluid is injected to progressively expand the envelope.

C. Expanders come in a multitude of sizes and shapes.

D. Textured expanders are generally favored and less prone to capsular contraction than the smooth variety.

II. HISTOPATHOLOGY OF TISSUE EXPANSION

A. Epidermis mitotic activity and thickness increases.

B. The dermis decreases in thickness.

C. Collagen deposition increases and fibers realign parallel to the surface. Elastic fibers become thicker and slightly fragmented.

D. Dermal appendages become separated from one another without significant morphologic changes.

E. Muscle layers atrophy and become thinner with abnormal sarcomeres and myofibrils.

F. Adipose cells atrophy with some permanent loss.

G. Vessels and nerves elongate and maintain diameter. Vascularity increases dramatically, particularly at the junction of the capsule and normal tissue. The number and caliber of capillaries increase. Vascular endothelial growth factor (VEGF) production increases.

H. Excessively rapid or overaggressive expansion can result in irreversible damage to tissue.

I. A cellular and connective tissue, multilayered capsule forms around the expander.

J. Most histologic changes are reversed 2 years after expander removal.

III. BASIC TECHNIQUES

A. The underlying principal is to expand donor-site tissue that will be moved as a flap to reconstruct a defect.

B. The anticipated reconstructive procedure must be planned prior to the surgical procedure. The need to provide sufficient surface area should be balanced with the need to match the skin color and hair quality of the expanded tissue to the future recipient site.

C. The expanded tissue should be mobilized by incisions that can be concealed in the best manner possible, preferably along a border of an aesthetic unit. The incision lines used to place the expander should ideally be reused as part of the future flap incisions.

D. After expansion and during the flap procedure, backcuts made at the base of the flap can minimize the amount of tissue wasted after elevation of the flap.

E. A wide area of dissection is used to place the expander so that it does not underlay suture lines. If the expander is placed under an incision, the tension delivered by the expansion can lead to wound dehiscence or an unfavorable scar.

F. After a postplacement interval, the expander is inflated in 3- to 7-day intervals. Using a small needle (23 gauge), saline is injected into the port of the expander. Patient discomfort is an indication to end an expansion session. The complete expansion process is stopped once the surface area is deemed to be large enough to create the desired flap to resurface the defect. Overexpansion is the rule to ensure minimal tension at final closure.

G. Repeated expansion and flap procedures may be required for large lesions, such as congenital giant nevi or burn scars.

IV. SCALP

A. Male-pattern baldness, traumatic alopecia, and burns can be treated with tissue expansion.

B. The scalp can be expanded by a factor of two without obvious hair thinning.

C. Expanders are placed deep to the galea and over the periosteum of the calvarium. The expanders are then inflated over subsequent weeks. Scoring the galea at the time of expander placement can facilitate subsequent scalp expansions.

D. Bilateral temporo-parietal-occipital **Juri flaps** with hair can be expanded and rotated on branches of the superficial temporal artery to cover midline hairless regions (see Chapter 33). Expansion is continued until the arc of the tissue mound overlying the expander equals the sum of the width of the planned flap and width of the expander.

E. Alternatively, a midline sagittal incision can be used to place the bilateral expanders, and the bald area is closed in a V-Y manner.

F. Finally, hair plug grafts can augment the hairline.

V. FOREHEAD

A. Expanders are placed beneath the frontalis (galea counterpart) muscle. If possible, two expanders on opposite sides of the defect allow for symmetric medial advancement over the defect.

B. The planned flap procedure should preserve the normal brow position, frontalis function, and forehead sensory innervation.

VI. NOSE

A. Forehead expansion can also be used to expand forehead skin to allow primary closure of forehead flap donor sites.

B. Secondary contracture of the expanded tissue covering the nose can be a problems (see Chapter 37).

VII. EAR

Custom-shaped expanders in the hairless mastoid region are used.

VIII. FACE AND NECK

A. The ideal reconstructive procedure should use scarless expanded tissue from the face and neck to rotate over the defects of the face. The incision lines should be at the margins of aesthetic units. Using this approach, the surgeon replaces "like with like" tissue.

B. Traction on the lower eyelid from the rotated flap should be minimized, or an ectropion can occur.

C. In the lateral face, a **Mustarde**-type cervicofacial flap can be created from expanded lateral neck tissue.

D. In the lower face, multiple expanders on the neck are well tolerated and provide adequate tissue for flaps in this region. The opposite forces to the outward expansion might also cause mandibular occlusal disturbances and should be monitored.

IX. CRANIOFACIAL DISORDERS

A. Orbits of congenital anophthalmos and a small bony orbit can be expanded.

B. For soft tissue, primary closure of soft tissue over Tessier lateral facial clefts can be accomplished with less tension after expansion.

X. IMMEDIATE POSTMASTECTOMY BREAST RECONSTRUCTION (SEE ALSO CHAPTER 100)

A. Tissue expansion followed by implant placement is one of the most frequently used breast reconstruction methods.

B. Textured expanders are preferred.

C. The expander is ideally placed immediately after mastectomy. For immediate reconstruction, the expander should be covered by pectoralis and/or serratus anterior muscle in the area of the skin incision.

D. Tissue expanders enlarge the skin envelope, permitting the insertion of permanent implants to restore breast mound symmetry.

XI. CONGENITAL OR ACQUIRED BREAST ASYMMETRY

See Chapter 100.

XII. TRUNK

A. Traditional myocutaneous flaps used for reconstruction in the region can be augmented by preexpansion.

B. Multiple expanders are placed radially above the fascia.

XIII. EXTREMITIES

A. Multiple expanders are best placed radially to the defect rather than axially.

B. Endoscopy can facilitate pocket dissection for expansion placement.

C. Expansion below the knee is predisposed to infection and extrusion.

XIV. PREEXPANSION OF FULL-THICKNESS SKIN GRAFTS

A. Full-thickness grafts provide better aesthetic defect coverage, but the drawbacks are primary graft contraction and donor-site morbidity.

B. Preexpansion of the donor site facilitates primary closure of the donor site and provides a larger surface area of the graft.

XV. COMPLICATIONS OF TISSUE EXPANSION

A. **Infection** can occur from contamination during placement, from retrograde contamination from an external port, or after an expander extrudes. Early infections often require implant removal. Late implant infections are often limited by the capsular formation and the tissue can be used for the planned flap with minor risk. However, permanent implants should not be placed in the same contaminated areas.

B. **Extrusion** is usually due to inadequate placement technique, infection, or overaggressive expansion. After late extrusion, the expanded tissue can often be salvaged.

C. **Pain** and numbness during expansion are the best indicators of excessive intraluminal pressure of overaggressive expansion. Volume reduction is possible by withdrawing saline from the port. In contrast, mild discomfort is a reliable indicator of the volume limit during an expansion session.

10

Musculocutaneous Flaps

Delora L. Mount, M.D., and Stephen J. Mathes, M.D.
University of California, San Francisco, San Francisco, California, U.S.A.

I. INTRODUCTION

A. Musculocutaneous flap reconstruction is one of the most important reconstructive procedures available.

B. Advantages of reconstructing a defect with en bloc muscle and skin flap are numerous. Studies have demonstrated that the muscle portion of the flap provides reliable well-vascularized tissue, enhancing oxygen delivery to the healing reconstructed bed. Additional studies have shown enhanced resistance to infection compared to fascial and skin flaps. Additionally, muscle flaps have been used effectively to treat osteomyelitis. Muscle bulk provides stable obliteration of large dead spaces and can be designed for aesthetic contour.

C. Inclusion of the skin and subcutaneous tissue with the muscle flap provides complete reconstruction of a composite defect, often obviating the need for a skin graft. The skin and subcutaneous territory, when taken in continuity with muscle, can provide durable cutaneous coverage that can sustain pressure and postoperative field radiation. The cutaneous portion can serve a specialized function such as mucosal substitution of alimentary and genitourinary tracts. It also serves as a well-vascularized malleable scaffolding upon which secondary surgical aesthetic refinements such as nipple reconstruction can be performed.

D. This chapter will focus on the indications, applications, and technical and anatomic considerations of successful musculocutaneous flap reconstruction.

II. ANALYSIS OF DEFECT

A. Analysis of the surgical defect is of foremost importance in selecting the optimal reconstructive plan.

B. Defects following trauma or surgical extirpation are complex defects requiring composite tissue replacement. For example, following resection of oropharyngeal tumors, both soft tissue bulk and mucosal lining of the alimentary tract are absent. In this case, muscle provides the bulk and the skin territory provides functional lining of the oropharynx.

C. Factors important in the analysis of surgical defects include:

- Depth of the defect
- Surface size of the defect
- Location of the defect
- Underlying structures exposed, i.e., heart, bone, brain
- Local tissue factors, i.e., radiation, perfusion
- Function of missing or deficient tissues
- Contour of missing or deficient tissues

D. Once analysis of the defect has been accurately assessed, the surgeon can proceed with selection of the appropriate optimal flap for reconstruction.

III. ANATOMY/CLASSIFICATION

A. Successful myocutaneous transfer requires complete understanding of vascular anatomy and the microrelationships of muscle perfusion to the overlying skin paddle.

B. The vascular patterns of muscle circulation have been extensively studied and are classified into five subtypes by Mathes and Nahai (Fig. 1).

C. Careful dissection during flap harvest and transfer is necessary for sufficient flap perfusion after inset. Adequate muscle perfusion is paramount not only to survival of the muscle flap, but indirectly to the cutaneous components.

D. Muscle sustains skin perfusion through distinct musculocutaneous perforating vessels to distinct territorial distributions (Fig. 2). Based on the number and territorial distribution of perforator circulation, large areas of skin may be transferred reliably with the muscle, either as a rotational or free microvascular transfer.

E. Numbers and territories of musculocutaneous perforators vary considerably with the muscle being transferred (Fig. 3). Success in musculocutaneous flap transfer is dependent on careful, knowledgeable dissection of muscle vasculature and avoidance of injury to the musculocutaneous perforators to the corresponding skin/subcutaneous territory.

IV. TECHNICAL CONSIDERATIONS

A. Tissue Preparation

1. Careful dissection of muscle vascular pedicles is required. Injury can occur from Bovie cautery current or heat, excessive dissection of the vessels resulting in arterial spasm, and kinking or stretching of the vessels with inset.
2. Venous outflow of the pedicle is particularly vulnerable to positional or rotational kinking. In fact, many flap losses can be attributed to venous outflow problems.
3. Following musculocutaneous flap dissection, prior to transfer, several techniques can be used to protect both the vascular pedicle as well as the musculocutaneous perforators. To protect the vascular pedicle, a small cuff of areolar tissue around the vessels should be present so that with rotation or free transfer the pedicle will be protected from kinking and stretching. Musculocutaneous perforators can be protected from

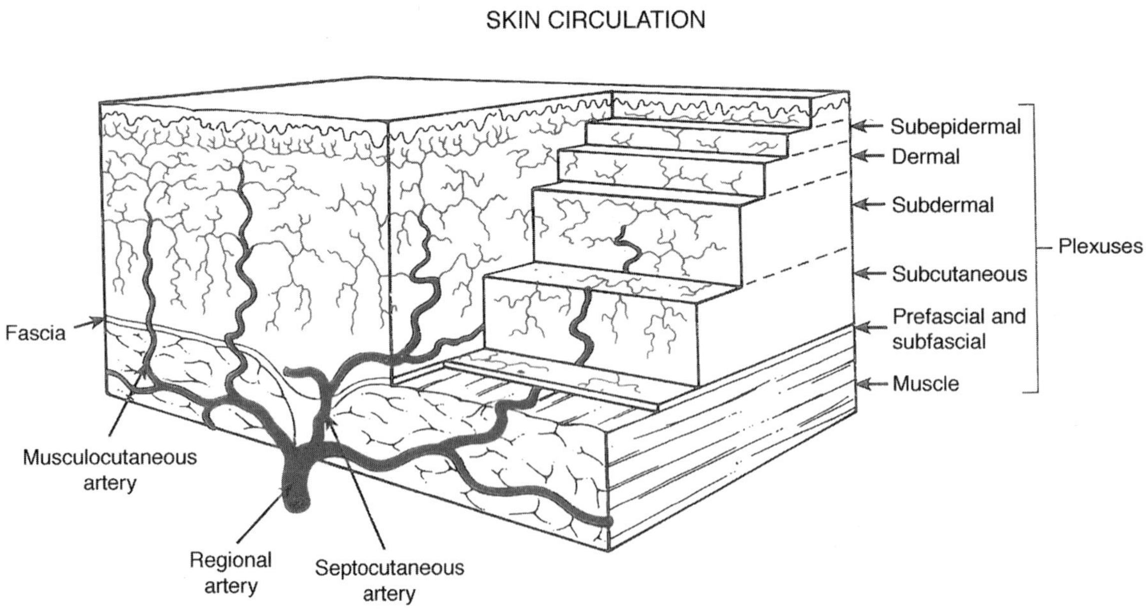

Figure 1 Skin circulation.

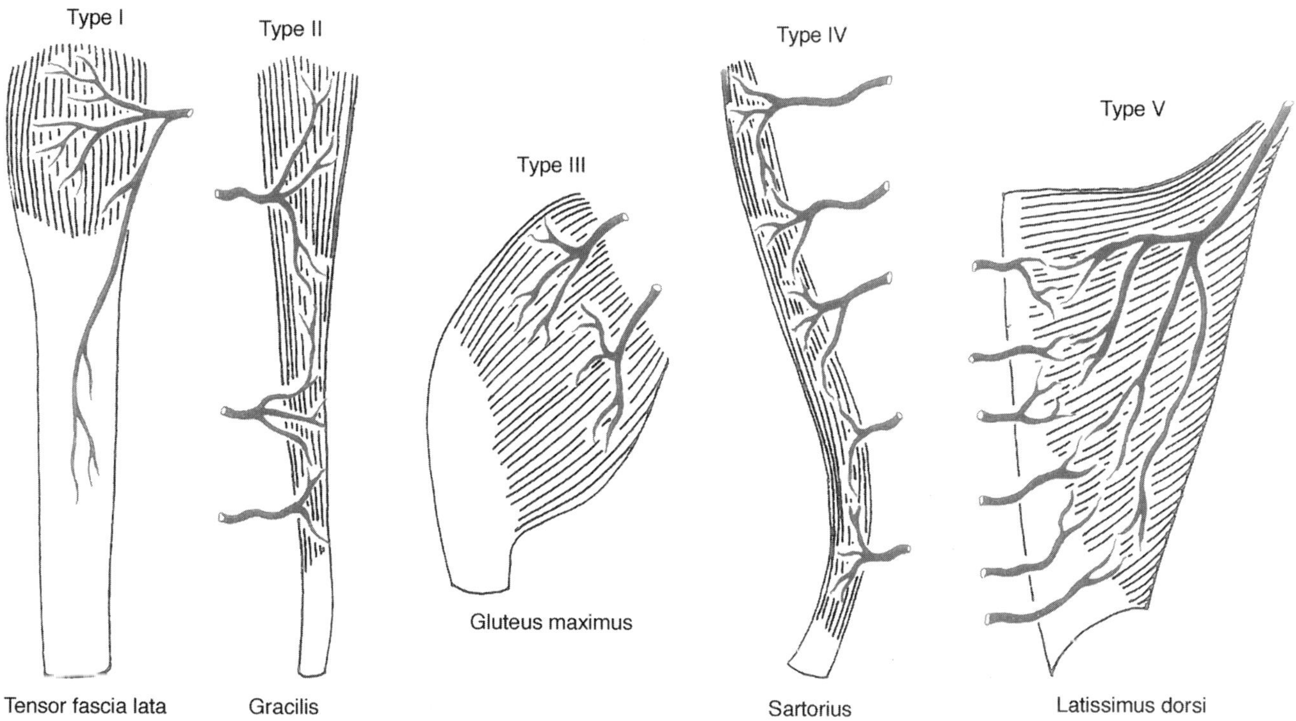

Figure 2 Classification of muscle/musculocutaneous flaps. Patterns of vascular anatomy: type I, one vascular pedicle; type II, dominant pedicle(s) and minor pedicle(s); type III, two dominant pedicles; type IV, segmental vascular pedicles; type V, one dominant pedicle and secondary segmental pedicles. (From Mathes SJ; Nahai F: Classification of the vascular anatomy of muscles: experimental and clinical correlation. *Plast. Reconstr. Surg*. 67:177, 1981.)

shear forces by suturing the muscle fascia to the muscle edges. This prevents traumatic separation of the fascia from the muscle during transfer, preventing disruption of the musculocutaneous and septocutaneous perforators.

4. Free microvascular transfer of musculocutaneous flaps requires additional care in atraumatic vessel handling and suture techniques. The addition of topical vasodilators, administration of systemic anticoagulation and warm operating room temperature have been shown to improve success of free microvascular transfer.

B. The Delay Principle

1. When greater areas of skin and soft tissue are needed, a technique of delay can be used to increase the skin territory safely transferred.
2. This is a two-stage technique by which a secondary vascular pedicle is ligated during the first stage, rendering the corresponding skin territory ischemic. Circulation is resultantly increased to supply the ischemic area by the primary pedicles.
3. When actual transfer of the flap is done in the second stage, the enlarged skin territory is more reliably transferred.

C. Preexpansion

1. Placement of submuscular tissue expanders can be used to both increase the size of a musculocutaneous flap and allow for primary closure of the donor site.
2. This is particularly useful in the tensor fascia lata flap, where preexpansion allows a larger flap to be transferred and often allows the donor defect to be closed primarily.

D. Supercharging

1. Improved circulation in a musculocutaneous flap can be produced by supercharging. This is a technique by which a microsurgical anastomosis

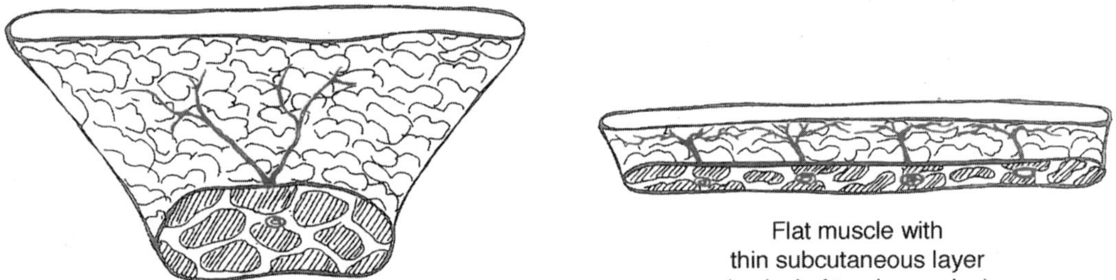

Narrow muscle with
thick layer of subcutaneous fat
(typical of limb muscles)

Flat muscle with
thin subcutaneous layer
(typical of trunk muscles)

Figure 3

is performed to a secondary vascular pedicle of a rotational flap.

2. An example would be a supercharged TRAM (transverse rectus abdominis musculocutaneous) flap where the flap is rotated for inset based on the superior epigastric vessels, and the inferior epigastric vessels undergo microvascular anastomoses to vessels in the axilla.

E. Innervated Flap

1. Flaps can be transferred with motor and/or sensory innervation.
2. An important example of this is tongue reconstruction with a motor-innervated musculocutaneous flap. Motor nerves, which usually accompany the vascular pedicle, are anastomosed during transfer for postoperative motor reinnervation and tongue motor function.

V. FLAP DESIGN

Musculocutaneous flaps can be fashioned into many functional and aesthetic units. The following are common uses for various musculocutaneous flaps:

A. Breast Reconstruction

1. Muscle and subcutaneous tissue provides bulk and aesthetic contour.
2. Skin provides new breast skin and a scaffold for nipple reconstruction.
3. Examples:
   - TRAM
   - Latissimus dorsi musculocutaneous flap

B. Oropharynx and Tongue

1. Muscle and subcutaneous tissue provides bulk, aesthetic contour, and functional motor activity (e.g., tongue).
2. Skin provides mucosal substitution for floor of mouth, tongue, and hypopharynx.
3. Examples:
   - Rectus abdominis
   - Gracilis
   - Latissimus dorsi

C. Scalp/Craniofacial Defects

1. Muscle provides neo-dura mater and fills dead space of composite wounds.
2. Skin provides cutaneous coverage.
3. Examples:
   - Rectus abdominis
   - Gracilis
   - Latissimus dorsi
   - Trapezius

D. Vaginal/Perineal

1. Muscle and subcutaneous tissue provides obliteration of large post-extirpative defects
2. Skin territory provides skin replacement and mucosal substitution (e.g., vaginal wall lining)
3. Examples:
   - Rectus abdominis
   - Gracilis

E. Trunk/Back

1. Muscle and subcutaneous tissue provides dead space obliteration.
2. Skin territory provides skin replacement.
3. Examples:
    - Pectoralis major
    - Rectus abdominis
    - Latissimus dorsi
    - Gluteus maximus
    - Gracilis

F. Extremity

1. Muscle provides vascularized tissue for treatment of ischemic areas/infected wound/coverage of orthopedic hardware.
2. Skin territory provides stable skin coverage.
3. Examples:
    - Rectus abdominis
    - Latissimus dorsi
    - Gracilis

VI. SUMMARY

1. Musculocutaneous flaps, whether transferred as a pedicled rotational or free microvascular transfer, are technically dependent on knowledge of anatomic relationships, flap design, and accurate assessment of the composite defect.
2. These flaps, when successfully harvested and inset, provide a versatile, reliable, and malleable flap choice for reconstruction of major composite defects.

11

Transplantation in Plastic Surgery

Maria Siemionow, M.D., Ph.D., and Omar F. Ahmed, M.D.
Cleveland Clinic Foundation, Cleveland, Ohio, U.S.A.

Carrel's landmark developments in vascular anastomosis technique (1902) helped thrust transplantation to the forefront of scientific innovation. With further surgical and antirejection advances (Fig. 1), increased orthotopic and heterotopic transplantation to anatomically similar and different recipients sites, respectively, will signal the next revolution in plastic surgery.

I. AUTOGRAFT TRANSPLANTATION

A. **Background**

- An **autograft** is a tissue or organ transferred from one location to another on the same individual.
- Sushruta Samhita in India (700 B.C.) was the first to report an autogenous tissue transfer, using a forehead flap for nose reconstruction.
- The first Western report by Tagliacozzi was a forearm flap for nose reconstruction in Italy (1597).
- Thiersch revolutionized the use of free full-thickness skin grafts.

B. **Skin autografts** include full-thickness skin grafts (low contracture, better cosmesis) and split-thickness skin grafts (better take and availability).

C. **Bone autografts** include nonvascularized and vascularized bone grafts. Vascularized bone grafts have a dual blood supply of periosteal covering and endosteal blood vessels and are thus transferred in a pedicled or microvascular manner.

D. **Cartilage autografts**, used in craniofacial reconstruction, have limited donor sites (conchal, nasal septal, and costal regions).

E. **Nerve autografts** (e.g., sural nerve) degenerate, leaving the remaining myelin sheath as a conduit for regenerating axons where the injured nerve cannot be coapted without tension.

II. ALLOGRAFT TRANSPLANTATION

A. Background

1. An **allograft** is a tissue or organ transferred between unrelated individuals of the same species.
2. An **isograft** is tissue transferred between genetically identical individuals (e.g., monozygotic twins).
3. According to legend, the earliest allograft transplantation involved skin donated from a slave for reconstruction of the master's nose in Italy (1503).
4. Skin allografts were increasingly used in the nineteenth century, with Winston Churchill donating to a fellow wounded officer in 1898.

B. Immunology

1. Allografts are rejected by recipient immunocompetent cells reacting to donor cell antigens. Donor cell antigens are termed major histocompatibility complex (MHC) antigens in non-

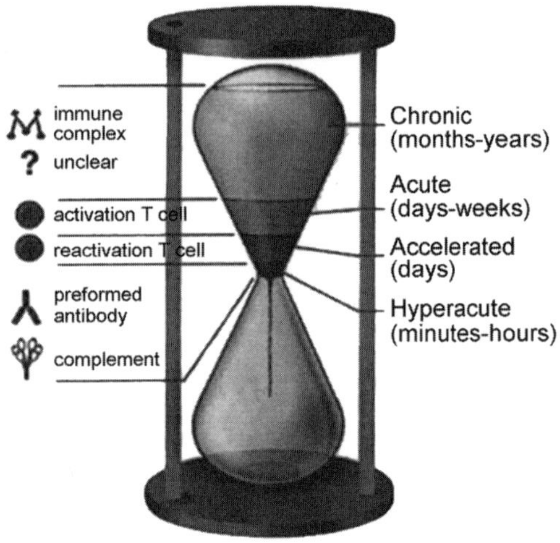

Figure 1 Clinical rejection syndromes. The mechanisms of rejection can be described based upon the speed of transplant damage. Preformed antibodies and presensitized lymphocytes cause rapid rejection compared with primary and slowly evolving responses.

humans and human leukocyte antigens (HLAs) in humans.

2. Three classes of MHC antigens have been identified, of which MHC class I and class II antigens are capable of triggering lymphocytes. Although MHC class I antigens are found on all somatic cells, MHC class II antigens are found only on certain lymphocytes (B cells, monocytes, macrophages, dendritic cells, Langerhans cells) and vascular endothelium.
3. MHC antigens are presented to the host immune system by antigen-presenting cells (APCs). APCs stimulate both helper T cells via cytokines (IL-1, IL-6) and tumor necrosis factor (TNF) and B cells via IL-1 and IL-4.
4. Helper T cells provide class II–restricted rejection and stimulate cytotoxic T cells and large granular lymphocytes that provide class I–restricted rejection.
5. Secondarily, B-cell antibodies provide indirect rejection.

C. Therapy

1. Tissue matching is often used in blood and solid organ transfer.
2. Nonspecific or specific immunosuppression can be used in allograft transplantation.
3. *Nonspecific immunosuppression* includes total lymphoid irradiation and pharmacologic agents.
   - Steroids (e.g., prednisone) inhibit IL-1.
   - Cyclosporin is a fungal (*Tolypocladium*) metabolite that inhibits helper T-cell IL-2 synthesis with a relatively low therapeutic/toxic ratio. Major toxicities are renal failure and hypertension.
   - Newer agents include FK-506 (tacrolimus; an IL-2 mRNA synthesis inhibitor), rapamycin (cytokine signal transduction inhibitor), and the antimetabolites Brequiner sodium and mycophenolate mofetil.
   - Immunosuppression side effects include infection, nephrotoxicity, bone marrow suppression, and tumor formation. The most common tumors are skin cancer, lymphomas, and lung carcinoma.
4. *Specific immunosuppression* includes monoclonal antibodies (e.g., anti-ICAM-1).

D. Skin Allografts

1. Survival is prolonged in severely burned (i.e., immunocompromised) patients.
2. Skin allografts have the highest rejection profile secondary to high vascularity and MHC expression. They also carry a risk of disease transmission.
3. Cultured keratinocytes provide temporary coverage with immunosuppression.

E. Bone Allografts

1. Bone allografts are nonvascularized, readily banked, and reconstituted with saline.
2. After donor cells are rejected, a scaffold for creeping substitution remains.
3. Bone allografts can be used with autograft or in osteotomy sites (with long-term internal fixation).

F. Cartilage Allografts

1. Cartilage allografts are used as readily as autograft since chondrocytes are immunologically shielded by matrix.
2. Preserved cartilage is more abundant and less infective.
3. Problems include resorption and potential warping.

G. Nerve Allografts

1. Nerve allografts are used in carefully selected patients with severe nerve injury.
2. Antigenicity can be reduced with warm and cold temperature preservation.
3. Cyclosporin, FK-506, and anti-ICAM-1/LFA-1 antibodies can prolong survival.

H. Muscle Allografts

1. Survival has been demonstrated clinically using prednisone and cyclosporin immunosuppression.
2. Muscle allografts have limited clinical use at this point.

III. XENOGRAFT TRANSPLANTATION

A. Background

1. A **xenograft** is transferred between individuals of different species.
2. Xenograft transplantation was performed throughout the nineteenth century, but Bert first differentiated autograft, allograft, and xenograft behavior (1863).

B. Immunology/Therapy

1. Xenogeneic tissue can be strongly antigenic because of high levels of recipient preformed antibodies; it is discordant when natural antibodies are present or concordant when absent.
2. Increased therapeutic levels are necessary to counteract rapid hyperacute rejection, precluding xenografts from most species (e.g., pig to human).

C. Skin Xenografts (Porcine)

1. Skin xenografts can serve as temporary biologic dressings.
2. Xenogeneic dermis can prepare wounds for grafting.

D. Cartilage Xenografts (Bovine)

Cartilage xenografts have been used in temporomandibular joint repair with minimal postoperative morbidity.

IV. COMPOSITE TISSUE ALLOGRAFT (CTA) TRANSPLANTATION

A. Background

1. A CTA is a neurovascularized, nonvital allograft composed of functional integumentary and aesthetic musculoskeletal elements.
2. According to legend, Saints Cosmas and Damian performed the first human leg transplantation in Syria (348 A.D.).
3. Gilbert (1964) was the first to perform a cadaveric hand transplant, but this survived only 3 weeks.
4. Dubernard performed the first modern human hand transplantation in Lyon, France (1998).

B. Immunology/Therapy

1. Rejection of an individual CTA component is proportional to its relative antigenicity (Fig. 2).
2. Elements with higher relative antigenicity have increased vascular supply.

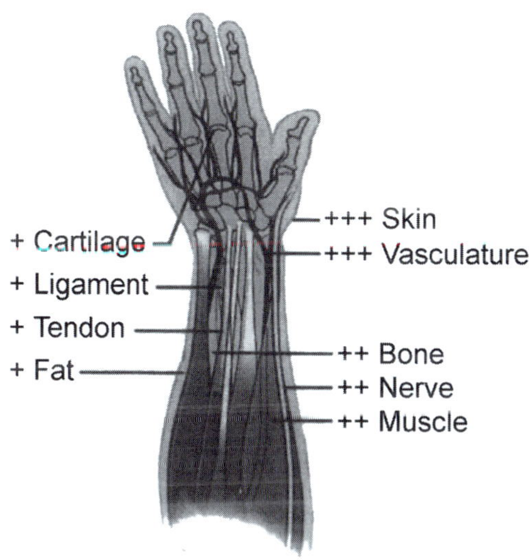

Figure 2 Relative antigenicity of individual components of CTAs (limb). Skin has high MHC expression and donor-derived (passenger) leukocytes. Bone itself has low MHC expression, but marrow has high expression and passenger leukocytes. Vasculature is unique since it has intermediate MHC expression and can be rejected via humoral mechanisms. Overall component antigenicity is also affected by its vascular supply requirements.

3. Staged immunosuppression strategies may protect components with high functional return potential while minimizing host exposure.

C. Limb CTA

1. Limb CTA may be preferred to autoreconstruction because the repair is immediate, orthotopic, neurotized, and not associated with donor-site morbidity.
2. Transplantation is technically achievable, and normal healing has been observed.
3. Limb CTA is still controversial secondary to use of life-long immunosuppression (and its associated morbidities) for a non–life-threatening problem.

V. THERAPEUTIC TRENDS IN REJECTION PREVENTION

A. The future includes development of new pharmacologic agents, multiple therapy protocols, and tolerance induction.

B. Tolerance (immunologic unresponsiveness to donor tissue) was first described by Nobel laureate Medawar and may replace prolonged immunosuppression.

C. Experimentally, tolerance can be induced centrally or peripherally. Central tolerance creates chimerism (donor and recipient antigen tolerance) or mixed chimerism (recipient T-cell protection).

D. Tolerance principles have been applied in solid organ transfer and hold promise for transplantation in plastic surgery.

12

Tissue Engineering and Biomaterials

Michael J. Yaremchuk, M.D., and J. Peter Rubin, M.D.*
Massachusetts General Hospital, Boston, Massachusetts, U.S.A.

I. TISSUE ENGINEERING

Three possible strategies are under laboratory investigation.

A. Isolated Cell or Cell Substitutes

1. Example—stereotactic infusion of fetal dopamine-producing cells into the brain for the treatment of Parkinson's disease.
2. Obstacles—immunologic rejection, cell function failure.

B. Tissue-Inducing Substances

1. Example—polymer membranes with growth factor impregnation for nerve conduits.
2. Obstacles—availability and delivery of appropriate biological signal molecules.

C. Cells Placed in or Within Matrices

Matrices may be autologous materials such as fibrin glue or synthetic polymers. Cells may be autologous and expanded in culture, or allogeneic.

1. Examples—osteoblasts, chondrocytes, hepatocytes, enterocytes, and urothelial cells have been seeded into various polymers to create neotissue.
2. Obstacles—reactivity of host to polymers and implanted cells. Limitation of tissue culture to expand cell number.

II. CLINICALLY AVAILABLE PRODUCTS

A. Dermal Replacements

1. Integra (Integra Life Sciences, Plainsboro, NJ).
2. Bovine collagen and shark glycosaminoglycan provide a scaffold for host fibroblast and endothelial cell ingrowth. This new dermis is later covered with epithelial grafts.

B. Cultured Epithelial Cells

Small skin biopsies can be expanded in tissue culture up to 10,000-fold for burn wound resurfacing.

III. ALLOPLASTIC MATERIALS

A. Government Regulation

1. FDA regulates implant devices.
2. Implant materials are not approved by FDA; only devices are approved.

B. Characteristics of Ideal Implant Material

1. Biologically inert
2. Easily shapeable
3. Maintains form and consistency

* *Current affiliation*: University of Pittsburgh, Pittsburgh, Pennsylvania, U.S.A.

4. Nontoxic
5. Nonimmunogenic

C. Biocompatibility

Biocompatibility, a favorable interaction between the implanted material and the host, is influenced by three factors:

1. Physical qualities of the material: surface texture and charge, firmness, toxicity of breakdown products.
2. Surgical technique: asepsis, handling of implant, extent of pocket dissection, choice of implant bed, implant dimensions relative to site, method of fixation.
3. Host response: soft tissue vascularity, thickness of soft tissue coverage, tension, bacterial contamination of implant site, past or future radiation exposure, systemic disease affecting wound healing (e.g., diabetes), immunosuppression.

D. Natural Response to Implanted Materials

1. Smooth-surfaced implants are encapsulated.
2. Porous implants may allow for incorporation by soft tissue and bony ingrowth.
   - Better fixation but more difficult to remove
   - Theoretical resistance to infection because host defenses are within the device
3. Implants placed under soft tissue that is too thin or under tension will be extruded.

E. Specific Materials

Metals

Stainless steel

Vitallium (cobalt-chromium alloy)

- More resistant to corrosion than steel
- Lower incidence of hypersensitivity

Titanium: favored material for craniofacial plating systems

- Either pure or in alloy with aluminum and vanadium (Ti-6Al-4V)
- Very resistant to corrosion
- Lowest artifact in CT and MRI imaging studies

F. Resorbable Plates and Screws

1. Usually copolymer of polylactic and polyglycolic acids
2. Degrade by hydrolysis and debris cleared by macrophages
3. Useful for the pediatric craniofacial skeleton to avoid potential complications of growth restriction and plate translocation

G. Hydroxyapatite

1. Form of calcium phosphate found in bone matrix.
2. Can be produced as dense granules, porous form (based on the calcium carbonate skeleton of marine coral), or powdered cement mix.
3. Although bony ingrowth possible, material is too brittle to bear loads.

H. Polysiloxane (Silicone) (Fig. 1)

1. Polymer with noncarbon backbone.
2. Can be produced in consistencies ranging from liquid to hard solid.
3. Liquid silicone is not approved by the FDA for injection.

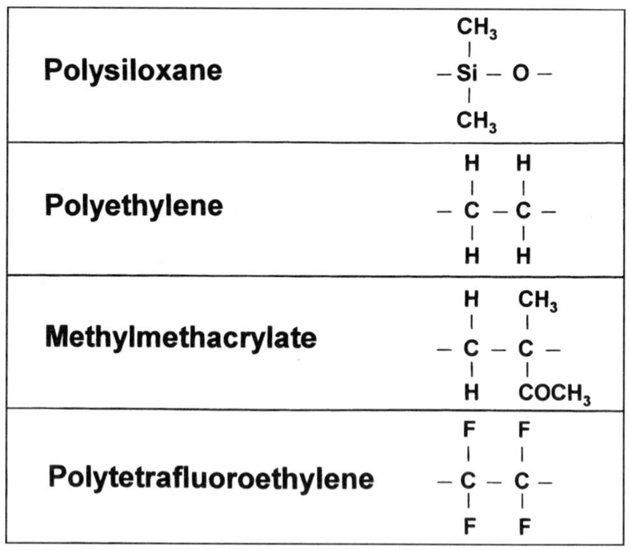

Figure 1 Molecular structure of common polymer biomaterials. (From Rubin JP; Yaremchuk MJ: Complications and toxicities of implantable biomaterials used in facial aesthetic and reconstructive surgery. *Plastic. Reconstr. Surg.* 100(5):1336, 1997.)

I. Polyethylene (Medpor)

1. Simple carbon chain backbone.
2. Like silicone, can be produced in a variety of consistencies; high density is preferred for facial implants.
3. Porous form is most commonly used.
   - 125–250 μm pores allow soft tissue and limited bony ingrowth
   - Easily carved in operating room and holds screws for fixation

J. Polytetrafluoroethylene (GoreTex)

1. Frequently used for vascular grafts.
2. Flexible and pliable, easily cut to shape.
3. Composed of fibrils with 30 μm pores; allows limited tissue in growth.

K. Acrylic/Methylmethacrylate

1. Long history of use as bone cement in orthopedics.
2. Polymer powder mixed with monomer to harden material; easily shaped.
   - Reaction highly exothermic—potential injury to underlying brain
   - Monomer toxic to both patient and operating room staff (need good ventilation)
3. Variation is preformed implant known as hard tissue replacement (HTR).
   - Porous implant
   - Negatively charged calcium hydroxide coating to encourage bone growth

L. IMPLANT COMPLICATIONS

A. Infection—mandates removal of the device.

B. Exposure—can be related to inadequate soft tissue cover or infection.

C. Displacement/migration—related to device fixation.

D. Hypersensitivity is rare for metals and almost unheard of for polymers.

13

Anatomy and Embryology of the Skin

Chia Soo, M.D.
David Geffen School of Medicine at UCLA, Los Angeles, California, U.S.A.
H. Peter Lorenz, M.D.
Stanford University Medical Center, Stanford, California, U.S.A.

The skin or integument consists of two distinct embryological tissue layers: ectoderm and mesoderm. The surface ectoderm gives rise to the epidermis and epidermal derivatives such as glands, hairs, and nails, while the mesoderm gives rise to the dermis.

I. EPIDERMIS

A. The initial **ectoderm** layer covering the embryo is only one cell thick.

B. After neurulation in the 4th week of gestation, the ectoderm proliferates to form an outer protective layer of simple squamous epithelium called **periderm** and an inner **basal layer** of proliferating cells.

C. At 11 weeks of gestation, proliferation of the basal layer (now designated the **germinative layer or stratum germinativum**) produces a new **intermediate layer** just deep to the periderm. The intermediate layer cells produce keratin and are called **keratinocytes**.

D. At approximately 21 weeks of gestation, the periderm is shed and the intermediate layer keratinocytes differentiate into three distinct layers: the inner **stratum spinosum**, the middle **stratum granulosum**, and the outer **stratum corneum (horny layer)** (Fig. 1). Only the stem cell-containing stratum germinativum is capable of cell division in the epidermis.

II. KERATINOCYTE DIFFERENTIATION

A. Stratum germinativum cells migrating through the stratum spinosum produce large amounts of **keratin** and **envelope proteins**. Upon reaching the stratum granulosum layer, keratinocytes stop production of keratin and envelope proteins and begin production of **filagrin**, a protein for bundling intracellular keratin filaments, and **transglutaminase**, an enzyme for cross-linking envelope proteins.

B. Next, intracellular release of lytic enzymes produces the **terminally differentiated**, cornified, enucleated keratinocytes that enter the stratum corneum.

III. REGULATION OF KERATINOCYTE DIFFERENTIATION

A. Various growth factors and cytokines regulate epidermal proliferation and differentiation, including epidermal growth factor, transforming growth factor-α, transforming growth factor-β, keratinocyte growth factor, interleukin-1, and interleukin-6.

B. Excessive transforming growth factor-α can result in psoriasis and other hyperproliferative skin diseases.

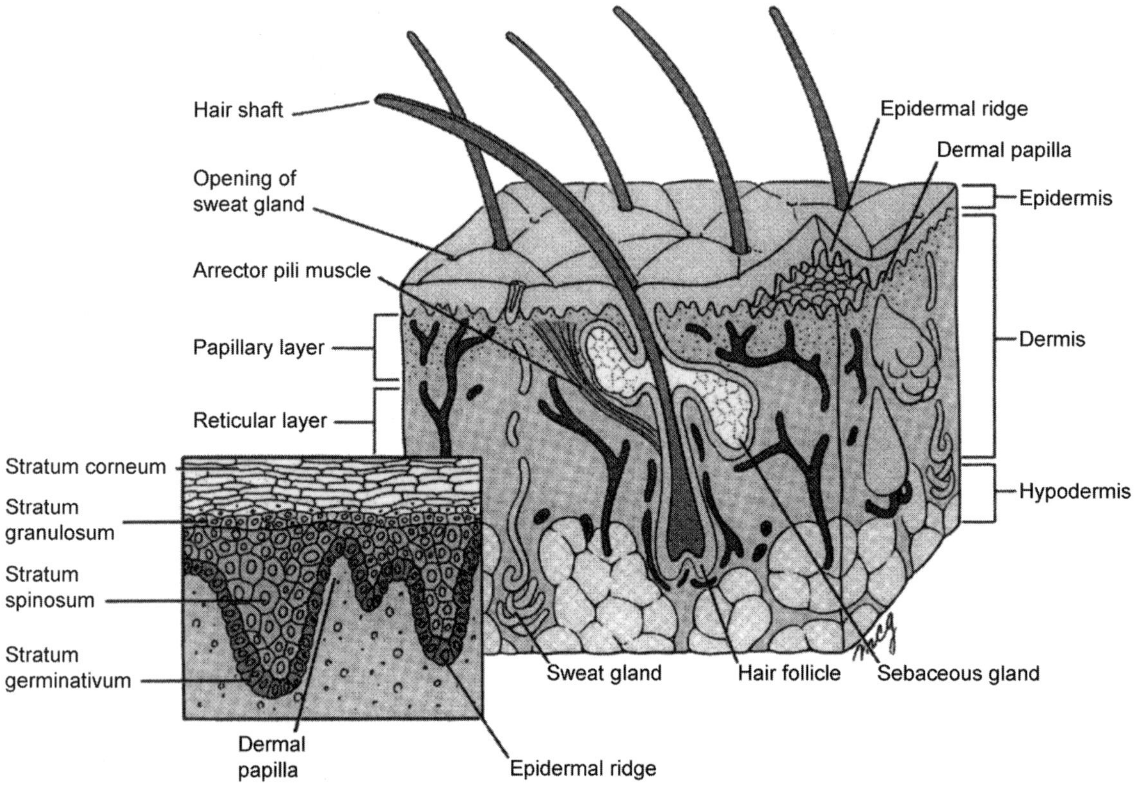

Figure 1 Organization of the dermis and epidermis. The patterns of interdigitating dermal papillae and epidermal ridges first develops during the third month of gestation. Sebaceous glands develop from the epidermal lining of the hair follicles, appearing about 1 month after a given hair bud is formed. (From Larsen WJ: *Human Embryology*. Churchill Livingstone, New York, 1993.)

C. **Ichthyosis** is a general term for disorders characterized by excessive keratinization that results in dryness and fish-like scaling of the skin. It is treated with topical medications and careful skin maintenance.

D. **Harlequin fetus** is a rare, generally lethal, autosomal recessive disorder in which stratum granulosum cells exhibit defective keratin fiber bundling. This leads to abnormal keratinocyte maturation and inability of stratum corneum keratinocytes to slough properly.

IV. OTHER EPIDERMAL CELLS

A. Besides keratinocytes, the epidermis also contains melanocytes, Langerhans cells, and Merkel cells.

B. Skin **melanocytes** are derived from neural crest cells that detach at 6–7 weeks gestation from the neural tube, migrate into the dermis, and differentiate into **melanoblasts**. The melanoblasts then enter the developing epidermis and differentiate into melanocytes at the epidermal-dermal junction. Melanocytes produce **melanin**, a pigment that functions as a barrier to solar radiation. In adults, approximately 5–10% of epidermal cells are melanocytes.

C. **Langerhans cells** are skin macrophages that originate from bone marrow and first appear in the epidermis at 7 weeks. Langerhans cells perform various immunological functions that range from prevention of cutaneous carcinogenesis to mediation of contact allergy.

D. Lastly, **Merkel cells** are mechanoreceptors of possible neural crest or epidermal origin. They first appear in the epidermal base at 4–6 months gestation and interact with underlying dermal nerve endings. They are only found in plantar and palmar regions.

V. DERMIS

A. The dermis originates from two embryonic sources of mesoderm. The majority is derived from the somatopleuric layer of the lateral plate mesoderm, but the dermatomal divisions of the somites also contribute.

B. During the third month, the outer dermal layer proliferates and protrudes into the epidermis to form **dermal papillae** (Fig. 1).

C. In between the dermal papillae are the **epidermal ridges**.

D. At about 4 months, the dermis divides into a more superficial **papillary layer** and a deeper, denser **reticular layer**.

E. By mid-gestation, the **hypodermis**, or subcutaneous fatty layer, develops.

F. The dermal papillae determine the variability of surface skin patterns. The first patterns to arise are whorls on the palmar and plantar surfaces of the digits at 11–12 weeks. By the fifth month, the entire cutaneous surface pattern is established and retained for life.

VI. VASCULATURE

A. The organization of the dermal vasculature is already defined by the end of the first trimester. By 6–7 weeks, a single layer of vessels is present in the dermis, to be followed by two parallel layers of capillary plexuses between 7 to 11 weeks. These capillaries are present only within the dermis, since epidermal metabolism is entirely dependent on diffusion of gases and nutrients.

B. Neonatal skin has approximately 20 times more vasculature than needed for skin metabolism. The excess vasculature is necessary for thermal regulation.

C. Dermal nerve development coincides with vascularization.

VII. HAIR DEVELOPMENT

A. Hair follicle development begins in the primitive two-layer epidermis with the formation of **hair buds (hair germs)** by cells in the basal layer (stratum germinativum) (Fig. 2).

B. Next, these cells multiply and grow downward into the dermis to form **hair nodules (hair pegs)**, followed by **hair bulbs (bulbous hair pegs)** with **dermal papillae**.

C. The epithelial cells of the hair bulb overlying the dermal papilla form the **germinal matrix** that later gives rise to the hair shaft. Proliferating germinal matrix cells undergo keratinization and are incorporated into the developing **hair shaft**.

D. Pigments from hair bulb melanocytes are incorporated into the maturing keratinocyte.

E. The peripheral epithelial cells (ectoderm derived) of the hair bulb develop into the **inner and outer**

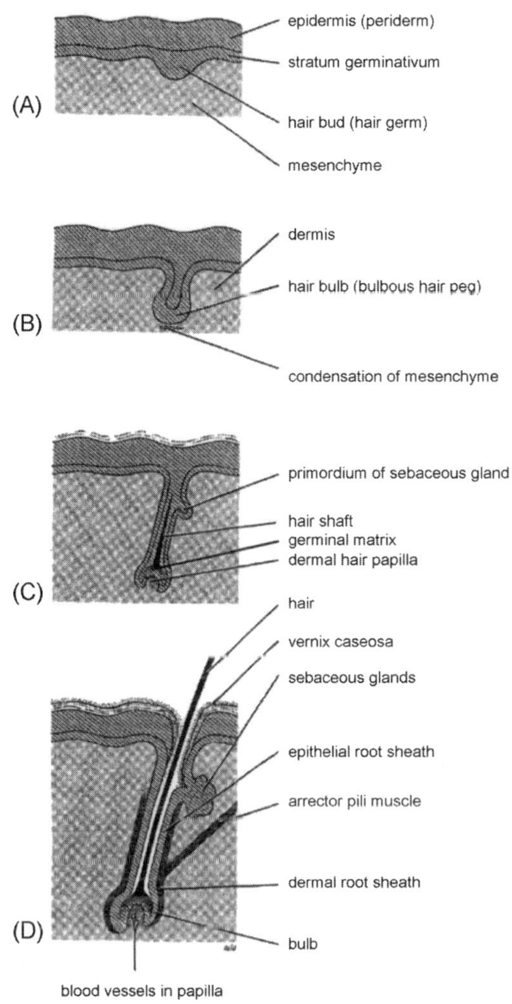

Figure 2 Successive stages in hair and sebaceous gland development: (A) 12 weeks; (B) 14 weeks; (C) 16 weeks; (D) 18 weeks. Note that the sebaceous gland develops as an outgrowth from the side of the hair follicle. (Modified from Moore KL: *Before We Are Born; Basic Embryology and Birth Defects*. Saunders, Philadelphia, 1974.)

epidermal root sheath, while the surrounding dermal cells (mesoderm derived) develop into the **dermal root sheath**. Except for eyebrow and eyelash follicles, all follicular dermal root sheaths associate with smooth muscle cells of the arrector pili muscle that functions to erect hair, creating a "gooseflesh" appearance.

F. An average man or woman has approximately 5 million hair follicles.

G. The first hair follicles appear on the eyebrows, eyelids, upper lip, and chin at about 2 months gestation. By 5 months of gestation, the majority of hair follicles are developed, and it is likely that new hair follicle formation does not occur after birth.

H. The first generation of hairs is called **lanugo** and consists of fine, unpigmented hairs that are generally shed at birth.

VIII. GLAND DEVELOPMENT

Like the hair follicle, sebaceous, apocrine, and sweat glands are also produced by epidermal downgrowth.

A. Sebaceous Glands

1. Sebaceous glands develop as diverticulae from the sides of the hair follicle. However, in hairless areas of the body, such as the glans penis and labia minora, sebaceous glands develop as autonomous epidermal downgrowths.
2. The diverticulae then branch into the surrounding dermis to form ducts and secretory acini (alveoli). These acini utilize a **holocrine** mechanism by which entire cells filled with secretory products are broken down and shed into the ducts.
3. By 6 months gestation, mature facial sebaceous glands are present.
4. During fetal development, the sebaceous glands actively produce **sebum**, an oily substance that lubricates hair and skin. The fetal sebum then combines with desquamated epithelial cells and periderm remnants to form the **vernix caseosa**, a protective waterproof covering for the fetus.
5. After birth the sebaceous glands are relatively dormant and remain that way until hormonal activation during puberty.

B. Apocrine Glands

1. Apocrine glands are coiled, unbranched glands that initially develop all over the body in association with hair follicles. By late gestation, however, the apocrine glands disappear except in specific areas such as the axilla, mons pubis, prepuce, scrotum, and labia minora.
2. In contrast to the sebaceous glands, the apocrine glands secrete by an apocrine mechanism in which small portions of cytoplasm containing secretory vesicles are released into the gland lumen.
3. **Hidradenitis suppurativa** is a chronic condition characterized by recurrent bacterial infections of the apocrine glands.

C. Sweat Glands

1. Sweat glands begin development at 20 weeks of gestation as solid, coiled, unbranched downgrowths of the stratum germinativum.
2. The central cells degenerate to form the gland lumen while the peripheral cells differentiate into an inner **secretory cell** layer and an outer **myoepithelial cell** layer. The secretory cells secrete via an **eccrine** mechanism in which fluids are secreted directly across the plasma membrane into the gland lumen.
3. Once in the lumen, the sweat is expelled by contraction of the sympathetically innervated myoepithelial cells.
4. Sweat glands are present in all cutaneous areas except for a few areas such as the nipples.
5. **Large sweat glands** develop in association with hair follicles of the axilla, pubic, and areola regions. Because of this, their ducts do not open directly onto the skin surfaces as do ordinary sweat glands, but rather into hair follicles just superficial to the sebaceous gland openings.

14

Normal Scars, Hypertrophic Scars, and Keloids

Chia Soo, M.D.
David Geffen School of Medicine at UCLA, Los Angeles, California, U.S.A.

H. Peter Lorenz, M.D.
Stanford University Medical Center, Stanford, California, U.S.A.

From an evolutionary perspective, the replacement of injured areas with fast-growing "scar" tissue is beneficial in that it rapidly reestablishes cutaneous integrity of the organism. However, in certain individuals and under certain conditions, the protective repair response can become pathologic and lead to the formation of hypertrophic scars or keloids. Although frequently discussed together, the current evidence suggests that hypertrophic scars and keloids are different entities with different etiologies.

I. NORMAL SCAR TISSUE

A. Definition

1. From a clinical standpoint, a normal scar remains within the confines of the original wound, is not elevated above skin level, and continues to soften and become less prominent with time.
2. Histology reveals replacement of the normal dermal collagen architecture with a relatively avascular compact collection of collagen bundles and a few scattered fibroblasts.
3. No hair follicles are present in scar tissue.

B. Etiology

After injury, repair occurs through a series of overlapping phases: inflammation, proliferation, and remodeling, with an end result of scar formation.

II. HYPERTROPHIC SCAR

A. Definition

1. Clinically, hypertrophic scars are confined within original wound margins, but are elevated above the skin level. Many will partially regress with time.
2. Unlike normal scars and keloids, hypertrophic scars are commonly associated with contractures (e.g., wound contraction over a joint space).
3. Histology reveals increased blood vessels and cells relative to normal scar, as well as distinct connective tissue nodules containing myofibroblasts.
4. Collagen fibrils in hypertrophic scars are also finer, more organized, and with larger interfibrillar distances than keloid collagen fibrils.

B. Etiology

1. The exact etiology is unknown, but both intrinsic factors and exogenous stimuli may be involved.
2. Risks factors include those that can potentially delay wound coverage longer than 2–3 weeks (e.g., increased wound depth, size, tension, or infection). Delayed wound closure may prolong the inflammatory phase of repair, which results

in the release of more pro-fibrotic growth factors and cytokines.

C. Biologic Characteristics

1. Hypertrophic scars contain higher numbers of Langerhans cells, T lymphocytes, and keratinocytes with enhanced antigen presentation properties to T lymphocytes. In addition, keratinocytes from hypertrophic scars display a more "activated phenotype" than normal scar keratinocytes, with elaboration of more pro-fibrotic growth factors such as PDGF and TGF-β.
2. Besides a prolonged inflammatory phase, the granulation phase of hypertrophic scars is also abnormal. Excessive numbers of nonfunctional microvessels with occluded lumens are present, which may result in tissue hypoxia that further stimulates angiogenesis and fibroplasia.
3. Fibroblasts from hypertrophic scars are more sensitive to TGF-β. The normal proteoglycan ratio is altered in hypertrophic scars—decorin is decreased and biglycan increased—with possible effects on collagen deposition pattern.
4. Increased cellularity is also noted, especially of myofibroblasts, indicating a possible defect in apoptosis.
5. Increased wound tension in hypertrophic scars may transmit extracellular matrix forces to the cell membrane with further elaboration of fibrogenic factors.

D. Treatment

The best therapy for hypertrophic scars is prevention by early coverage of open wounds with either autologous tissue or biologic skin equivalents. A wide variety of treatment modalities have been developed, but satisfactory outcomes are difficult to obtain. Conservative management includes pressure garments, silicone gel sheets, laser, cryotherapy, serial casting, splints, and corticosteroid injections.

1. Pressure therapy begins immediately after complete reepithelialization and is continuously applied until complete scar maturation (at least 4–6 months). Recommended pressure level is above 24 mmHg (inherent capillary pressure) but below 30 mmHg (capillary perfusion pressure). Response rates from 60 to 80% have been reported, but there have been no conclusive randomized studies. Pressure therapy is recommended for wounds requiring more than 10–14 days for coverage (e.g., reepithelialization, grafting) and strongly indicated for wound requiring greater than 21 days for coverage.
2. Silicone sheets may increase local skin temperature by 1–2°F, which can increase the activity of collagenases severalfold. Silicone sheets are also applied continuously for at least 3 months.
3. Previous trials with CO_2, argon, and neodymium:yttrium-aluminum-garnet (Nd:YAG) lasers were disappointing with recurrence rates from 0 to 100%. However, the 585 nm flash-pumped pulse dye laser is selectively absorbed by hemoglobin and, thus, more specific for vascular structures. The photothermolysis of capillaries results in cutaneous hypoxia that facilitates tissue necrosis and sloughing. Some studies have shown up to ~80% improvement, while others have shown no improvement of hypertrophic lesions.
4. Cryotherapy results in superficial tissue necrosis, and response rates of 51–76% have been reported after repeated treatments.
5. Serial casting and splints are used for management of contractures across joints.
6. Corticosteroid injections, either as primary therapy (intralesional) or as intraoperative and postoperative (wound margin) adjuvant therapy, have been used for hypertrophic scars. They are most effective for small, recent lesions. The large surface area of many burn hypertrophic scars makes this approach impractical.
7. Surgical management is indicated for hypertrophic scars refractory to conservative treatment. In such cases, surgical excision is usually followed by some form of surgical skin coverage (e.g., primary closure, skin graft, flap) and adjuvant corticosteroid, pressure, or silicone therapy. Simple excision alone without wound coverage has a high recurrence rate that ranges from 50 to 80%. For management of contractures, appropriate tension release by Z-plasties or tissue excision followed by concomitant tissue coverage can be effective without additional adjuvant therapy. In designing skin coverage, the presence of dermal tissue is important. For instance, keratinocyte sheets alone have similar contraction rates to uncovered skin, while the contrac-

tion rates for skin grafts and flaps is as follows: split thickness skin grafts > full thickness skin grafts > flaps.

8. Other management options, more commonly utilized for keloids than hypertrophic scars, include pharmacologic intervention to increase collagenase activity and inhibit collagen cross-linking.
9. Radiation has also been applied to refractory hypertrophic scars, but it is less effective as a primary treatment modality than as an adjuvant following surgery. The risk of subsequent malignant tissue degeneration, although generally considered low, precludes the widespread use of radiation.

III. KELOIDS

A. Definition

1. Keloids extend beyond the original wound margins and are elevated above skin level.
2. Spontaneous regression is rare.
3. Like hypertrophic scars, keloids also exhibit increased vascularity and cellularity relative to normal scar. However, unlike hypertrophic scars, keloids have thicker, less organized collagen fibrils and few, if any, connective tissue nodules with myofibroblasts.
4. The lack of collagen organization in keloids may account, in part, for the lack of keloid-associated contractures.

B. Etiology

1. In contrast to hypertrophic scars, intrinsic factors appear to play a greater role in keloid development than extrinsic factors. Genetic, anatomic, endocrine, and immune factors have all been implicated, but the definitive etiology is unknown.
2. Keloids have been reported in nearly all races except albinos. Increased skin pigmentation is a risk factor. The incidence of keloids is increased in African American, Hispanic, and Asian populations (up to 16% incidence in African Americans).
3. In addition, skin with modified dermal layers (e.g., eyelid, areola, and genitalia) or skin lacking melanocytes (e.g., palms, soles) is rarely affected by keloids.
4. Familial cases of keloids have also been described with autosomal dominant and recessive patterns of inheritance.
5. Since most keloids arise between ages 10 to 30, appear to develop more rapidly during puberty and pregnancy, and seem to regress with menopause and advanced age, a sex hormone association has been suggested.
6. Alternatively, an immune mechanism for keloid formation has also been proposed. Keloid patients have a higher incidence of allergic symptoms than hypertrophic scar patients, and keloid incidence directly correlates with serum IgE levels. IgE can stimulate mast cell degranulation of profibrotic factors such as histamine. Histamine increases fibroblast collagen synthesis; increased histamine levels are found in keloid tissue.
7. Finally, persistent inflammation from scalp cellulitis, acne vulgaris, or hidradenitis suppurativa may trigger keloid formation.

C. Treatment

Keloids, more so than hypertrophic scars, are often refractory to conservative measures or surgery alone. Surgery combined with some form of adjuvant therapy generally achieves the best response rates.

1. Conservative management is similar to hypertrophic scars. Monotherapy with pressure garments, silicone materials, and cryotherapy have been used on keloids with less success than with hypertrophic scars.
2. Intralesional corticosteroids have been used as initial therapy with a 50% response over 5 years. Light cryosurgery prior to steroid injection creates tissue edema and collagen disruption and may allow better steroid dispersal. Corticosteroids alone, however, can only soften and flatten keloids, but not make them disappear. Corticosteroids induce collagen, fibronectin, TGF β, and collagenase inhibitor mRNA down-regulation, and thus may shift the balance toward matrix degradation in keloids. Adverse effects include localized skin atrophy, depigmentation, telangiectasia, necrosis, ulceration, as well as (rarely) systemic effects such as Cushingoid habitus.

Table 1 Features of Normal Scars, Hypertrophic Scars, and Keloids

	Normal scar	Hypertrophic scar	Keloid
Definition:			
Beyond confines of original wound	No	No	Yes
Relative position to skin level after remodeling	Not elevated	Elevated	Elevated
Histology (after reepithelialization):			
Nonvascular α-smooth muscle staining	Absent	Present (myofibroblasts)	Rare
Cellularity and vascularity	Normal	Increased	Increased
Connective tissue nodules	Absent	Present	Rare
Collagen fibers	Fine, basket-like weave	Fine (inside nodules) Thicker (outside nodules)	Thick, parallel arrays
Natural history:			
Emergence after injury	<4 weeks	<4 weeks	3 months to years
Clinical course without treatment	Not applicable	Partial resolution	No resolution
Association with contractures	Rare	Common	None
Epidemiology:			
Risk factors	Not applicable	Increased wound depth Increased wound size Increased wound tension Wound infection Delayed wound coverage (>2–3 weeks)	Dark skin Family history Blood type A Increased sex hormones Increased IgE levels Prolonged inflammation Location of injury[a]
Incidence	Not applicable	Unknown	6–16% in Africans
Peak age of onset	Not applicable	Unknown	10–30 years

[a] Shoulders, anterior chest, upper arms, mandibular angle >> cheeks, ear lobes, neck >> eyelids, genitalia, palms, soles, cornea, mucous membranes, umbilical cord.
Source: Data compiled from Refs. 1–13.

Table 2 Pathogenesis of Normal Scars, Hypertrophic Scars, and Keloids

	Normal scar	Hypertrophic scar	Keloid
Inflammation phase:			
Duration	Normal	Prolonged	Normal to prolonged
Mast cells	Normal	Increased	Increased
Keratinocyte phenotype	Normal	Abnormal ("activated")	(Unknown)
Granulation phase:			
Fibroblast proliferation	Normal	Normal	Normal
Fibroblast extracellular matrix production	Normal	Increased	Increased
Extracellular matrix protease activity	Normal	Decreased	Decreased
Pro-fibrotic growth factors	Normal	Increased	Increased
Neovascularization	Normal	Abnormal	Abnormal
Remodeling phase:			
Myofibroblasts upon reepithelialization	Disappear	Persist	Generally absent
Decorin	Normal	Decreased	Decreased
Biglycan, versican	Normal	Increased	Normal
Growth factors and cytokines:			
TGF-β, PDGF, IGF-I	Normal	Increased	Increased
IFN-α	Normal	(Unknown)	Decreased
IFN-γ	Normal	Increased	Decreased
IL-1	Normal	Increased	Normal

Source: Data compiled from Refs. 1–13.

3. Surgical management goals are to remove inflamed keloid tissue with minimal iatrogenic tissue trauma, since trauma can lead to further inflammation and keloid formation. Resection of all inflamed areas including trapped hair follicles, epithelial cysts, or tracts should be accomplished with minimal tissue undermining. Wound repair conditions are optimized by minimizing dead space, hematoma formation, foreign materials, and wound tension. For large flat keloids, the excised keloid tissue may be debulked and autografted to avoid new donor site trauma. The presence of residual keloid tissue after excision does not increase the recurrence rate. However, surgical excision alone, even with skin graft resurfacing, still results in unacceptable recurrence rates of up to 80% at 2 years. Laser surgery appears to have similar recurrence rates as conventional surgery.
4. Because of these recognized inadequacies of conventional therapeutic modalities, postoperative adjuvant therapy utilizing pressure, silicone materials, corticosteroids, radiation, interferon, and oral medications has been described. For specific areas such as the ear lobe, keloid excision followed by corticosteroid therapy and compression have recurrence rates of ~10%. For other areas, excision followed by adjuvant corticosteroids has average recurrence rates of ~50%. Low-dose radiation following excision is effective with ~10–20% recurrence rates. A typical regimen consists of 400–500 cGy per treatment given once a week starting the day of excision for 3 weeks (total dose = 1200–1500 cGy). Radiation is generally reserved for older patients with severely symptomatic and debilitating keloids because of the potential carcinogenic effects of radiation. However, the total surface area and dose is so low that many radiation oncologists consider the risk for malignant transformation negligible.
5. Interferon-α2b injection after surgery was associated with ~20% recurrence rate in a small series of patients. Clearly, more studies and longer follow-up on interferon application are required.
6. Various oral medications aimed at decreasing overall extracellular matrix deposition have been advocated but are not widely accepted in keloid management. Examples include:
    - colchicine—increases tissue collagenase activity
    - penicillamine and s-aminopropionitrile—lysyl oxidase (collagen cross-linking) inhibitors
    - pentoxifylline—decreases fibroblast proliferation and decreases glycosaminoglycan and fibronectin production.

REFERENCES

1. Bermann B, Biely HC. Adjunct therapies to surgical management of keloids. *Dermatol. Surg.* 1996; 22:126–130.
2. Clark RAF: The Molecular and Cellular Biology of Wound Repair. Vol. xxiii. New York: Plenum Press, 1996.
3. Ehrlich HP, Desmouliere A, Diegelmann RF, Cohen IK, Compton CC, Garner WL, Kapanci Y, Gabbiani G: Morphological and immunochemical differences between keloid and hypertrophic scar. *Am. J. Pathol.* 1994; 145:105–113.
4. Ladin DA, Hou Z, Patel D, McPhail M, Olson JC, Saed GM, Fivenson DP: p53 and apoptosis alterations in keloids and keloid fibrolasts. *Wound Repair Regen.* 1998; 6:28–37.
5. Machesney M, Tidman N, Waseem A, Kirby L, Leigh I: Activated keratinocytes in the epidermis of hypertrophic scars. *Am. J. Pathol.* 1998; 152:1133–1141.
6. Madden JW, Peacock EE Jr: Studies on the biology of collagen during wound healing. 3. Dynamic metabolism of scar collagen and remodeling of dermal wounds. *Ann. Surg.* 1971; 174:511–520.
7. McCauley RL, Chopra V, Li YY, Herndon DN, Robson MC: Altered cytokine production in black patients with keloids. *J. Clin. Immunol.* 1992; 12(4):300–308.
8. Nemeth AJ: Keloids and hypertrophic scars. *J. Dermatol. Surg. Oncol.* 1993; 19(8):738–746.
9. Niessen FB, Spauwen PH, Schalkwijk J, Kon M: On the nature of hypertrophic scars and keloids: a review. *Plast. Reconstr. Surg.* 1999; 104(5):1435–1458.
10. Placik OJ, Lewis VL Jr: Immunologic associations of keloids. *Surg. Gynecol. Obstet.* 1992; 175(2):185–193.
11. Saed GM, Ladin D, Olson J, Han X, Hou Z, Fivenson D: Analysis of p53 gene mutations in keloids using polymerase chain reaction-based single-strand conformational polymorphism and DNA sequencing [see comments]. *Arch. Dermatol.* 1998; 134(8):963–967.
12. Tan EM, Hoffren J, Rouda S, Greenbaum S, Fox IWt, Moore JH Jr, Dodge GR: Decorin, versican, and biglycan gene expression by keloid and normal dermal fibrolasts: differential regulation by basic fibroblast growth factor. *Exp. Cell. Res.* 1993; 209(2):200–207.
13. Tredget EE, Nedelec B, Scott PG, Ghahary A: Hypertrophic scars, keloids, and contractures. The cellular and molecular basis for therapy. *Surg. Clin. North Am* .1997; 77(3):701–730.

15

Bites and Stings

Andrew D. Smith, M.D., and Marc H. Hedrick, M.D.
David Geffen School of Medicine at UCLA, Los Angeles, California, U.S.A.

Bites and stings are common problems in medical practice. Dog bites account for 60–80% of this type of injury. Although the true incidence is difficult to determine, it is estimated that 1–3 million dog bites occur each year. Urban expansion into the wilderness will only increase the incidence of animal encounters in the future. Tetanus prophylaxis should be addressed for all bite and sting wounds.

I. MAMMALIAN BITES

A. Human Bites

1. The main clinical problem with human bites is infection. Human saliva contains up to 1011 bacteria/mL, and plaque on teeth has an even greater bacterial concentration.
2. Organisms include *Eikenella corrodens*, *Staphylococcus* species, *Streptococcus viridans*, *Bacteroides* species, and microaerophilic streptococci.
3. Many serious bite wound infections occur when the joint capsule is penetrated, as in a fistfight. These wounds must be specifically sought because they are readily missed.
4. Treatment should include wound irrigation, joint irrigation if necessary, intravenous antibiotics, and elevation. In almost all instances human bites should not be closed except when on the face.
5. Antibiotic treatment of human bite wounds involves the use of penicillin or ampicillin plus a β-lactamase inhibitor (amoxicillin/clavulanic acid or ampicillin/sulbactam).

B. Cat Bites

1. Cat bites often leave deeply penetrating wounds that are heavily contaminated. These wounds may even penetrate into underlying bone.
2. Organisms include *Pasteurella multocida* and *Staphylococcus* species.
3. Antibiotic treatment also consists of penicillin plus a first-generation cephalosporin or amoxicillin plus a β-lactamase inhibitor.

C. Dog Bites

1. Dogs can generate massive force with their muscles of mastication and can cause extensive soft-tissue injury. Soft-tissue infection, however, is not as common in dog bites, but prophylaxis is still recommended.
2. Infecting organisms include *Pasteurella multocida*, *Bacteroides* species, *Streptococcus viridans*, *Fusobacterium*, and *Capnocytophaga*.
3. Antibiotic treatment again consists of penicillin plus a first-generation cephalosporin or amoxicillin plus a β-lactamase inhibitor.

D. Rabies Prophylaxis

1. All animal wounds should be irrigated and cleansed with detergent.

2. The chance of an animal having rabies is increased if the animal was behaving abnormally or if it was an unprovoked attack.
3. Dogs and cats may be observed for 10 days if they are healthy. Previously immunized animals should be considered low risk.
4. Skunks, bats, raccoons, and other wild carnivores should be considered rabid.
5. Rodents, rabbits, and livestock rarely ever carry the rabies virus.
6. Current treatment recommendations by the U.S. Centers for Disease Control (CDC) are summarized in Table 1.

II. SNAKE BITES

A. Snake Identification

1. The majority of snake bites in the United States are nonvenomous.
2. A thorough attempt at snake identification should be undertaken.
3. Venomous snakes indigenous to the United States are either crotalids (rattlesnakes, copperheads, cottonmouths) or elapids (coral snakes).
4. There are three important species of *Crotalidae* in the United States, which include *Crotalus* and *Sistrurus* (rattlesnakes) and *Agkistrodon* (copperheads and water moccasins). These snakes have a thick body, triangular head, elliptical pupils, and facial pits.
5. Elapids, or coral snakes, are brightly colored and have a distinctive red band adjacent to a yellow band. "Red on yellow, kill a fellow; red on black, venom lack."

B. Assessment of Envenomation

1. This determination is important because treatment of envenomation carries a significant risk. If there are no fang marks, then there is no envenomation. Even with fang marks, about one fourth are not envenomed and another one half will be only mild.
2. The best marker of envenomation is local tissue destruction by the venom (mixture of enzymes and peptides with broad actions). Pain, edema, discoloration, or bullae at the site are good markers.
3. Rattlesnake bites tend to be more severe than *Agkistrodon* bites.

C. Treatment

1. Immobilization, extremity neutral positioning, a compression dressing, and rapid transport to a hospital are recommended. Tourniquets, ice immersion, and incision and suction are not recommended.
2. Mild cases of envenomation can be treated with observation and supportive care.
3. Antivenin therapy is recommended for treatment of severe cases.
4. Early surgical debridement to remove venom is not advocated by most authors.
5. Fasciotomy for compartment syndrome is reserved for the usual indications.

Table 1 Rabies Treatment Recommendations

Animal	Condition of attack	Treatment
Domestic animals (dogs and cats)	Healthy and available for observation (10 days)	None, unless animal develops rabies
	Rabid or suspect	RIG and HDCV
	Unknown	Consider RIG and HDCV
Wild animals (bats, foxes, coyotes, other carnivores)	Regard as rabid; kill and test animal	RIG and HDCV
Others (livestock, rodents, lagomorphs)	Consider individually	Consult local public health officials

Human rabies immune globulin (RIG): 20 IU/kg; 50% into wound and 50% given IM.
Human diploid cell rabies vaccine (HDCV): given on days 0, 3, 7, 14, and 28.

6. Organisms present in rattlesnake mouths include *Pseudomonas* species, *Staphylococcus* species, clostridia, and Enterobacteraciae.
7. Empiric coverage is usually begun using ticarcillin with clavulanic acid.
8. Severe cases of envenomation can induce coagulopathy; these are treated with fresh-frozen plasma and cryoprecipitate.
9. Tetanus prophylaxis is indicated.

D. Antivenin Therapy

1. A polyvalent equine antivenin is commercially available to treat bites. The antivenin is obtained by immunizing horses to crotalid venom and then pooling the globulin fraction of the horse serum.
2. Therapy is most effective if started immediately. Therapy is recommended for use in life-threatening envenomation for up to 24 h following a bite.
3. Risks of treatment include anaphylaxis (1–39%) and a dose-dependent, delayed-type serum sickness. It is best to start the infusion slowly to attempt to avoid complications of antivenin use.
4. The dose depends on the amount of venom to be neutralized (not the weight of the patient). Treatment of severe bites can be started with 5–10 vials.
5. Coral snake venom produces respiratory depression and alteration in central nervous system function. An antivenin is commercially available and treatment should be started with 3–5 vials of antivenin.

III. INSECT BITES AND STINGS

A. Fire Ants

1. The red fire ant (*Solenopsis invicta*) is an aggressive species that tends to inflict multiple bites.
2. The bites are usually limited, but near-fatal cases have been documented. Anaphylaxis is the major problem with their bites.
3. The bite has a characteristic appearance with an initial vesicle followed by a sterile pustule.
4. The venom is unique in that it consists of 95% nonprotein alkaloid.
5. The treatment is mechanical scrubbing with soap and water to remove the venom. Anaphylaxis is treated in the standard fashion.

B. Spiders

1. Two common species are dangerous to humans.
2. The **brown recluse spider** (*Loxosceles reclusa*) has three pairs of eyes and a violin-shaped carapace on its body.
   - There is minimal pain at the site, but a hemorrhagic blister commonly develops and progresses to necrosis.
   - Systemic symptoms are mild.
   - Treatment is supportive. If started early, dapsone may prevent ulceration.
3. The **black widow spider** (*Lactrodectus macrotans*) has a black body with a red hourglass on its underbelly.
   - Its bite causes a systemic reaction, which has a rapid onset and up to 5% mortality.
   - Treatment is supportive and an antivenin is available for severe cases.
   - Dantrolene, calcium, and methacarbamol are second-line agents.

C. Bees and Wasps

1. The most important consequence of bee and wasp stings is anaphylaxis. In fact, this is responsible for more deaths than all other venomous animal bites and stings.
2. Bees leave a stinger in the wound, which kills the bee. The stinging apparatus should be scraped with a knife to remove it.
3. Individuals with a known sensitivity should wear a warning bracelet and carry an epinephrine antianphylaxis kit for injection.

IV. BITES AND STINGS BY MARINE ANIMALS

A. Marine Invertebrates

1. Three major groups are *Schyphozoa* (jellyfish), *Hydrozoa* (Portuguese man-of-war and hydras),

and *Anthozoa* (corals and anemones). These animals have nematocysts for poisoning and capturing prey.

2. Cutaneous contact generates a painful skin reaction and occasionally anaphylaxis. Full-thickness penetration by nematocysts can be fatal.
3. Treatment consists of removing all tentacles and deactivating unexploded nematocysts with a baking soda slurry, papain, or vinegar. Systemic side effects are managed supportively.

B. Venomous Fish

1. Stingrays can envenomate, usually when stepped on by a swimmer.
2. Treatment consists of irrigation and soaking the affected part.

C. Sharks

1. Usual wound management principles should be followed along with tetanus prophylaxis.

16

Lacerations

Chi Y. Chung, M.D., and George H. Rudkin, M.D.
David Geffen School of Medicine at UCLA, Los Angeles, California, U.S.A.

I. DEFINITION

A laceration is a wound created by the tearing of tissue during blunt or penetrating trauma. Lacerations may be divided into simple, beveled, tearing, and burst or stellate types. This chapter describes the evaluation and treatment of skin and soft tissue lacerations commonly encountered in plastic surgery, with special emphasis on facial trauma.

II. PATIENT EVALUATION

A. Life Support Protocols

1. The principles of basic life support (BLS), advanced cardiac life support (ACLS), and advanced trauma life support (ATLS) are of utmost importance in the evaluation of patients with lacerations, since there may be associated life-threatening injuries.
2. The "ABCs" of life support protocols state that a patient must first have a secure airway, effective spontaneous breathing or mechanical ventilation, and confirmed circulation.
3. The ACLS protocol adds a "D" for defibrillation of lethal cardiac arrhythmias, and the ATLS protocol includes control of hemorrhage and the treatment of shock.

B. Evaluation of Injuries

1. After the "ABCs," cardiac arrhythmias, hemorrhage, and shock have been appropriately assessed and treated, the patient should be evaluated for associated injuries and lacerations.
2. Bleeding from lacerations can almost always be controlled temporarily with direct pressure. Clamps should never be applied blindly into a wound. Uncontrollable bleeding from wounds should be treated appropriately with prompt surgical or angiographic intervention.
3. Bleeding of the head and neck warrants prompt attention to avoid possible upper airway obstruction. Significant hemorrhage from facial injuries is usually due to injury of the external maxillary artery, superficial temporal artery, or angular artery.

III. WOUND EVALUATION AND DEBRIDEMENT

A. Evaluation

1. When evaluating lacerations, it is important to understand the mechanism and depth of injury. Stellate lacerations result from compression forces and have extensive damage of the wound edges with abrasion of the surrounding skin. They are much more susceptible to infection than are simple lacerations.
2. Lacerations must be evaluated for possible bony, neurovascular, muscle, or tendon injury deep to the skin wound. Complex wounds should be evaluated in the operating room

where there is better lighting, hemostasis control, and surgical assistance. Tissue often appears to be missing, but usually is not. A photographic record of injuries may be helpful for surgical planning, teaching purposes, and possible medicolegal documentation.

B. Cleaning

1. All embedded dirt and debris must be removed promptly to avoid an accidental tattoo (particles fixed in the dermis) and to decrease the risk of infection from foreign bodies, especially organic materials. Once anesthetized, the wound may be scrubbed effectively with sterile gauze or a scrub brush moistened with sterile saline and mild soap. Oil substances can be removed with a small amount of ether, acetone, or xylol prior to scrubbing.
2. Injuries to hair-bearing regions of the head and face may be shaved to facilitate proper cleaning and closure. An exception is the eyebrow, which should not be shaved since misalignment of this hair-bearing area is obvious and difficult to correct.
3. High-pressure irrigation (>8 psi) decreases wound infection rates as compared to low-pressure irrigation. Sterile saline can be forced through a syringe fitted with a 19 gauge needle in order to achieve the necessary pressure to remove additional debris.

C. Sharp Debridement

1. Wound edges must be trimmed sharply to remove devitalized tissue and debris. Wound edges are best trimmed perpendicular to the skin, except in hair-bearing regions, where the edges may be beveled in the direction of the hair follicles.
2. Sharp debridement helps to reorient lacerations for optimal skin closure.

D. Hemostasis

1. Most minor bleeding from lacerations will stop spontaneously with applied pressure in a patient with a normal temperature, an adequate platelet count, and normal coagulation parameters. Bleeding small vessels may be carefully cauterized or ligated.
2. Major vascular injuries may require consultation with a vascular surgical team.

E. Antimicrobial Therapy

1. Patients with lacerations or puncture wounds should receive treatment for possible inoculation of *Clostridium tetani.*
2. Tetanus prophylaxis guidelines from the Immunization Practices Advisory Committee of the Centers for Disease Control (CDC) are shown in Table 1.
3. In most clean lacerations, antibiotics covering Gram-positive skin flora are sufficient. A dirty wound or laceration by unknown mechanism should be treated with antibiotics effective against both Gram-positive and Gram-negative organisms. Antibiotics are an adjunct to proper wound care and must not replace appropriate wound cleaning and debridement.
4. Closure of wounds with $>10^5$ organisms per gram of tissue will fail 70–100% of the time. Closure of wounds contaminated with β-hemolytic streptococci may fail with even fewer organisms. Lacerations with a high level of bacterial contamination or a crush component may require debridement and open wound care prior to consideration of delayed primary closure. This is rarely indicated for facial lacerations.

IV. WOUND CLOSURE

Simple lacerations may require only debridement of ragged edges and devitalized tissue, followed by atraumatic wound closure. Complicated lacerations, including those that involve deeper structures, may be dressed or closed temporarily pending definitive management in the operating room. In general, complex tissue rearrangement should be avoided in the setting of acute trauma.

A. Anesthesia

1. Most uncomplicated lacerations are amenable to the use of local anesthesia or regional blocks. Local anesthetic is injected slowly with a small-bore needle (25 gauge or smaller) in the surrounding tissues.
2. The addition of epinephrine (1:100,000) to the local anesthetic helps decrease bleeding due to a vasoconstrictive effect. Epinephrine should not be used near end arteries, as in the digits, to avoid potential ischemia and necrosis. Epinephrine should also be avoided or sparingly used in

Table 1 Tetanus Prophylaxis Guidelines

Hx of adsorbed tetanus toxoid (doses)	Clean, minor wounds		All other wounds[a]	
	Td[b]	TIG[c]	Td[b]	TIG[c]
Unknown or less than 3 doses	Yes	No	Yes	Yes
Greater than or equal to 3 doses	No	No	No	No
If only 3 doses of fluid toxoid have been received, then a 4th dose of toxoid, preferably an adsorbed toxoid, should be given.	Yes, if >10 years since last dose		Yes, if >5 years since last dose	

DT: diphtheria and tetanus toxoids adsorbed (for pediatric use); DTP: diphtheria and tetanus toxoids and pertussis vaccine adsorbed; T: tetanus toxoid adsorbed; Td: tetanus and diphtheria toxoids adsorbed (for adult use); TIG: tetanus immune globulin.

[a] Such as, but not limited to, wounds contaminated with dirt, feces, soil, and saliva; puncture wounds; avulsions; and wounds resulting from missiles, crushing, burns, and frostbite.

[b] For children <7 years old; DTP (DT, if pertussis vaccine is contraindicated) is preferred to tetanus toxoid alone. For persons >7 years of age, Td is preferred to tetanus toxoid alone.

[c] If passive immunization is needed, human tetanus immune globulin (TIG) is the product of choice. The currently recommended prophylactic dose of TIG for wounds of average severity is 250 units IM. When T or Td and TIG are given concurrently, separate syringes and separate injection sites should be used. Most experts consider the use of adsorbed toxoid mandatory in this situation.

The recommended pediatric schedule for DTP includes a booster dose at age 4–6 years. The first Td booster is recommended at age 14–16 years (10 years after the dose at age 4–6 years).

stellate lacerations, where blood flow may be compromised, or in contaminated lacerations since decreased blood flow diminishes local wound defenses against infection.

3. Lacerations of the digits can be approached with a digital block, which involves the infiltration of local anesthetic (no epinephrine) into the adjacent web spaces and across the dorsum of the digit at its base.
4. Facial lacerations can be anesthetized with field blocks or facial blocks, based on the sensory distribution of the trigeminal nerve.
5. Nasal mucous membranes are best anesthetized with 4% topical cocaine solution, applied with cotton-tipped applicators. Cardiac monitoring is appropriate when using cocaine.
6. Topical anesthetics may be helpful especially in the treatment of pediatric patients. EMLA cream (eutectic mixture of local anesthetics; 2.5% lidocaine, 2.5% prilocaine) has been used most often for local anesthesia prior to injection or intravenous catheter insertion. LET gel (4% lidocaine, 1:2000 epinephrine, 1% tetracaine) has been shown to be safe and effective for anesthesia prior to suture repair of simple facial and scalp lacerations in children. These topical agents are most effective when applied under an occlusive dressing at least 30 minutes prior to the procedure.

B. Layered Repair

1. Subsequent to appropriate osseous stabilization, revascularization, or nerve or tendon repair, each underlying layer must be reapproximated carefully to eliminate dead space and reduce tension across the wound margins prior to skin closure.
2. The use of fascial, subcutaneous, and deep dermal closures assists in decreasing tension across the skin edges.

C. Suturing Techniques

Proper suturing technique involves approximation, alignment, and eversion of the skin edges. Basic techniques are shown in Table 2.

V. POSTOPERATIVE CARE

A. Wound Care

1. Wounds must be kept clean and observed for infection. The wound may be cleansed daily with cotton applicators moistened with hydrogen peroxide, followed by application of topical antibacterial ointment.

Table 2 Suturing Techniques

Suture	Technique	Advantages	Disadvantages
Simple interrupted	Series of single loops of suture taking equal bites of dermis, knotted to one side	Can remove individual sutures for wound inspection without unraveling entire length	Slower placement and removal
Simple running	Single suture taking series of bites along the length of wound	Rapid placement and removal, hemostasis	Cannot remove single segment in cases of infection
Vertical mattress	Series of wide deep sutures alternating with narrow superficial bites; may be interrupted or running	Effective approximation and eversion	More time consuming
Horizontal mattress	Single suture in a box forming two parallel loops along and across the wound	Effective approximation with eversion, effective hemostasis	May cause tissue ischemia
Running subcuticular	Single running intradermal suture along length of wound	No visible suture, easy removal if monofilament suture, no removal if absorbable suture	More time consuming; slow-absorbing suture may expose
Skin staples	Approximate wound edges with surgical stapler	Rapid placement, can remove individual staples for inspection	May leave marks on skin, appears noncosmetic
Tissue adhesives	Apply adhesive "glue," e.g., butylcyanoacrylates	Use without anesthesia, especially in children, no removal necessary	Not for use over mobile areas

2. Ophthalmic ointment should be used on wounds around the orbit.
3. Wounds that develop erythema or suppuration are managed with suture removal and drainage of pus. The infected wound is then treated with wet to dry dressings three times per day and allowed to granulate and close by secondary intention.
4. Nonabsorbable sutures are usually removed within 5 days on the face, 7–10 days on the trunk, and may be left for 10–14 days or more on the extremities.

B. Scar Maturation

1. Sun exposure should be avoided for 6 months after closure to avoid hyperpigmentation and reddening of the scar. Sunblock should be applied if sun exposure cannot be avoided.
2. Scars should be allowed to fade, soften, and flatten prior to consideration for revision. Scar maturation may take 6 months to a year or more.

C. Scar Revision

1. Linear scars that cross skin folds may be improved with Z-plasty, W-plasty, or V–Y techniques, which attempt to lengthen, stagger, and change the direction of a scar.
2. Relatively small scars with one side higher than the other or depressed scars from avulsion flaps may excised and reapproximated with improved results.

VI. SPECIAL CONSIDERATIONS

A. Facial Lacerations

1. Lacerations are the most common injury to the face.
2. Repair of lacerations involving the **eyebrows** should include evaluation for any fractures of the supraorbital ridge or frontal sinuses and repair of any divided muscle underneath the brow.

3. Full-thickness lacerations of the **eyelid** require careful closure of the conjunctiva and reapproximation of the tarsal plate and ciliary margin, which allows for proper alignment of the lid margin and skin. Injury of the lacrimal system may require repair with very fine sutures after cannulation with a fine polyethylene catheter.
4. **Nasal lacerations** are approximated after evaluation of the bony and cartilaginous framework. The nose is subject to shear forces during trauma and can hide intranasal soft tissue lacerations. Careful inspection and repair will decrease scar formation at critical areas such as the internal valve and help to prevent stenosis or synechiae. Septal hematomas must be evacuated through a small mucosal incision to minimize the risk of chondromalacia with loss of septal cartilage and resultant saddle nose deformity. Nasal ala or tip avulsion may be replaced with a composite graft.
5. Lacerations of the **ear** should be debrided conservatively, with an attempt to return tissue to its original position. Sutures in the cartilage are often unnecessary, especially if the skin sutures provide adequate support. Sutures on the ear are usually removed in 10–14 days.
6. **Perioral lacerations** require precise alignment of the vermilion cutaneous junction, which should be carefully marked prior to the instillation of local anesthesia. Lip lacerations may be reapproximated using rapidly absorbing surgical gut sutures.

B. Lacerations Involving Nerves

1. Any suspected nerve injury should be evaluated thoroughly in the operating room with the assistance of magnifying loupes or a microscope, but need not be repaired immediately.
2. Complex repairs, including free nerve grafts, should be avoided in the setting of acute trauma.
3. Severe functional deficits of the face occur with injuries to the facial nerve branches. For example, injury to the temporal branches causes paralysis of the eyebrow and brow ptosis. Clean, sharp injuries are carefully reapproximated in fascicular units. Blunt injuries often require sharp debridement prior to nerve repair.

C. Tendon Lacerations

1. Even with near-normal function of the digit, any possible tendon laceration warrants consultation from the hand surgery team. Such injuries should be explored within 5 days, as missed partial tendon lacerations can lead to tendon rupture, triggering within the tendon sheath, or entrapment of the tendon flap in the sheath opening.
2. The treatment of upper extremity lacerations is discussed in detail in Chapter 71.

17

Skin and Soft Tissue Grafts

Chi Y. Chung, M.D., and George H. Rudkin, M.D.
University of California, Los Angeles (UCLA), Division of Plastic and Reconstructive Surgery, Los Angeles, California, U.S.A.

I. HISTORY

A. The origin of skin and soft tissue grafts dates back 3000 years.

B. Sanskrit texts record the use of free skin grafts to repair mutilations of the nose, ear, and lip.

C. In 1823, Buenger recorded the first successful free skin autograft in Europe.

D. The current technique of skin grafting is attributed largely to Reverdin, who published a paper describing small autogenous skin grafts or pinch grafts in 1869 and described homografts in 1872. His reports were followed by Ollier and Thiersch, who described the thin split-thickness skin graft in 1872 and 1886, respectively.

E. The full-thickness skin graft was reported by Wolfe in 1875 and Krause in 1893.

II. TYPES OF SKIN GRAFTS

Skin grafting involves the free transfer of epidermis with varying amounts of the underlying dermis to cover and heal an open wound.

A. Full- vs. Split-Thickness

1. Full-thickness skin grafts contain the entire dermis, while split-thickness grafts contain varying portions of the dermis.
2. Split-thickness grafts measure 12/1000 inch (thin) to 18/1000 inch (thick) in thickness, and contain a variable percentage of dermis, since the measurable thickness of the dermal layer varies in different areas of the body.
3. Primary contraction describes the immediate recoil of a harvested skin graft due to the elastin in the dermis. Secondary contraction is the contracture of a healing wound due to the presence of myofibroblasts. The number of these modified smooth muscle–like fibroblasts within a wound is directly proportional to the rate of contraction.
4. Open wounds left to heal secondarily exhibit marked skin contracture. Skin grafts inhibit wound contracture in proportion to the percentage of dermis transferred. Full-thickness skin grafts exhibit more primary contraction, but less secondary contraction, and therefore are better suited for wounds of the hands, areas of flexion, and the face. In addition, full-thickness grafts are better suited for the face because they exhibit less discoloration over time than split-thickness skin grafts.
5. Full-thickness and thick split-thickness grafts contain more of the dermal layer with its nerve endings, hair follicles, and secretory glands than thin split-thickness grafts. Therefore, thick grafts have better reinnervation from the wound bed, more hair growth, and more secretion from sweat and sebaceous glands. Sweat gland secretion

depends on sympathetic reinnervation of the skin graft, while sebaceous glands secrete independently of graft reinnervation.

B. Sheet vs. Meshed

1. Harvested skin grafts can be used as a continuous sheet or incised to provide a meshed graft. Meshed grafts may be applied either expanded or unexpanded. A sheet graft provdes an uninterrupted surface that produces a better aesthetic appearance, but it does not allow for drainage of blood and serum from under the graft. A sheet graft requires more donor skin harvesting than an expanded meshed graft to cover an equal wound area.
2. A meshed graft allows for drainage of wound fluid through its perforations and allows access to the wound base should infection occur. Although an expanded meshed graft can cover a larger wound, it heals by contraction and epithelialization, resulting in a "waffle" pattern that is not aesthetically pleasing.

III. OTHER SOFT TISSUE GRAFTS

A. The successful transfer of mucosa, fascia, and fat has been described for reconstructive and aesthetic procedures.

B. Full or split-thickness mucosal grafts can be obtained from the mouth, conjunctiva, and nasal septum to reconstruct lining for missing mucosal surfaces.

C. Harvested fascia has been described for use as a sling or for soft tissue augmentation, as in the lip.

D. Grafts for augmentation are limited by resorption over time.

E. Fat may be harvested and injected to fill soft tissue defects, although its survival is variable. The quantity of soft tissue successfully transferred is limited, as large volumes of tissue are unlikely to be revascularized.

IV. TECHNIQUE

Successful skin grafting requires the preparation of a clean vascular bed, harvest of the skin graft, immobilization of the graft onto the recipient bed, and appropriate wound care to the donor site.

A. Skin Graft Harvest

1. Skin grafts can be harvested from essentially anywhere on the body, using a variety of techniques.
2. Skin grafts may be excised with a mechanical power or drum-type dermatome, or freehand with a Weck knife or scalpel.
3. Common donor sites for full-thickness skin grafts include the upper eyelids, post-auricular region, supraclavicular area, and groin.
4. Split-thickness grafts are commonly taken from the abdominal wall, thigh, and buttocks.
5. Skin grafts can be meshed with a mechanical skin mesher or incised by hand, also called "pie-crusting." Mesh expansion ratios greater than 1.5:1.0 are used only in situations where wounds are very large and donor sites are limited, such as in burn patients with large-area burns.

B. Skin Graft Adherence

1. Skin grafts require a clean and vascular recipient bed. Therefore, they do not take well on bone, cartilage, nerve, or tendon, especially without their respective periosteum, perichondrium, epineurium, or paratenon.
2. Immobilization is essential to prevent shearing between the graft and the recipient bed. Skin grafts are sutured or stapled to the wound surface and a dressing is applied to prevent movement and trauma.
3. A tie-over bolster dressing may be used to apply the graft to convex or concave surfaces or areas of movement.
4. Splints or casts help immobilize skin grafts on the extremities.
5. In order for a skin graft to survive, it must undergo serum imbibition, inosculation, and revascularization—processes where the graft adheres to the recipient bed and vascular communication is reestablished.

Phase	Postop days	Biological processes
Serum imbibition	1–2	Fibrin deposition causes graft adherence to recipient bed Skin graft is sustained by nutrients absorbed by diffusion

Phase	Postop days	Biological processes
Inosculation	3–7	Reestablishment of blood flow between preexisting graft and recipient end capillaries
Revascularization	>4	Revascularization by ingrowth of new vessels

6. Graft circulation becomes essentially normal by postoperative day 7.
7. Lymphatic drainage occurs at a similar rate, allowing the graft to resume its normal weight by postoperative day 9.

C. Postoperative Care

1. Skin graft dressings should remain in place for at least 5–7 days while graft adherence takes place. Graft viability is optimized by immobilization with bolsters and splints during this time.
2. Dressings must be removed earlier if there is evidence of fluid accumulation or infection.
3. Grafts are covered with moist gauze dressings, such as Xeroform, to prevent desiccation.
4. Full-thickness donor sites are usually closed primarily, but may be covered with an additional split-thickness skin graft.
5. Split-thickness donor sites are treated with an occlusive dressing such as DuoDerm or Opsite. By keeping the skin moist and clean until reepithelialization occurs, these semipermeable polyurethane dressings allow the wound to heal more rapidly, and with fewer infections and less pain, compared to the alternate method of allowing the wound to desiccate.
6. Complete reepithelialization of donor sites occurs within 7–10 days for thin split-thickness skin grafts, and after 10–17 days for thicker split-thickness grafts.

V. COMPLICATIONS

A. Hematoma or Seroma

1. The collection of blood or serous fluid underneath the graft is the most common cause of skin graft failure. Shearing forces between the graft and the recipient bed allow the collection of fluid and prevent graft adherence, serum imbibition, and inosculation.
2. Meticulous preparation of the recipient site and strict immobilization of the graft can prevent or minimize the formation of hematomas or seromas.
3. If a fluid collection is identified very early, it may be "rolled out" with cotton swabs or evacuated with a needle puncture in order to salvage the graft.

B. Infection

1. Infection is the second most common cause of skin graft failure.
2. Bacteria produce plasmin and other proteolytic enzymes that destroy the fibrin layer between the graft and recipient bed.
3. Bacterial counts in the wound must be less than 10^5 per gram for skin graft survival. Quantitative wound cultures may be useful prior to grafting if contamination is a concern. Wounds contaminated with β-hemolytic streptococci require fewer organisms to produce failure of wound closure.
4. Donor sites must also be kept clean to prevent infection and additional skin loss at these sites.
5. Development of erythema or suppuration requires removal of bolsters or dressings and wound care with wet dressings three times a day.

VI. SKIN GRAFT SUBSTITUTES

In certain situations, particularly large burns, there may be inadequate donor skin to cover a large surface area, necessitating alternatives to traditional skin grafting.

A. Delayed Autografts

Autologous skin may be harvested and preserved up to 3 weeks in solution before application to a wound.

B. Allografts and Xenografts

1. Allografts and xenografts have been used for temporary wound coverage. Human cadaveric allograft skin (HCAS) will "take," but is rejected at approximately 10 days or later if the patient is immunosuppressed, such as in severe burns.

2. Xenografts such as porcine skin are usually rejected prior to vascularization.

C. Synthetic and Bioengineered Skin Substitutes

1. Silicone polymers and composite membranes have been developed for the temporary coverage of large excised burn wounds.
2. Biobrane (Dow B. Hickam, Inc.) consists of a thin silicone rubber membrane bonded to nylon mesh.
3. More recently, human neonatal fibroblasts have been cultured onto Biobrane to yield TransCyte (Advanced Tissue Sciences), formerly marketed as Dermagraft-Transitional Covering, in an attempt to place living cells in a wound with a biosynthetic epidermal "barrier."
4. Integra artificial skin (Integra Lifesciences Corp.) is a bilayer membrane consisting of a three-dimensional porous matrix of cross-linked bovine tendon collagen and chondroitin-6-sulfate in the dermal replacement layer combined with a removable silicone layer for temporary epidermal replacement.
5. Apligraf (Novartis Corp.) is a living skin equivalent with a bilayer of human keratinocytes and fibroblasts seeded on a bovine collagen matrix.
6. Human keratinocytes have been cultured to yield sheets of epithelium to provide wound coverage. This type of coverage is fragile since it lacks dermis, and the harvesting of these cells requires time and expense. Recent research suggests that the grafting of cultured keratinocytes may be enhanced in the presence of a dermal layer, using either an acellular human dermal matrix or a "neodermis" from artificial skin.

18

General Dermatology

Stefani R. Takahashi M.D.
David Geffen School of Medicine at UCLA, Los Angeles, California, U.S.A.

I. ACNEIFORM DISORDERS

A. Acne Vulgaris

1. Epidemiology and Pathogenesis

a. Acne is an inflammatory disorder of the pilosebaceous unit.

b. The primary cause of acne is unknown.

c. While most patients present during preadolescence or adolescence, acne may present in early childhood or later adulthood.

d. The pathogenesis involves the interaction of hormones, bacteria, and hyperkeratinization of the hair follicle. Abnormal keratinization of the hair follicle results in obstruction of sebum flow, producing the comedone.

e. Hormonal factors, including androgenic production, stimulate sebaceous gland development and activity.

f. The anaerobic diphtheroid *Propionibacterium acnes* releases free fatty acids from the sebum via lipases. These free fatty acids are important causes of inflammation. Resultant rupture within the pilosebaceous unit causes further inflammation as a foreign body reaction that clinically appears as a pustule or nodule.

g. Extrinsic causes of acne include occupational exposure to comedogenic substances, such as cutting oils and chlorinated hydrocarbons, some cosmetic products, physical trauma to the skin from clothing, sports equipment or excessive washing, and certain medications including corticosteroids, lithium carbonate, barbiturates, diphenylhydantoin, and oral contraceptives.

2. Clinical Findings

a. The primary, noninflammatory lesions of acne are the open (blackhead) and closed (whitehead) comedones.

b. Inflammatory lesions include papules, pustules, and cystic nodules. Severe inflammation may result in the formation of sinus tracts and both atrophic and hypertrophic scars.

3. Laboratory Findings

a. In women with acne and hirsutism with or without menstrual irregularity, evaluation for hormonal abnormalities of adrenal and ovarian origin should be considered.

b. Laboratory evaluation includes free testosterone, luteinizing hormone, follicle-stimulating hormone, DHEAS-S, and 17-hydroxy progesterone.

4. Treatment

a. Mild acne may be managed with topical agents. Benzoyl peroxide preparations are available as washes, gels, and lotions in 2.5–10% concentrations. Benzoyl peroxide has strong antibacterial effects without induction of resistance. It may be drying, and care must be taken to avoid bleaching by contact with hair, clothing, and linens.

b. Topical antibiotics including erythromycin and clindamycin may be applied as gel, lotion, or solution.

c. Benzoyl peroxide and topical antibiotics are usually applied once or twice daily.

d. Topical retinoid products such as tretinoin, adapalene, and tazarotene provide comedolytic activity. These products may cause irritation, increase sensitivity to sunlight, and are usually applied in the evening.

e. Moderate acne often requires the use of oral antibiotics, which have both anti-bacterial and anti-inflammatory effects. Tetracyclines, including tetracycline, minocycline, and doxycycline, are usually the first line of treatment. Erythromycin, ampicillin, and Bactrim may be considered in recalcitrant cases.

f. The use of oral contraceptives may be considered in female patients with moderate acne.

g. Individual acne cysts may be treated with intralesional triamcinolone injection at concentrations of 1–2.5 mg/mL. There is a risk of subcutaneous tissue atrophy with this procedure.

h. Superficial chemical peels have also been used to reduce comedones, pustules, and mild acne scarring.

i. Use of the synthetic oral retinoid isotretinoin is reserved for those with severe, recalcitrant nodulo-cystic acne. Isotretinoin affects keratinization and reduces sebaceous gland size and activity. Isotretinoin is a teratogenic drug and requires extensive counseling and use of contraception by females of childbearing age as well as monthly pregnancy testing. In 2001, the FDA developed a program to increase the safe and effective use of Isotretinoin. Prescribers must study the program developed by the FDA in conjunction with pharmaceutical companies, e.g., the S.M.A.R.T. "Guide to Best Practices" provided by Roche, and then sign and return to Roche the Letter of Understanding certifying their knowledge of the measures to minimize fetal exposures to Isotretinoin. Prescribers then receive special self-adhesive qualification stickers from the pharmaceutical company. All prescriptions for Isotretinoin must have the special sticker attached to the prescriber's regular prescription form in order for the prescription to be filled. This sticker will indicate to the pharmacist that the patient is "qualified" according to the new package insert, which means that the female patient has had negative pregnancy tests, as well as education and counseling about pregnancy prevention. The pregnancy test will be repeated every month throughout the Accutane treatment course, and no prescriptions should be given for more than a 1 month supply of Accutane at a time. Baseline liver function tests, complete blood count and serum lipid levels, as well as follow-up after 3 and 6 weeks of therapy, are recommended.

B. Rosacea

1. Etiology and Pathogenesis

a. Rosacea is an acneiform inflammatory disorder of the pilosebaceous unit with a component of vascular instability resulting in flushing and telangiectasias.

b. Rosacea is generally a disease of adulthood that affects the central face.

c. It is more common in fair-skinned individuals.

d. The cause of rosacea is unknown.

2. Clinical Findings

a. Individuals with rosacea are predisposed to flushing and blushing. Exposure to sun, heat, cold, emotional stimuli, spicy foods, hot beverages, and alcoholic beverages may evoke this reaction. Recurrent flushing and blushing leads to persistent erythema with telangiectasias.

b. Inflammatory papules and pustules may be present in rosacea. Comedones are absent. Inflammatory nodules and centrofacial edema occur in severe forms of the disease.

c. Chronic inflammation causes hyperplasia of connective tissue, sebaceous glands, and blood vessels most commonly seen on the nose as rhinophyma.

d. Signs of ocular rosacea include blepharitis, conjunctivitis, iritis, and keratitis.

3. Treatment

a. Preventive treatment in individuals predisposed to or with rosacea includes reduction or avoidance of trigger factors such as excessive heat or cold, alcoholic beverages, and spicy foods. Daily use of sun-protective measures is essential. Emotional stress may also affect some individuals.

b. Topical therapy is useful in treatment of papules and pustules. Topical metronidazole applied once or twice daily is usually effective. Topical antibiotics such as erythromycin, clindamycin, or topical antifungal agents of the imidazole class may be alternative methods of treatment.

c. Oral antibiotics may be required in moderate to severe disease. Tetracycline, minocycline, and doxycycline are usually effective in the treatment of papules and pustules and occasionally reduce erythema. Oral erythromycin may be tried in patients who do not respond to the tetracyclines.

d. In severe or recalcitrant cases, use of isotretinoin may be considered. Treatment of rosacea with isotretinoin often requires a lower dosage than that required by acne vulgaris. Counseling and laboratory monitoring are required as discussed in the acne treatment section above.

e. Telangiectasias may be destroyed by light electrodessication or laser surgery.

f. Techniques for treatment of rhinophyma include CO_2 laser ablation, hot wire loop or shaw scalpel excision, and dermabrasion.

C. Perioral Dermatitis

1. Epidemiology and Pathogenesis

a. Perioral dermatitis is considered by some as a variant of rosacea.

b. Women of childbearing age are primarily affected.

c. Although the pathogenesis is unknown, perioral dermatitis is often preceded or aggravated by the use of potent, fluorinated topical steriods. Use of potent steriods on the face should therefore be avoided.

d. Many other factors, including ultraviolet light, bacteria, Demodex infestation, contact irritants, and hormones, have been suggested.

2. Clinical Findings

a. Micropapules on an erythematous, finely scaly background are usually found in a perioral distribution. Although the nasolabial folds, chin, and upper lip are most often involved, the periorbital involvement also occurs.

b. A rim of sparing around the vermillion border of the lip is classically found.

3. Treatment

a. Discontinuation or weaning of topical steriod use is essential but may result in an initial exacerbation of disease.

b. Topical antibiotics such as metronidazole or erythromycin applied twice daily may be useful.

c. A 1- to 2-month course of oral antibiotics of the tetracycline category is usually required. Oral erythromycin may be used as an alternative.

II. ECZEMATOUS DERMATITIS

A. Contact Dermatitis

1. Etiology and Pathogenesis

a. Contact dermatitis is an acute or chronic inflammatory skin reaction to a substance that has come into contact with the skin. Reactions fall into two categories: allergic and nonallergic.

b. Primary irritant contact dermatitis is a nonallergic reaction that may occur upon the first exposure to a substance such as soaps, detergents, and solvents.

c. Allergic contact dermatitis is a classic delayed hypersensitivity reaction to a substance. Common contact allergens include:

- Neomycin
- Local anesthetics (procaine and benzocaine)
- Nickel
- Lanolin
- Thiuram mix (present in rubber products)
- Formaldehyde (preservative in many materials)
- Epoxy resin
- Imidazolidinyl urea (preservative)
- Pentadecacatechol (poison oak, poison ivy)
- Latex
- Benadryl
- Thimerisol
- Para-amino benzoic acid (PABA)
- Povidone-iodine
- Chlorhexidine
- Methylmethacrylate

2. Clinical Findings

a. Acute contact dermatitis presents as pruritic, well-demarcated erythematous plaques. Vesiculation and crusting may occur.

b. The pattern of the lesion may reflect the shape of the contact substance (e.g., tape) or may be linear (poison oak).

c. Chronic contact dermatitis results in thick, hyperpigmented plaques.

3. Laboratory Findings

a. Patch testing involves application of the allergen to the skin to check for an allergic inflammatory response. Patch testing should not be performed during an acute reaction due to the potential for nonspecific, false-positive reactions under those circumstances. This phenomenon is known as the excited skin syndrome.

b. The standard patch test that is currently available tests for 24 of the most common contact allergens.

4. Treatment

a. Avoidance of the primary irritant or primary allergen is the mainstay of treatment.

b. Acute contact dermatitis is treated symptomatically:

- Wet dressings to dry weeping lesions
- Potent topical steroid application
- Oral antihistamines for pruritus
- A 2-week taper of systemic steroids for severe cases

c. Chronic contact dermatitis is treated symptomatically with topical steroid application and antihistamines for itch.

III. PSORIASIS

A. Psoriasis Vulgaris

1. Etiology and Pathogenesis

a. Psoriasis is a common skin disorder affecting 1–3% of the population in the United States.

b. There is a wide range of clinical presentation in those who are genetically predisposed.

c. The cause of psoriasis is unknown.

d. Most patients develop psoriasis in the third decade of life.

e. Psoriasis exhibits the Koebner phenomenon, which is the development of psoriasis lesions in areas of trauma, including a surgical wound, sunburn, and scratching or rubbing.

f. Other triggers for psoriasis include stress, infection (especially acute streptococcal infection), and medications (e.g., β-blockers, lithium, systemic corticosteroids, and antimalarial agents).

2. Clinical Findings

a. Primary lesions of psoriasis are well-demarcated, erythematous papules and plaques with thick, micaceous (silvery) scale.

b. Nail changes include pitting of the nail plate, yellowish macules beneath the nail plate ("oil spots"), and distal onycholysis (separation of the nail plate from the nail bed).

c. Psoriatic arthritis occurs in 5–8% of patients.

d. Less common severe forms of psoriasis include generalized pustular psoriasis and diffuse erythrodermic psoriasis.

3. Laboratory Findings

Skin biopsy may be performed for diagnosis.

4. Treatment

a. There is a wide variety of treatments for psoriasis.

b. Topical treatments include topical corticosteroids, calcipotriene (vitamin D_3 analog), tazarotene (retinoid), anthralin, and coal tar.

c. Phototherapy with UVB radiation and photochemotherapy with use of systemic psoralen plus UVA are often used.

d. Systemic treatment for severe psoriasis includes anti-TNF agents and anti-T-cell, e.g., Etanercept, Alefacept, Efalizumab and Infliximab, methotrexate, cyclosporine, and acitretin.

IV. INFECTIONS OF THE SKIN

A. Impetigo

1. Etiology and Pathogenesis

a. Impetigo is a superficial bacterial infection of the skin. *Staphylococcus aureus* and group A β-hemolytic *Streptococcus pyogenes* are the most common causes.

b. Impetigo primarily affects infants and children, but adults may be affected. It is highly contagious in children.

c. Nasopharyngeal infections are often the source of the bacteria.

d. Impetigo may secondarily infect preexisting skin lesions, including eczema, contact dermatitis, stasis ulcers, varicella, tinea, and traumatic lesions.

2. Clinical Findings

a. Initial lesions are superficial vesicles or pustules that easily rupture to produce erosions with honey-like serous crusts. Bullae may also occur. Lesions often spread rapidly by autoinoculation.

b. The most common site of involvement is the face, but any site may be affected.

3. Laboratory Findings

a. Gram's stain of vesicle fluid reveals Gram-positive cocci.

b. Bacterial culture of lesional fluid can be performed to identify the causative agent.

4. Treatment

a. Oral antibiotic therapy with penicillin or erythromycin for 10 days is generally effective. Systemic antibiotics should always be used in cases caused by *Streptococcus* due to the risk of postinfectious glomerulonephritis. Culture-based bacterial sensitivities may be useful in guiding therapy for resistant cases.

b. Topical antibiotic therapy is a useful adjunctive therapy. Topical ointments containing muripurocin, bacitracin, and/or polymyxin are applied twice daily.

B. Cellulitis

1. Etiology and Pathogenesis

a. Cellulitis is an acute dermal and subcutaneous infection.

b. Children and older adults are at increased risk.

c. Additional risk factors include diabetes mellitus, immunosuppression by disease or medication, and drug or alcohol abuse.

d. Group A β-hemolytic *Streptococcus pyogenes* and *Staphylococcus aureus* are the most common etiologic agents in adults. Many other bacteria have been isolated, especially group B streptococci in newborns and *Haemophilus influenzae* in children.

e. Cellulitis usually occurs by a portal of entry such as an underlying skin disease, ulcer, traumatic lesion, surgical wound, or mucosal infection. Rarely, hematogenous spread to skin may cause cellulitis.

2. Clinical Findings

a. Prodromal features include fever, chills, and malaise.

b. Erythema usually develops at the site of entry and expands rapidly to produce a hot, tender, indurated plaque. Vesicles, bullae, pustules, erosions, ecchymoses, and hemorrhage may occur within the plaque.

c. Regional lymphadenopathy is common.

3. Laboratory Findings

a. Leukocytosis is usually present.

b. Cultures of skin lesions and blood are usually performed but are positive in only approximately 25% of cases.

4. Treatment

a. Organism-appropriate systemic antimicrobial therapy is essential in the treatment of cellulitis.

b. In most cases, first-generation cephalosporins are appropriate.

C. Dermatophytoses of the Skin

1. Etiology and Pathogenesis

a. Dermatophytoses are superficial fungal infections of the skin.

b. The most common causes of tinea pedis (athlete's foot), tinea corporis (ringworm), tinea cruris (jock itch), tinea manum, and tinea faciale are *Trichophyton rubrum* and *Trichophyton mentagrophytes*. Infections by the *Epidermophyton* and *Microsporum* genera of dermatophytes are less common.

c. Predisposing factors include immunosuppression by disease or by medication, perspiration, and warm, humid climate.

2. Clinical Findings

a. Skin lesions consist of well-demarcated erythematous, scaly patches, and plaques. Central clearing may be present in large plaques, producing the annular lesions that led to the commonly used misnomer of "ringworm."

b. Annular lesions are most common in tinea corporis.

c. Inflammatory variants of tinea on the feet and hands may contain vesicles, bullae, or pustules within the plaques.

d. Interdigital maceration and peeling between the toes are also common.

e. Lesions of tinea may or may not be accompanied by pruritus.

3. Laboratory Findings

a. Demonstration of fungal hyphae may be done by microscopic evaluation of potassium hydroxide (KOH) mounting of scale.

b. Fungal culture may be performed to isolate the causative organism.

4. Treatment

a. Topical antifungal agents of the imidazole (e.g., clotrimazole, miconazole, ketoconazole, econazole) and allylamine (e.g., naftifine, terbinafine) classes are most frequently used. Twice-daily application is usually continued for 2–4 weeks.

b. Systemic antifungal agents such as griseofulvin, itraconazole, and terbinafine may be required for recalcitrant or extensive disease.

c. Antifungal powders may be applied to susceptible areas after bathing as a preventive measure.

D. Herpes Simplex Virus

1. Etiology and Pathogenesis

a. Herpes simplex virus type 1 (HSV-1) and herpes simplex virus type 2 (HSV-2) cause mucocutaneous oral, facial, and genital infections.

b. Primary infection occurs by direct contact with the virus.

c. Following primary infection, the virus may remain latent in the dorsal root ganglion. Recurrence may be triggered by sun exposure, fever, trauma, illness, stress, and immunosuppression. Recurrence may also be spontaneous.

d. Disseminated disease may occur in the setting of immunosuppression.

2. Clinical Findings

a. Primary HSV infection is often asymptomatic or has minimal symptoms. It may occasionally be accompanied by fever, malaise, and regional lymphadenopathy.

b. The average incubation period from time of exposure to onset of clinical disease is 5–10 days.

c. Classic lesions are painful, grouped vesicles on an erythematous base resembling "dewdrops on a rose petal." Erosions and ulcerations may follow.

d. Recurrent HSV is often heralded by symptoms of itching and burning. An erythematous patch develops in the area followed by the development of grouped vesicles.

e. Fever and regional lymphadenopathy may occur.

3. Laboratory Findings

a. A Tzanck preparation may be easily performed by smearing cells from the base of a vesicle onto a glass slide and staining with Wright's or Giemsa stain. Multinucleated giant cells are seen in both HSV and varicella zoster virus infections.

b. Direct antigen testing using monoclonal antibodies against HSV-1 and HSV-2 proteins may be performed on smeared lesional preparations.

c. While direct antigen testing is more rapid, viral culture is more sensitive in confirming the diagnosis. Viral culture is also helpful in acyclovir-resistant cases.

d. Serology for circulating HSV antibodies may be useful in distinguishing primary versus recurrent attacks. Since 85% of the adult population worldwide is seropositive for HSV antibodies, serology is most helpful when it is negative.

e. Polymerase chain reaction (PCR) and immunoperoxidase staining are specialized tests that may be useful on tissue samples.

4. Treatment

a. Inoculation of HSV may be prevented by avoidance of direct contact with active lesions.

b. Treatment of acute and recurrent HSV infection with oral antiviral agents such as acyclovir, valacyclovir, and famcyclovir is effective in shortening the course of disease and reduction of viral shedding.

c. Intravenous acyclovir should be used in severe disease and in immunocompromised patients.

d. For those patients with frequent recurrences (>6 per year), daily suppressive therapy with oral antiviral agents may be indicated.

e. Reactivation of HSV has been reported with procedures such as chemical peels, dermabrasion, laser resurfacing, and collagen implantation. In patients with a history of HSV, prophylactic oral antiviral therapy should be instituted for such procedures.

19

Congenital Melanocytic Nevi

Peter J. Taub, M.D., H. Peter Lorenz, M.D., and Malcolm Lesavoy, M.D.
Stanford University Medical Center, Stanford, California, U.S.A.

I. HISTORY

A. 1832—Alibert describes a giant "waistcoat and drawers" nevus

B. 1878—Baker reports staged excision of giant congenital melanocytic nevi (CMN)

C. 1897—Jablokoff and Klein report on the malignant potential of giant CMN

II. INCIDENCE

A. A pigmented lesion occurs in at least 2.5% of newborns.

B. Only 1% of newborns have biopsy-proven melanocytic nevi.

C. In the general population, incidence is 1–4%. The incidence is lower in Latin America (0.2%) and higher in Japan (2.1%).

D. Very large nevi are present in only 1 in 2,000–20,000 newborns and constitute 0.1% of all cutaneous melanomas

III. CLASSIFICATION

CMN may be classified according to size (although this is arbitrary):

A. Small CNV are less than 1.5 cm in diameter.

B. Medium CNV are between 1.5 and 20 cm in diameter.

C. Large or giant CNV are greater than 20 cm in diameter.

D. Others have classified these lesions based on treatment options:

- Small lesions may be easily closed primarily.
- Large lesions require other closure options.
- Giant lesions occupy a significant proportion of the affected anatomic site. Some use the size of the patient's palm when describing lesions of the head and neck and twice that for other anatomic sites.

E. Most are small and singular.

IV. HISTOLOGY

A. CMN are characterized by nevus cells arranged in sheets or nests within the epidermis or dermis. The cells often exhibit neural differentiation that resembles neurofibromas or schwannomas.

B. Histologic types include superficial and thick.

- Superficial types are:
  - Most common
  - Well-differentiated lesions confined to the epidermis and upper dermis
  - Lighter in color as the mature melanocytes are confined to the epidermis
  - Found on the face, torso, and extremities

- Thick types are:
  - Irregular lesions that extend into deeper layers and structures, including nerves, vessels, and muscle
  - Darker lesions that appear most often on the back, scalp, and buttocks

C. CMN may involve epithelial structures such as lymphatic vessels or arrector pili muscles. Only in very large CMN are nevus cells found in muscle or bone.

D. Larger CMN may be associated with other abnormalities:

- Ocular manifestations
- Spina bifida occulta
- Neurofibromatosis
- Leptomeningeal melanocytosis:
  - These may be asymptomatic or may give rise to obstructive hydrocephalus, seizures, focal neurologic deficits, or melanoma.
  - Diagnosis requires meningeal biopsy.
  - MRI can detect asymptomatic cases.
  - Symptomatic cases have a poor prognosis.
  - Risk factors for leptomeningeal melanocytosis include large or multiple CMN, midline back location, and no evidence of cutaneous melanoma.

V. ASSOCIATED TUMORS

Tumors that arise in conjunction with CMN include:

A. Schwannomas

B. Neurofibromas

C. Hemangiomas

D. Wilms' tumors

E. Melanoma

- Disagreement exists over the exact relationship to melanoma. It appears that the risk of developing melanoma by 10 years of age is 1 in 200,000, and the prognosis is very grave if melanoma develops.
- Less controversial is the general agreement that larger CMN are at greater risk for malignant degeneration than smaller lesions.

VI. GENETICS

A. Familial clusters of CMN have been reported.

B. There is an 11-fold increase in the rate of CMN among siblings of probands with small CMN.

VII. CLINICAL APPEARANCE

A. CMN are larger on average than acquired nevi.

B. Most are elevated; some can be flat and macular.

C. In contrast to acquired nevi, the borders are often irregular.

D. Surface may be smooth or lobular, but generally the skin markings are accentuated.

E. Pigmented lesions have a fine, speckled pattern.

F. In darker complectioned patients, the nevi can have a blue tone.

G. CMN may be hairless, but more often contain large coarse hairs.

H. Very dark pigmentation is rare in white infants but relatively common in darkly pigmented infants.

I. CMN do not remain static after birth, but grow in proportion to the overall increase in body size.

VIII. DIAGNOSIS

A. Requires confirmation that the lesion was present at birth

B. Often made clinically without the need for biopsy

C. Differential diagnosis includes:

- Epidermal nevus—usually linear without plaques or hair
- Café au lait spot—do not distort the skin or display speckling
- Mongolian spot—blue/gray in color and do not distort the skin surface or display speckling
- Pigmented arrector pili hamartoma—lightly pigmented and associated with prominent hair. May become indurated with massage
- Congenital Baker's melanosis—appears later in childhood with coarse, long hairs

D. In the neonatal period, the appearance of an enlarging nodular mass warrants open biopsy to differentiate the lesion from common hyperplastic nodules.

E. Multiple punch biopsies may help in deciding which are high-risk areas.

IX. TREATMENT

A. Excision may be considered as early as possible, while retaining function and cosmesis.

B. The reported risk of developing melanoma within a CMN ranges from 0 to 40%. However, recent studies report the risk of developing melanoma within a very large CMN is in the range of 3–5% in the pediatric population. With age, lifetime risk likely increases to 5–10%.

C. Specific indications for excision include:

- Midline back location
- Ulceration
- Pruritis
- Infection

D. Treatment principles are as follows:

- All lesions should be photographed and measured at birth.
- Family history of CMN should be obtained.
- Small, benign-appearing lesions do not need to be excised in infancy if general anesthesia is required.
- Atypical lesions require immediate excision.
- All small lesions should be considered for prophylactic excision before the age of 12 years (when the risk of melanoma increases more rapidly).
- Dominant nodules may be present that may represent a variant of sarcoma, which requires immediate treatment.
- Incomplete excision often results in recurrence.

E. Surgical techniques include:

- Direct closure after excision
- Excision and split thickness skin grafts
- Serial staged excisions
- Tissue expansion
- Excision and free flap closure
- Combinations of the above

20

Benign Cutaneous Neoplasms

Kathleen Behr, M.D.
David Geffen School of Medicine at UCLA, Los Angeles, California, U.S.A.

Benign cutaneous tumors are exceedingly common. Many can be diagnosed clinically, although some need a biopsy for diagnosis. The neoplasms can be divided into epithelial, dermal, appendageal, melanocytic, mesenchymal, and neural tumors. Clinical presentation, course, and treatment for the most common tumors in each group will be discussed.

I. EPITHELIAL NEOPLASMS

A. Epidermal Nevus

1. Clinical: A hamartomatous tumor of closely set flesh-colored or brown verrucous papules that are often linear. The lesion is present at or shortly after birth.
2. Course: If the lesion is extensive, developmental abnormalities in other systems may be present.
3. Treatment: Excision is most reliable. Epidermal nevi must be excised below the deep dermis to prevent recurrence.

B. Nevus Sebaceous

1. Clinical: A solitary lesion present at birth as a yellowish patch or plaque with predilection for the scalp. The lesion is raised at birth, then flattens until puberty, when it becomes verrucous.
2. Course: If multiple nevus sebaceous lesions are present, systemic abnormalities may coexist. Secondary tumors often develop in this lesion, such as steatocystoma papilliferum (8–19%) and basal cell carcinoma (5–7%).
3. Treatment: Surgical excision before puberty is recommended due to the potential development of basal cell carcinoma.

C. Seborrheic Keratosis

1. Clinical: Extremely common. Lesions are flesh-colored to dark brown rough warty papules that are well demarcated and have a "stuck-on" appearance. Variants include dermatosis papulosa nigrans, which are small facial papules in darker-skinned individuals, and stucco keratosis, which are gray-white papules on the legs.
2. Course: Benign lesions often increase in number with age.
3. Treatment: Cryotherapy in fair-skinned individuals only, otherwise secondary pigmentation change develops in darker skin types. Other therapies include electrodessication, curettage, laser, and excision. If the lesion is shaved, the specimen should be sent for pathology.

II. DERMAL NEOPLASMS

A. Acrochordon ("Skin Tag")

1. Clinical: Very common tumors that present as flesh-colored pedunculated papules.
2. Course: Common in body folds, especially in obese individuals.

3. Treatment: Irritated lesions are treated by cryotherapy, electrodesiccation, or snip excision.

B. Angiofibroma

1. Clinical: Small 1–3 mm reddish-brown or flesh-colored smooth shiny papules on the sides of the nose, medial cheeks, and chin.
2. Course: Isolated lesions are common in middle age. Multiple lesions are seen in tuberous sclerosis complex.
3. Treatment: For isolated lesions, shave biopsy or cautery is curative. For multiple lesions, dermabrasion or laser is palliative.

C. Dermatofibroma

1. Clinical: Common papule on lower extremity. Presents as firm reddish-brown papule that dimples when pinched.
2. Course: Benign growth secondary to arthropod bite or ingrown hair.
3. Treatment: No therapy needed. Surgery is avoided since the scar is often more apparent than the original lesion.

D. Keloid

1. Clinical: Firm, tender, pink to purple scar beyond the border of the original area of trauma or surgery. Common on the shoulders, upper back, and chest.
2. Course: Lesions are often tender and pruritic and often recur with excision.
3. Therapy: Recurrences are common with all therapy. Intralesional Kenalog 10–40 mg/cc every 3–4 weeks is the mainstay of treatment. Topical silicone dressings are reported to be helpful. For larger lesions, excisions may be performed but should be combined with postoperative intralesional steroids, interferon-α 2b or radiation therapy.

E. Pyogenic Granuloma

1. Clinical: Rapidly developing vascular lesion that arises at the site of trauma. Common on the face, fingers, toes, and trunk.
2. Course: Bleeds spontaneously after minor trauma.
3. Treatment: Shave excision and electrodesiccation of the base to prevent recurrence.

III. APPENDAGEAL TUMORS

A. Hair Differentiation

1. Epidermal Inclusion Cyst

a. Clinical: Firm, intradermal, freely mobile tumor often with a visible puncta in the epidermis.

b. Course: Benign lesion, but significant foreign body reaction develops if the cyst wall ruptures.

c. Treatment: Inflamed cysts are incised and drained. Noninflamed cysts can be removed through excision. The entire capsule must be removed to prevent recurrence.

2. Milia

a. Clinical: Small 1–2 mm white superficial cyst common on face.

b. Course: Benign; common after laser or dermabrasion.

c. Treatment: Epidermis is nicked with a #11 scalpel blade, and the cyst is extracted.

3. Pilomatricoma (Calcifying Epithelioma of Malherbe)

a. Clinical: Firm, deep-seated nodule, often disc-shaped, under the epidermis. Most common on the face or upper extremities in childhood.

b. Course: Benign, slowly growing.

c. Treatment: Excision.

4. Steatocystoma Multiplex

a. Clinical: Multiple, slow-growing, 0.5–3 cm yellowish cysts. Common on the sternal areas, axillae, neck, and scrotum.

b. Course: Autosomal dominant condition.

c. Treatment: No good therapy. Larger lesions can be excised or drained.

5. Trichoepithelioma

a. Clinical: Single or multiple flesh-colored papules or nodules on the face.

b. Course: Solitary lesions must be clinically and histologically differentiated from basal cell carcinoma. Multiple lesions are often inherited as an autosomal dominant trait.

c. Treatment: Solitary lesions are excised. Multiple lesions are palliatively treated with shave excisions, dermabrasion, or laser.

B. Eccrine

1. Eccrine Hidrocystoma

a. Clinical: Solitary or multiple 1–3 mm translucent bluish cyst on the face.

b. Course: Benign. Number and size may increase in summer.

c. Treatment: Lesions are nicked with a #11 scalpel blade, and the surface is lightly electrocauterized.

2. Eccrine Poroma

a. Clinical: Solitary, pink or flesh-colored sessile or slightly pedunculated papule. Most common on the sole of the foot.

b. Course: Rarely, a malignant eccrine poroma develops from long-standing benign eccrine poroma.

c. Treatment: Excision.

3. Syringoma

a. Clinical: Single or multiple 1–3 mm slightly yellowish papules common on eyelids, axillae, umbilicus, and pubic area. Can be eruptive on neck, axilla, chest, or abdomen.

b. Course: Benign.

c. Treatment: Cosmetic therapy includes electrodesiccation or laser.

C. Apocrine: Apocrine Hidrocystoma

a. Clinical: Solitary or multiple bluish cystic nodules, ranging in size from a few millimeters to 1.5 cm. Most common on the face.

b. Course: Benign.

c. Treatment: Nick with a #11 scalpel blade and cauterize.

D. Sebaceous: Sebaceous Hyperplasia

a. Clinical: Yellowish papule 1–4 mm on face with central del. Lesions increase with age.

b. Course: Benign. Must differentiate from basal cell carcinoma.

c. Treatment: Cosmetic therapy includes electrodessication or laser, but lesions often recur.

IV. MELANOCYTIC

A. Café Au Lait

1. Clinical: Discrete pale brown macules, 2–20 mm in diameter, with serrated or irregular margins.
2. Course: Isolated lesions occur in 10–20% of the normal population. Multiple lesions (six or more) may be a marker of multisystem disease such as neurofibromatosis.
3. Treatment: None; can be treated with laser, but they often recur.

B. Lentigo

1. Clinical: Acquired, circumscribed, light-brown macule induced by ultraviolet light.
2. Course: Persists indefinitely even in the absence of light.
3. Treatment: Includes sunblock, bleaching creams, light liquid nitrogen, or laser.

C. Nevi

1. Clinical: A junctional nevus is a flat brown macule. An intradermal nevus is a fleshy papule. A compound nevus appears as a brown papule.
2. Course: Nevi should be removed if irritated, itchy, changing in size/shape/color/depth/borders, or atypical in appearance to rule out atypical histology or melanoma.
3. Treatment: Lesions can be shaved for cosmetic purposes. If the appearance is atypical, nevi should be excised. All specimens should be sent for pathologic evaluation.

D. Becker's Nevus

1. Clinical: Brown macule or plaque measuring several centimeters in size and often acquired near puberty. Most often found on the shoulders and back. Five times more common in men than in women. Hypertrichosis is variable.
2. Course: Benign.

3. Treatment: Nd:Yag laser therapy for brown component and hair removal laser for hypertrichosis.

V. MESENCHYMAL: LIPOMA

1. Clinical: Dermal, soft, well-circumscribed nodules.
2. Course: Benign. Angiolipomas can be painful.
3. Treatment: Excision can be performed through small incision or punch.

VI. NEURAL: NEUROFIBROMA

1. Clinical: Protuberant to pedunculated flesh-colored papules or nodules that are soft to palpation.
2. Course: If multiple, rule out neurofibromatosis.
3. Treatment: Excision.

21

Basal Cell and Squamous Cell Carcinomas of the Skin

H. Peter Lorenz, M.D.
Stanford University Medical Center, Stanford, California, U.S.A.
Marc H. Hedrick, M.D., and Timothy A. Miller, M.D.
David Geffen School of Medicine at UCLA, Los Angeles, California, U.S.A.

I. INCIDENCE

A. Skin cancer is the most common human cancer.

B. Over 700,000 new cases are diagnosed annually.

C. Approximately 77% are basal cell carcinomas, 20% are squamous cell carcinomas, and 3% are melanomas or rare tumors.

D. The incidence and mortality rates are increasing in the United States, with an annual increase of 3–7% in Caucasians.

II. ETIOLOGY

A. Squamous Cell Carcinoma

1. Sun exposure has been shown to be the major environmental cause of both basal and squamous cell carcinomas (Table 1). Greater than 80% of nonmelanoma skin cancers are found on sun-exposed areas such as the head, arms, and hands.
2. In addition to UVB radiation from sunlight, a past history of therapeutic radiation treatment has been associated with the development of cutaneous malignancies. Patients with chronic radiation dermatitis (erythema, atrophy, alopecia, telangiectasia, pigmentation change, and actinic keratosis) may develop squamous cell carcinoma.
3. Squamous cell carcinoma can also develop at sites of chronic inflammation such as nonhealing ulcers (burn scars, pressure sores, venous or arterial insufficiency ulcers) and chronic sinus sites due to osteomyelitis. These cancers commonly occur on nonexposed areas and present many years after the start of the original process. When squamous cell carcinoma is present in a chronic burn ulcer, it is termed a Marjolin's ulcer.
4. Although mainly of historic interest, chemical exposure (coal tar, petroleum products, or arsenic exposure) can occasionally predispose exposed individuals to squamous carcinoma.

B. Basal Cell Carcinoma

1. Several genetic and biophysical traits are associated with an increased susceptibility to developing basal cell cancer (Table 2). The presence of melanin granules in the skin or dark skin coloring appears to be photoprotective. UV-related mutations have been linked to mutations of the p53 tumor suppressor gene. These have been noted in 56% of basal cell carcinomas.
2. Basal cell carcinoma typically presents as a sporadically occurring tumor. However, several syndromic causes of basal cell carcinoma have also been described. Nevoid basal cell carcinoma

Table 1 Etiologic Factors for Squamous Carcinoma of the Skin

Sun exposure (UVB radiation)
Previous radiation therapy with radiation dermatitis
Chemical exposure (coal tar, petroleum products, arsenic)
Chronic ulceration/inflammation
Genetic predisposition (fair skin)
Xeroderma pigmentosum
Immunosuppression

syndrome (NBCCS), or Gorlin's syndrome, is a disorder transmitted in an autosomal dominant fashion with a low penetrance. Its cause has been traced to a mutation in a putative tumor suppressor gene located at 9q23.1-q31. Mutations at this locus may have implications for sporadic basal cell carcinoma as well. In fact, 50% of nonsyndromic basal cell carcinomas exhibit a mutation at this locus. The primary manifestations of NBCCS, in addition to basal cell carcinoma, are odontogenic keratocysts, dyskeratosis, pitting of the palms and soles, and intracranial calcifications. The average age of onset is 20 years, and the face and back are the locations primarily affected.

3. Bazex's syndrome is also an autosomal dominant disorder resulting in multiple small basal cell carcinomas of the face, usually first noticed in adolescence or young adulthood. It may also result in "ice pick" marks on the extremities and hypotrichosis.
4. Rombo syndrome is an autosomally inherited disorder that has also been found to be associated with basal cell carcinoma. These tend to occur later in life, around 35 years of age, and are associated with other skin conditions and hypotrichosis.
5. Finally, other inherited disorders such as xeroderma pigmentosum, albinism, linear unilateral basal cell nevus, and nevus sebaceous of Jadassohn have been associated with an increased risk of developing basal cell carcinoma.

III. PATHOLOGY OF SQUAMOUS CELL CARCINOMAS

A. Squamous cell carcinoma has uniform gross and microscopic morphology, unlike that of basal cell carcinoma. Squamous cell carcinoma appears as sharply defined erythematous plaques with elevated borders. As invasion deepens, the borders elevate further and the lesions appear as painless, firm, red nodules with scaling, ulceration, and/or horn formation.

B. Carcinoma in situ lesions are reddish in color with slightly raised borders.

C. Histologically, squamous carcinoma in situ is characterized by atypical squamous cells completely replacing the epidermis. In actinic keratosis, the atypical cells only partially replace the epidermis. A lymphocytic infiltrate is usually present in the superficial dermis.

D. Invasion is defined as atypical keratinocyte migration through the basement membrane into the dermis.

E. These cells are pleomorphic, have multiple mitoses, and are dyskeratotic with horn pearls consisting of concentric layers of squamous cells with central keratinization. They range in histologic grade from well differentiated to poorly differentiated, depending on their resemblance to normal cells. In addition, histologic evidence of perineural invasion may herald a more aggressive lesion.

F. The pseudoglandular types and the spindle cell types are variants of squamous cell carcinoma.

G. Verrucous carcinomas are a slow-growing variant characterized by their fungating appearance and can be deeply invasive without metastasis.

IV. PATHOLOGY OF BASAL CELL CARCINOMAS

A. The gross and microscopic morphology of basal cell carcinoma is varied. Five major gross morphologic types of basal cell carcinoma exist: (1) nodulo-ulcerative, (2) pigmented, (3) superficial, (4) morpheaform, and (5) fibroepithelio-

Table 2 Biophysical Risk Factors for Basal Cell Carcinoma

Male sex
White race
Celtic origin
Easily sunburned
Increasing age
Blue eyes
Fair complexion

ma. In addition, numerous rarer variants have also been reported (Table 3).

- The nodulo-ulcerative variety is most common and begins as a small, slowly enlarging papule with pearly edges and telangiectasias. Central ulceration (rodent ulcer) may occur when the tumor grows and replaces the epidermis. Most nodulo-ulcerative tumors behave predictably and exhibit slow growth.
- The pigmented basal cell carcinoma is similar to the nodulo-ulcerative type, but differs in its brown pigmentation and is often misdiagnosed grossly as malignant melanoma.
- Superficial basal cell carcinoma occurs as single or multiple patches that are indurated and scaly. Grossly, they may be ringed by a raised pearly border that slowly expands. Superficial ulceration or crusting may occur centrally, resembling eczema, psoriasis, or tinea.
- The morpheaform or sclerosing form is the most aggressive of the clinical subtypes of basal cell carcinoma. These lesions appear as flat or slightly depressed yellowish plaques with indistinct borders. Ulceration is rare and is typically located on the face. A dense desmoplastic reaction is present.
- Fibroepithelioma variants are typically raised and moderately firm with an erythematous and smooth surface. This type occurs commonly on the lower trunk, especially on the lumbosacral region.

B. Histologically, basal cell carcinoma exhibits lobules, nests, cords, or strands of tumor cells extending from the basal layer of the epidermis. The classic histologic pattern is cellular with peripheral palisading of cells that are clustered and separate from the stroma. The tumor cells contain large hyperchromatic nuclei that are nonanaplastic in appearance and resemble the nuclei of basal cells of the epidermis. They may have a large ratio of nucleus to cytoplasm.

C. Basal cell carcinomas can also be histologically divided into differentiated and undifferentiated subtypes (Table 3). Several histologic patterns may exist in a single tumor. There are two major factors that influence the histologic appearance of basal cell carcinomas: (1) the relative differentiation and proliferating ability of its cells, and (2) the nature of the stromal response evoked.

Table 3 Histologic Patterns and Variants of Basal Cell Carcinoma

Undifferentiated	Differentiated	Uncertain differentiation
Nodular	Adenoid	Adamantinoid
Superficial	Basosquamous	Granular cell
Pigmented	Keratotic	
Morpheaform	Clear cell	
Fibroepithelioma	Infundibulocystic	
Giant cell	Glandular differentiated subtypes	

V. PRECURSOR LESIONS

These lesions help identify patients at risk for later development of basal cell carcinoma, squamous cell carcinoma, or melanoma.

A. Actinic Keratoses

1. These present as rough, scaly, erythematous plaques present on chronically exposed skin: forehead, nose, cheeks, neck, and superior pinna. Usually, mild tenderness is present.
2. Because they represent a risk factor for nonmelanoma skin cancer (basal or squamous cell), these patients should be closely followed. The progression rate for a single actinic keratotic lesion to squamous cell carcinoma is estimated to be 1 in 1000 per year. Signs of conversion to carcinoma include an increase in thickness, induration, ulceration, and rapid increase in size.
3. These lesions may also spontaneously regress if the patient limits sun exposure: up to 25% per year may regress. However, they commonly recur at the same site after substantial reexposure.
4. Treatment ranges from continued observation to destructive ablation. Single lesions can be destroyed with liquid nitrogen cryotherapy. Diffuse involvement is best treated with topical medications such as 5-fluorouracil (5-FU), masoprocol, or retinoids.
5. Treatment with isotretinoin (Retin-A®), chemical peeling, and CO_2 laser resurfacing may reduce the risk of further development of cutaneous malignancy in these sun-damaged individuals.

B. Squamous Cell Carcinoma In Situ

This has been referred to as Bowen's disease and occurs predominantly in older patients.

1. These lesions are erythematous with raised, well-defined borders and a scaly appearance that may be confused with psoriasis.
2. They present with an indolent history, having been present for years with slow growth.
3. When located on the penis, this lesion is termed erythroplasia of Queyrat.
4. Histopathologically, there is atypia of the full thickness of the epidermis without dermal invasion.
5. Progression to squamous carcinoma is slow, but 5% ultimately develop dermal invasion.
6. Treatment generally requires complete excision for both definitive diagnosis to rule out invasion and cure. If surgical excision is not performed after biopsy, ablation can be done with cryotherapy or electrodesiccation and curettage.

C. Keratoacanthoma

This is a rapidly growing lesion that may have either a benign or malignant phenotype.

1. Grossly and histologically, it resembles squamous cell carcinoma, but its ambivalent nature is manifested by rapid initial growth over a several week period that is typically followed by a latent period, then a period of regression, each lasting several weeks.
2. These lesions have been termed "deficient squamous cell carcinomas" because of their tendency to regress spontaneously, but they may occasionally progress to invasive or metastatic squamous cell carcinoma. The cause of this regression is unknown but may be immunologically mediated.
3. Because of its clear malignant potential and its frequent confusion with squamous cell carcinoma, complete excision and histologic evaluation are recommended.

D. Human Papillomavirus

1. Human papillomavirus (HPV) has been found in association with Bowen's disease and with epidermodysplasia verruciformis, both of which are associated with squamous carcinoma.
2. Immunocompromised HIV patients and immunosuppressed transplant patients have an association between HPV and squamous carcinoma. These groups require aggressive sun protection and frequent surveillance.

VI. TREATMENT

A. Surgical Excision

1. Surgical excision is the most common technique used for treating basal and squamous cell carcinoma. Since approximately 80% of basal and squamous cell carcinomas are small with excisional wounds that can be closed primarily, excisional biopsy and primary closure is frequently appropriate for both biopsy and treatment and can be performed in a single office visit. The lesion should be resected as an ellipse with its long axis along Langer's lines. The tissue specimen should be marked according to its original orientation in situ and sent to the pathologist for evaluation of margins.
2. For larger lesions or lesions where the diagnosis is in question, punch or shave biopsies may be appropriate.
3. For pigmented lesions where malignant melanoma is included in the differential diagnosis, a complete excisional biopsy to allow proper histologic staging should be performed.

Clear surgical margins are essential for both squamous and basal cell carcinomas.

1. Multiple frozen sections should be utilized on all but the most straightforward lesions to ensure complete excision. After excising the specimen, we obtain additional margin(s) of 1–2 mm in all directions and submit them for frozen section evaluation. These fragments of tissue can be excised at the margin of resection, identified at specific points based on their orientation relative to an imaginary clock placed onto the wound (i.e., 12–3 o'clock, 3–6 o'clock, etc.). The deep margin should also be marked separately and submitted. We use silver nitrate rather than ink to mark the border of interest in all our specimens. It leaves a thin layer of red-brown pigment that will not wash off and that is easily visible histologically. Further resection can be

performed in precise locations as indicated by the frozen section results.

3. The optimal surgical margin is not known. Authors have recommended a minimum margin of 4 mm to eradicate > 95% of tumors > 2 cm in diameter. While the planned surgical margin is an important consideration, it is nevertheless arbitrary. A histologically clear margin must be obtained for cure.

B. Mohs Surgery

1. Mohs chemosurgery was first described by Frederic Mohs.
2. After the specimen is excised and oriented, a surgical map of the tissue is made on a card to document orientation of the specimen. The edges of the specimen are marked with zinc chloride paste to facilitate identification of the surgical margins.
3. This technique is particularly useful for infiltrative basal cell carcinomas that have finger-like projections emanating from the tumor. These projections may be missed by less directed excision of tissue.
4. Mohs surgery also gives excellent results with recurrent tumors. Furthermore, tumors with an aggressive histologic subtype or those tumors in critical anatomic locations may be best treated with Mohs.
5. Lesions where the risk of significant functional loss increases with each 1 mm of margin taken are those that benefit the most from Mohs surgery. These include medial canthal and alar rim lesions.

VII. NONOPERATIVE THERAPY

A. Radiation Therapy

Radiation therapy may be an effective treatment for some patients with diffuse areas of basal cell and squamous cell carcinomas.

1. It is used predominantly in older patients who may be too ill to tolerate a general anesthetic and in whom there is little concern for late development of radiation-induced skin cancers.
2. The potential complications of radiation such as dry eye, xerostomia, epilation, lacrimal duct scarring, skin necrosis, and poor wound healing should also be considered.
3. The treatment regime generally utilizes 4000–6000 cGy in 10–30 fractions, depending on the specific characteristics of the tumor.

B. Chemotherapy

Chemotherapy is useful for basal cell carcinoma only.

1. 5-Fluorouracil (5-FU) is a chemotherapeutic agent used topically for the treatment of basal cell carcinoma. Application is to the lesion and small margin of normal tissue. The treatment is typically performed nightly and continued for 4–12 weeks until the lesion becomes red and ulcerated. The lesion then sloughs and ultimately heals over the ensuing 1–2 months.
2. Isotretinoin and other vitamin A–based treatments have been shown in vivo to have antineoplastic effects. Topical retinoic acid treatment causes marked epithelial thickening with an increase in number of cell layers expressing markers of differentiation. Clinically, actinic keratoses regress with topical retinoid therapy. This effect may be enhanced by co-treatment with 5-FU. Topical retinoids may also be useful in the prevention of basal cell carcinoma.
3. Alpha-interferon has been shown in preliminary studies to be effective in the treatment of nodular and superficial basal cell carcinomas. The mechanism of action of alpha-interferon appears related to a nonspecific activation of macrophages and natural killer cells in the area of the tumor, increasing the magnitude of their hosts' antineoplastic response.

C. Phototherapy

Phototherapy represents a relatively new modality for the treatment of basal cell carcinoma.

1. An inactive photosensitizer is administered, which accumulates in the tissue of interest. Light is then administered to the tumor, photoactivating the sensitizer, which in turn converts molecular oxygen to free radicals with tumoricidal activity.
2. Because of the widespread photosensitization in the patient, this form of therapy is not currently useful for treating isolated tumors.
3. It may have a role in the treatment of patients with widespread disease such as those with Gorlin's syndrome.

Table 4 Characteristics of Basal Cell Carcinomas Associated with High Recurrence Risk

Long duration
High-risk area (midface, ear)
Large size
Aggressive histologic features (morpheaform, perineural invasion)
Neglected tumor
Inadequately treated or recurrent disease
History of radiation exposure

D. Cryosurgery and Electrosurgery

1. The use of physical energy to treat basal cell carcinoma may yield excellent cure rates in properly selected tumors. Patients with nodular or superficial tumors that are small (5–15 mm) with well-defined borders are good candidates for cryosurgery or electrosurgery if the location is such that wound contraction will give an acceptable functional and aesthetic outcome. Cryosurgery typically utilizes liquid nitrogen (temperature −195.6°C) applied rapidly with the use of a spray device or wand. An intracellular temperature of −40°C is required for cell destruction.
2. Electrosurgery uses manual curettage of the tumor followed by the application of one of several forms of electrical energy, such as electrocautery. When using either of these techniques, the wounds are covered with antibiotic ointment and allowed to heal by secondary intention. Margins cannot be inspected for residual cancer using these methods.

VIII. TREATMENT OUTCOME

A. Since basal and squamous cell carcinomas are rarely fatal, survival should not be the sole criterion for treatment success. Rather, complete tumor eradication and functional and aesthetic reconstruction should be the goals of treatment. Tumor control is best determined by recurrence rate, but, unfortunately, there are several factors that make this parameter difficult to evaluate.

B. Several tumor characteristics of high recurrence risk have been identified (Table 4). Skin cancers that occur on the midface, particularly around the nose and ears, are more likely to recur. This is thought to be due to the location of these tumors near the embryonic lines of fusion, which may facilitate deeper tumor spread. Furthermore, surgeons are less willing to obtain wide margins in these areas. Large cancers, often an indication of neglect and denial, are also more likely to recur.

C. The morpheaform variety of basal cell carcinoma behaves much more aggressively and clearly has the greatest recurrence rate of the various histologic subtypes. Subclinical tumor extension in morpheaform basal cell carcinoma has been noted to be three times that in nodular forms. Recurrence rates of tumors with histologic features of sclerosis (morpheaform) and infiltration, as well as features of both basal and squa-

Table 5 Planning Surgical Margins for Primary Excision of Basal Cell Carcinoma

Tumor type	Area	Anticipated margin (mm)	Frozen section
Solid—circumscribed			
<2 cm	Noncritical[a]	5–10	No
>2 cm	Noncritical	5–10	Yes
<1 cm	Critical[b]	2–3	Yes
>1 and <2 cm	Critical	3–5	Yes
>2 cm	Critical	5–10	Yes
Morpheaform or aggressive subtype	Any	7–10	Yes
Other histologic subtypes	Individualized	Individualized	

[a] Noncritical areas include the trunk, upper arms, and legs.
[b] Critical areas include the face, head, hands, feet, and perineum.

mous carcinoma, are several times higher than nodular forms (12–30% vs. 1–6%). This is due to the finger-like projections emanating from the central tumor mass, which may extend several millimeters into surrounding normal tissue.

D. Table 5 details a reasonable approach to estimating margins preoperatively. Squamous cell carcinoma lesions larger than 3 cm and/or with anaplasia are substantially more difficult to cure due to the tendency for lymphatic spread and distant metastases. Some authors recommend at least 3 cm margins for these lesions, especially if located on the trunk or extremities, which is common.

E Careful histologic examination of the margins and reexcision of positive margins yield cure rates of approximately 95% for primary nonmelanoma skin tumors. However, acceptable cure rates can be obtained with other forms of therapy. For example, a small truncal lesion can be adequately treated with cryotherapy or curettage and electrosurgery.

F. If a reconstructed patient is found to have had an untreated positive margin, we recommend reexcision. However, some authors recommend observation because only 30% grossly recur. Each case must be individualized, based on the patient's age, comorbidities, lesion type, grade, depth, and location.

G. Recurrence typically occurs within the first 2 years after the initial resection. If recurrent tumor is present grossly, larger margins are indicated, which may include tissue previously used to reconstruct the defect.

22

Malignant Melanoma

Richard L. Shapiro, M.D., F.A.C.S.
New York University School of Medicine, New York, New York, U.S.A.

The incidence of cutaneous malignant melanoma has been rising steadily over the last century throughout the world. In the year 2000, approximately 1 in 75 Americans was diagnosed with melanoma, in comparison to 1 in 1500 in 1935. Although accounting for only 5% of all skin cancers diagnosed annually, over 75% of all skin cancer deaths are due to melanoma. In 2003, 54,200 new cases were reported in the United States and 7600 patients died of melanoma. Fortunately, due to a heightened awareness of the early cutaneous manifestations of melanoma, the majority (>80%) of patients are diagnosed when the primary tumor is confined to the skin. Early diagnosis correlates significantly with increased survival. Five-year survival rates exceeding 90% are achieved in patients with localized disease in comparison to rates of approximately 60% and 5% in those with regional lymph node and distant metastases, respectively.

I. EPIDEMIOLOGY AND RISK FACTORS

A. Incidence—Equal numbers of men and woman are diagnosed within a broad range of ages, beginning in the third decade of life.

B. Location—Melanoma most commonly arises on the skin for:

- Men—on the back
- Women—on the lower extremities
- Dark-skinned ethnic groups (African American, Asian, and Hispanic)—in the palmar and plantar skin (acral) or in the nailbed (subungual)
- Other locations—while over 95% of melanomas arise in the skin, these tumors also arise in other anatomic locations such as the eye, mucous membranes, and anus.
- Occult primary lesion—approximately 3% of patients who present with metastatic disease have an absence of a clinically demonstrated primary lesion. Patients with metastases from an occult primary melanoma have the same prognosis and management as patients with known primary lesions.

C. The typical patient with melanoma has light-colored eyes, blonde to red hair, and a fair complexion that tans poorly and burns easily during brief periods of intense sun exposure.

D. Risk factors

- A single, blistering sunburn sustained as a child or teenager is a significant risk factor for the development of melanoma and is more deleterious than prolonged exposure to the sun in the later years.
- The development of atypical (dysplastic) nevi is another significant risk factor. While patients with greater than 100 dysplastic nevi (atypical mole syndrome) have a 10–15% incidence of melanoma in their lifetime, the presence of even a single atypical mole also increases the

risk. The prophylactic excision of all dysplastic nevi is *not* justified, however, as melanoma in the majority of patients arises de novo from normal skin as opposed to from a preexisting nevus. However, complete excisional biopsy of any preexisting mole that has changed in appearance, itches, or bleeds is recommended.

- Children with giant (>14–20 cm) congenital nevi are also at increased risk for melanoma, although this occurs uncommonly (<10%) and usually only in patients with truncal lesions within the first decade of life.
- Any patient who has been diagnosed previously with a melanoma has an 8–12% risk of developing a second primary cutaneous melanoma in the course of their lifetime.
- Familial—there is a 10% incidence of melanoma in first-degree family members. This underscores the need for lifelong total cutaneous surveillance of all melanoma patients and their immediate families.

II. DIAGNOSIS AND PROPER BIOPSY TECHNIQUE

A. A thorough physical examination includes an inspection of the *entire* cutaneous surface (including the palmar and plantar sin, web spaces, and mucous membranes) of a completely undressed patient under appropriate lighting conditions.

B. The ABCD rule helps to identify those pigmented lesions most likely to be melanoma. Lesions that are **a**symmetric, with irregular **b**orders, **c**olor variation, and **d**iameters exceeding 6 mm (the size of a pencil eraser) are considered to be suspicious. In addition, any pigmented lesion that becomes darker or lighter in color, increases in size, becomes raised, itches, or bleeds should immediately arouse suspicion.

C. Complete surgical excision is the biopsy method of choice for all cutaneous lesions suspected of being melanoma.

- Punch and shave biopsies are sometimes performed on less suspicious lesions but are suboptimal techniques as tumor thickness may be underestimated. In such situations, complete excisional biopsy should be performed subsequently to more accurately assess tumor thickness.
- Incisional biopsy of larger, more cumbersome lesions is acceptable if tumor thickness is accurately assessed.
- For extremity lesions, surgical biopsy incisions should always be oriented vertically as to not interfere with or complicate subsequent definitive excision and reconstruction.

D. Immunohistochemistry is utilized routinely to complement standard histopathologic techniques in confirming the diagnosis of melanoma.

- The monoclonal antibody HMB-45 and the polyvalent antibody recognizing the S-100 antigen are used most extensively. While a combination of the two may improve the histopathologic characterization of difficult lesions, neither has proved to be completely reliable. For example, the S-100 protein, although expressed in almost all melanomas, is also detected in other tissues of neural crest derivation.
- Although HMB-45 staining may be used to distinguish unusual melanomas from unusual benign nevi, it is often not identified in metastatic lesions or in amelanotic or desmoplastic melanomas.

III. ASSESSMENT OF TUMOR THICKNESS AND STAGING

A. Tumor thickness is a measure of the vertical growth phase of melanoma and is the most powerful prognostic indicator of the potential for local recurrence, metastases, and death. Melanoma thickness is assessed in millimeters by ocular microscopy as described by Breslow or by increasing levels of dermal penetration in the manner described by Clark.

B. Melanoma is staged according to published American Joint Committee on Cancer (AJCC) guidelines utilizing the TNM system (Table 1). This system incorporates Breslow and Clark levels within the T classification. When Breslow and Clark levels are in discordance, the thicker assessment predominates. Patients seeking an opinion after lesion excision at another institution must provide their reports and biopsy slides for in-house review to confirm the diagnosis of melanoma and tumor thickness prior to planning definitive surgery.

Table 1 Melanoma Staging and Prognosis

Stage	Criteria	TNM	5-year survival (%)
IA	Breslow ≤ 0.75 mm or Clark level II	T1 N0 M0	93
IB	Breslow > 0.75–1.5 mm or Clark level III	T2 N0 M0	87
IIA	Breslow > 1.5–4 mm or Clark level IV	T3 N0 M0	66
IIB	Breslow > 4 mm or Clark level V	T4 N0 M0	50
III	Regional lymph node metastasis or in-transit metastasis	Any T, N1 or 2, M0	40
IV	Distant metastasis[a]	Any T, any N, M1	<10

[a] Includes metastasis to skin, subcutaneous tissues, or lymph nodes beyond the regional nodes (M1a) and visceral metastasis (M1b).
Source: American Joint Committee on Cancer. Manual for Staging of Cancer. Beahrs OH, Henson DE, Hutter RVP, et al., eds. 4th ed. Philadelphia: Lippincott, 1992.

IV. PREOPERATIVE METASTATIC WORKUP

A. The degree of suspicion with which ambiguous radiological findings are viewed is dependent on the risk for metastases as assessed by physical examination, melanoma thickness, and disease stage (Table 2). Findings suspicious for metastases on CT scan may be further investigated using more advanced imaging techniques such as MRI or PET scanning.

B. Cytological confirmation of metastatic disease is essential and is almost always possible via fine needle aspiration biopsy performed under radiological (CT or ultrasound) guidance.

V. EXCISION MARGINS

A. The propensity of melanoma to recur locally is well documented and has historically influenced the surgical approach to this tumor. However, the surgical treatment of melanoma in terms of excision margin width (Table 2) has been studied extensively in prospectively randomized trials and has become increasingly more conservative over the past several decades.

Table 2 Surgical Treatment of Primary Cutaneous Malignant Melanoma (Clinically Negative Regional Lymph Nodes[a])

Thickness	Preop workup[b]	Excision margins	Rx—Regional nodes
in situ		5 mm	
<1 mm	CXR; LDH	1 cm	
1–3.9 mm	CXR; LDH CT (chest, abd, pelvis) CT/MRI (brain)	2 cm	Sentinel lymphadenectomy[c]
≥4 mm	CXR; LDH CT (chest, abd, pelvis) CT/MRI (brain)	≥2 cm[d]	Sentinel lymphadenectomy[c]

[a] Patients with biopsy-proven (FNA) regional lymph node metastases (AJCC stage III) undergo formal (complete) lymph node dissection at the time of wide and deep excision of the primary lesion. Patients presenting with biopsy proven distant metastases (AJCC stage IV) undergo wide and deep excision of the primary lesion without sentinel lymphadenectomy. Patients presenting with palpable regional lymph node metastases and distant metastases are candidates for palliative formal lymph node dissection only in the setting of minimal stage IV disease.
[b] CT scans are performed with intravenous contrast in patients with melanoma; MRI scanning is more sensitive in the detection of CNS metastases; MRI and/or PET scanning may be useful in cases in which CT scan findings are indeterminate.
[c] Formal (complete) lymph node dissection is performed immediately if intraoperative microscopic analysis (touch prep, frozen section, rapid immunostain) of the sentinel lymph node(s) reveals evidence of metastatic melanoma. If sentinel node metastases are confirmed later on final pathology, formal (complete) lymphadenectomy is performed as a second procedure.
[d] Minimal excision margins of 2 cm advised for melanomas ≥4 mm in thickness. Wider (3 cm) margins are often performed for these thick lesions, although no prospectively randomized data support this practice.

B. Excision sites are most often closed primarily, although split or full thickness skin grafting and/or flap closure may be required for the reconstruction of larger defects. In patients requiring skin grafting for closure of a wound located on the extremity, skin should never be harvested from that limb to avoid reintroducing melanoma cells into the wound.

C. Similarly, the changing of gloves and surgical instruments should be performed routinely after melanoma excision to avoid wound contamination.

VI. TREATMENT OF THE REGIONAL LYMPH NODES

A. Elective Lymph Node Dissection (ELND)

1. Prospectively randomized studies have consistently failed to demonstrate a significant survival advantage with ELND.
2. Therefore, at the present time, the excision of clinically negative, microscopically positive lymph nodes in patients with melanoma is generally not performed to enhance survival but is primarily performed to identify those patients at high risk for systemic disease.

B. Sentinel Lymphadenectomy

1. As proposed by Morton and associates, sentinel lymphadenectomy provides an alternative to routine ELND in patients who are at risk (>1 mm thick) for subclinical micrometastases but have no clinical evidence of regional nodal disease.
2. Cutaneous lymphoscintigraphy is a method for defining the primary lymphatic drainage of cutaneous melanomas and identifying a lymph node in the regional lymph node basin, termed the sentinel node, most likely to contain micrometastases. Intraoperative lymphatic mapping facilitates the selective identification and excision of the sentinel lymph nodes.
3. Rapid histopathologic staging is performed intraoperatively by microscopic examination of the sentinel node. Immediate therapeutic dissection of the regional nodes is performed if metastases are noted in the sentinel lymph node.
4. A large multi-institutional randomized study (Multicenter Selective Lymphadenectomy Trial, MSLT) has been carefully designed to confirm the accuracy of this technique and the hypothesis that regional lymph node metastases occur rarely in the absence of metastasis to the sentinel node.
5. Sentinel lymphadenectomy is most accurately and easily performed at the time of wide and deep excision of the primary melanoma. Consequently, patients who have already undergone definitive wide and deep excision of the primary lesion are not ideal candidates for sentinel lymphadenectomy as lymphatic flow and drainage patterns may have been altered by that prior surgery.
6. Several hours prior to surgery, the site of the primary lesion is injected with 800 μCI Tc-99M filtered sulfur colloid in four divided doses. After the induction of anesthesia, isosulfan blue dye (2 cc) is injected intradermally at the site of the melanoma to stain the afferent lymphatics and sentinel node blue. The site is massaged manually for 20 minutes prior to incision in the skin overlying the sentinel lymph node as identified preoperatively by lymphoscintigraphy and confirmed intraoperatively with a hand held gamma detector (Neoprobe).
7. Intraoperatively, the sentinel lymph node is identified visually by the appearance of blue stain in the node and/or in the afferent lymphatics and by confirming the gamma signal with the hand-held probe.
8. After the sentinel lymph node has been removed from the field, no evidence of blue dye should be apparent, nor should there be any residual radioactivity (exceeding background) detected with the gamma probe.
9. The sentinel node is taken immediately to surgical pathology for rapid microscopic examination utilizing touch prep, frozen section analysis, and/or rapid immunostains. If no definitive evidence of metastatic melanoma is noted, wide and deep excision is performed and the procedure is terminated. If micrometastases are confirmed in the sentinel lymph node, then formal (therapeutic) lymphadenectomy is performed at that time.
10. Postoperatively, the sentinel lymph node is serially sectioned and meticulously examined utilizing H&E staining and S-100 and HMB-45 immunostaining. Patients with confirmed mi-

crometastases in the sentinel node undergo complete lymph node dissection as a second procedure.

C. Clinically Negative Regional Lymph Nodes

The vast majority of patients with malignant melanoma are diagnosed with no clinical evidence of regional lymph node metastases. The potential for regional lymph node metastases is most accurately assessed by tumor thickness.

1. In situ—by definition, has no real potential for lymph node metastases. Nodal treatment is not indicated.
2. Thin melanomas (<1 mm)—the risk of regional lymph node metastases is minimal (<5%), therefore treatment of the regional lymph nodes is not indicated.
3. Intermediate thickness lesions (1–4 mm)—have a 20–25% incidence of microscopic regional disease and a 3–5% risk of distant metastases. These patients should theoretically derive the greatest therapeutic benefit from elective lymph node dissection (ELND).
4. Thick primary melanomas (>4 mm)—with no clinical evidence of regional lymph node metastases or radiological evidence of distant disease, these patients are still at high (50–75%) risk to have microscopic nodal metastases and are therefore also appropriate candidates for intraoperative lymphatic mapping and sentinel lymphadenectomy.

D. Clinically Positive Lymph Node Metastases

Any palpable lymph node in a patient with melanoma should be considered metastatic until proven otherwise. Fine needle aspiration biopsy (FNA) is an accurate, reliable method of confirming metastatic melanoma. If FNA is not available or results are indeterminate, excisional biopsy of the lymph node is performed. Patients presenting with or subsequently developing regional lymph node metastases are at high risk for distant metastases and should therefore undergo CT scanning of the chest, abdomen, and pelvis with intravenous contrast and CT or MRI scanning of the brain.

1. No distant metastasis—in patients with cytologically or histologically proven regional nodal metastases, formal (complete) lymph node dissection is performed. The development of palpable lymph node metastases is correlated significantly with substantially diminished survival (10–50%) and is influenced strongly by the number of and the extent to which the lymph nodes are involved. Adjuvant radiation therapy may play a role in reducing the likelihood of regional recurrence rates in patients after resection of extensive lymph node metastases or in controlling bleeding from bulky inoperable metastases.
2. Distant metastasis or lymph node metastases fixed to adjacent structures—regional lymph node dissection should *not* be performed routinely in these cases. Radiation therapy provides palliation. Prognosis is poor.

VII. ADJUVANT IMMUNOTHERAPY

A. The rationale for using immunotherapy to treat patients with melanoma is based in part on the observation that evidence of partial regression is seen histologically in up to 20% of primary melanomas.

B. Patients at high risk for distant metastasis such as those with thick primary melanomas greater than 4 mm (Stage IIB) or regional lymph node metastases (Stage III) are appropriately offered interferon 2-alpha immunotherapy. However, despite a modest survival benefit, treatment-limiting side effects (severe flu-like syndrome) occur commonly in the majority of patients and can be life-threatening (cardiovascular and hepatic toxicity).

C. Melanoma antigen vaccines may alternatively be offered to this cohort of patients with a relative absence of side effects. Although as yet unproved, clinical results are encouraging.

VIII. POSTOPERATIVE FOLLOW-UP

The risk of developing a second primary melanoma necessitates that all patients, irrespective of lesion thickness, continue life-long follow up with their dermatologist for total cutaneous examination, as should all of their first-degree relatives.

A. In situ—routine dermatological surveillance is sufficient.

B. Thin melanomas (<1 mm)—follow-up at 3- to 6-month intervals for 2 years and at 6- to 12-month intervals thereafter. A CXR and routine blood chemistries are obtained on a yearly basis.

C. Intermediate thickness—return at 3-month intervals for 2 years and at 6-month intervals thereafter. Chest x-ray and LDH levels are performed each year as are CT scans for 2–5 years after surgery.

D. Thick primary lesions (>4 mm)/lymph node metastases—will ultimately develop systemic disease. Follow-up physical examination occurs at 3- to 6-month intervals for life with CT scanning performed on at least a yearly basis.

IX. TREATMENT OF LOCAL RECURRENCE

A. Local recurrence in a patient with malignant melanoma is an ominous clinical event and is almost always associated with the development of systemic metastases. The survival of these patients is extremely poor, averaging less than 5% at 10 years.

B. Local recurrence most often appears clinically as a blue-tinged subcutaneous nodule arising in close proximity (within 2–5 cm) to an excision site of a primary melanoma (satellite metastasis) or en route to the regional lymph node basin (in-transit metastasis). Any subcutaneous nodule arising in the vicinity of a melanoma excision site should be considered to be disease recurrence or progression until proven otherwise.

C. Diagnosis is rapidly and accurately accomplished by FNA. Excisional biopsy may sometimes be required for confirmation. A complete metastatic survey should then be performed.

D. For single lesions, wide local excision with a generous rim of normal tissue is essily performed. Patients with multiple satellite and/or extensive in-transit metastases of the extremity are candidates for isolated limb perfusion with melphalan-containing chemotherapeutic regimens. This procedure is technically difficult and should therefore only be performed in dedicated centers. Despite the considerable technical difficulties and potential for local morbidity, isolated limb perfusion is the treatment of choice for patients with extensive local recurrence confined to a single extremity. Although no significant benefit in survival has been demonstrated, satisfactory palliation can often be achieved.

E. In patients for whom isolated limb profusion is not appropriate, significant palliation may be obtained through the direct injection of metastatic nodules with cytokine immunomodulators such as BCG or interleukin-2, or investigational chemotherapeutic agents such as cisplatin-containing gel.

23

Mohs Micrographic Surgery

Kathleen Behr, M.D.
David Geffen School of Medicine at UCLA, Los Angeles, California, U.S.A.

I. INTRODUCTION

Mohs micrographic surgery is a meticulous tissue-sparing technique that results in a high cure rate for removal of cancerous tissue.

II. HISTORY

A. Dr. Frederic Mohs developed the concept of micrographic surgery and first used the technique for cancer removal in 1936.

B. He originally used a fixed technique applying zinc chloride fixative prior to surgical excision. In 1953 he first used the fresh technique on an eyelid tumor because he was being filmed and had a time constraint. It worked so well that he continued to use the fresh technique on all eyelid tumors. In 1969 he presented a series of 60 cases with a 5-year cure rate of 100%.

C. The technique was then rapidly expanded. Clinical series with high cure rates for tumors in many different locations were published by Tromovitch and Stegman in 1974 and Mohs in 1976.

D. In 1986 the technique was renamed Mohs micrographic surgery.

III. PROCEDURE

A. Excision of Tissue

1. After proper explanation of the procedure to the patient, including risks and treatment options, the Mohs procedure is begun on the biopsy-proven tumor.
2. The clinically involved area is marked out and cleansed with alcohol or betadine. Anesthesia is given with 1% lidocaine and epinephrine (except digits, where epinephrine is excluded).
3. The tumor is debulked with a curette or scalpel. The tumor is then removed with a 1–3 mm margin. The blade is angled to cause a 45 degree beveled cut at all skin edges, and a smooth level cut is made under the tumor. Nicks are often made in the skin edge at three points such as 9, 12, and 3 o'clock for orientation. The saucerized specimen should be continuous, smooth, and thin with appropriate orientation.
4. The wound is then cauterized for hemostasis. A pressure bandage is placed, and patients are placed in a waiting room.

B. Lab Processing

1. Proper processing is critical and is done within the Mohs unit.
2. The technician takes the specimen and draws a surgical map of the tissue on a card showing orientation of anatomic features and nicks.
3. Specimens are processed whole or divided into sections.
4. The edges are marked with dye for color coding on the tissue and also on the map. The tissue specimen is then mounted deep side up on the

cryostat. The outermost deep side is flattened with a slide.

5. The tissue block is frozen and then a microtome shaves a horizontal section that includes the entire base of the specimen as well as a continuous epidermal margin.
6. This thin ribbon section is mounted on a slide and stained, usually with hematoxylin and eosin stain or with toluidine blue.

C. Microscopic Examination

1. Interpretation of the slides is performed by the Mohs surgeon. The Mohs surgeon checks to make sure all the skin edge and the entire base in present on pathology. If not, more tissue is cut from the block or excised from the patient until this is achieved.
2. If tumor is present, the location is marked in red ink on the map. Any positive areas are excised from the patient, and the Mohs process is repeated until the patient is free of tumor.

D. Repair

1. Repair depends on many factors such as location, defect size, and patient health.
2. Often, a multidisciplinary approach is taken with involvement of plastic or oculoplastic surgeons.

IV. INDICATIONS

A. Primary indications include:

- Recurrent or persistent tumor.
- Aggressive growth patterns (i.e., morpheaform pattern, basosquamous cell carcinoma, and perineural involvement).
- Tumors located in embryonic fusion planes of the face.
- Areas that desire maximum preservation of tissue (eyelids, nose, ear, digits, and lips).
- Large or deeply penetrating tumors (>1 cm nose, >2 cm elsewhere).
- Other tumors successfully treated by Mohs include Bowen's disease, verrucous carcinoma, atypical fibroxanthoma, malignant fibrous histiocytoma, extramammary Paget's disease, lentigo maligna, Merkel cell carcinoma, sebaceous carcinoma, leiomyosarcoma, sweat gland tumor, keratoacanthoma and dermatofibroma sarcoma protuberans (DFSP).

V. ADVANTAGES

A. High cure rate with maximal tissue preservation

B. Outpatient procedure performed under local anesthesia has rapid specimen processing

C. Cost effective when compared to inpatient surgery

VI. RESULTS

The results are excellent, which is to be expected from a procedure in which 100% of the margin is examined, especially in contiguously spread tumors.

A. Basal cell carcinoma—Cure rates of 99% in all primary basal cell carcinomas and 94.4% for recurrent basal cell carcinomas.

B. Squamous cell carcinoma—The 5-year cure rate is 97.5% for primary tumors and 81.9% for recurrent tumors.

C. Melanoma—The 5-year cure rate Mohs reported from 200 patients was 65.2%. This included thick and thin lesions. Reports of 5-year survivals as high as 96% for thin lesions exist. Many surgeons use Mohs for lentigo maligna and lentigo maligna melanoma but use standard excisions for other types.

VII. TRAINING

Mohs training often involves a 1- or 2-year fellowship after completion of residency.

24

Soft Tissue Sarcomas

Steven R. Beanes, M.D., and Frederick R. Eilber, M.D.
David Geffen School of Medicine at UCLA, Los Angeles, California, U.S.A.

I. BACKGROUND

A. Sarcomas are a heterogeneous group of malignant neoplasms that arise from the mesoderm.

B. Sarcomas are rare and unusual neoplasms, despite being derived from tissue that comprises two-thirds of the mass of the human body.

C. They typically behave in a similar fashion wherever they arise: local mass at the primary tumor site and hematogenous metastasis.

D. The site of origin of a sarcoma affects the biologic characteristic of the tumor.

II. EPIDEMIOLOGY

A. Occur in all age groups

B. Comprise 1% of adult malignancies: 5000–6000 new cases in the United States per year

C. Comprise 15% of pediatric malignancies

D. Fifty percent of all sarcomas develop in the extremities

III. PREDISPOSING FACTORS

A. Most sarcomas occur in patients without an identifiable predisposing factor.

B. Multiple risk factors have been associated with development of sarcomas, including both genetic factors:

- Neurofibromatosis
- Retinoblastoma
- Li-Fraumeni syndrome
- Gardner's syndrome and environmental factors:
  - Radiation exposure
  - Lymphedema

IV. PATHOLOGY

A. Sarcomas are classified by the histologic type of tissue formed by the tumor.

B. Specific chromosomal translocations are associated with soft tissue sarcomas:

- Synovial sarcoma: associated with t(X;18)
- Myxoid liposarcoma: associated with t(12;16)
- Rhabdomyosarcoma: associated with t(2;13)

C. Most common histologic types are:

- Liposarcoma (22%)
- Leiomyosarcoma (19%)
- Malignant fibrous histiocytoma (MFH) (17%)
- Synovial sarcoma (12%)

D. Although the exact histologic type is an important piece of data in the evaluation of the sarcoma patient, it is not as influential in terms of prognosis and therapy as histologic grade.

Biologic behavior is currently best predicted based on histologic grade (I, II, III), as determined by:

- Mitotic index
- Cellularity
- Necrosis
- Degree of nuclear anaplasia

E. Increasing use of molecular and tissue-specific immunohistochemistry may better define the histologic subtypes of soft tissue sarcomas (S-100, cytokeratins, CA-115, actin, myosin).

F. Low-grade lesions have a low risk of metastasis (<5%)

G. Intermediate-grade lesions have an intermediate risk of metastasis (20–30%)

H. High-grade lesions have a high risk of metastasis (>50%)

I. For lesions in which disparate regions of histologic grades exist, the highest grade encountered is used to categorize the tumor. This pattern of mixed histologic grades is most often encountered in liposarcoma

J. Prognostic factors:

- Favorable factors: size < 5 cm, superficial lesions, low grade
- Unfavorable factors: size > 5 cm, deep lesion, high grade

K. Staging

- The American Joint Committee on Cancer Staging System uses the TNM classification method, with the addition of G for the histologic grade.
- The Memorial Sloan-Kettering Cancer Center Staging System:

Stage	Number of unfavorable factors
0	0
I	1
II	2
III	3
IV	Metastasis

L. Chemotherapy-responsive sarcomas

- Liposarcoma
- Malignant fibrous histiocytoma
- Synovial sarcoma
- Malignant peripheral nerve sheath tumor (MPNST)

M. Chemotherapy-resistant sarcomas

- Alveolar sarcoma
- Epithelioid sarcomas
- Leiomyosarcoma
- Hemangiopericytoma

V. DIAGNOSIS

Soft tissue sarcomas frequently present as painless solid masses. Thorough history and physical examination can facilitate the diagnosis.

A. Biopsy

1. Biopsy should be performed in:
   - All adults with any soft tissue masses that are symptomatic or enlarging
   - Any new mass that persists beyond 4 weeks or a mass that results after local trauma that persists for 6 weeks
   - Any mass that is larger than 5 cm
2. Masses larger than 5 cm should have a CT-guided core biopsy performed.
   - If CT-guided biopsy is not adequate for histology/grade, then open biopsy should be performed.
   - Open biopsy should be conducted with a longitudinal incision centered over the mass in its most superficial location.
3. Fine-needle aspiration is:
   - Not an appropriate diagnostic modality in extremity soft tissue sarcoma evaluation, since the tissue histology is disrupted, not allowing for grading of the tumor.
   - Possibly helpful in diagnosing intraabdominal and retroperitoneal tumors.

B. Evaluation of Local and Distant Disease

1. CT Scan vs. MRI

A. Both studies are sufficient in defining the tumor's relation to surrounding bone, muscle, neurovascular structures, and adjacent organs.

B. Final choice depends upon availability, cost, and experience.

2. Evaluation of Metastasis

1. Lung is the principal site of distant metastasis in extremity soft tissue tumors.
2. Liver is the principal site of distant metastasis in visceral soft tissue tumors.
3. Subsequently, extremity lesions require chest imaging (chest x-ray for low-grade lesions or chest CT scan for high-grade lesions), while visceral lesions require abdominal CT scan or MRI (which can be performed during initial imaging of the primary tumor).

VI. MANAGEMENT OF EXTREMITY SOFT TISSUE SARCOMAS

A. Surgical Excision

Surgical excision remains the primary modality of curative therapy for all soft tissue sarcomas.

1. Surgical aim is complete removal of the tumor with maximal preservation of limb function. Sacrifice of major neurovascular structures can be avoided with careful dissection through normal tissue planes.
2. Tumors should be resected with a rim of normal tissue (minimum 0.5 cm).
3. Pathologic confirmation of tumor-free margins is imperative.

B. Lesions < 5 cm

1. Complete excision of the primary tumor with negative margins
2. Postoperative external beam radiation therapy:
   - Recommended for high-grade tumors
   - Optional for low grade tumors

C. Low-Grade Lesions > 5 cm

1. Complete excision of the primary tumor
2. Postoperative external beam radiation therapy

D. High-Grade Lesion > 5 cm

1. +/− preoperative chemotherapy
2. Complete excision of the primary tumor
3. Perioperative brachytherapy or postoperative external beam radiation therapy. Brachytherapy is the technique of radiation delivered to the tumor bed by means of an implantable radioactive source.
4. Postoperative chemotherapy considered for chemo-responsive tumors (MFH, liposarcoma, synovial, and MPNST).

VII. MANAGEMENT OF RETROPERITONEAL OR VISCERAL SOFT TISSUE SARCOMAS

A. Surgery is the main form of therapy:

- Chemotherapy has not been shown to be efficacious.
- It is not possible to deliver adequate levels of external beam radiation without damaging normal tissue.

B. It is necessary to distinguish sarcoma from lymphoma. CT-guided core needle biopsy is used in cases of:

- Sarcoma: surgical resection with postoperative external beam radiation therapy
- Lymphoma: chemotherapy

VIII. RECURRENT DISEASE

A. Approximately 33% of patients develop local recurrence, with a median disease-free interval of 18 months. Recurrence varies with anatomic site and surgical margins:

- Extremity = 20%
- Head and neck = 50%
- Retroperitoneal ≥ 80%

B. A sarcoma recurrence usually presents as a nodular mass or a series of nodules arising in the surgical scar.

C. Patients with isolated local recurrence should undergo re-resection with postoperative adjuvant therapy

D. Distant metastasis:

- Extremity lesions most commonly metastasize to the lung.
- If the primary tumor is controlled, thoracotomy with the purpose of total resection of all

metastatic disease should be performed in all patients who could tolerate the thoracotomy.

IX. RESULTS

A. Survival is significantly dependent upon the grade of the tumor:

- Ten-year survival for low-grade extremity soft tissue sarcomas is approximately 90%, while 10-year survival for high-grade extremity soft tissue sarcomas is 50–60%.
- Ten-year survival for low-grade retroperitoneal sarcomas is 50–60%, while the 10-year survival for high-grade retroperitoneal sarcomas is 20–30%.

B. The main prognostic factors that determine the outcomes of distant metastasis and disease-specific mortality include:

- High histologic grade
- Deep location
- Size > 5 cm

25

Burns

Arvind N. Padubidri, M.D., F.R.C.S., and Maria Siemionow, M.D., Ph.D.
The Cleveland Clinic, Cleveland, Ohio, U.S.A.

I. EPIDEMIOLOGY OF BURNS

A. Between 2 and 2.5 million persons each year sustain burns in the United States.

B. Of these patients, 100,000 receive hospital treatment.

C. Burns at the extremes of age carry a greater morbidity and mortality.

D. Scalds are the most frequent form of burn injury.

II. PATHOPHYSIOLOGIC CHANGES IN BURN PATIENTS

A. Thermal injury causes coagulation necrosis of the skin and underlying tissues to a variable depth. Burn injury also exerts deleterious effects on all other organ systems.

B. Hemodynamic—The first 24-h postburn are characterized by decreased blood volume, increased blood viscosity, and depressed cardiac output. Microvascular permeability is increased directly by heat and indirectly by endogenous mediators. The diminished blood volume and cardiac output cause oliguria, which may progress to acute renal failure. Numerous factors have been reported to increase vascular permeability and leukocyte infiltration:

- Histamine
- Arachidonic acid metabolites (principally thromboxane A_2 and the leukotrienes)
- Substance P
- Fibrin degradation product D
- Activated proteases
- Platelet-activating factor (PAF)
- Cytokines such as interleukin-1 (IL-1) and tumor necrosis factor (TNF)

C. Immune system—Humoral and cell-mediated immunity are both impaired and are manifested as depressed levels of immunoglobulin, reduced activation of complement, and diminished stimulation of lymphocyte proliferation and response.

D. Hematologic—There is immediate red blood cell destruction in direct proportion to the extent of the burn, particularly third-degree burns. Endothelial injury may lead to release of thromboplastins and to collagen exposure; the latter then initiates platelet adhesion, aggregation, and contact activation of factor XII. Severe full-thickness burns induce consumption of coagulation factors at the burn site, which contributes to the development of disseminated intravascular coagulation (DIC).

E. Gastrointestinal—Ileus is universal in patients with burns of more than 25% total body surface area (TBSA). Gastric and duodenal mucosal damage, secondary to focal ischemia, can be observed as early as 3–5 h postburn. If the mucosa is unprotected, the early erosions may progress to frank ulceration.

F. Endocrine—In the early postburn period, a *catabolic endocrine* pattern develops that is characterized by elevated glucagon, cortisol, and catecholamine levels with depressed insulin and triiodothyronine levels. These effect an increase in metabolic rate, glucose flow, and a negative nitrogen balance. Their magnitude correlates with the size of the burn area.

III. INITIAL MANAGEMENT

A. Indications for hospital admission: The following are the admission criteria for all patients with burn injuries according to the American Burn Association.

- Second- and third-degree burns greater than 10% of TBSA in patients under 10 or over 50 years of age
- Second-degree burns greater than 20% TBSA in other ages
- Third-degree burns greater than 5% TBSA in any age
- Significant burns of the face, hands, feet, genitalia, or perineum
- Significant electrical/lightning injuries
- Significant chemical burns
- Associated inhalation injury, concomitant mechanical trauma, or significant preexisting medical illnesses
- Burns requiring special social, emotional, or long-term rehabilitative support, including cases of suspected or actual child abuse

B. Initial care: ABCDEF (A = airway, B = breathing, C = circulation, D = disability, E = expose, F = fluids). As with all trauma patients, the first priority is maintenance of airway. Associated injuries and comorbid conditions are noted.

C. Evaluation of burn involves:

- Extent of burns: Although the classic "Rule of 9" is still followed in many centers, it is not accurate. The Lund and Browder chart is easier to use and is corrected for age (Fig. 1).
- Depth of burn injury is generally difficult to assess initially. It is sufficient to distinguish between erythema and actual skin damage at the initial examination.
- First-degree burn—superficial burn that involves only the epidermis. The area is erythematous, tender, and usually heals in less than 7 days.
- Second-degree burn—destruction of the epidermis and upper dermal layer. The skin is red, blistered, and sensory nerve damage causes extreme pain.
- Third-degree burn—destruction of the epidermis and dermis. The area is white, leathery, charred, and pain is absent due to destruction of sensory nerves
- Fourth-degree burn—destruction of skin, muscle, and bone.

D. Fluid resuscitation:

- Fluid resuscitation should be started in all patients with burns with TBSA >15%. The goal is to restore and maintain adequate tissue perfusion and prevent organ ischemia. The resuscitation formulas are to be used as guidelines only. In the United States, the Baxter or Parkland formula (4 mL of Ringer's lactate/kg/% TBSA over the first 24 h) is widely used. Half this volume is infused in the first 8 h post-burn, and the remaining half over the next 16 h. Colloids are usually given in the second 24 h, after the massive fluid shifts occur.
- Blood—for full thickness burns of more than 10% TBSA, the whole blood requirement is estimated at 1% of the patient's normal blood volume for each 1% deep burn.
- Monitoring of fluid resuscitation—urine output 0.5–1 cc/kg/h is the most accurate parameter for resuscitation. Invasive measurement techniques (central venous pressure/pulmonary capillary wedge pressure) should be avoided whenever possible.

E. Medications: Narcotic pain medication is administered intravenously for major burns. Patient-controlled analgesia (PCA) may be advised if the patient is conscious and oriented.

F. Routine tetanus prophylaxis is employed. There is no role for prophylactic antibiotic therapy.

G. Escharotomy and fasciotomy may be needed for circumferential constricting burns. Both are useful to treat distal ischemia in the extremities. Escharotomy is used in the chest to prevent

CHART FOR ESTIMATING SEVERITY OF BURN WOUND

Name ____________ Ward __________ Number _______ Date ____
Age _____ Admission weight ___________

Lund and Browder charts

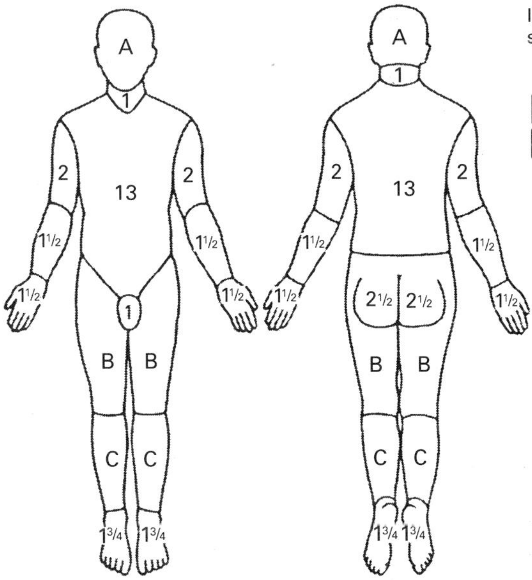

Ignore simple erythema

Partial thickness loss (PTL)

Full thickness loss (FTL)

Region	% PTL	% FTL
Head		
Neck		
Ant. trunk		
Post. trunk		
Right arm		
Left arm		
Buttocks		
Genitalia		
Right leg		
Left leg		
Total burn		

Relative percentage of body surface area affected by growth

Area	Age 0	1	5	10	15	Adult
A = ½ of head	9½	8½	6½	5½	4½	3½
B = ½ of one thigh	2¾	3¼	4	4½	4½	4¾
C = ½ of one leg	2½	2½	2¾	3	3¼	3½

Figure 1 The Lund and Browder chart used to assess total body surface area of burns. Pediatric patients require a special chart (not shown).

respiratory embarrassment. Prompt recognition and release of the eschars should be performed.

H. Early burn eschar excision and skin grafting.

IV. INHALATION INJURY

Inhalation injury—a chemical tracheobronchitis and acute pneumonitis—is caused by the inhalation of smoke and other irritative products. In severe cases, it progresses to development of adult respiratory distress syndrome (ARDS).

A. Typical Signs of Significant Injury

1. Singeing of nasal hair
2. Significant facial burns
3. Carbonaceous sputum
4. Hoarseness
5. Stridor
6. Carboxyhemoglobin level of more than 15% at 3 h postexposure is strong evidence of smoke inhalation

B. Evaluation

1. Chest x-ray and arterial blood gases are routinely obtained.
2. Fiberoptic bronchoscopy may be performed at bedside.
3. Xenon ventilation/perfusion scanning has been reasonably accurate in diagnosing inhalation injury.

C. Treatment

Immediate treatment involves administering 100% oxygen. Endotracheal intubation is necessary in some cases. Hyperbaric oxygen has been used in some units.

V. ELECTRICAL INJURY

A. Electricity exerts its tissue-damaging effects by conversion to thermal energy.

B. Electric flash burns usually result in superficial burns. Hot element burns are pure heat burns and are usually full thickness. Arcing injuries are rare and may cause localized deep burns.

C. True electric burns are secondary to contact. The resultant damage is due to passage of electricity through the tissues. Tissue resistance to electrical current increases from nerve (least resistant) to vessel to muscle to skin to tendon to fat to bone (most resistant). Tissue damage occurs in tissues with the least resistance to electrical current, although the high heat generated by the high resistance in bone will cause secondary thermal damage to the adjacent musculature. Muscles that are closest to bone sustain a higher degree of secondary thermal damage than more superficial muscles. As a result, the full extent of the underlying tissue damage is not always evident by inspection.

D. Prompt fluid resuscitation is the keystone to prevent acute renal failure. Mannitol 25 g IV is given to increase renal perfusion.

E. Sodium bicarbonate is administered to alkalinize the urine to keep hemoglobin and myoglobin in a more soluble state.

F. Sulfamylon (with high eschar penetrability) is used for local burn care.

G. Technetium 99m muscle scans may be useful to evaluate muscle damage.

H. Electrical burns involving the extremities are observed closely for compartment syndrome.

I. Early excision and skin grafting are advocated.

J. Oral commissure burns are managed conservatively and monitored for bleeding from the labial artery, which is seen in about 10% of cases.

VI. BURN WOUND CARE

Ideally, a burn dressing should be absorbent, nonadherent, and should act as a barrier to prevent colonization of the wound by pathogenic bacteria.

A. Local Management

1. Initial care involves debridement of necrotic tissue and open blisters, protection from the environment, and edema reduction.
2. Enzymatic debridement is practiced in some centers.
3. Early tangential excision of burn tissue provides better functional and aesthetic results. The postexcision wound is ideally covered with meshed split thickness autografts.

B. Topical Agents

- Silver sulfadiazine (1% Silvadene)—most commonly used agent. Active against most Gram-positive and Gram-negative organisms. The "pseudoeschar" that forms over the burn can confuse the inexperienced observer. Leukopenia can occur.
- Sulfamylon (Mafenide acetate)—has superior eschar penetration. Excellent choice for ears, noses, and some electrical burns. It has the disadvantage of causing intense pain on application and is associated with metabolic acidosis.
- Silver nitrate (0.5%)—effective as a prophylactic against *Pseudomonas* colonization. Disadvantages include production of black stains, hyponatremia, and methemoglobinemia.
- Povidone iodine—not effective, inactivated by wound exudate

C. Skin Substitutes/Artificial Skin (See Chapter 17)

1. Integra® bovine collagen and chondroitin-6-sulfate dermal matrix with a silicone rubber "epidermal" layer.
2. AlloDerm®—an acellular, immunologically inert dermal transplant. Allows the successful use of ultrathin autografts while maximizing the amount of dermis delivered to the wound site. These autografts leave thin donor sites that heal faster and with fewer complications.

3. Apligraf®—a novel bi-layered living skin equivalent; derived from neonatal foreskin; has been used in acute wounds and partial thickness donor sites. Apligraf behaves similar to a partial thickness autograft, and is safe and effective (see Chapter 7).
4. Cultured epidermal autografts (CEA) are used in extensive burns wherein there is a shortage of donor sites. Cultured CEA lack durability and barrier function.
5. Other biologic dressings include homografts (cadaver skin), xenografts (pig skin), or amnion. These are used in some centers.
6. Biobrane is a custom-knit nylon fabric bonded to an ultrathin silicone rubber membrane that is covalently bonded to collagenous peptides from porcine skin. It is transparent, flexible, stretchable, conforms to the wound, and is simple to store. It can be used effectively on partial thickness burns, especially in outpatient management.

VII. SUPPORTIVE CARE

A. The metabolic response following burn injury increases in magnitude as the extent of burn increases. Postburn hypermetabolism is manifested by increased oxygen consumption, elevated cardiac output and minute ventilation, increased core temperature, wasting of lean body mass, and increased urinary nitrogen excretion. The daily caloric requirement is estimated by the Curreri formula:
   - Adults: (25 kcal/kg) + (40 kcal/% TBSA)
   - Children: (60 kcal/kg) + (35 kcal/% TBSA)

B. Burn management includes several other disciplines, such as physical and occupational therapy, social services, and psychology.

VIII. COMPLICATIONS

The most common cause of death is bronchopneumonia (2%). Sepsis is responsible for 0.7%; inadequate fluid resuscitation, 1%; inhalation injury, 1%; and GI hem orrhage, 0.1%.

A. Burn Infections

1. Burn wound infections can be classified on the basis of the causative organism, the depth of invasion, and the tissue response. Burn wound sepsis is defined as $> 10^5$ organisms per gram of tissue. Biopsies for quantitative and qualitative bacteriology are routinely obtained. Histologic examination of the biopsy specimen, which permits staging of the invasive process, is the only reliable means of differentiating wound colonization from invasive infection. Appropriate broad-spectrum antibiotics are administered to treat the infection. The clinical signs of burn wound sepsis are:
   - Conversion of second-degree burn to full-thickness necrosis
   - Focal black or dark brown discoloration of wound
   - Degeneration of wound with formation of new eschar
   - Hemorrhagic discoloration of subeschar fat
   - Erythematous and edematous wound margin
2. Candidal (yeast) and noncandidal (filamentous) fungal wound infections have become an increasingly important cause of burn-associated morbidity and mortality.
3. Pneumonia—The most common site of infection in the burn patient is the lungs. Pneumonia is considered to be the primary cause of death in over half of fatal burns. Bronchopneumonia is commonly caused by *Staphylococcus aureus* and Gram-negative opportunistic bacteria. Hematogenous pneumonia commonly begins relatively late in the postburn course. An infected wound or a vein harboring a focus of intraluminal suppuration is the source of infection in the vast majority of cases.
4. Suppurative thrombophlebitis can occur in any previously cannulated peripheral or even central vein. Strict limitation of cannula residence to 3 days or less in burn patients has been associated with a reduction in the incidence of this complication from 4.3% to 2.5%. Treatment involves surgical excision of the entire length of vein involved in the suppurative process and the systemic administration of antibiotics.
5. Acute endocarditis—Identification of characteristic murmurs is difficult in burn patients because of their hyperdynamic circulation. Two-dimensional echocardiographic examination may detect valvular lesions, but small vegetations may remain undetected. *Staphylococcus aureus* is the

most common causative agent. Systemic maximum-dose antibiotic therapy is prescribed for at least 3 weeks.

6. Suppurative sinusitis is most likely to occur in patients who require long-term transnasal intubation, particularly those with tubes in both the airway and the gastrointestinal tract. CT scan is useful as a diagnostic test. Therapy is initiated with broad-spectrum antibiotics, but surgical drainage of the involved sinuses may be necessary.
7. Bacteremia and septicemia—To minimize the development of antibiotic-resistant bacteria, systemic antibiotics should not be given prophylactically. They are administered only on the basis of a secure clinical or laboratory diagnosis of infection. Antibiotics are generally given perioperatively to patients undergoing debridement of burn wounds.
8. In burn patients with septicemia, initial antibiotic therapy should be based on the results of the institution's microbial surveillance program and on the histologic findings of burn wound biopsy specimens or Gram-stained preparations of secretions and other infected material.

B. Gastrointestinal

1. Ulcerations of the gastrointestinal tract— Acute ulceration of the stomach and duodenum (Curling's ulcer) is now effectively controlled by prophylactic antacid or H2-receptor antagonist therapy.
2. Acalculous cholecystitis
3. Pancreatitis
4. Acute dilatation of the colon (Ogilvie's syndrome) may occur in burn patients who develop sepsis.
5. The use of early enteral feeding improves mucosal blood flow, and reduces mucosal atrophy and subsequent bacterial translocation.

C. Hypertrophic Scars/Keloids

1. These scars are red, thick, hard, pruritic, and dry.
2. Treatment begins conservatively with massage, moisturizers, antihistamines, pressure garments, and silicone sheet therapy.
3. Intralesional injections of triamcinolone are also used.
4. Scar revision with Z-plasty, V-Y plasty, or W-plasty may be required.

D. Contractures

1. Every effort is made in the initial care of a burn patient to prevent contractures. When contractures develop, they are released and reconstructed with skin grafts or flaps depending on the aesthetic and functional needs of the area.
2. Tissue expanders may be used to provide tissue with the closest match.
3. Occasionally, free tissue transfers have been used to resurface large defects.

E. Heterotopic Bone Formation

1. This can occur around joints and in soft tissues, usually in areas of burn.
2. This appears to be secondary to the immobilization that occurs, whether secondary to pain, splinting, or contracture.

F. Marjolin's Ulcer

1. Squamous cell carcinoma arises in the chronic burn scar after a latency period of approximately 35 years.
2. These tumors are highly invasive, and regional node metastases are present in 35% of cases.

IX. BURNS OF SPECIAL AREAS

A. Eyelids

1. Eyelids are treated by early excision and skin grafting to prevent corneal exposure and ulceration.
2. There is no role for tarsorrhaphy.

B. Ears

1. Topical mafenide acetate (Sulfamylon) is used for better eschar penetration.
2. Bulky dressings are provided and patients are told to avoid pillows.
3. Suppurative chondritis is treated by prompt debridement of necrotic cartilage.

C. Face

1. Most surgeons wait 10–21 days before excising and grafting facial burns. Forehead and neck

tissue provides the best color match for facial burns.

2. Grafts are applied to conform to the aesthetic units of the face.
3. Facemasks are worn for several months for pressure to reduce hypertrophic scar formation.

D. Breasts

1. Scarring of the chest wall following a burn during childhood inhibits normal breast development.
2. If the nipple-areola complex is intact, constricted breast tissue is likely present underneath and can be released and grafted prior to the placement of a tissue expander.

E. Hands

1. Sheet grafts are preferred over meshed grafts on the hand to minimize graft contracture.
2. The hand is immobilized with wrist in 15–20° extension, metacarpal-phalangeal joints in 75–80° flexion, and the interphalangeal joints in full extension.

F. Axillary Contractures

1. Solitary anterior or posterior webs may be released by employing Z-plasties, multiple V-Y plasties, or local flaps.
2. Parascapular fasciocutaneous flaps are useful for reconstruction of axillary defects.

G. Perineum

1. Burn scar contracture is frequent.
2. Multiple V-Y plasties and local flaps can release these contractures.

X. OUTPATIENT CARE

A. Prompt initial attention is given to all minor burns.

B. Burned areas are thoroughly washed, blisters debrided, and dressings applied. Patients are regularly seen in the burn clinic to monitor the progress of healing.

C. Any full-thickness burn area greater than a square inch should be grafted.

D. Application of Unna boot compression dressings to lower extremity skin grafts provides excellent protection of both meshed and non-meshed grafts and allows immediate ambulation and range of motion.

XI. FROSTBITE

With frostbite, the skin and subcutaneous tissue of exposed body parts, especially the hands, feet, nose, and ears, are most often affected. Intracellular ice crystallization and microvascular occlusion have been implicated as the basic pathophysiologic consequence of frostbite injury.

A. Degrees of Frostbite

1. 1st degree—White hard plaque
2. 2nd degree—Clear fluid, superficial blisters
3. 3rd degree—Purple fluid, deep blisters, discolored skin

B. Treatment

Rapid warming of the affected part in a water bath (40–44°C) for those presenting within 24 h is recommended. Dermal microcirculation is improved with aspirin (prostaglandin synthesis inhibitor).

XII. CHEMICAL BURNS

The severity of tissue damage from acids, alkali, and other chemicals is related to the concentration of the agent, the amount of agent in contact with tissue, and the duration of contact. They are usually deeper than they initially appear and may progress with time. The initial treatment is lavage with copious amounts of water or saline.

A. Hydrofluoric acid burns are treated with the application of 10% calcium gluconate paste over the affected area. Subcutaneous injections may be required for more extensive burns.

B. Phenol burns are treated with topical application of propylethylene glycol (PEG).

C. Phosphorus burns require continuous application of saline dressings because residual phosphorus will ignite when dry. Topical copper sulfate (1%) stains the phosphorus particles dark, which facilitates debridement.

D. Tar burns respond well to application of bacitracin or neomycin ointment for 12 h, at which time the ointment is washed off and silver sulfadiazine is applied.

26

Radiation and Plastic Surgery

Maria Siemionow, M.D., Ph.D., and Arvind N. Padubidri, M.D., F.R.C.S.
The Cleveland Clinic, Cleveland, Ohio, U.S.A.

Radiation therapy is a common treatment modality for a variety of medical conditions but it often negatively impacts plastic surgery procedures because of its detrimental effects upon tissues and wound healing. An understanding of its physics and tissue effects are critical to optimal patient management.

I. PHYSICS OF RADIATION THERAPY

Ionizing radiation may be classified as either electromagnetic or particulate.

A. Electromagnetic radiation consists of a wave of electrical and magnetic energy, characterized by emissions of varying wavelengths, from the very short wavelengths (x-rays and gamma rays) to the longer wavelengths (microwaves and radiowaves).

B. Particulate radiation consists of particles such as electrons, protons, alpha particles, and neutrons. Radiation may be delivered either locally by placing sources directly on or in the patient (brachytherapy) or by using external beam sources (teletherapy).

C. Radiation dose is the amount of radiation energy absorbed per unit mass of tissue irradiated.

- Radiation dose is measured in scientific international units of the gray (Gy), equal to 1 joule per kilogram. Doses are usually expressed in hundredths of a Gy, the centigray (cGy). The rad is the outdated non-SI unit of dose and is equivalent to 1 cGy.
- A typical pelvic plain film x-ray delivers a gonadal organ dose that averages 0.1–0.2 cGy, and a lower abdominal CT scan delivers a radiation dose of 2–4 cGy. Skin entrance doses are higher. Doses ranging from 5 to 15 cGy have been shown to be teratogenic. Therefore, the typical diagnostic study delivers far less radiation than this threshold.
- Microcephaly and mental retardation are the most common complications of in utero radiation exposure.
- Organs most sensitive to developing cancer in response to radiation are the breast, thyroid, GI tract, and bone marrow. Pediatric radiology studies, as well as those on the fetus, should be minimized.
- A typical radiation dose for treatment of a head and neck neoplasm would be in the range of 5000–7000 cGy. A standard dose fractionation scheme for a curative course of external radiation is one 180–200 cGy treatment per day, 5 treatments per week.
- The higher the beam energy, the more penetrating the beam is into tissue. In the treatment of most cancers, low-energy x-ray beams have

been largely replaced by high-energy beams delivered by megavoltage machines. High-energy beams both penetrate deeper and spare the skin and superficial tissues from the full dose of radiation.

II. CELL AND TISSUE EFFECTS OF RADIATION

A. Classification

1. Lethal damage is irreversible, irreparable, and leads irrevocably to cell death.
2. Sublethal damage, under normal circumstances, can be repaired by the cell in hours, unless a second dose leads to lethal damage.
3. Potentially lethal damage is damage that can be modified by changing the cell's environment after the delivery of the radiation. The effects of ionizing radiation on normal tissues depend on four treatment-related factors: total dose, dose fraction size, total volume treated, and elapsed time during irradiation. Injury to normal tissues may be caused by radiation effects on the microvasculature or the support tissues. Most clinical radiotherapy is delivered in daily fractions to minimize adverse effects on normal tissue.

B. Specific Cellular and Tissue Responses

1. Skin

Radiation-damaged skin heals poorly. The effect of radiation on the skin can be classified into acute effects, occurring in the first 6 months, and late effects, occurring beyond 6 months. Acute effects occur predominantly in tissues with a high level of mitotic activity. They include three classic signs: erythema, dry desquamation, and moist desquamation. Typically, acute effects are self-limiting and resolve within 2–4 weeks after completion of radiation. Late effects are thought to be secondary to vascular compromise from radiation-induced end arteritis and stromal fibrosis. Late effects include increased or decreased skin pigmentation, thickening and fibrosis of the skin and subcutaneous tissues, telangiectasia, and dysfunction of the sebaceous and sweat glands. Dose-dependent changes are as follows:

- 100 cGy—threshold for radiation-induced skin damage
- 200–600 cGy—temporary erythema and hair loss occurs
- 1500 cGy—dry desquamation
- >4000 cGy—permanent hair loss, dermal hypoplasia, fibrosis, edema, moist desquamation, intense erythema, and possible cancerous changes
- 200–1000 cGy—appear to be more carcinogenic than larger doses. Basal cell and squamous cell carcinomas are the most frequent skin cancers arising in irradiated skin.

2. Keratinocytes

In general, cells are most sensitive in the G2 (post-DNA synthesis) and M (mitosis) stages, and most resistant in late S (DNA synthesis) phase. Basal cell keratinocytes, like all rapidly dividing cell populations, are sensitive to radiation. The main erythematous reaction is usually seen 8 days after the radiation dose and represents an inflammatory reaction. Late radiation changes produce an irregular epidermis with areas of atrophy alternating with variable hyperplasia.

3. Melanocytes

Stimulation of melanocytes after radiation may result in increased pigmentation of irradiated skin.

4. Collagen and Fibroblasts

Acute radiation damage results in dermal inflammation and edema of collagen bundles. Radiation decreases the proliferative ability of fibroblasts. Late effects manifest clinically as cutaneous atrophy and fibrosis resulting in contraction.

5. Cutaneous Adnexal Structures

The most sensitive structures in the skin are the germinal epithelium, sebaceous glands, and hair follicles. Hair follicles in the mitotically anagen phase are particularly sensitive to ionizing radiation. Radiation may cause hair dysplasia or alopecia, depending on the dose. This may affect healing of epidermal injury and skin graft donor sites. Sebaceous glands are also destroyed by chronic radiation exposure. Eccrine glands are the most radioresistant, and generally some survive radiation therapy.

6. Bone

Radiation may disturb bone growth in the immature axial or appendicular skeleton. Complications in the mature skeleton include osteoradionecrosis, pathologic fracture, and radiation-induced neoplasms.

7. Bone Marrow

Bone marrow is the tissue most sensitive to radiation exposure. Whole-body irradiation halts bone marrow cellular proliferation, and the resulting bone marrow depletion is an important cause of death from the procedure. Leukemia can be a common complication.

8. Blood Vessels

Radiation-induced erythema is due to dilation of superficial blood vessels of the dermis. In the acute phase, vascular permeability increases and degenerative changes in basement membrane develop. Radiation also impairs endothelial cell proliferation, produces vascular wall edema, and enhances thrombosis. Late effects include a variety of responses in arteries, such as ulceration, thrombosis, medial fibrosis, and necrosis. The venous drainage is also compromised by the radiation-induced fibrosis and constriction of the veins. All these changes result in impaired blood inflow, drainage, or both, and consequently in tissue hypoxia and severe delay of healing.

9. Microcirculation

Radiation causes progressive injury to the microcirculation. Siemionow et al. (1999) showed that muscle flaps irradiated with 800 cGy had hemodynamic characteristics and leukocyte-endothelial interactions similar to those of nonirradiated flaps, suggesting minimal damage to microvessels and the endothelial cell lining.

10. Wound Healing

Wound healing is a complex, proliferative process that is profoundly impaired by radiation. The negative influences of radiation on wound repair include decreased vascularity, hypoxia, and impairment of the proliferative capacities of local tissues. In addition, ionizing radiation is directly toxic to fibroblasts, which are the most important connective tissue cells involved in repair. Radiation often affects fibroblasts permanently.

III. PLASTIC AND RECONSTRUCTIVE SURGERY ON IRRADIATED AREAS

A. Skin Grafts and Flaps

1. Rudolph et al. (1982) noted a complication rate (defined as the need for further surgery) of 100% for thin split-thickness skin grafts for radiation ulcers in an analysis of 200 previously irradiated patients who had skin graft or flap reconstruction. Several medical centers currently use preoperative subatmospheric pressure dressing therapy to improve the wound bed granulation tissue and decrease infection prior to skin grafting.
2. Kurul et al. (1997) concluded that reconstructive surgery in previously irradiated areas is more difficult than in nonirradiated cases.
3. Fascia/muscle or myocutaneous flaps have several advantages for reconstruction in previously irradiated areas. They are more resistant to bacteria inoculation and provide better vascularized tissue and volume replacement for contour defects. In reconstructing radiation ulcers, omental flaps and myocutaneous flaps are especially useful, particularly if the radiation damage can be fully excised. Surgical manipulation of the vessels in the irradiated area can lead to intramural wall dissection and formation of red and white thrombi—unless the donor vessels are limited, most surgeons would prefer to carry out the anastomosis outside the radiation field.

B. Breast Cancer and Reconstruction

1. Plastic surgeons frequently deal with irradiated tissue in the breast, where radiation has a definite role both in the local control and in the treatment of metastatic disease.
2. The typical radiation dose for breast cancer is five 180–200 cGy treatments per week for several weeks, totaling approximately 5000–6000 cGy. Radiation is delivered either preoperatively or postoperatively depending on the stage of disease.
3. Irradiated breast tissue often becomes firm, with telangiectasia and other signs of skin atrophy appearing in time. Although tissue expanders and implants are used for breast reconstruction in irradiated patients, they are associated with significant complications. Less problematic is autogenous reconstruction with either a latissimus dorsi flap or a transverse rectus abdominis myocutaneous (TRAM) flap. However, radiation therapy after a TRAM flap can result in increased fat necrosis, causing a firm breast with loss of volume, contour, and symmetry.

IV. IMPROVING HEALING IN IRRADIATED TISSUE

Plastic and reconstructive surgeons should be aware of a number of measures that have been shown to improve the healing of irradiated tissue.

A. Therapeutic measures: Growth factors, most notably PDGF, TGF-β, and bFGF, have been shown to accelerate healing in radiated wounds in animal models. Electrical stimulation enhances the healing of wounds in human and animal models. Hyperbaric oxygen (HBO) is a new therapy for managing radiation necrosis. HBO has gained widespread use, particularly in the management of osteoradionecrosis of the mandible. Subatmospheric pressure dressing is the latest tool that has shown promise. However, prospective randomized studies are needed to support the use of many of these treatment modalities.

B. Careful wound care: Meticulous debridement, pulsatile water irrigation, and aggressive local and systemic antibiotic therapy are essential. Even a small nidus of devascularized tissue will allow bacterial overgrowth, with potential progressive necrosis.

C. General measures: Anabolic metabolism and optimal nutrition are of major importance in irradiated patients.

D. Treating radiation changes in skin: Skin changes due to acute effects are treated with supportive topical care. Hypopigmentation is protected by the use of adequate sunblocks. Contractures secondary to fibrosis are prevented by appropriate physical therapy.

V. RADIATION THERAPY OF SKIN CANCERS AND OTHER LESIONS

A. Radiation therapy is effective in treating many skin lesions, including Kaposi's sarcoma, mycosis fungoides, lymphoma cutis, squamous cell carcinoma, basal cell carcinoma, and metastatic melanomas.

B. The recommended dose may vary from 2000 to 6000 cGy, depending on the size of the lesion. In general, treatment of most skin cancers requires doses and fractionation schemes that destroy the basal layers of the epidermis but spare the underlying dermis. Radiation necrosis can occur in patients receiving large doses.

27

Soft Tissue Injuries to the Face

Eric J. Stelnicki, M.D.
Hollywood, Florida, U.S.A.

I. DOG BITES

Dog bites are becoming an epidemic problem in the United States.

A. Although dog bites can occur anywhere on the body, they are particularly troubling when they involve the face. The soft tissue injuries resulting from a bite vary from partial-thickness lacerations to avulsions with loss of muscle and bone.

B. Dog breeds most commonly involved include the pit bull terrier, aikita, chow, doberman, and rottweiler. The best treatment is primary prevention; care should be taken in handling any of these breeds. Particular attention should be given when young children are around these dogs.

C. Treatment of dog bites depends on the severity of the injury.

- Because the face is such a cosmetically sensitive area, all dog bites here should be closed primarily. However, no skin grafts or rotation-advancement flaps should be attempted in the acute care setting.
- The edges of stellate lacerations created by a bite should be sharpened with a scalpel to allow for accurate closure of the wound.
- Any devitalized tissue should also be debrided.
- Prior to closure, the wound should be irrigated with Betadine and saline solutions. A layered or simple closure should be performed using monofilament sutures.
- Antibiotic coverage for *Pasteurella* is essential.

D. If there is a large area of soft tissue loss or underlying bone injury, the patient should be taken to the operating room for copious irrigation and wound debridment. Then, within 24 h, the patient should undergo further debridement and secondary reconstruction of the injury. All patients should receive antibiotics.

E. Local skin flaps provide well-vascularized coverage of the wound. Skin grafts are rarely used because of the risk of postoperative infection.

- Suggested flaps on the cheek include: nasolabial advancement flaps, Limberg flaps, and cervical-facial flaps.
- Bites to the eyelid should be accompanied by a careful ophthalmologic examination to rule out corneal abrasion or a penetrating injury to the globe.
- Full-thickness defects into the lip require careful closure of the oral mucosa to prevent contamination of the wound by oral flora. Absorbable sutures are recommended.

Patients should rinse their mouths 5 times a day with a peroxide-based antimicrobial mouthwash.

Care must be taken to align three important labial structures: the orbicularis oris muscle, the white roll, and the red line. The pars marginalis of the orbicularis oris must be closed with interrupted or figure-of-8 monofilament absorbable sutures. Failure to properly realign this muscle will lead to abnormal lip movement and appearance characterized by abnormal muscle bulging lateral to the bite area.

The white roll marks the border between the red lip vermilion and the normal skin of the lip. This must be exactly reapproximated. Failure to properly do this result in a noticeable deformity in the lip margin. This should therefore be the first area precisely realigned and closed in the epidermal closure of the lip.

The second area to be realigned and closed should be at the red line, which forms the junction between the wet and dry mucosae of the lip. Failure to reapproximate this line leaves a vertical distortion in the lip vermilion. It also results in chapping and scabbing of the lip postoperatively due to eversion of wet mucosa into the dry mucosa zone.

- Defects of greater than one-third of the eyelid, lip, or ear should have a delayed closure following complete debridment of the wound, using reconstructive principles for these areas described later in this text.

II. BLUNT TRAUMA

A. Abrasions

1. Skin abrasions of the face vary in thickness, similar to burns. The depth of abrasions should be carefully analyzed in order to determine the appropriate treatment plan.
2. Superficial abrasions should be scrubbed clean under local anesthesia and covered 4 times a day with a petroleum-based ointment in order to keep the wound moist and clean.
   - The goal should be to prevent scab formation on the surface of the wound. The abrasion should be cleaned twice daily with water and soap.
   - Parenteral antibiotics are usually not required.
3. Partial-thickness abrasions, like partial-thickness burns, extend into the dermis.
   - Stellate edges of the wound should be sharply debrided.
   - The wound should be scrubbed clean with a sterile scrub brush and antimicrobial soap under local anesthesia.
   - Conservative management of these injuries is paramount. Many large wounds will heal without scar or with a much-diminished scar over time. Like a superficial abrasion, the wound should be kept moist with a petroleum ointment, covered by a nonabsorptive dressing such as telfa, four times a day.
   - Twice-per-day cleansing to prevent scab formation improves the final result.
   - After 2–3 weeks, scarring from partial-thickness abrasions can be decreased by using pressure massage and silicone sheeting.
   - Hypertrophic scars can be decreased by intralesional injection of steroids that are thought to increase collagenase activity within the wound.
   - If, after 6–12 months, the scar is red and raised, then it may be effectively treated with a tunable dye laser to decreased vascularity.
   - Local scar excision and reconstruction of the area should be delayed for 1 year to allow the scar to mature fully.
4. Full-thickness abrasions
   - Full thickness abrasions are caused by a significant amount of blunt trauma. Therefore, the evaluating physician must be alerted to the presence of other secondary injuries. Monitoring of Glasgow coma score, visual exam, and careful neurologic exam and evaluation of the cervical spine to rule out injury are mandatory.
   - All stellate and devitalized edges of the abrasion are sharply debrided.
   - Primary closure of the wound is performed when possible. However, local advancement flaps are often needed to close the defect. These should be not done at the time of the initial debridment and repair.
5. Traumatic tattooing
   - This is frequently seen in conjunction with abrasions.

- Particulate matter of wood, concrete, asphalt, soil, etc. are frequently embedded in the dermis. The depth of penetration varies with the depth of the abrasion.
- When traumatic tattoing is noted, it is essential to completely remove these particles at the time of treatment. Failure to do so increases the risk of infection and can lead to permanent pigmented scarring in the area of the abrasion. General or regional anesthesia is frequently required. A sterile scrub brush, a soft tissue rasp, and a 10-blade scalpel are effective tools in removing these particles.
- Postoperative antibiotic coverage is recommended.
- If a patient presents with a healed abrasion containing traumatic tattooing, there are two treatment options. Small areas can be excised and closed primarily with a local flap. Larger areas, such as an entire forearm, are best treated with a combination of laser and direct particle excision. Large particles can be extracted with a tip of an 18-gauge needle. Small-pigmented particles can be obliterated via repeat use of a Q-switched laser. The type of Q-switched laser used depends on the pigment of the tattoo. CO_2 laser can also be used to bring deep particles closer to the surface and convert the healed abrasion back into an acute wound. Once this occurs, dermabrasion and a scrub brush can be used for debridement.

B. Hematomas

1. Isolated hematomas can occur after blunt or penetrating trauma.
2. Hematomas may represent soft tissue injury with a rupturing of dermal or subdermal blood vessels secondary to the injury. In this scenario, treatment with a warm compress and conservative observation is all that is required. In the case of a large hematoma, the mass may be aspirated with a needle 7–10 days postinjury, once the hematoma liquefies.
3. Hematomas are often indicators of underlying bony injury. Examples include the "raccoon eyes" of a basilar skull fracture, isolated periorbital hematoma seen in orbital floor fractures, or sublingual hematomas present following mandibular fractures.
4. Cauliflower ear
   - A cauliflower ear is the delayed consequence of repeated blunt trauma to the auricle that produces recurrent, subperichondral hematomas.
   - These hematomas create a chondroinductive matrix for chondroblasts contained within elevated perichondrium. The chondroblasts migrate into the hematoma and form ectopic cartilage in this area, inducing significant deformation in the shape of the ear's helical structure.
   - The cauliflower ear is typically seen in professional boxers, but it can be seen following any blunt trauma to the ear or in patients who habitually rub and squeeze their ear helices.
   - Acute treatment involves immediate incision and drainage of any auricular hematomas. Meticulous homeostasis should be obtained, followed by a layered primary closure. In the case of large hematomas, a suction drain should be left in place for several days.
   - Delayed treatment: The heterotopic cartilage can be directly excised through a postauricular approach. The deformity is over-corrected using a fine diamond rasp to shave down the cartilage. A compression dressing is then used to redrape the skin.

C. Avulsions

Blunt trauma resulting in the full-thickness loss of skin and all underlying tissue constitutes an avulsion. Certain sites require a variety of reconstructive techniques for their restoration.

1. Ear

A. A complete ear avulsion or amputation requires immediate microvascular reconstruction. Microvascular reconstruction using vein grafts to anastomose at least one ear artery and two ear veins to either the superficial temporal or occipital vessels is required. When successful, complete normal restoration of external ear structure can be achieved.

B. Delayed treatment of avulsed ears requires total ear reconstruction using either a costochondral graft or a Medpor implant covered with skin or temporal parietal fascia.

C. Partial avulsions are treated with sharp debridement of wound edges followed by local advancement flaps, such as the Antia-Buch advancement flap. Larger defects require harvesting cartilage from the contralateral ear and covering this free cartilage graft with a temporal parietal flap and a full-thickness skin graft.

2. Eyelids

A. Avulsions of eyelids is a true medical emergency because lack of coverage puts the underlying globe at risk from exposure keratopathy. Immediate coverage is needed to prevent corneal damage and decreased visual acuity.

B. Acute care involves assessing the extent of the avulsion, obtaining an ophthalmology consult to document visual acuity, placing ophthalmic antibiotic ointment on the cornea, and covering the eye with a nonpermeable occlusive eye shield. This traps moisture around the eye, preventing dryness and protecting the ocular surface.

C. The lid is reconstructed using a variety of techniques. Care must be taken to replace each of the three lamellar layers to the eye.

- Conjunctiva can be replaced with adjacent or cross-lid conjunctiva. Free conjunctiva grafts made of oral mucosa or palatal mucosa are also an effective replacement.
- The middle lamella or tarsus is reconstructed using non-vascularized cartilage grafts or via some form of tarsal plate advancement.
- Skin is replaced via local flap advancement or full-thickness skin grafting. Importantly, non-vascularized grafts need to be in contact with vascularized tissue (i.e., advancement flap as opposed to another graft) to survive.

III. PENETRATING TRAUMA

A. Lacerations

1. Lips

A. Lip lacerations are treated similar to full-thickness abrasions.

B. A three-layered closure must be performed in order to seal the laceration off from the oral cavity and reconstitute the orbicularis oris muscle.

C. It is essential to align the white roll and the red line properly in these patients in order to restore normal lip contour.

2. Cheeks

A. Deep cheek lacerations require a layered closure.

B. These lacerations can penetrate into the oral cavity, and the wound should be carefully irrigated prior to closure to explore this possibility. If the oral cavity is breached, a separate closure must be performed.

C. Cheek lacerations also run the risk of injuring branches of the facial nerve. A full facial nerve exam should be performed prior to anesthetizing the area for closure. If the nerve is lacerated, then a primary nerve anastomosis should be performed at the time of laceration repair.

3. Eyelids

A. The repair of eyelid lacerations also involves a careful three-layered closure.

B. A few buried absorbable gut sutures should be used in the conjunctiva. The gray line at the tarsal margin must be carefully reapproximated to restore the normal curvature of the eyelid margin. The borders of the tarsal plate must also be carefully realigned.

C. **Ptosis**—Lacerations to the upper lid can damage the insertions of the levator aponeurosis or Müller's muscle onto the tarsal plate. These cases should be identified preoperatively so that the detached eyelid elevators can be properly advanced to the tarsal plate at the time of primary laceration repair.

D. **Ectropion**—Any injury to the lower lid heightens the risk of increased sclera show and lid pulldown (ectropion). The risk of developing an ectropion is decreased by proper realignment of the injured lid structures. However, in some cases, cartilage grafting, lateral canthopexy, or tarsal strip advancement is required to provide additional support to the damaged lower lid and correct lower eyelid malposition.

4. Ears

A. Ear lacerations require acute debridment of injured cartilage followed by the placement of perichondral sutures to support the cartilage.

B. The cartilage repair is then followed by a layered skin closure.

B. Gunshot Wound

1. Any gunshot wound requires a complete head/neck exam and neurological evaluation.
2. Injuries to soft tissue, bone, teeth, and underlying neurovascular structures must be identified at the time of initial presentation.
3. Patients may require triple endoscopy, swallowing studies, arteriography, and/or CT scanning to rule out associated damage.
4. Low-velocity gunshot wounds involving soft tissue only can be debrided and closed primarily as described in the laceration section.
5. High-velocity gunshot wounds require serial debridements prior to closure. The patient should be seen initially and stabilized. The wound should be debrided serially over 48 h to determine the complete extent of the injury. At that point, primary closure is advocated.

IV. BURNS

A. Acute management of burns will be covered in the section on burn therapy. However, it is worth mentioning here that most second-degree facial burns are treated with antibiotic ointment and subsequently covered with a moist, semi-occlusive dressing. Third-degree facial burns should be treated early by debridement and skin grafting in order to decrease scar formation.

B. Second- and third-degree auricular burns are best treated with Sulfamylon, which penetrates down to the cartilage and gives excellent coverage against pseudomonas infections.

C. Delayed reconstruction:

- Neck

  Severe burns of the neck require excision and reconstruction in order to prevent scar contraction that limits neck mobility.

  Skin grafts have been used successfully in the past.

  However, for large burns involving greater than half the skin on the neck, a deltopectoral flap reconstruction with or without tissue expansion has been advocated.

- Cheeks

  Burns to the cheeks are best reconstructed with a cervicofacial flap with or without associated tissue expansion in the neck.

  If skin grafting is required, split-thickness scalp grafts leave minimal donor site morbidity and provide grafts with a similar color match.

- Lips

  Complete restoration of burned lips is difficult.

  The best methods available today involve mucosal advancement flaps of buccal mucosa, advancement of tissue from the opposite lip (if available), or free microvascular tissue transfer.

- Nose

  Full-thickness burns to the nose require a three-layered reconstruction.

  Mucosal lining must be achieved with a local mucosal advancement flaps or grafts.

  The cartilage must be reconstructed using auricular, septal, or costochondral cartilage.

  The skin is resurfaced preferably with local vascularized advancement flaps. In most cases, unburned forehead skin (forehead flap) is the best choice for reconstruction.

- Ears

  Burned ears are reconstructed by excising the burn, covering the cartilage with a temporal parietal fascia flap, and then resurfacing the ear with a skin graft.

- Hair

  Focal burn allopecia can be repaired through a combination of serial burn excision, tissue expansion, and micrografting of hair implants.

28

Infections of the Face

Eric J. Stelnicki, M.D.
Hollywood, Florida, U.S.A.

Due to the hypervascular nature of facial tissue, it is rare for facial infections to occur. When they do, there is usually an underlying cause, which must be discovered in order to eradicate the noxious process. It is rare for a simple laceration to result in infection, unless one is dealing with an immunocompromised host. A careful history and physical is, therefore, essential in the evaluation of any facial infection.

I. DENTAL ABSCESS AND FACIAL CELLULITIS

One of the most common causes of facial cellulitis is a dental abscess. The collection of purulent material in this closed space can cause cellulitis in the overlying gingiva. Often it is easier for a dental infection to extend into the soft tissues of the face rather than around the adjacent gum line.

A. History

1. In working up a patient with facial cellulitis, a complete dental exam and history are mandatory. The history should include any mention of recent dental work or facial trauma.
2. The number of teeth present in the mouth should also be carefully documented.

B. Treatment

1. If a dental abscess is discovered, immediate relief can be obtained by incising the gingiva and periosteum directly surrounding the infection and creating a window for open drainage.
2. In order to accomplish adequate drainage, a regional anesthetic block involving the infraorbital nerve, greater palatine nerve, lesser palatine nerve, or inferior alveolar nerve is required, depending on the site of infection.
3. Local injections around the infected abscess are very painful and give poor relief due to the surrounding inflammation and acidic microenvironment, and therefore should only be given as a supplement to a regional anesthetic block.
4. Following drainage, the patient should rinse four times per day with peroxide-based antimicrobial mouthwash.
5. Parenteral antibiotic coverage should provide coverage for *Staphylococcus*, *Streptococcus*, *Eikenella*, Gram-negative rods, and anaerobes. Penicillin derivatives, such as Augmentin, are good initial therapies. Patients with penicillin allergies should receive alternative medications such as clindamycin.
6. The underlying dental infection then needs to be addressed. In some cases this necessitates tooth extraction, and the patient should be referred to a local dentist as soon as possible.
7. If there is concern about a deep underlying facial abscess, an MRI scan should be obtained.

II. AURICULAR PERICHONDRITIS

A. Deep infections of the auricular perichondrium are most commonly caused by lacerations to the ear that extend down to the cartilage. If not properly debrided and covered with antibiotics, this type of injury opens a portal to a relatively avascular space in the facial soft tissue that is easy for bacteria to colonize.

B. Rarely, auricular perichondritis develops from an overlying skin infection such as an infected sebaceous cyst or nevus.

C. Perichondritis is diagnosed by the presence of pain, cellulitis, swelling, and soft tissue fluctuance in the ear. The extent of the infection should be clearly marked with permanent marker to document the progression of the infection

D. Treatment is primarily surgical.

- Any lacerations should be opened and extended as needed to drain the abscess. The perichondrium itself must be incised, but the underlying cartilage is left untouched.
- Following copious irrigation, the wound should be packed open for several days with Betadine-soaked gauze.
- Broad-spectrum parenteral antibiotic coverage should be instituted.
- Once the cellulitis has decreased, the wound may be allowed to heal by secondary intention or can be covered with local flaps of postauricular skin or temporal parietal fascia.
- Often the underlying cartilage will have to be debrided.

III. MASTOIDITIS AND CHOLESTEATOMA

A. Acute Mastoiditis

1. Acute mastoiditis is characterized by necrosis of the mastoid air cells, mastoid antrum, and their bony partitions. It usually develops as a complication of chronic otitis media.
2. Patients with acute mastoiditis present with headache, pain on direct mastoid palpation, fever, otorrhea, conductive hearing loss, and posterior auricular erythema.
3. A CT scan will show bone destruction and fluid in the air cells.
4. Treatment involves intravenous vancomycin, gentamicin, and metronidazole for 2 weeks. A myringotomy tube is placed if there is fluid behind the tympanic membrane. A mastoidectomy is performed in the presence of an abscess.

B. Cholesteatomas

1. Cholesteatomas develop in patients with chronic otitis media that has been left untreated.
2. Squamous epithelium piles up in the middle ear and forms a mass of infected cellular debris that destroys the ear canal and the middle ear ossicles.
3. If untreated, a cholesteatoma will progress to purulent labyrinthitis, facial paralysis, and intracranial infection.
4. Cholesteatomas are diagnosed in patients with chronic otitis media by CT scan or MRI, which demonstrate a soft tissue mass in the middle ear and associated destruction of the ossicles.
5. Bacteria present in the mass include *Pseudomonas*, *Staphylococcus*, and *Proteus*.
6. Treatment involves treating the otitis media and radial mastoidectomy.

IV. SIALOADENITIS

A. Infection of the salivary glands involves *Staphylococcus aureus* and mixed Gram-negative organisms that multiple in the salivary glands as a result of ductal obstruction or decreased salivary production secondary to dehydration.

B. Untreated, the infection will spread throughout the facial soft tissue.

C. Symptoms include facial pain, swelling over the gland, fever, and erythema.

D. Intraoral examination may reveal a purulent discharge from a duct orifice.

E. CT scans are useful in ruling out an underlying abscess.

F. Treatment involves intravenous antibiotics, sialagogues such as lemon drops to increase saliva production, hydration, and hot compresses over the gland. Incision and drainage is required if an abscess develops.

V. INFECTED BITES

A. If a bite from any source becomes infected, it must be drained immediately. It is the mistake of the novice surgeon to attempt to treat a bite wound infection with antibiotics alone. Any success without debridment would constitute an exception rather than the rule.

B. Infected bites must be distinguished from reddened wounds that are in the early phases of wound healing. Purulent discharge, increasing pain, fever, or expanding cellulitis are all ominous signs.

C. Treatment involves opening the bite incision, wound irrigation, debridement of devitalized tissue, and closure by secondary wound healing.

D. Antibiotics specific to the bite source should be instituted.

E. Once epithelialization is complete, pressure massage and nightly silicon sheeting are often recommended to decrease the degree of scar formation.

29

Pharyngeal Tumors

Suzanne K. Doud Galli, M.D., Ph.D.,* **and Mark D. DeLacure, M.D., F.A.C.S**
New York University School of Medicine, New York, New York, U.S.A.

Despite treatment advances, there has been little improvement in survival for patients with pharyngeal carcinomas. A multidisciplinary approach involving oncologists, dentists, nutritionists, speech pathologists, and surgeons is required for the management of these patients.

I. STAGING

A. Oropharynx Tumor (T) Staging

1. T1 tumor is 2 cm or less in diameter.
2. T2 tumor is more than 2 cm but less than 4 cm in diameter.
3. T3 tumor is more than 4 cm in diameter.

4a. Tumor invades larynx, extrinsic muscles of tongue, medial pterygoid, hard palate, or mandible.

4b. Tumor invades lateral pterygoid, pterygoid plate, lateral nasopharynx or skull base, or encases carotid.

B. Hypopharynx Tumor (T) Staging

1. T1 tumor is less than 2 cm in diameter and is limited to one subsite.
2. T2 tumor is greater than 2 cm and less than 4 cm in diameter or involves more than 1 subsite.
3. T3 tumor is more than 4 cm in diameter or involves fixation of the hemilarynx.

4a. Tumor invades thyroid/cricoid cartilage, hyoid bone, thyropid gland, esophagus, or central compartment soft tissue.

4b. Tumor invades prevertebral fascia, encases carotid artery, or involves mediastinal structures.

C. Nasopharynx Tumor (T) Staging

1. T1 tumor is confined to the nasopharynx.
2. T2A tumor has no parapharyngeal extension; T2B tumor has parapharyngeal extension.
3. T3 tumor extends to the oropharynx or nasal fossa.
4. T4 tumor has intracranial extension or cranial nerve or orbital involvement.

D. Regional Nodal Disease (N)

1. NX lymph nodes—cannot be assessed
2. N0—no lymph node metastases
3. N1—single ipsilateral node metastasis that is 3 cm or less in diameter
4. N2A—single ipsilateral lymph node metastasis more than 3 cm and less than 6 cm in diameter
5. N2B—multiple ipsilateral node metastases less than 6 cm in diameter
6. N2C—bilateral or contralateral node metastases less than 6 cm in diameter
7. N3—lymph node metastasis greater than 6 cm in diameter

**Current affiliation*: Fairfax Hospital, Fairfax, Virginia, U.S.A.

E. Distant Metastasis (M)

1. MX—distant metastasis cannot be assessed
2. M0—no distant metastasis
3. M1—distant metastasis

F. Staging

General pattern of staging
  Stage 0: TisN0M0
  Stage I: T1N0M0
Unique staging for oropharynx and hypopharynx
  Stage II: T2N0M0
  Stage III: T3N0M0 or T1,T2,T3N1M0
  Stage IV: T4N0,N1M0 or any T,N2,N3,M0 or any T, any N,M1
Unique staging for nasopharynx
  Stage II: T2N0M0 or T1T2,N1M0
  Stage III: T1,T2,T3N2M0 or T3N0,N1M0
  Stage IV: T4N0,N1,N2M0 or any T,N3M0 or any T, any N,M1

II. INCIDENCE

A. All Pharyngeal Tumors

1. Male:female incidence = 2.5:1
2. Black > white

B. Oropharynx

1. Male:female incidence = 4:1
2. Usually presents in 4th to 5th decade
3. Tonsils are the most common site of malignancy

C. Hypopharynx

1. Male:female incidence = 2:1
2. Usually presents in the 6th to 8th decade
3. 95% of cases are squamous cell carcinomas
4. Pyriform sinus is the most frequent site

D. Nasopharynx

1. Infrequent in the United States
2. More frequent in China
3. Usually presents in the 5th to 6th decade

III. ANATOMIC CONSIDERATIONS

A. Anatomic Boundaries (Fig. 1)

1. Oropharynx
   - Soft palate, tongue base, tonsils, tonsillar fossae and pillars, and the posterior pharyngeal wall from the level of the vallecula to the level of the soft palate

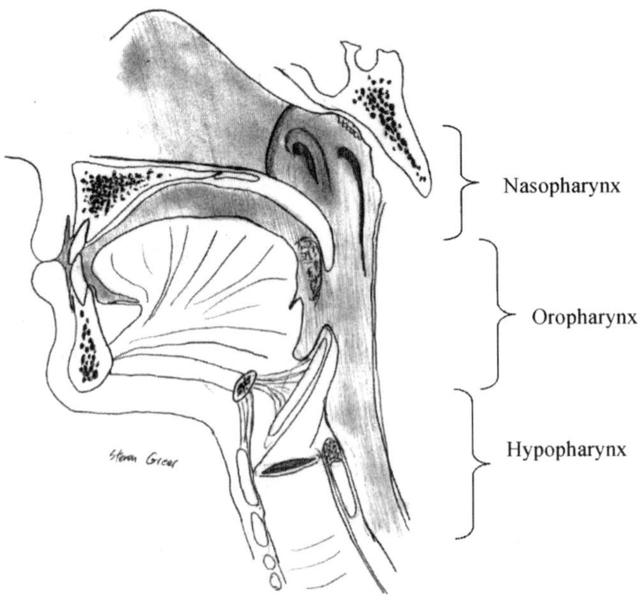

Figure 1 Anatomic boundaries.

2. Hypopharynx
   - Postericoid area, pyriform sinus, and posterior pharyngeal wall
   - Extends from the vallecula to the lower border of the cricoid cartilage
3. Nasopharynx
   - Posterosuperior wall from junction of the hard and soft palate to the skull base
   - Lateral wall including fossa of Rosenmüller, torus, and orifice of the Eustachian tube
   - Inferior wall at superior surface of the soft palate

B. Most Frequent Sites of Tumor Involvement

1. Oropharynx—tonsils, then base of tongue
2. Hypopharynx—pyriform sinus
3. Nasopharynx—posterior

C. Lymphatic Drainage

1. Oropharynx—upper deep cervical chain, posterior triangle, and retropharyngeal nodes can be involved
2. Hypopharynx—jugulodigastic nodes, posterior triangle, and retropharyngeal nodes can be involved
3. Nasopharynx—retropharyngeal nodes

D. Neural Involvement

1. Otalgia is secondary to referred pain from the lingual, glossopharyngeal, or vagus nerves
2. Cavernous sinus extension of nasopharyngeal mass with cranial nerve II, IV, V, VI effects
3. Horner's syndrome with involvement of the cervical sympathetic chain

IV. DIAGNOSIS

A. Physical Exam

1. Thorough head and neck exam
2. Biopsy of mass or fine needle aspiration of lymph node
3. Panendoscopy to rule out synchronous primaries

B. Radiographic Evaluation

CT scan to determine extent of disease and to provide radiographic diagnosis of nonpalpable adenopathy

C. Oropharynx Cancers

Present with neck mass, odynophagia, or otalgia

D. Hypopharynx Cancers

Present with neck mass, throat pain, odynophagia, or otalgia

E. Nasopharynx Cancers

Present with neck mass, otologic symptoms or nasal symptoms, cranial nerve involvement at advanced stages

V. ETIOLOGY

A. Oropharynx

Associated with tobacco and alcohol use and Plummer-Vinson syndrome

B. Hypopharynx

Associated with tobacco and alcohol use, gastric reflux

C. Nasopharynx

Associated with Epstein-Barr virus and environmental factors like nitrosamines, polycyclic hydrocarbons, and nickel

VI. HISTOLOGY

A. Oropharynx and Hypopharynx

95% are squamous cell carcinomas (SCC)

B. Nasopharynx

Histologic types are:

- SCC
- Nonkeratinizing
- Undifferentiated

VII. TREATMENT

A. Oropharynx

1. Radiation therapy, including necks for T1 and T2 tumors
2. Surgery and radiation for T3 and T4 tumors
3. Surgical approaches include transoral, mandibular swing, composite resection, and pharyngotomy; glossectomy with laryngectomy, laryngoplasty, or suspension to prevent aspiration

B. Hypopharynx

1. Radiation therapy or partial laryngopharyngectomy for T1 and T2 tumors
2. Combined surgery and radiation with total laryngectomy/partial pharyngectomy for T3 and T4 tumors
3. Esophagectomy required if esophageal involvement is present

C. Nasopharynx

1. Chemotherapy and radiation therapy
2. Neck dissection for persistent neck disease
3. Surgical resection is via a craniofacial approach for persistent disease, with application of brachytherapy

VIII. 5-YEAR SURVIVAL

A. Oropharynx

1. Stage I and II—80%
2. Stage III—50%; base of tongue carries worse prognosis

B. Hypopharynx

Overall survival is 40%

C. Nasopharynx

1. Poor survival with SCC type and skull base involvement—10%
2. Nonkeratinizing and undifferentiated cancers—50%

30

Laryngeal Tumors

Suzanne K. Doud Galli, M.D., Ph.D.,* and Mark D. DeLacure, M.D., F.A.C.S.
New York University School of Medicine, New York, New York, U.S.A.

The larynx is the second most common site for malignancies in the head and neck region. Two percent of all malignancies are found in the larynx. Because of the important functional aspects of the larynx, alternatives to radical surgical procedures have been investigated to allow for organ preservation. As with other tumors of the upper aerodigestive system, a multidisciplinary team comprised of surgeons, oncologists, dentists, nutritionists, and speech pathologists is required for the optimal management of these patients.

I. TNM STAGING

A. Primary Tumor (T)

1. Supraglottis
   - Tis—carcinoma in situ
   - T1—limited to one subsite with normal vocal cord mobility
   - T2—greater than one subsite, or with glottic extension
2. Glottis
   - Tis—carcinoma in situ
   - T1—confined to vocal cord with normal mobility (T1a—one cord; T1b—both cords)
   - T2—extends to the supraglottis or subglottis
3. Subglottis
   - Tis—carcinoma in situ
   - T1—limited to the subglottis
   - T2—extends to the glottis
4. In general
   - T2a—normal vocal cord mobility
   - T2b—impaired vocal cord mobility
   - T3—confined to larynx with vocal cord fixation, invades paraglottic space, and/or minor cartilage erosion
   - T4a—invades thyroid cartilage or soft tissue beyond larynx
   - T4b—invades prevertebral space, encases carotid artery and/or invades mediastinum

B. Regional Nodal Disease (N)

1. Nx—lymph nodes cannot be assessed
2. N0—no lymph nodes involved
3. N1—single ipsilateral node metastasis with diameter <3 cm
4. N2a—single ipsilateral node metastasis >3 cm and <6 cm in diameter
5. N2b—multiple ipsilateral node metastases <6 cm in diameter
6. N2c—bilateral or contralateral node metastases <6 cm in diameter
7. N3—nodal metastasis greater than 6 cm

*Current affiliation: Fairfax Hospital, Fairfax, Virginia, U.S.A.

C. Distant Metastasis (M)

1. Mx—distant metastasis cannot be assessed
2. M0—no distant metastasis
3. M1—distant metastasis

D. Staging

Stage 0: TisN0M0

Stage I: T1N0M0

Stage II: T2N0M0

Stage III: T3N0M0 or T1,T2,T3N1M0

Stage IV: T4N0,N1M0 or any T,N2,N3M0 or any T, and N, M1

II. INCIDENCE

A. Male:female = 6:1

B. Usually presents in the 5th to 7th decade of life

C. Incidence is 2.7 cases per 100,000 people

III. ANATOMIC CONSIDERATIONS

A. Anatomic Boundaries

1. Larynx in general
    - Anteriorly: the lingual epiglottis, thyrohyoid membrane, anterior commissure, thyroid cartilage, cricothyroid membrane, anterior cricoid cartilage
    - Posteriorly and laterally: the aryepiglottic folds, arytenoids and intraarytenoid space, mucous membrane of cricoid cartilage, vestibule, ventricle, and subglottic space
2. Supraglottis
    - Extends from the vallecula to the laryngeal ventricle
    - Epiglottis, aryepiglottic folds, arytenoids, false cords
3. Glottis
    - True vocal cords
    - Anterior and posterior commissures
4. Subglottis—10 mm below the true cords

B. Most Frequent Sites of Tumor Involvement

1. Glottis—most common site
2. Subglottis location represents <2% of all laryngeal tumors

C. Lymphatic Drainage

1. Supraglottis—drains into levels I, II, III
2. Glottis
    - Drains into levels II, III, IV, Delphian (pretracheal)
    - True vocal cords are devoid of lymphatic vessels
    - Metastasis as a late phenomenon
3. Subglottis—drains into levels II, III, IV
4. Bilateral drainage of supraglottis and subglottis
5. Adjacent tissue spread from glottis and subglottis

D. Anatomic Factors Pertinent to Tumor Spread

1. Broyle's ligament
    - Attaches the vocalis tendon to the thyroid cartilage
    - Potential site of tumor spread through the fenestrations in the cartilage
2. Elastic membranes
    - Prevent early tumor spread between compartments
    - Act as a relative barrier to early cartilage invasion
    - Conus elasticus and/or quadrangular membrane
3. Potential spaces
    - Allow spread of tumor outside the larynx
    - Pre-epiglottic space and paraglottic space

E. Vocal Cord Fixation

1. Invasion of the vocal cord proper, cricoarytenoid muscle or joint, or recurrent laryngeal nerve
2. May be mimicked by tumor mass on adjacent structures (aryepiglottic folds)

IV. DIAGNOSIS

A. Physical Examination

1. Thorough exam of head and neck
2. Evaluation of all mucosal surfaces
3. Palpation for cervical adenopathy
4. Flexible laryngoscopy
5. Panendoscopy and biopsy

B. Radiographic Studies

1. CT for advanced lesions prior to endoscopy and biopsies and for nodal staging
2. MRI may add complementary information regarding cartilage invasion

C. Symptoms

1. Supraglottis
   - Early: neck mass, dysphagia, odynophagia, globus sensation, referred otalgia
   - Late: hoarseness, stridor, "hot potato" voice
2. Glottis
   - Early: hoarseness
   - Late: dysphagia, odynophagia, globus sensation, referred otalgia, cough, hemoptysis, stridor
3. Subglottis—dyspnea, stridor (late presentation)

V. ETIOLOGY

A. Social habits—cigarette smoking and alcohol abuse

B. Viral agent—laryngeal papillomatosis

C. Occupational exposure—asbestos, nickel and fossil fuels

VI. HISTOPATHOLOGY

A. Squamous Cell Carcinoma

1. Accounts for >90% of all laryngeal tumors
2. Grading:
   - Gx—Grade not assessed
   - G1—well differentiated
   - G2—moderately differentiated
   - G3—poorly differentiated

B. Verrucous Carcinoma

Accounts for 2% of vocal cord cancers

VII. TREATMENT

A. Carcinoma In Situ

Vocal cord stripping during microlaryngoscopy

B. Supraglottis and Glottis

1. T1 and T2: radiation *or* partial laryngectomy
2. Advanced disease: total laryngectomy, combined therapy, and organ sparing protocols
3. Radiation for N1 tumors
4. Surgery for N2–3 tumors
5. Relative contraindications to partial laryngectomy include vocal cord fixation, invasion of the thyroid cartilage, and invasion of the intra-arytenoid space

C. Subglottis

Radiation therapy, laryngectomy, and neck management

D. Organ-Sparing Therapy

1. Radiation therapy in smaller tumor
2. Laryngectomy for salvage of T3, T4 failures
3. Role of chemotherapy is still under investigation
4. Neoadjuvant (anterior) chemotherapy
   - Three cycles of chemotherapy followed by radiotherapy for major or complete responders (e.g., >70%)
   - Poor responders (e.g., <70%) go on to surgical arm with postoperative adjuvant radiation therapy

31

Salivary Gland Tumors

Daniel Grinberg, M.D. and Mark D. DeLacure, M.D., F.A.C.S.
New York University School of Medicine, New York, New York, U.S.A.

I. INTRODUCTION

A. Salivary glands are ectodermal in origin and begin as solid ingrowths from the oral epithelium.

B. Salivary glands have two types of secretory cells (serous and mucous) that are arranged into acini. These acini drain through a series of ducts: intercalated ducts, then into striated ducts, and ending in excretory ducts.

C. Tumors of the salivary glands have specific cellular origins; e.g., mucoepidermoid carcinoma arises from excretory ducts while an oncocytoma arises from striated ducts.

II. INCIDENCE

A. Salivary gland tumors represent 3–4% of all head and neck neoplasms

B. Location:

- 80% parotid
- 12% submandibular
- 8% sublingual and minor salivary glands

C. Benign tumors

- 75% of parotid tumors
- 50% of submandibular tumors
- 25% of minor salivary glands

D. Most common tumor: pleomorphic adenoma (45% of all tumors and 84% of benign neoplasms)

E. Most common malignant tumor: mucoepidermoid carcinoma (30–50% of malignant neoplasms)

F. Risk factors: only established cause is prior exposure to radiation

III. BENIGN TUMORS

A. Pleomorphic Adenoma (Benign Mixed Tumor)

1. Most common tumor of the salivary glands
2. Most originate in the parotid gland
3. Are usually slow-growing and painless
4. Multilobular and encapsulated
5. Epithelial and mesenchymal elements arise from the myoepithelial cells
6. Slight female preponderance
7. Onset usually in the fifth decade
8. Small percentage (3–15%) undergo malignant transformation after an average of 10 years
9. Treatment: superficial parotidectomy
10. Recurrence is unusual, but when it happens, it is often multicentric and difficult to treat

B. Warthin's Tumor

1. Papillary cystadenoma lymphomatosum
2. Well-encapsulated
3. Oncocytes are found in Warthin's tumor, which appears as a hot spot on radionucleotide scan (same as oncocytoma)
4. 6% of all salivary gland tumors
5. Almost exclusively in the parotid gland
6. 2:1 male predominance, with onset usually occurring between the 40s and 70s
7. Bilateral in about 10% of patients
8. Treatment: superficial parotidectomy

C. Oncocytoma

1. Oncocytes are round granular eosinophilic cells with an excessive quantity of mitochondria
2. Less than 1% of parotid tumors
3. Appears as "hot" nodule on nuclear scans
4. May be multiple and bilateral
5. Most people are 55–70 years of age at diagnosis
6. Indistinguishable from oncocytic carcinoma by pathology. Differentiated by clinical behavior
7. Treatment: parotidectomy

D. Basal Cell Adenoma

1. 2% of all parotid tumors
2. Can be confused with adenoid cystic carcinoma
3. Most commonly seen in minor salivary glands of the upper lip or in the parotid gland
4. Treatment: surgical excision

E. Hemangioma

1. Most common parotid tumor found in children
2. Capillary hemangiomas are more common than cavernous type of hemangioma
3. Rapid growth phase is usually seen at 1–6 months, with gradual involution over the next 1–12 years
4. 50–90% regress within the first 5 years of life
5. Slight female predilection
6. If complications (e.g., bleeding, high-output heart failure, or airway compromise), treatment may be necessary
    - Steroids 2–4 mg/kg per day orally with a 40–60% response rate
    - Interferon should be reserved for life-threatening situations due to its toxicity
    - Surgical excision and laser treatment may be used in select circumstances

F. Benign Lymphoepithelial Lesion (BLEL)

1. Not a neoplasm
2. Pathologic architecture: lymph node enlargement within the parotid gland blocks salivary ducts, resulting in multicystic swelling of gland
3. Unilateral, bilateral or even successive enlargements of the salivary glands
4. May be secondary to chronic parotitis or an autoimmune disease (most commonly in HIV-positive patients)
5. Treatment is primarily symptomatic

IV. MALIGNANT TUMORS

A. Adenoid Cystic Carcinoma

1. 4–6% of all neoplasms of the major salivary glands
2. Most common malignancy in submandibular and minor salivary glands
3. Three histologic characteristics
    - Cribiform
    - Tubular
    - Solid—worst prognosis
4. Slow-growing mass
5. Usually asymptomatic
6. Perineural invasion and extension is common (20–80%, according to different series)
7. There is a lifelong risk of local recurrence, with 48% recurrence after 20 years
8. Lymphatic spread is uncommon
9. 90% of patients with distant metastasis had local-regional failure
10. 90% of systemic disease involves the lung
11. Survival: 65% at 10 years, 20% at 30 years

12. Tumor is radiosensitive but generally not radiocurable
13. Treatment: wide excision, including adjacent muscles and nerves, is advocated

B. Mucoepidermoid Carcinoma

1. Two components are involved: epidermoid cells and mucous cells. The more prevalent the mucous cells, the lower the grade and the better the prognosis.
2. Most common carcinoma of the parotid and second-most prevalent carcinoma of the submandibular gland
3. Most common salivary gland carcinoma in children
4. 75% of mucoepidermoid carcinomas are low grade
5. Low grade:
   - Low recurrence rate
   - Greater than 90% 5-year survival rate
   - Treatment: wide resection
6. High grade:
   - 5-year survival varies from 35 to 60%
   - Treatment: Wide excision with postoperative radiation therapy

C. Acinous Cell Carcinoma

1. 90% occur in the parotid. Oral cavity is the second most common location
2. 3% are bilateral (second to Warthin's tumors)
3. Usually present in the third or fourth decade of life
4. 2:1 female predominance
5. Four histologic patterns: solid, microcystic, papillary-cystic, and follicular
6. Most behave as low-grade malignancies—prognosis is therefore favorable
7. Seldom metastasize, with recurrences usually occurring if they are incomplete excised
8. Treatment: wide excision. Radiation therapy appears particularly ineffective against this tumor.
9. 80–90% 5-year survival; 80% 10-year survival

D. Malignant Pleomorphic Adenoma (Carcinoma Ex-Pleomorphic Adenoma)

1. Also known as "malignant mixed tumor"
2. 75% occur in the parotid gland
3. Two types:
   - Carcinoma ex-pleomorphic adenoma—most common type with malignant component comprised of only the epithelial cell component
   - Carcinosarcoma with malignant mesenchymal and epithelial components
4. Usually in long-standing tumors (10–19 years) with rapid increase in rate of tumor growth after steady growth for many years
5. Usually invasive at the time of diagnosis with poor prognosis
6. High rate of regional (25%) and distant (33%) metastasis
7. Treatment: wide excision with postoperative radiation therapy
8. 5-year survival rate: 48–77%; 20-year survival approaches zero

E. Adenocarcinoma

1. Group of neoplasms originating from glandular units
2. These tumors are now classified in more homogeneous subgroups, such as salivary duct carcinoma, terminal duct carcinoma, myoepithelial carcinoma, and adenocarcinoma; not otherwise specified
3. Can vary from well differentiated to poorly differentiated, low to high grade, and invasive lesions
4. Poor prognosticators are advanced stage, high grade, and invasive pattern
5. Treatment: wide excision with postoperative radiation therapy, since recurrence carries a grave prognosis
6. 70% 5-year survival

F. Squamous Cell Carcinoma

1. Very unusual salivary tumor
2. Must exclude:
   - High-grade mucoepidermoid carcinoma
   - Metastatic cutaneous carcinoma from other

sites, such as scalp, face, and, less likely, oral cavity and oropharynx

- Invasion of the gland from contiguous structures
- Squamous metaplasia within the gland

3. 2:1 male predominance
4. Most patients are over 60 when diagnosed
5. Treatment: parotidectomy followed by postoperative radiation therapy
6. 5- and 10-year survival rates: 83% and 75% for stage I; 14% and 11% for stage II and stage III disease, respectively

G. Undifferentiated Carcinoma

1. Epithelial malignancy that lacks distinguishable histologic characteristics
2. Treatment: wide excision followed by radiation therapy
3. Worst prognosis of all salivary gland tumors

H. Lymphoma

1. Originate from intraglandular lymph nodes dispersed within the salivary gland parenchyma. Embryologically, the intraglandular lymph nodes become entrapped in the developing salivary gland
2. Most originate in the parotid gland due to its abundance of lymphoid tissue
3. 85% of salivary gland lymphomas are of the non-Hodgkin's variety
4. Primary lymphoma usually associated with chronic autoimmune sialoadenitis
5. Patients with Sjögren's syndrome have a 44-fold higher chance than a healthy individual of developing lymphoma. Prognosis is also much worse for lymphomas associated with Sjögren's syndrome
6. Treatment: chemotherapy

V. STAGING (TABLE 1)

A. Major Salivary Glands

1. Primary tumor is staged according to size
2. Two subcategories reflecting the presence or absence of local extension

B. Minor Salivary Glands

1. Staged according to the particular site of origin: oral cavity, oropharynx, etc.

Table 1 Staging System for Major Salivary Gland Cancer

T stage	Extent of tumor
Tx	Primary tumor cannot be assessed
T0	No evidence of primary tumor
T1	Tumor < 2 cm in greatest dimension
T2	Tumor 2–4 cm in greatest dimension
T3	Tumor 4–6 cm in greatest dimension
T4	Tumor >6 cm in greatest dimension

All categories are subdivided:
(a) No local extension.
(b) Local extension—clinical or macroscopic invasion of skin, soft tissue, bone, or nerve.

32

Tumors of the Skull Base

Daniel Grinberg, M.D., and Mark D. DeLacure, M.D., F.A.C.S.
New York University School of Medicine, New York, New York, U.S.A.

I. INTRODUCTION

A. Skull base surgery was pioneered by the three specialties of neurosurgery, neuro-otology, and craniofacial plastic surgery.

B. Plastic surgeons can be involved either in the initial treatment of the tumors and malformations or in the craniofacial reconstruction after tumor removal. Plastic surgeons, therefore, should be familiar with the unique diseases in this region.

C. The skull base is one of the most challenging areas of the human anatomy. Surgery of this area is complex due to the restricted access and the proximity of vital structures. Thus, good command of this anatomy is essential to safe and effective surgery in this area.

D. The tumors are commonly benign and locally destructive (meningioma, schwannoma) due to compression.

F. The skull base is divided into three subdivisions: anterior, middle (lateral), and posterior fossae.

II. TUMORS OF THE ANTERIOR SKULL BASE

A. Midline

1. Congenital encephaloceles
2. Craniofacial clefts
3. Pituitary tumors
4. Craniopharyngiomas

B. Paramedian

1. Orbital tumors
2. Extensions of sinus tumors and other adjacent tumors

III. TUMORS OF THE MIDDLE (LATERAL) SKULL BASE

A. Glomus jugulare

B. Lower clival tumors

C. Extensions of cholesteotomas

D. Juvenile angiofibromas

E. Nasopharyngeal carcinoma

F. Sphenoid wing meningiomas

G. Neuromas of the trigeminal nerve

H. Carotid artery aneurysms

IV. TUMORS OF THE POSTERIOR SKULL BASE

A. Acoustic neuromas

B. Various cranial nerve compressions

C. Meningiomas

D. Lesions of the craniocervical junction

V. BENIGN SKULL BASE TUMORS

A. Fibrous Dysplasia

1. Also known as ossifying fibroma.
2. Caused by the replacement of normal bone with fibrous connective tissue.
3. Women are affected more than men, with the peak incidence in those aged 20–40 years.
4. Occurs most commonly in the calvarium and maxilla, which can result in gross cosmetic deformity.
5. Treatment is indicated only for cosmesis or for symptomatic disease (e.g., nerve compression).
6. Malignant degeneration to osteosarcoma is rare, but has been reported, especially after radiation therapy.

B. Juvenile Angiofibroma

1. Benign, highly vascular tumor with a propensity for locally aggressive behavior.
2. Occurs almost exclusively in adolescent males. Believed to correlate with increase in testosterone levels.
3. Rare.
4. Usually originates in the sphenopalatine foramen.
5. At diagnosis, 75% have localized disease, while 20% have intracranial extension, involving the anterior or middle cranial fossa and extending into the cavernous sinus.
6. Presents as nasal obstruction with recurrent, brisk epistaxis. Biopsy is not recommended since it could be life-threatening due to severe hemorrhage.
7. Angiography reveals multiple tortuous vessels with a dense blush in the capillary phase. Embolization can decrease intraoperative blood loss.
8. Treatment is surgery with 10% recurrence after surgical resection.
9. Radiation therapy can be used for recurrences or inoperable tumors.

C. Meningioma

1. Slow-growing tumors that compress rather than invade critical structures.
2. Female predominance (2–4:1), with mean age of presentation at 45 years.
3. Skull base involvement is rare. Most common location is intracranial in the parasagittal region.
4. Meningiomas extend along planes of least resistance and into bones along haversian canals.
5. Treatment is complete surgical excision. Prognosis is excellent.
6. Five-year recurrence rate is 10–15%.

D. Paraganglioma

1. Arise from chemoreceptor systems.
2. Commonly referred to as *glomus tumors*, even though they have little in common with true glomus tumors.
3. Carotid body tumors are the most common type (60%), followed by jugulotympanic and vagal tumors.
4. 3:1 female predominance, with presentation usually between 40–60 years of age.
5. Familial in 10% of cases, expressed as an autosomal dominant trait with variable penetrance.
6. Two to 3% are secretory tumors with increased levels of norepinephrine.
7. Ten percent of tumors are multifocal (more common among familial cases).
8. Characteristic pathologic finding is Zellballen, which are compact nests of chief cells surrounded by modified Schwann cells.
9. Treatment is surgical excision. Some authors advocate embolization 24–48 hours preoperatively to decrease intraoperative blood loss.
10. Radiation therapy may be used to arrest growth, but is not likely to be curative.

E. Pituitary Adenoma

1. Usually originate from the anterior lobe of the pituitary gland.
2. Twenty to 40% are nonfunctioning adenomas.
3. Most common hormone-producing tumor secretes prolactin.

4. Most common presentation is with bilateral hemianopsia secondary to compression of the optic chiasm.
5. Treatment: transsphenoidal surgical resection.

F. Chordoma

1. Slow-growing, locally aggressive benign tumor derived from vestigial remnants of the notochord.
2. Diplopia from cranial nerve VI involvement is the most common presenting symptom.
3. Affects both sexes, with peak incidence of 20–29 years.
4. Treatment is surgical excision.
5. Overall survival is 4–8 years.
6. Local recurrences are common. Distant metastasis is unusual.

VI. MALIGNANT SKULL BASE TUMORS

A. Olfactory Neuroblastoma

1. Uncommon neuroendocrine tumor arising from the nasal olfactory epithelium.
2. No sexual predilection, occurring in all ages.
3. Usually presents with nasal obstruction and epistaxis.
4. At time of diagnosis, an olfactory neuroblastoma usually has intracranial and dural involvement.
5. Lymphatic metastasis occurs 10–30% of the time.
6. Treatment has involved various sequences of surgery, radiation, and chemotherapy.
7. Recurrence occurs in 30–40% of patients.

B. Chondrosarcoma

1. Seventy-five percent occur at the middle fossa skull base.
2. Affects both sexes, with peak incidence of 30–50 years of age.
3. Pain is prominent secondary to bone destruction.
4. Treatment is surgical excision.
5. Frequent local recurrence with rare systemic metastasis.
6. Five-year survival is 50%.

C. Nasopharyngeal Carcinoma

1. Squamous cell carcinoma of the nasopharynx.
2. Strong association with Epstein-Barr virus.
3. Especially common in China and Southeast Asia.
4. Male:female preponderance is 3:1.
5. Most common site is at the fossa of Rosenmüller—present with serous otitis media, nasal obstruction, and/or epistaxis.
6. Most common presentation: asymptomatic cervical adenopathy.
7. Commonly involves the cavernous sinus, cranial nerves VI, IV, III, II, I (in decreasing order).
8. Prognosis is best with undifferentiated type (60% 5-year survival) and worse with well-differentiated squamous cell (20% 5-year survival).
9. Treatment: radiation therapy with chemotherapy.

D. Orbital Rhabdomyosarcoma

1. Most common head and neck soft tissue malignancy in children.
2. Peak incidence around age 5 with a slight male predominance.
3. Caucasian children affected 3 times as often as other races.
4. Usually presents as rapidly progressive unilateral proptosis.
5. Treatment: chemotherapy and radiation therapy.
6. Cure is achievable in up to 80% of cases; recurrence is often fatal.

VII. SURGICAL APPROACHES

The surgery should accomplish the following goals:

A. Complete removal of disease.
B. Protection of vital structures.
C. Restoration of anatomical barriers to isolate intracranial from extracranial environments.
D. Creation of a functional and aesthetically acceptable reconstruction.

33

Reconstruction of the Forehead, Scalp, and Calvarium

Randy B. Miller, M.D.
Baylor College of Medicine, Houston, Texas, U.S.A.

Larry H. Hollier, M.D.
Texas Children's Hospital and Baylor College of Medicine, Houston, Texas, U.S.A.

I. SCALP

A. Layers of the Scalp (Fig. 1)

The acronym SCALP is a good way to remember the layers:

1. S—skin
2. C—connective tissue
3. A—(galea) aponeurotica
4. L—loose areolar tissue
5. P—pericranium

B. Anatomic Pearls of the Scalp

1. Thickest skin in the body (3–8 mm)
2. Galea aponeurotica is continuous with the frontalis muscle anteriorly and the occipitalis muscle posteriorly
3. Subgaleal fascia (subaponeurotic/subepicranium) has intracranial connections via emissary veins
4. Galea fuses with the temporo-parietal fascia at the superior temporal crest
5. Pericranium fuses with the deep temporal fascia
6. Scalp blood supply—blood vessels run above the galea in subcutaneous tissue

C. Scalp Vascular Supply—Four Territories (Fig. 2)

1. Internal carotid artery—supraorbital and supratrochlear artery
2. External carotid artery
   - Temporal—superficial temporal artery
   - Occipital—occipital artery
   - Postauricular—posterior auricular artery

D. Nerve Supply

1. Ophthalmic division of cranial nerve five (V1)—anterior sensation
2. Occipital division of the second cervical nerve (C2)—posterior sensation
3. Great auricular nerve—postauricular sensation
4. Auriculotemporal/maxillary nerve (V2)—temporal sensation

E. Lymphatics

1. No distinct lymphatic drainage patterns in the scalp
2. No barriers to lymphatic flow
3. Lymphatics run in the subdermal and subcutaneous level

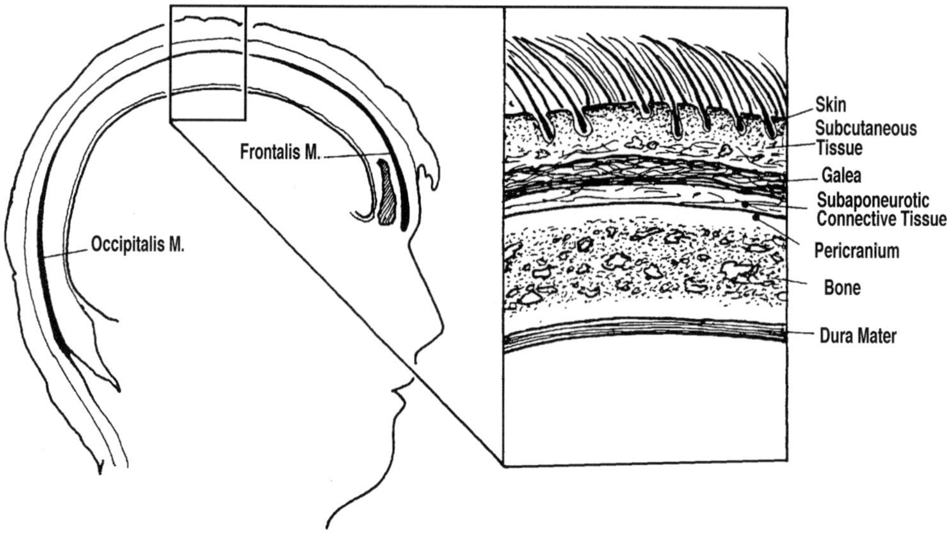

Figure 1 Layers of the scalp. (From Panje WR; et al.: *Local Flaps in Facial Reconstruction*. New York: Mosby-Year Book, 1995.)

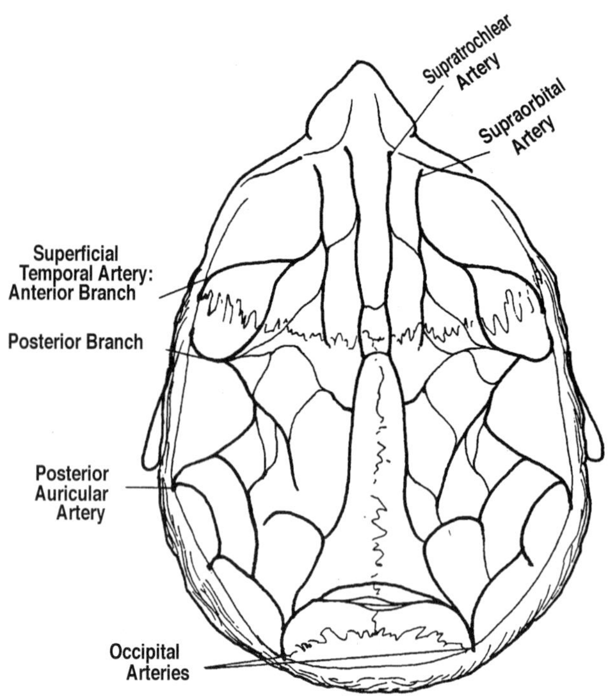

Figure 2 Vascular anatomy of the scalp. (From Panje WR; et al.: *Local Flaps in Facial Reconstruction*. New York: Mosby-Year Book, 1995.)

4. Drainage routes—parotid, preauricular, postauricular, upper cervical, occipital
5. Neck dissection indicated with regionally aggressive disease of the scalp and forehead

II. TRAUMATIC SCALP DEFECTS

A. Skin Grafting (Vascularized Bed Necessary)

1. Pericranium intact—skin graft can be applied directly to the defect.
2. If pericranium has been removed, galea frontalis, pericranial, or temporo-parietal fascial flaps can be rotated to cover exposed bone prior to skin grafting.
   - The outer table can be burred down to bleeding diploe to create a vascularized surface prior to grafting.
   - Subatmospheric pressure dressing can facilitate one-stage grafting, obviating the wait for granulation tissue to form over burred calvarium.

B. Local Flaps

1. Cranial convexity limits usable flap length.
2. Galea scoring increases the length of flaps. The blood vessels run in the subcutaneous tissue

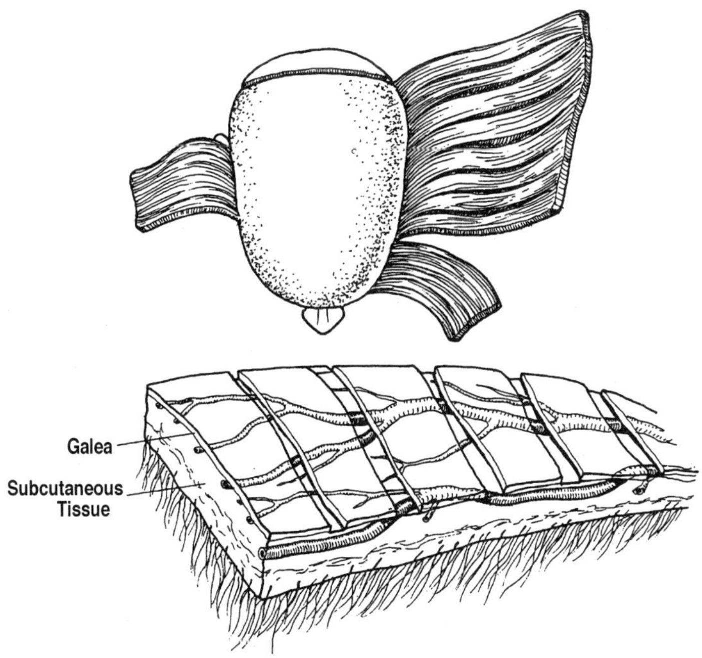

Figure 3 Scoring of the galea to increase usable scalp flap surface area. (From Panje WR; et al.: *Local Flaps in Facial Reconstruction.* New York: Mosby-Year Book, 1995.)

above the galea. Scoring too deeply can result in transection of these vessels and compromise of flap viability (Fig. 3).

3. Up to approximately 30% of the surface area (10 cm^2) of the scalp can be covered with adjacent tissue. This should be expected to be less in cases with a history of irradiation or previous surgery.
4. Rotational flaps
   - Opposing flaps work well.
   - Posterior flap of the reconstruction should be designed with its base in the occipital region to take advantage of the skin laxity in this region.
   - A skin graft may be necessary in a portion of the donor site if the flap cannot be expanded adequately to cover both recipient and donor sites.
5. Orticochea flap (Fig. 4) three or four flap designs have been described based on the major vessels of the scalp (supratrochlear, superficial temporal, etc.) to cover defects up to 20 cm^2.
6. Juri flap (temporo-parieto-occipital flap) (Fig. 5)—most extensively used for anterior hairline and most reliable distally when delayed once or twice.

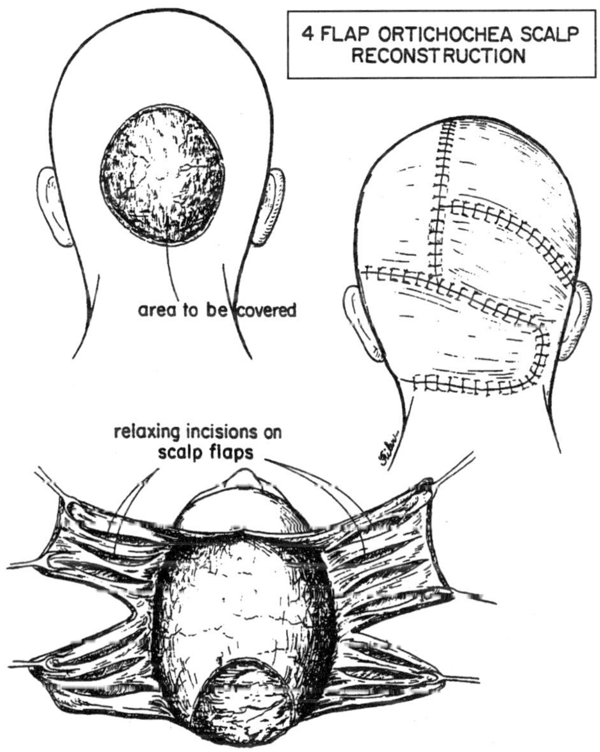

Figure 4 Ortichochea four-flap scalp reconstruction technique. (From Shestak KC; et al.: *Reconstruction of Defects of the Scalp and Skull.* Boston: Little Brown, 1994.)

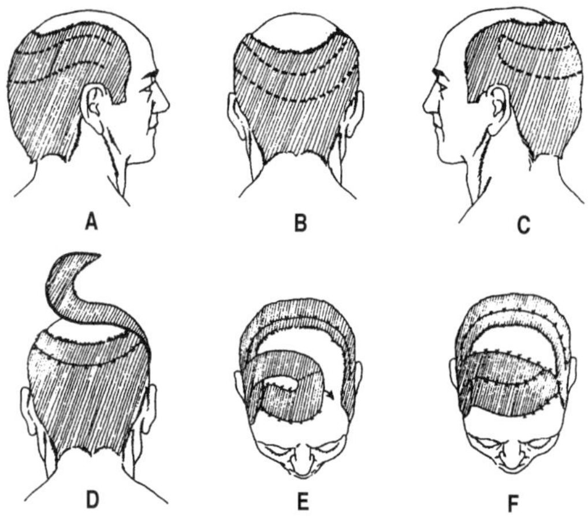

Figure 5 Temporo-parieto-occipital monopedicled flap. (From Juri J; et al.: Aesthetic aspects of reconstructive scalp surgery. *Clin. Plastic Surg.* 1981;8(2):243-254.)

C. Tissue Expansion (See Also Chapter 9)

1. Can resurface up to 50% of the scalp using tissue expansion techniques.
2. May result in significant molding of the skull (particularly in children). This generally remodels spontaneously, however.
3. Not used for open wounds. In these cases, a skin graft is generally placed initially followed by tissue expansion at a later date.

D. Microvascular Free Tissue Transfer

1. Latissimus dorsi muscle flap and skin graft are commonly used for coverage of large scalp defects.
2. The superficial temporal vessels are most frequently used recipient vessels. The temporal region should be explored first because of variability in the anatomy of the veins of this area.
3. Use of the facial or external carotid vessels usually requires that the flap be positioned at least partly in a preauricular location. Vein grafts may be needed in these situations.
4. The use of a skin paddle with the free tissue transfer in these cases is generally too bulky, and a skin graft is preferred.

E. Scalp Avulsions

1. Most frequently result from hair becoming caught in machinery; incidence has female predominance.
2. Avulsions occur at the level of the loose areolar plane along bony prominences (supraorbital/temporal).
3. Microvascular replantation is the treatment of choice, given that the avulsed scalp is often in good condition and amenable to replantation. For near-total avulsions, replantation is best, but acceptable vessels are difficult to find. Replantation should still be attempted if only an artery is found, and leeches can be used for venous drainage. The superficial temporal system is good to suture the replant into, but frequently vein grafts will be necessary.
4. The avulsed flap may be converted into a skin graft if replantation is not possible. Hair-bearing tissue is very unique and valuable, and should not be discarded. Definitive reconstruction should be delayed in these situations.

III. CALVARIUM

A. Calvarial Development and Growth

1. Intramembranous ossification—frontal, parietal, and temporal bones.
2. Endochondral ossification—occipital and sphenoid bones.
3. Cranium doubles in volume in the first year of life and triples in volume by 3 years of age.
4. Ninety percent of calvarial growth is complete by age 7.

B. Calvarial Anatomy

1. Three layers are present in the adult calvarium—outer table, diploe, and inner table. These are not present in the neonatal period but develop during early childhood.
2. Parietal cranium is on average the thickest (good for calvarial bone harvest site).

IV. CALVARIAL DEFECTS

A. Factors Influencing Need for Reconstruction

1. Size—smaller defects are less likely to require reconstruction as they are less noticeable and do not compromise protection of the underlying brain. There is, however, no single critical-size

defect that always requires reconstruction. Each case must be individualized.

2. Non–hair-bearing areas of scalp (i.e., forehead) tolerate even small defects poorly. The underlying contour irregularity tends to be very noticeable.

B. Autogenous Reconstruction

Autogenous reconstruction is dependent upon the take of bone grafts. The margins of the defect should always be debrided back to bleeding bone.

1. Rib
   - Large volume is available, particularly as each rib may be split in two, doubling the graft volume.
   - Rib harvest should be accomplished using an incision between the anterior and posterior axillary lines.
   - No more than two adjacent ribs should be excised to prevent instability of the chest wall.
   - The ribs should be harvested subperiosteally to promote bone regeneration.
   - Ribs are similar in contour to the skull, so little shaping is required.
   - "Washboard effect" may occur in rib cranioplasty due to the seams between adjacent ribs. As such, this form of reconstruction is generally a poor choice in cranioplasties involving the forehead.
2. Calvarium (Fig. 6)—parietal skull posterior to the coronal suture and away from the midline (to avoid the sagittal sinus) is generally the preferred site for harvest.
   - In situ harvest

     Preferred for small grafts.

     Harvest is accomplished by burring a trough around graft site into the diploe. This allows the osteotome to be used at the appropriate angle and minimizes the step-off between the donor site and the surrounding skull. The most common error at this point is the failure to burr deeply enough, resulting in too superficial a graft harvest.

     Once the trough is completed, a side-cutting burr is used to undermine the edges of the graft and facilitate the placement of a 20-mm curved osteotome, which is slowly worked around the periphery of the graft until the harvest is complete.

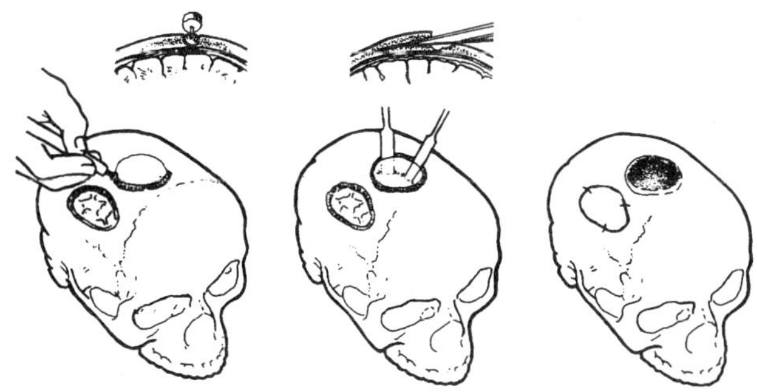

Figure 6 Technique for in situ harvest of calvarial bone graft. (Left) High-speed burr outlines the limits of the graft. (Middle) Osteotome separating the outer and inner cortex. (Right) Outer cortex graft used to cover lateral defect. (From Shestak KC; et al.: *Reconstruction of Defects of the Scalp and Skull*. Boston: Little Brown, 1994.)

   - Extracranial harvest

     Preferred for large grafts.

     A craniotomy is performed, and the outer and inner tables of the skull are split from one another ex vivo.

     The inner table is placed back into the donor site, and the outer table is used for graft material.
3. Iliac crest
   - Potential source for cranioplasty grafts, but generally not used due to relatively limited volume, contour mismatch, and abdominal morbidity (e.g., herniation).
   - Iliac crest is more useful as a source of cancellous bone.
4. Alloplastic cranioplasty
   - Only used in defects without a history of infection.
   - Great care should be used when placed in proximity to the frontal sinus.
   - Smooth contour and the absence of a donor site are the primary advantages.
   - Soft tissue envelope overlying the reconstruction should be without significant scarring or a history of irradiation.
   - Materials (see also Chapter 12)

Methylmethacrylate (acrylic)—least expensive material. The hardening process is exothermic and may generate significant heat. As such, an irrigation of cool saline should be used during this time. The acrylic used should be large enough to cover the entire defect. Additional acrylic added onto the initial reconstruction often forms seams that are prone to fragmentation. Wires should be used to span the cranial defect prior to placement of the acrylic to act as scaffolding and increase the stability of the reconstruction.

Calcium phosphate cements (bioceramics)—these are the most expensive of all options in cranioplasty. They are generally packaged as powders that are mixed with solution to form a paste, which hardens in an isothermic reaction. Osteoconductivity or bony ingrowth into the material has been demonstrated in some cases as the calcium cement is resorbed. These materials are highly biocompatible, with little evidence of tissue reaction.

V. FOREHEAD RECONSTRUCTION

A. Aesthetic Subunit Principle

Reconstruction should be accomplished as a single subunit if possible. In defects greater than 50% of the forehead, the remainder of the forehead may be excised and incorporated into the reconstruction.

B. Surgical Options

1. Skin grafting
   - Full-thickness donor sites superior (cephalad) to the clavicle are preferred. The supraclavicular area is a good choice in older patients.
   - Pericranium or another vascularized bed must be present to allow for successful grafting. Temporoparietal fascia flaps or galeafrontalis flaps may be used to provide a vascularized bed, if necessary.
2. Local flaps
   - Generally limited to the reconstruction of small defects in the forehead due to the lack of suitable adjacent tissue for transfer.
   - A medial skin island can be created by undermining the lateral skin from the frontalis muscle.
3. Tissue expansion
   - Can be utilized if sufficient forehead remains to be expanded for coverage.
   - Provides the best color and texture match for forehead defects, but requires a two-stage procedure.
4. Free tissue transfer
   - Capable of providing single-stage coverage of large forehead defects.
   - Choices for donor site are limited, with radial forearm flap often the best option to provide a large volume of skin in a thin flap with a long pedicle.
   - Color match is problematic.

34

Orbital Surgery

Peter J. Taub, M.D., and H. Peter Lorenz, M.D.
David Geffen School of Medicine at UCLA, Los Angeles, California, U.S.A.

I. NORMAL ANATOMIC RELATIONSHIPS

A. Eye fissure follows the pattern of the eyebrow (desirable angle off the horizontal is approximately 2° lateral elevation)

B. Intercanthal distance (ICD)—distance between the medial canthi. Normal is 28–32 mm (which roughly equals the orbital fissure distance from medial to lateral canthus).

C. Interorbital distance (IOD)—distance between the lacrimal crests as measured on a posteroanterior cephalogram. Normal is 24–32 mm in males and 22–28 in females.

D. Interpupillary distance (IPD)—distance between the pupils. Normal is 55–65 mm.

E. Upper eyelid overlaps the iris by 1–2 mm.

II. PREOPERATIVE EVALUATION

Preoperative evaluation includes a thorough history and physical examination, cephalogram, and computed tomography (CT) scan of the head with three dimensional reconstruction. Patients should also have a full ophthalmologic examination. The following cephalometric lines may be traced on a posteroanterior cephalogram (Fig. 1):

A. D-D line—line between the lacrimal crests.

B. T-T line—line between the temporal crests 1 cm above the supraorbital rim. Also measured is the optimal distance to the midline (13 mm in adults).

C. I point—point between the superior central incisors.

D. LM point—lateral point of the posterior molar.

E. I-S line vertical midline from between the I point to the sella turcica.

F. M point—point found along a line parallel to LM-T and perpendicular to point T.

G. I-M line—line from the I point through the dacrion on each side to a point above the T-T line.

H. LM-I line—occlusal plane of the maxilla.

I. T-M line—line parallel to the LM-I line; passes through the lateral temporal crest (T) and perpendicularly intersects with line I-M.

III. SURGICAL APPROACHES

There are several surgical approaches to the orbit. They are used alone or in combination, depending on the area of the orbit undergoing surgery. They include:

A. Coronal incision—placed posterior to the anterior hairline.

B. Lateral upper blepharoplasty incision.

C. Lower blepharoplasty incision (transcutaneous or transconjunctival with or without lateral canthotomy).

D. Brow incision.

E. Maxillary gingivobuccal sulcus incision.

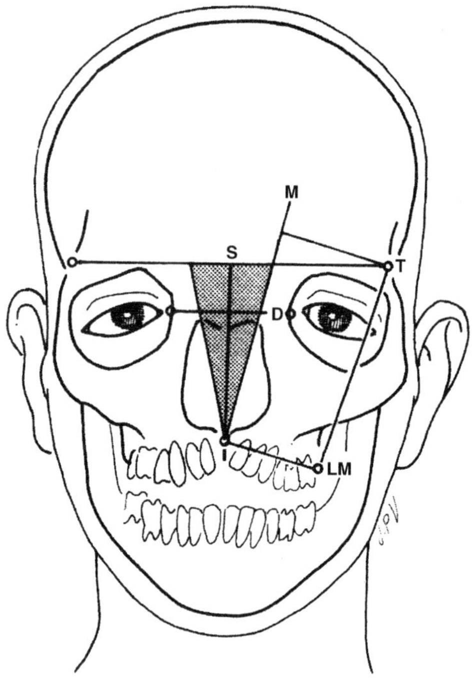

Figure 1 Orbital landmarks.

IV. POSTOPERATIVE COMPLICATIONS

A. Diplopia—usually due to acute globe repositioning or extraocular muscle imbalance.

B. Ectropion of the lower eyelid—often due to lower eyelid incisions.

C. Sinusitis.

V. ORBITAL HYPERTELORISM

A. Condition in which the distance between the orbital cavities is increased.

B. Seen with certain craniosynostosis syndromes, such as Apert and Crouzon's syndromes.

C. May be associated with premature fusion of the frontonasoethmoid complex, resulting in failure of the orbits to move toward the midline.

D. May be seen with various degrees and locations of facial clefting.

E. Severity is classified into three degrees:

- 1st degree—interorbital distance of 30–34 mm.
- 2nd degree—interorbital distance of 34–40 mm.
- 3rd degree—interorbital distance >40 mm.

F. Surgical correction

- Subperiosteal dissection within the orbit allows for mobilization of the bony structures.
- Osteotomies may be designed to advance the bony structures of the orbit uniformly toward the midline or to rotate the bony structures around a pivot point between the superior central incisors (right side of the midface rotates clockwise and the left side rotates counterclockwise).
- It is important to leave the medial canthal ligament attached to the orbital wall, while the lateral canthal ligament is left unattached to avoid tension across the aperture of the eye.
- It is necessary to evaluate and correct any associated nasal deformities.
- Nasal projection will be lost if bone is resected centrally and not replaced with adequate bone graft.

VI. ORBITAL DYSTOPIA

A. May occur in either the vertical or horizontal plane.

B. Must be distinguished from ocular dystopia, where portions of the orbit are displaced, as may occur following trauma.

VII. VERTICAL ORBITAL DYSTOPIA

A. Condition in which the orbital cavities do not lie in the same horizontal plane.

B. Etiologies of vertical orbital dystopia include:

- Craniofacial microsomia
- Craniosynostosis
- Facial clefting
- Hyperpneumatization of the frontal sinus
- Torticollis

VIII. HORIZONTAL ORBITAL DYSTOPIA

A. Condition in which the normal interorbital distance is altered.

B. In orbital hypertelorism, the orbits are displaced laterally. The orbits are diplaced medially in hypotelorism.

C. Surgical correction is through a box osteotomy, as described by Tessier.

D. Postoperative diplopia is more common with vertical manipulation of the orbit rather than horizontal manipulation.

IX. EXORBITISM

A. Condition in which there is a decrease in the volume of the bony orbit in the presence of normal soft tissue volume, resulting in forward protrusion of the globe.

B. Differs from exophthalmos, in which there is increased soft tissue volume in the presence of a normal bony orbit volume.

C. The eyelids may not close, leading to exposure keratitis of the cornea and loss of vision.

D. Herniation of the globe may occur with sneezing or coughing.

E. Etiologies include:

- Craniofacial dysostosis.
- Fibrous dysplasia.
- Frontal sinus mucocele.
- Osteoma.
- Traumatic disruption of the orbit.

F. When diagnosed in the neonatal period, temporizing maneuvers include topical lubricating agents and lateral tarsorrhaphy.

G. The distance from the lateral orbital rim to the cornea can be measured with a Hertel exophthalmometer (normal distance is 16–18 mm).

H. Reconstruction procedures currently include monobloc advancement, two-stage fronto-orbital advancement and LeFort III extracranial advancement, and/or outward rotation of the lateral wall combined with blowout of the medial and inferior walls of the orbit (described by Tessier).

X. POSTTRAUMATIC ENOPHTHALMOS

A. Enophthalmos is the posterior displacement of the globe into the bony orbit.

B. Clinically, the patient may show deepening of the supratarsal fold and malposition of the lateral canthus.

C. Etiologies include:

- Orbitozygomatic complex fracture, the most common cause, usually occurring with an orbital floor fracture.
- Globe immobilization following traumatic entrapment of the ocular musculature.
- Loss of orbital fat.
- Scarring of the retrobulbar tissue.

D. Mild deformity is corrected with autogenous bone graft (rib or calvarial) to increase the volume of the orbit. Prosthetic components (silicone, metal, or Medpore) are occasionally used.

35

Noncongenital Ear Reconstruction

Marc E. Mani, M.D.
Los Angeles, California, U.S.A.
Larry H. Hollier, M.D.
Texas Children's Hospital and Baylor College of Medicine, Houston, Texas, U.S.A.

Reconstruction of acquired ear deformities presents multiple challenges due to the complex cartilage structure, the thin skin coverage, and inconsistent blood supply. However, knowledge of the fundamental principles and a systematic approach can make ear reconstruction a rewarding experience for both surgeon and patient.

I. ANATOMY (FIG. 1)

A. Arterial Supply

1. The superficial temporal artery supplies the scapha and triangular fossa via a direct auricular branch.
2. The posterior auricular artery supplies the concha through perforators.

B. Venous Drainage

1. Retromandibular and posterior auricular veins.
2. These then drain into the external jugular system.

C. Nerve Supply

1. The great auricular nerve (C2-3) innervates the lower auricle, including both lateral (anterior branch) and medial (posterior branch) surfaces.
2. The auriculotemporal nerve (V3) innervates the superolateral surface of the ear.
3. The lesser occipital nerve supplies the superior aspect on the medial side.
4. The auricular branch of the vagus (nerve of Arnold) supplies the concha.

D. Aesthetic Relationships

1. The long axis of the ear is inclined at approximately 20°. In males, this varies between 10 and 30°, and in females between 2 and 20°.
2. The ear's vertical height roughly equals the distance between the lateral orbital rim and the root of the helix.
3. The width of the ear is 55% of the height.
4. The helical rim protrudes about 2 cm at the lobule and 1 cm at the apex.
5. The helical apex lies at the level of the eyebrow.

II. POSTTRAUMATIC RECONSTRUCTION

A. Exam

1. A full evaluation of the tympanic membrane for hemotympanum and the external auditory canal for lacerations and CSF leaks is imperative.
2. A thorough neurologic exam, including facial nerve function, should be performed.

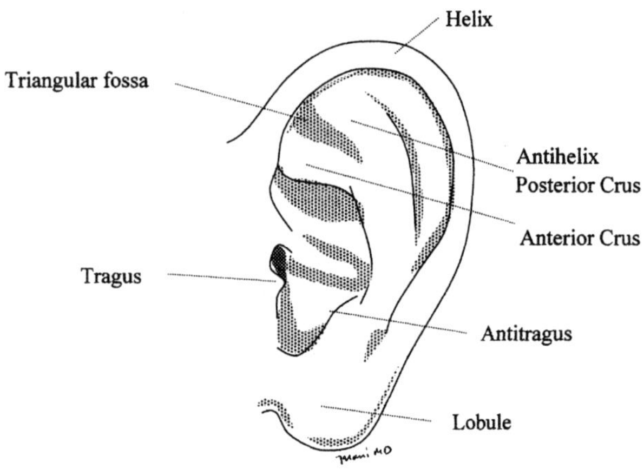

Figure 1 Anatomy of the auricle.

B. Debridement

1. Since the ear is highly vascular, minimal debridement is necessary following ear trauma. However, because of the risk of chondritis, all questionably viable and crushed cartilage should be removed.
2. Copious irrigation and prophylactic (broad-spectrum) antibiotics should be used.
3. Lacerations should be repaired within 12 h of injury.

C. Repair

1. A field block of local anesthesia at the base of the ear is adequate and preserves the structural relationships of the auricle itself.
2. For repair, suturing should begin at the depth of the wound and continue outward.
3. Cartilage sutures are rarely necessary and may increase the risk of chondritis. They should be used only when required to maintain the gross structure of the ear.
4. Nonadherent, conforming dressings without pressure points should be used.
5. The head is elevated for several days.

D. Otohematoma

1. Otohematoma is a collection of blood that accumulates between the perichondrium and cartilage.
2. A fibrotic, thickened clot distorts the cartilage.
3. It may manifest as severe pain in the post-operative period.
4. Early treatment consists of drainage and the use of conforming bolsters for approximately 7–10 days.
5. Late treatment may require carving of the cartilage to reestablish definition.

E. External Auditory Canal

1. Lacerations should be repaired and stented for 3–4 months.
2. Cicatricial stenosis may be treated by Z-plasty, scar excision, or skin grafting, followed by stenting.

F. Avulsions—Skin Loss with Exposed Cartilage

1. If the perichondrium is intact, a skin graft may be used.
2. If no perichondrium is present, methods that may be used include:
   - Wedge resection of the defect
   - Use of a postauricular flap to cover the defect
   - Removal of the cartilage and skin grafting the exposed raw surface of the postauricular skin
   - Healing by secondary intention

G. Avulsions—Full Thickness with Loss of Skin and Cartilage

1. Ear segment not available—one may use open treatment (as in human bites and gross contamination); for smaller defects, wedge excision and primary closure may be used.
2. Ear segment available
   - Small segments—may be directly reattached as a composite graft if treated within 12 h of injury.
   - Large segments

     Pocket principle—consists of dermabrasion of the skin of the amputated part, reattachment of the part to the ear base and burial under a retroauricular pocket of skin. The buried part is exteriorized 2 weeks later and allowed to reepithelialize or is skin grafted. A loss of ear definition is common with this method.

Fenestration—involves removing the skin from the posterior aspect of the amputated part, fenestration of the cartilage, and reattachment of the part of the ear base. This is then secured on a bed created in the retroauricular area. This is allowed to heal as a composite graft and later elevated with skin grafting of the post-auricular surface.

H. Near Total Avulsions

1. Microvascular replantation is the best option if donor and recipient vessels are available.
2. The superficial temporal artery is used as recipient vessel, and vein grafts are usually needed.
3. If no venous anastomosis is done, leeches may be employed.

III. BURN RECONSTRUCTION

A. Burns often present a greater reconstructive challenge, as the periauricular skin is often severely scarred and not usable in the reconstruction.

B. A rib cartilage framework is often necessary due to the extensive damage.

C. Coverage is most often accomplished with a temporoparietal fascia flap. However, the temporal vessels may have also been damaged by the burn injury, and preoperative Doppler examination should be done to ensure the availability of these vessels for the reconstruction.

IV. POSTONCOLOGIC RECONSTRUCTION

A. General Principles

1. Histological verification of complete excision should be confirmed on final pathology prior to any attempts at reconstruction. The visible margins of the tumor may be misleading as these cells may migrate along the plane of the auricular cartilage.
2. A CT scan of the temporal bone should be ordered if there is a question of extension to the bony canal or mastoid and for recurrent tumors.
3. For squamous cell carcinoma, wedge resection with cartilage excision is usually adequate
4. Skin resection alone may suffice for small basal cell carcinomas.

B. Tumors

1. May be benign (actinic keratosis, keratoacanthoma, sebaceous or keratinous cysts) or malignant.
2. Malignant tumors include squamous cell carcinoma (50–60%), basal cell carcinoma (30–40%), and melanoma (2–6%).

C. Lymph Node Evaluation

1. The concha and meatus drain to the parotid and infraauricular nodes.
2. The external canal and medial surface drain to the mastoid and infraauricular nodes.

V. RECONSTRUCTION BY REGION

In reconstructing the ear, it is important to remember that the majority of the conchal bowl may be harvested for grafting or resected without compromise of the structure of the ear.

A. Upper/Middle Third Defects

1. Wedge resection with primary closure (Fig. 2)
   - This may be done in the middle third of the helix, provided no more than 1 cm of conchal rim is resected.

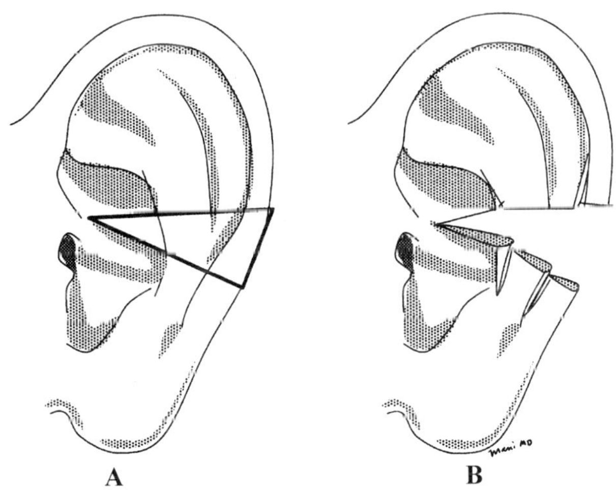

Figure 2 Wedge resection. (A) Resection is tapered anteriorly. (B) Full-thickness relaxing incisions allow closure without distortion of auricular shape.

- Relaxing incisions through lateral skin, cartilage, and medial skin inside the helical rim and at the conchal rim allow for the advancement of the helical rim, antihelical, and conchal sections.

2. "Tongue-and-groove" technique (Fig. 3)
   - This method involves staggering the lines of skin and cartilage incision so that a tongue of cartilage may be inserted between a groove of medial and lateral skin flaps.
   - Allows for a more structurally sound closure with less potential for notching of the reconstruction.
3. Antia-Buch flap (Fig. 4)
   - Can be used for helical defects less than 2 cm in both the upper and middle third of the ear.
   - Superior and inferior chondrocutaneous flaps are raised (Fig. 4B).
   - A V-Y advancement from the helical root is also created.
   - Dissection in the supra-perichondrial plane on the medial (posterior) aspect of the auricle is necessary to adequately mobilize the segments (Fig. 4C).
   - The margins of the flaps are then advanced and closed.

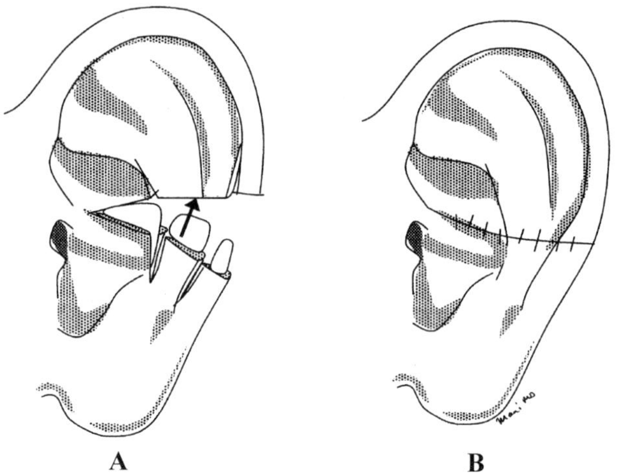

Figure 3 "Tongue-and-groove" technique (A) Incisions through skin and cartilage are staggered to leave cartilage "tongues." (B) Closure.

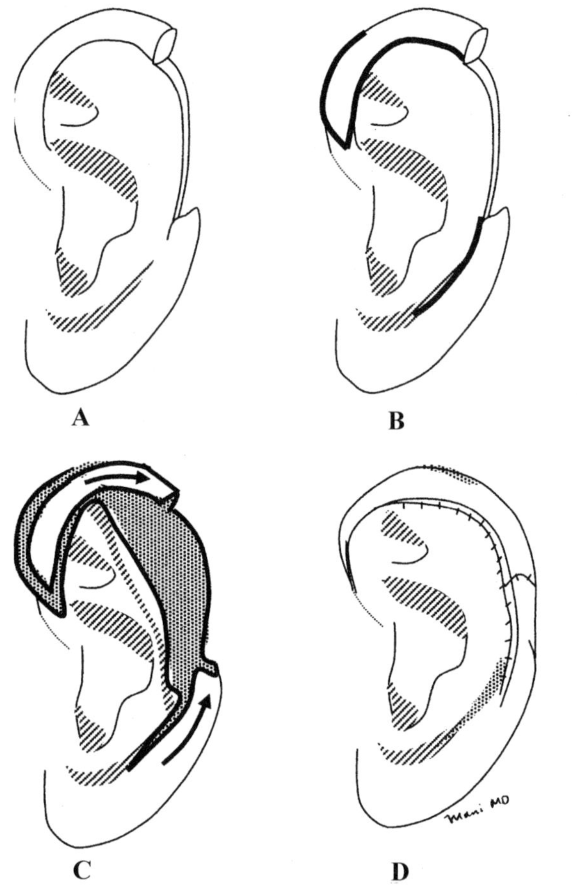

Figure 4 Antia-Buch flap. (A) Helical defect. (B) Lines of incision for flaps. (C) V-Y chondrocutaneous flap superiorly and advancement flap inferiorly (borrowing from the laxity of the lobule) are raised. (D) Resulting normal-appearing, slightly shortened ear.

4. Tubed flap (Fig. 5)
   - This technique should be used for helical rim defects only.
   - The skin flap is raised and tubed in the first stage (Fig. 5A). The tube may be raised in a pre- or postauricular position depending on the nature of the defect.
   - The tube is divided at one end at a second stage at least 7 days following the initial procedure (Fig. 5B). This is then inset to one end of the auricular helical defect (Fig. 5C).
   - Following another delay, the remaining tube is divided and inset to the ear (Fig. 5D).

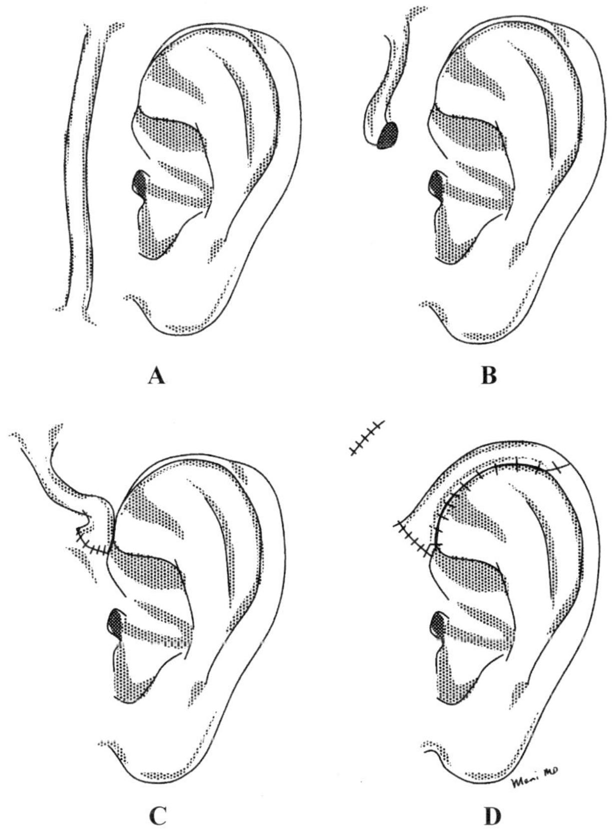

Figure 5 Tubed flap. (A) Superior helical rim defect with preauricular flap raised and tubed (Stage 1). (B) Caudal end of tube reelevated. (C) Caudal end of tube sutured to anterior helical root (Stage 2). (D) Cranial end of tube inset to remnant of helical rim (Stage 3).

5. Postauricular flap (Fig. 6)
   - A postauricular skin flap is raised and sutured to the lateral auricular skin at the margin of the defect.
   - After a delay of at least 7 days, the base of the postauricular flap is divided, turned under and inset to medial skin of the auricle to reform the helical rim.
   - Rib or other cartilage grafts may be incorporated into the flap at the time of final inset for structural support.
6. Composite grafts
   - These are useful for defects generally less than 1.5 cm in greatest diamter.
   - The contralateral ear is the most frequent donor site, particularly the helical root, where a small composite graft may be harvested and closed primarily.
   - The grafts work best if the wound is allowed to granulate for a short time preoperatively to improve the vascularity of the recipient bed.
   - Cooling of the graft in the early postoperative period (24 h) may improve survival of the graft by lowering its metabolic rate.
   - Prior to full revascularization, these composite grafts undergo a characteristic sequence of color changes, typically white to blue to pink.
7. Costal cartilage framework
   - Cartilage losses of greater than 2 cm may require a costal cartilage framework to replace the structural defect.
   - Autogenous costal cartilage can be harvested from any medial rib segment, but the synchon-

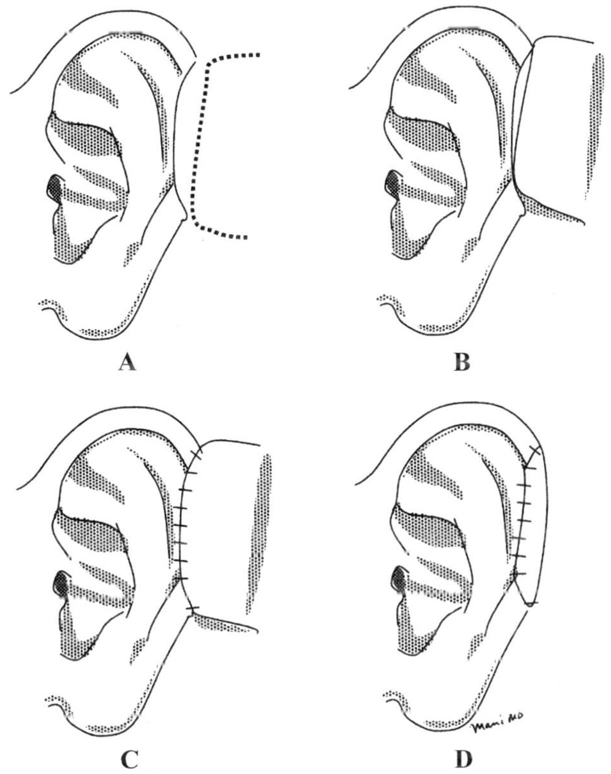

Figure 6 Postauricular flap. (A) Helical defect with flap outlined. (B) Flap raised. (C) Flap sutured to lateral auricular skin at defect margin (D) Flap base is divided, turned under and inset to medial skin of auricle to reform the helical rim.

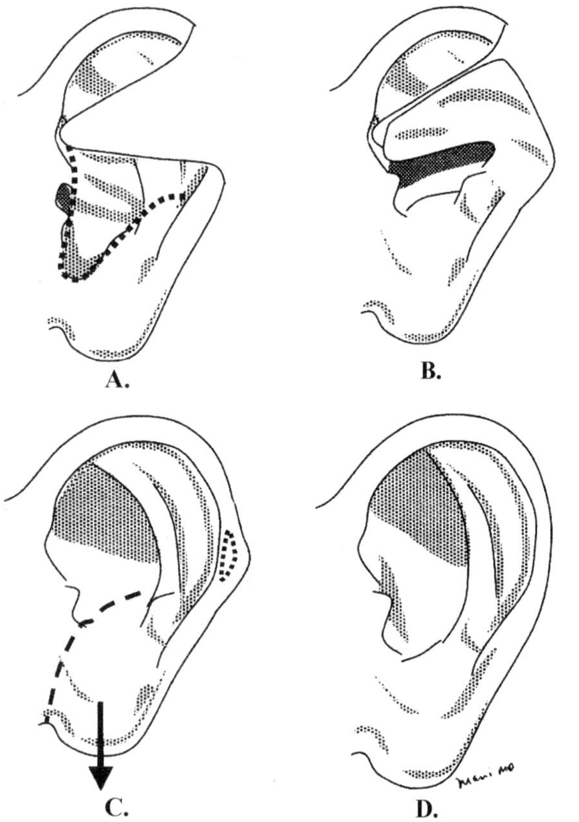

Figure 7 Orticochea flap. (A) Flap outlined. (B) Flap raised, containing the whole concha and carrying the lateral skin, cartilage, and medial skin with pedicle on the outer helix (at least 1 cm wide). (C) Pedicle is adjusted as outlined and the lobule pulled downward to make the auricle match the normal side in length.

drosis of the sixth and seventh ribs is preferred when large segments of cartilage are necessary.

- The medial aspect of the free-floating eighth rib is preferred for smaller segments and isolated helical support.
- These grafts may be carved based on a template fashioned from the normal contralateral ear.

8. Vascularized soft tissue coverage of the reconstruction usually requires a turn-down of the temporoparietal fascia pedicled on the superficial temporal vessels.
   - The superficial surface of the flap is developed in a plane just deep to the hair follicles in the subcutaneous tissue. Dissection too superficially will damage the follicles and result in alopecia. Dissection too deeply is usually manifest by bleeding from the veins on the superficial surface of the temporoparietal fascia.
   - Dissection should continue until the necessary length of flap has been elevated. However, it should be noted that the flap becomes random at a point approximately 12 cm above the helical root. Additional vascularized flap length is best achieved by posterior dissection.
9. Orticochea flap (Fig. 7)
   - This is a chondrocutaneous flap that is created by incising the concha (including the medial and lateral skin) and rotating this on a pedicle based on at least 1 cm of helical skin. The cartilage within the pedicle may be cut to improve the ease of rotation.
   - The flap is inset into the defect by sewing both skin layers, without need to suture the cartilage.
   - At a second stage (3 months later), the helix is corrected by adjustment of the pedicle, and the lobule is pulled down with releasing incisions through skin and cartilage.

B. Lower Third and Lobular Defects

1. Ear lobe
   - Half of the ear lobe may be excised as a wedge and closed primarily without resulting in a significant deformity.
   - Tears secondary to earrings pulling through ear lobe—these defects should be closed by exci-

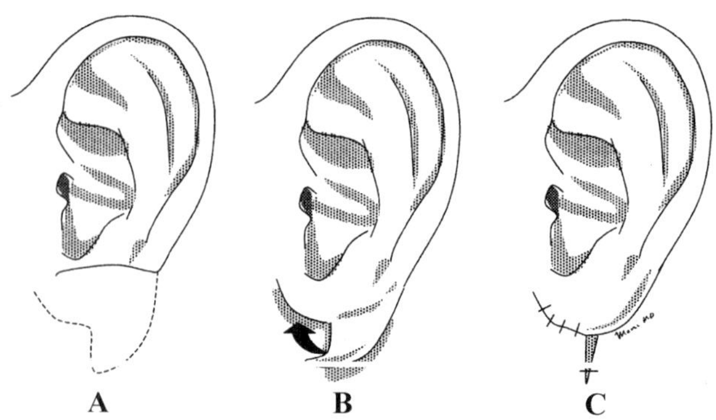

Figure 8 Rotation flap for lobule reconstruction. (A) Missing lobule. (B) Flap design, with posterior portion rotated under to form the medial skin. (C) Secondary defect closed primarily.

sing the epithelialized surfaces of the rent, and incorporating a Z-plasty such that a scar perpendicular to the lobule edge is avoided (since such a scar will contract and result in a notch in the earlobe).

- Missing ear lobe may be reconstructed using local skin flaps or contralateral conchal cartilage in a subcutaneous pocket.

An infra-auricular skin flap (Fig. 8) may be raised and turned under itself to recreate the lobule. The secondary defect is closed primarily.

Contralateral conchal cartilage may be placed in a subcutaneous pocket under the ear for 6 weeks, then raised as a composite flap (based superiorly on the auricle) and a skin graft placed on the medial aspect.

36

Cheek Reconstruction

Jamie P. Levine, M.D., and Barry M. Zide, M.D., D.M.D.
New York University Medical Center, New York, New York, U.S.A.

I. GENERAL CONSIDERATIONS

A. Small cheek defects can be closed primarily, after elliptical excision.

B. Keep the scar short and in the direction of skin lines.

C. When removing cancerous or precancerous lesions (melanoma in situ, etc.), consider delaying the reconstruction until all margins are proven histologically negative.

D. If the primary excision and closure leaves dog ears, these will not flatten out. One should plan on primary dog ear resection for a flat repair, or plan on revisions. The patient must be informed of this possibility.

E. If possible, avoid vertical incisions in the anterior and central cheek. These incisions should not be anterior to a line drawn vertically from the lateral canthus downward. These scars tend to be highly visible on direct (en face) view.

F. Large defects can occasionally be resurfaced with skin grafts, local flaps, or large transposition flaps from the neck and chest.

II. CHEEK ZONES

A. For larger defects, one can divide the cheek into aesthetic units to provide guidelines for reconstruction. These units have been separated into three overlapping aesthetic zones (Fig. 1):

- Zone 1—suborbital
- Zone 2—preauricular
- Zone 3—buccomandibular (includes oral lining when the defect is full thickness)

B. Each zone has specific reconstructive options, but smaller defects can be dealt with as described above.

C. One should avoid enlarging a defect into another zone for the best aesthetic outcome.

D. These zones do not have exact borders and overlap with each other to some degree. This allows for some flexibility when the reconstructive options are being planned.

III. ZONE 1—SUBORBITAL ZONE

A. Location

- The medial border is the nasolabial fold.
- The lateral border is the anterior sideburn.
- The inferior border is the gingival sulcus.
- The superior border is the lower eyelid skin.

B. Zone 1 is unique in that it can be further divided into three subunits—A, B, and C (Fig. 1). The main reason for this is the incorporation of the lower eyelid into Zone 1 territory. This area in itself has specific considerations that separate it from the rest of Zone 1.

- Subunit A and B—Full thickness skin grafts (FTSG) can be used, but this is discouraged if >5 mm depth. Full thickness skin grafting

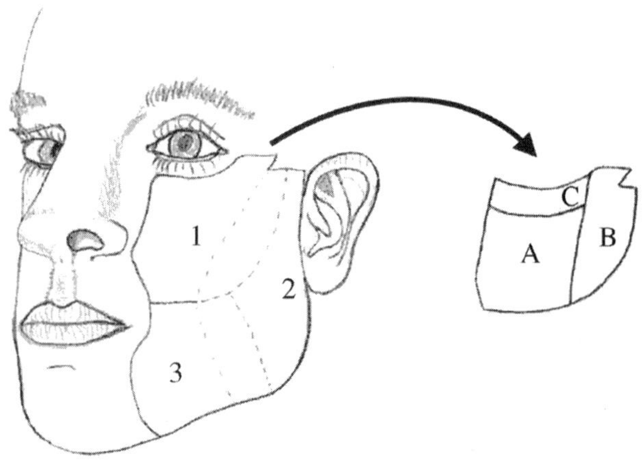

Figure 1 Line drawings of cheek aesthetic unit with three overlapping Zones 1, 2, and 3. Note that Zone 1 can be broken into three subunits: A, B, and C. (Adapted from Cabrera R; Zide BM: Cheek reconstruction. In: Aston SJ; Beasley RW; Thorne CHM, eds. *Grabb and Smith's Plastic Surgery*. Philadelphia: Lippincott-Raven Publishers, 1997.)

is best around the orbital margin. Patients can also disguise the graft with glasses.

- Subunit C—Location is the lower eyelid skin up to its junction with the cheek skin.
- Due to reasons of secondary contraction, split thickness skin grafts (STSG) tend to pull the lower lid inferiorly. Thus, FTSG in this region are required.
- Preferential skin graft harvest sites include preauricular, postauricular, or supraclavicular skin. These areas are more closely matched, for color and texture, to the native excised skin. Also, if there is excess, upper eyelid skin can be used.

C. When other closures, including direct closure and skin grafting, are considered either functionally or aesthetically undesirable, a local flap is the best option.

D. Even larger defects on the convex surface of the cheek will occasionally close secondarily with very little pull on the eyelid.

E. Rhomboid flap

- Very versatile flaps. Although each lesion has eight possible rhomboid flaps, the surgeon can usually find the optimal flap design for the given defect.
- Place donor site in relaxed skin tension lines.
- Best if based inferiorly to minimize edema and trap door effect.
- Flap design (Fig. 2):

  Place a circle around the defect, enough to include an acceptable margin.

  Lightly draw relaxed skin tension lines (RSTL) to encompass the defect.

  Draw darker lines of maximum extensibility (LME) to encompass the defect. The LME are perpendicular to the RSTL.

  Make the two possible rhomboids using the LME lines as two sides.

  Coming off the short rhomboid diagonal, draw the four possible flaps for each rhomboid.

  Choose the best ones based on the previously mentioned principles.

F. For smaller lesions up to 1.5 cm in size, a small posteriorly based rotation flap can be used for closure. This flap can be used with or without a backcut, depending on tension and overall flap rotation.

G. For larger Zone 1 cheek defects (> 3 cm), posteriorly based facial or cervicofacial flaps can be used.

- Cervicofacial flap dissection, in the subcutaneous plane, was first described in 1969. To improve blood supply and reliability, one can dissect in a deep plane (below SMAS) and incorporate this into the flap, similar to a deep-plane rhytidectomy.
- Posteriorly based facial and cervicofacial flaps survive better than anteriorly based flaps because the transverse branches of the facial and superficial temporal arteries are preserved.
- If a transposed flap, from below the lesion, crosses the inferior border of the mandible, the patient should be prepared for a subsequent W-plasty or Z-plasty revision. If possible, this can be done with the primary flap.
- If flap mobilization will leave a transverse incision on the cheek, this may be more noticeable aesthetically, especially in the younger patient, so the patient should be notified of this preoperatively.
- Deep-plane dissection allows for larger flaps to be taken. This is better for patients who

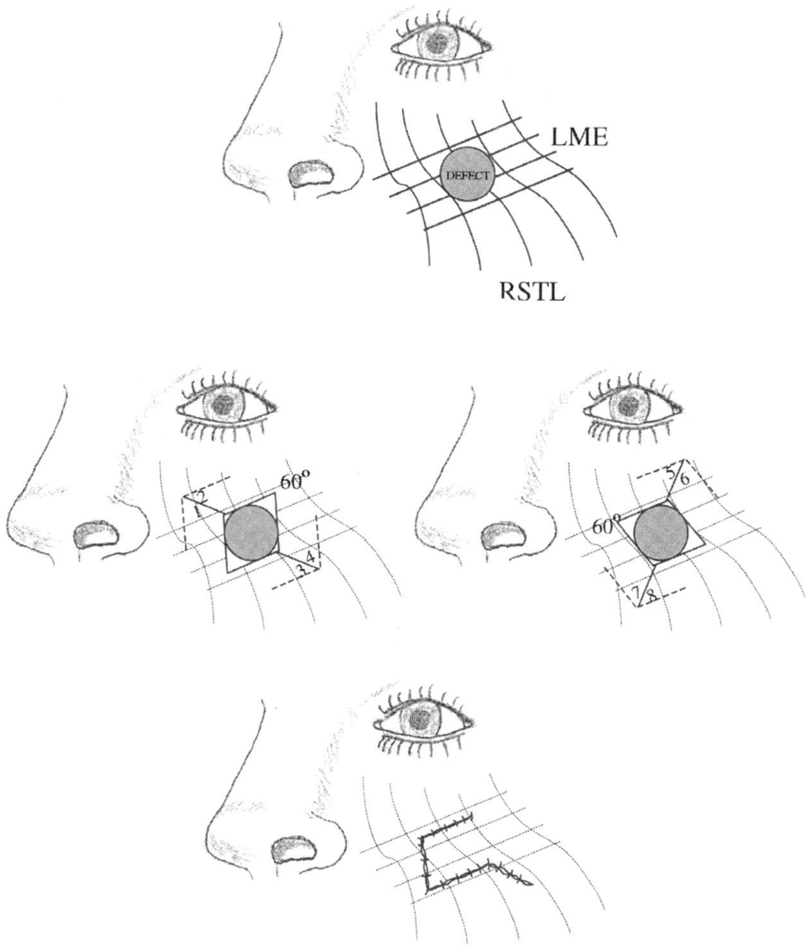

Figure 2 (Top) Note the orientation of the relaxed skin tension lines (RSTL) and the perpendicular orientation of the lines of maximum extensibility (LME). These are centered around the cheek defect. (Middle) The two proper rhomboids for this defect are shown and the associated flaps are noted (dashed lines). There are eight total possibilities for each defect. (Bottom) Although there are several choices for this defect, flap four satisfies the requirements discussed in the chapter and does not impinge on nearby structures. (Adapted from Cabrera R; Zide BM: Cheek reconstruction. In: Aston SJ; Beasley RW; Thorne CHM, eds. *Grabb and Smith's Plastic Surgery*. Philadelphia: Lippincott-Raven Publishers, 1997.)

are smokers and have a greater chance for distal flap loss.

- To prevent ectropion, the flap must be anchored to the periosteum of the anterior aspect of zygomatic arch and inferolateral orbital rim.
- Occasionally, fascia lata may be used along the lower eyelid to prevent ectropion.
- Lid-tightening procedures can be used any time the defect extends above the infraorbital rim. This decreases the postoperative risk of flap retraction and subsequent scleral show or ectropion.

H. If time constraints are not a problem, large tissue expanders can be placed via a remote face-lift or scalp incision, or within the lesion. The tissue expansion reservoirs can be placed behind the ear or under the scalp. Expansion continues for a 2- to 4-month period, or according to the patient's tolerance.

I. Serial excision is an excellent consideration for smaller lesions.

J. Some of these methods may require multiple operations and a long time period to complete the reconstruction. The plan should be discussed with the patient at length so that he or she understands what to expect and cooperation can be maximized.

IV. ZONE 2—PREAURICULAR ZONE

A. Location extends from the superolateral junction of helix and cheek, medially crosses from the sideburn to malar eminence, and inferiorly goes to the level of the mandible. All tissue over the parotid/masseteric fascia is included in this zone.

B. Skin grafting and local, primary closure techniques:

- Skin grafting in this zone may work well, especially in older patients. When skin grafts are used in this zone, however, they are relatively more hidden and less conspicuous than when used in the central face.
- Skin grafting has a limited application in the inferior part of Zone 2, except with squamous cell carcinoma (SCC), which may require an interval of observation.
- As there is usually skin excess in the preauricular region, elevation of this skin with advancement and subsequent closure is often a better choice than grafting. This advancement may be redone if required.
- The superior portion of Zone 2 may be amenable to horizontal resection, especially if it is posterior to the Z line. The horizontal dog ears can be carried medially and can be hidden in an upper blepharoplasty incision.
- Zone 2 defects should be reconstructed with flaps that are designed inferior to the lesion and posterior to the ear. Use anteriorly based cervicofacial flaps for this area.

C. Larger Zone 2 defects can be resurfaced with anterior based neck flaps.

- The primary flap can be delayed, which will help with the blood supply and overall reliability of the flap.
- The caudal platysma, if included, should be transected 4 cm below the mandible.
- Depending on the patient's needs, the lower level of the flap incision can be in the neck or below the clavicle. Neck incisions are visible. However, if the subplatysmal dissection is carried down posterior to the trapezial border and is below the clavicle when it is back-cut, the scar will be better hidden and the blood supply improved because of the subplatysmal dissection.

D. Large defects may require medially based cervicopectoral flaps. These flaps may extend onto the chest wall and receive additional blood supply from perforators coming from the internal mammary artery (IMA).

- Remain posterior to the trapezial border to avoid postoperative banding and scar contracture, which would require subsequent revision and/or Z-plasty.
- This flap can also be based laterally on thoracoacromial perforators and extended to include the anterior pectoral skin.

E. Other regional flaps include the deltopectoral, cervicohumeral, trapezius, pectoralis major, and latissimus dorsi flaps.

- The deltopectoral flap can be preexpanded, which can allow for primary closure and coverage of larger defects of the cheek.
- The trapezius flap can be used to provide bulk and can even be taken with bone if needed. The blood supply comes from the transverse cervical artery.
- The lower trapezius can even be elevated as an island flap and based on the above blood supply. A limited rotation arc can be present, due to variations in the venous drainage.
- The pectoralis major flap can provide both cheek coverage and lining if it is needed
- The latissimus dorsi flap has a long (8–12 cm in length) thoracodorsal vascular pedicle that allows for sufficient rotation to be used in the face. This flap has a relatively hidden donor site with minimal functional loss. The flap also provides soft tissue bulk from an area outside of the operative or irradiated field.
- Cervicohumeral flaps can be used for lower Zone 1 and 2 defects, and more recently it has been noted that an axial blood supply can be dissected out.

F. Microvascular free flaps may provide the best coverage for large full-thickness defects in these zones. They offer excellent versatility and have made some of the above-mentioned flaps historically important.

V. ZONE 3—BUCCOMANDIBULAR ZONE

A. Location

- Encompasses the lower anterior cheek area, inferior to suborbital Zone 1, and anterior to preauricular Zone 2.
- Reconstruction in this zone may require cheek skin and lining.
- This zone can also have associated/contiguous lip defects that require reconstruction.

B. On the central cheek, one can leave the wound to contract and granulate to help decrease the defect size. Scarring in this region will not cause an ectropion (unique to Zone 3). *Key point*: Mohs defects on convex surfaces will heal well in general.

C. Skin grafts are a poor choice for Zone 3 defects. The central cheek unit can be violated, and the wounds will then be visible on en face view. The graft's color mismatch will also be noticeable.

D. Vertical scars are preferred to horizontal scars in this zone. These scars are better positioned lateral to the Z line, where they will be less noticeable.

E. Lower Zone 3 scars are preferred to upper Zone 3 scars. Scars on the cheek prominence, as noted, are more noticeable. Nonbearded or upper malar eminence scars are more noticeable than on the lower, bearded (males) region that covers the scars.

F. Reconstruction can require intraoral lining and lip revision/functional restoration.

- Defects of the orbicularis oris or oral commissure will require functional sphincter reconstruction.
- Many of the previously mentioned flaps can be applied to these defects, either partially or alone.
- Small defects can be closed with simple transposition flaps or inferomedial-based cervicofacial flaps.
- Intraoral lining must be waterproof and saliva competent prior to external cheek closure.
- Tongue flaps are based on the paired axial lingual arteries. A tongue flap can help provide posterior oral lining, closure for cleft palate fistulas or floor of the mouth repair.
- Turnover or hinge flaps can provide lining for angle of the mouth defects. These flaps, along with the tongue flaps, require secondary coverage intraorally. Buccal fat pad, masseter crossover, and galeal flaps with periosteum do not require intraoral skin because they become quickly epithelialized. Muscle flaps will also reepithelialize spontaneously.
- Can fold or split many of above-mentioned flaps after delay, or two flaps can be used in combination.

G. These techniques (local or regional) have been mostly replaced with microvascular free flaps (MVFF).

- MVFF techniques can transfer large amounts of composite tissues needed for individualized reconstruction of various cheek defects. They are also distant from the area of excision or irradiation.
- Radial forearm free flaps can be harvested with a double skin paddle, vascularized palmaris longus, and antebranchial nerve if it is needed.
- In one step, this flap can provide both intraoral and cheek lining/coverage, static soft tissue support and sensation. Three-dimensional reconstruction of the defects can be matched.
- Tensor fascia lata (TFL) flap can also provide three-dimensional adaptability and provides a vascularized sling for missing soft tissue support.
- Parascapular free flap (fasciocutaneous) can be contoured to appropriately fill the soft issue defect. Vascularized bone can also be brought in with this free flap, if needed.

37

Nasal Reconstruction

Reza Sadrian, D.D.S., M.D.
San Diego, California, U.S.A.
Cynthia M. Goodman, M.D.
Greenbrae, California, U.S.A.
Larry H. Hollier, M.D.
Texas Children's Hospital and Baylor College of Medicine, Houston, Texas, U.S.A.

The nose is the most prominent facial feature and presents a reconstructive challenge because of its complex surface contour and composition. The choice of reconstructive method is based on the size, location, and depth of the defect.

I. ANATOMY

A. Components

1. Based on the underlying skeletal support, the nose can be divided into thirds.
   - The proximal third is supported by the bony nasal pyramid
   - The middle third is supported by the upper lateral cartilages
   - The distal third or lobule is supported by the alar (lower lateral) cartilages.
2. The septum is also critical to the support of the middle and distal third of the nose.

B. Layers

The nose is composed of three layers: skin, skeletal support, and mucosal lining. Each layer must be taken into consideration during reconstruction.

1. The skin is thick and sebaceous at the tip and alar rims.
2. The skin is relatively thin over the dorsum and sidewalls.

C. Aesthetic Subunits

1. The nose can be divided into the following aesthetic subunits: dorsum, sidewalls, tip, soft tissue triangles, columella, and alar-nostril sill (Fig. 1).
2. The borders between these subunits are transition areas where shadows from the contour of the nose fall. Incisions should be made along the subunit boundaries or in the midline of the nose to camouflage the scars. One should attempt to maintain the aesthetic subunits.

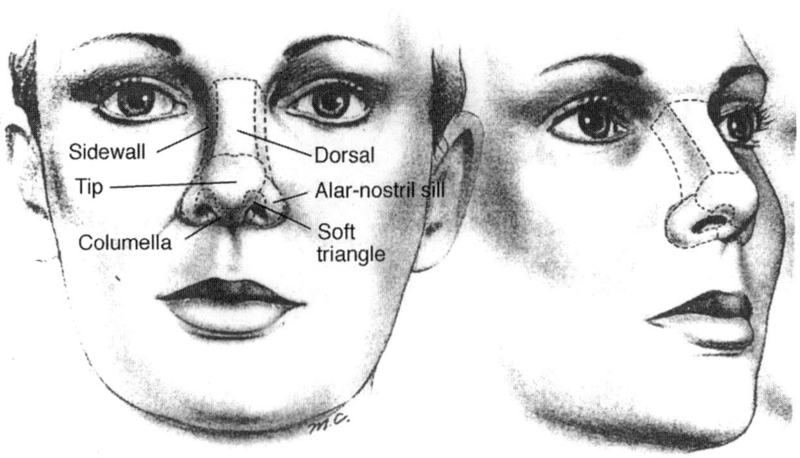

Figure 1 Nasal aesthetic subunits. (From Burget GC; Menick FI: *Aesthetic Reconstruction of the Nose*. St. Louis: Mosby, 1994.)

3. If the defect is greater than 50% of the subunit, the wound should be enlarged to include the entire subunit.

II. SKIN COVERAGE

A. Skin Grafts

1. Skin grafts are useful for partial-thickness defects on the dorsum or sidewall. This may be suboptimal since texture, thickness, and color need to match precisely or the reconstruction will look like a patch.
2. Common donor sites are the postauricular area for thin grafts and the supraclavicular area for thicker grafts.
3. The tip is not a good area for a skin graft due to the relatively thick sebaceous quality of the tissue in this location.

B. Composite Grafts

1. Full-thickness alar rim defects ≤1.5 cm in diameter may be reconstructed with auricular composite grafts consisting of skin and cartilage.
2. It is helpful to allow the margins of the wound to granulate to increase the take of these grafts.
3. It may also be helpful to cool the grafts postoperatively.
4. Composite grafts typically go through a characteristic color change from white to blue to pink over several days.
5. The graft may be harvested from the helical margin or the root of the helix.

III. LOCAL NASAL FLAPS

A. Rhomboid Flap (Fig. 2)

1. For small (<1.5 cm) dorsal and lateral sidewall defects, the rhomboid flap may be used in elderly patients with excess skin.
2. The donor defect should be designed so that its long axis is a line of minimal tension and along an aesthetic unit to camouflage the scar.

B. Bilobed Flap (Fig. 3)

1. Used for dorsal midline, tip, and adjacent supratip defects up to 2 cm in its greatest diameter.
2. Some of the dorsal hump may be shaved off to facilitate closure.
3. The second flap is used to close the donor defect.

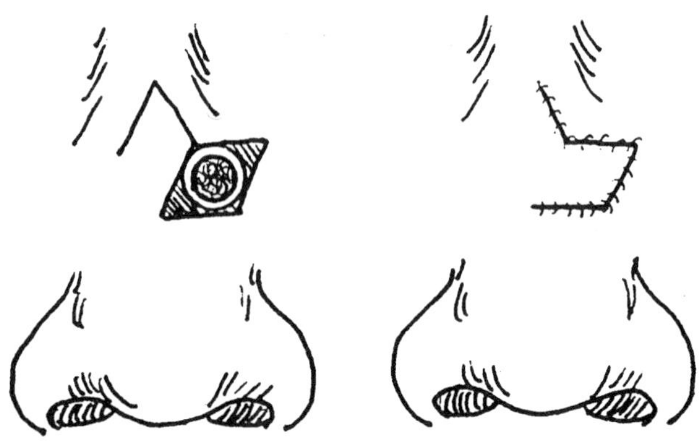

Figure 2 Rhomboid flap: defect and flap transfer.

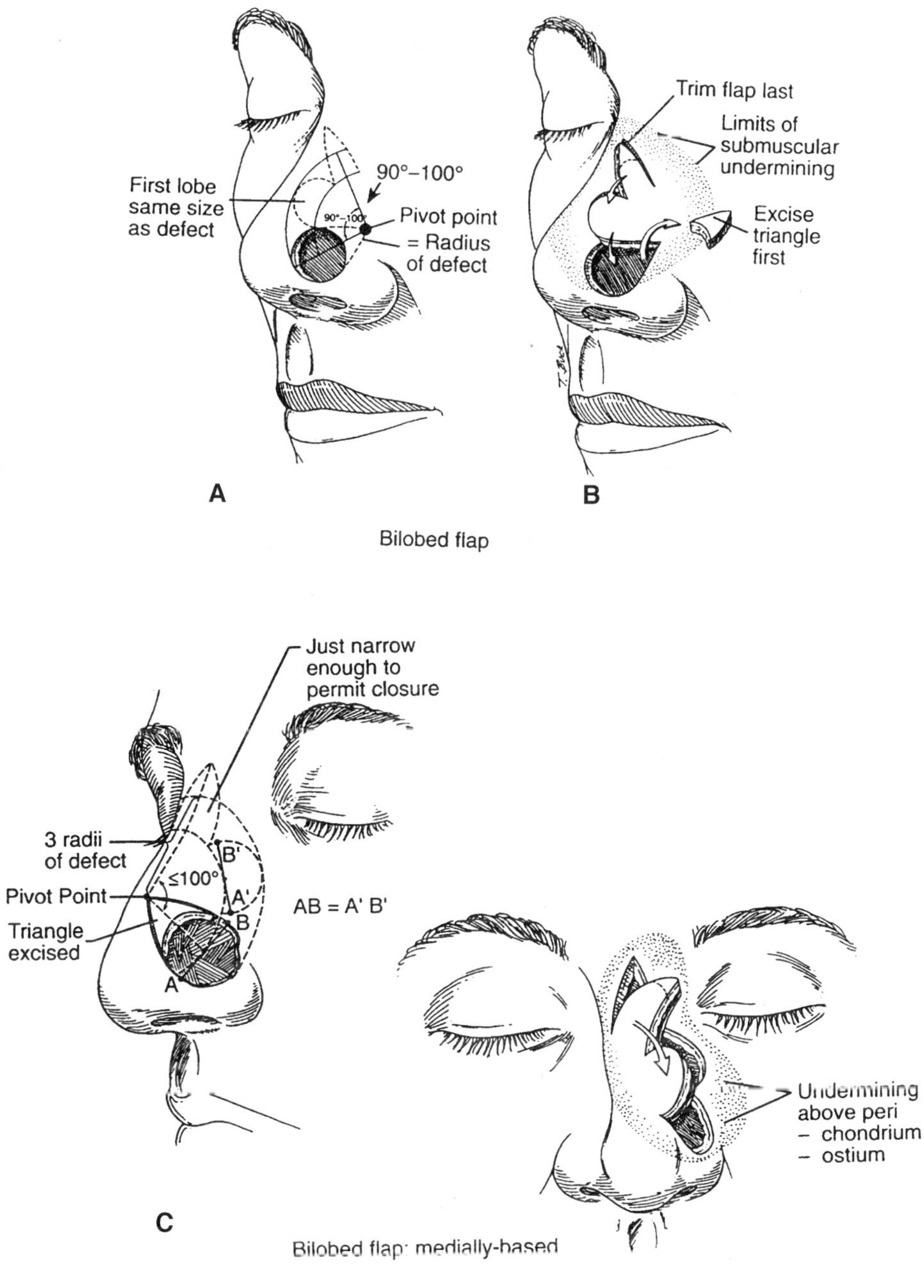

Figure 3 Design and transfer of bilobed flap. (From Burget GC, Menick FJ: *Aesthetic Reconstruction of the Nose*. St. Louis: Mosby, 1994.)

C. Dorsal Nasal Flap (Fig. 4)

1. Used for dorsal defects <2 cm and small supratip defects.
2. This is a rotation advancement flap of the dorsal nasal skin based laterally on the angular vessels and advanced caudally.
3. It may cause some cephalic tip rotation when used for larger defects close to the tip.

IV. REGIONAL FLAPS

A. Rotational/Advancement Cheek Flap

1. Dorsolateral nasal defects may be reconstructed with large rotational advancement cheek flaps.
2. This flap is based on the subdermal blood supply.
3. The inferior border of the incision is placed along the alar crease. A compensatory Burrow's tri-

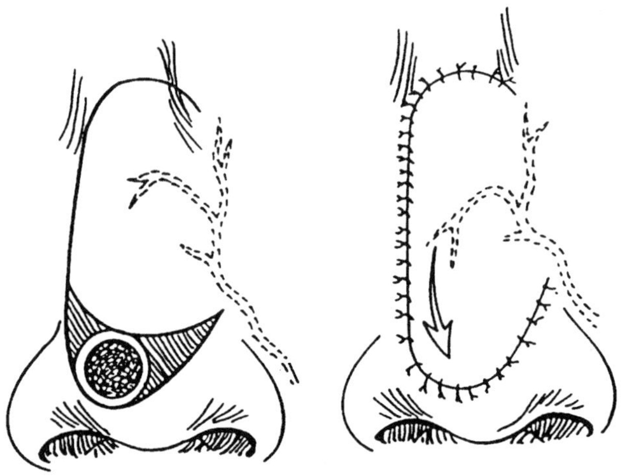

Figure 4 Dorsal nasal flap. (From Aston SJ; Beasley RW; Thorne CHM: *Grabb and Smith's Plastic Surgery*. 5th ed. Philadelphia: Lippincott-Raven, 1997.)

angle may be excised from the alar base and the nasolabial area.

4. In order to prevent flattening of the nasolabial groove, anchoring periosteal sutures to the deep dermis of the advanced flap may help recreate this angle.

B. Nasolabial Flap

1. Used for larger defects (≤2.5 cm) of the dorsum and sidewall.
2. This transposition flap can be based either superiorly or inferiorly.
3. The flap is elevated in the subcutaneous plane. This flap may also be based only on a subcutaneous pedicle to eliminate the dog-ear that results from flap transposition.

C. Glabellar Flap (Fig. 5)

1. Used for defects of the upper dorsum of the nose and medial canthus.
2. The glabellar skin can be transferred as a rotation, midline transposition flap, or an island flap. This flap is essentially a dorsal nasal flap with a prominent glabellar extension.

D. Paramedian Forehead Flap (Fig. 6)

1. Used for large defects encroaching on the columella, tip, or alar lobule and for subtotal and total nasal reconstruction.
2. This is an axial flap based on the supratrochlear artery, a terminal branch of the ophthalmic artery. The flap may also be based on the supraorbital or angular vessels.
3. To design the flap, a template of the defect is made and transposed onto the contralateral forehead, ensuring enough length to pivot on its vascular pedicle. To increase pedicle length, the flap can curve along the hairline or extend into the hairline and the hair secondarily removed.
4. The donor site may be closed primarily when the defect is ≤3 cm in size.
5. Preliminary forehead skin expansion will also help ease the close of the donor site. However, expanded skin has a tendency to contract and may deform the newly created nasal features when not anchored to the underlying skeletal support.

E. Gullwing Flap (Fig. 7)

1. Millard modified the paramedian forehead flap to include wide "wings" or transverse extensions over the natural horizontal furrows of the forehead.
2. This is useful for larger defects involving the nasal tip, infratip region, and lobule.

F. Scalping (Converse) Flap (Fig. 8)

1. For large total and near-total defects of the nose, the scalping flap may be used reliably.
2. It is elevated through a coronal incision behind the superficial temporal artery, extending to a skin paddle in the contralateral forehead. The frontalis muscle is not carried in the distal end of the flap.
3. The donor site on the forehead is closed with a full-thickness skin graft.

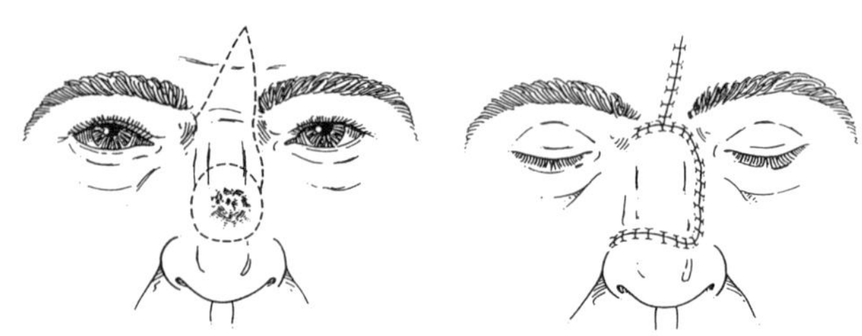

Figure 5 Glabellar flap. (From Jackson IT: *Local Flaps in Head and Neck Reconstruction*. St. Louis: Mosby, 1985.)

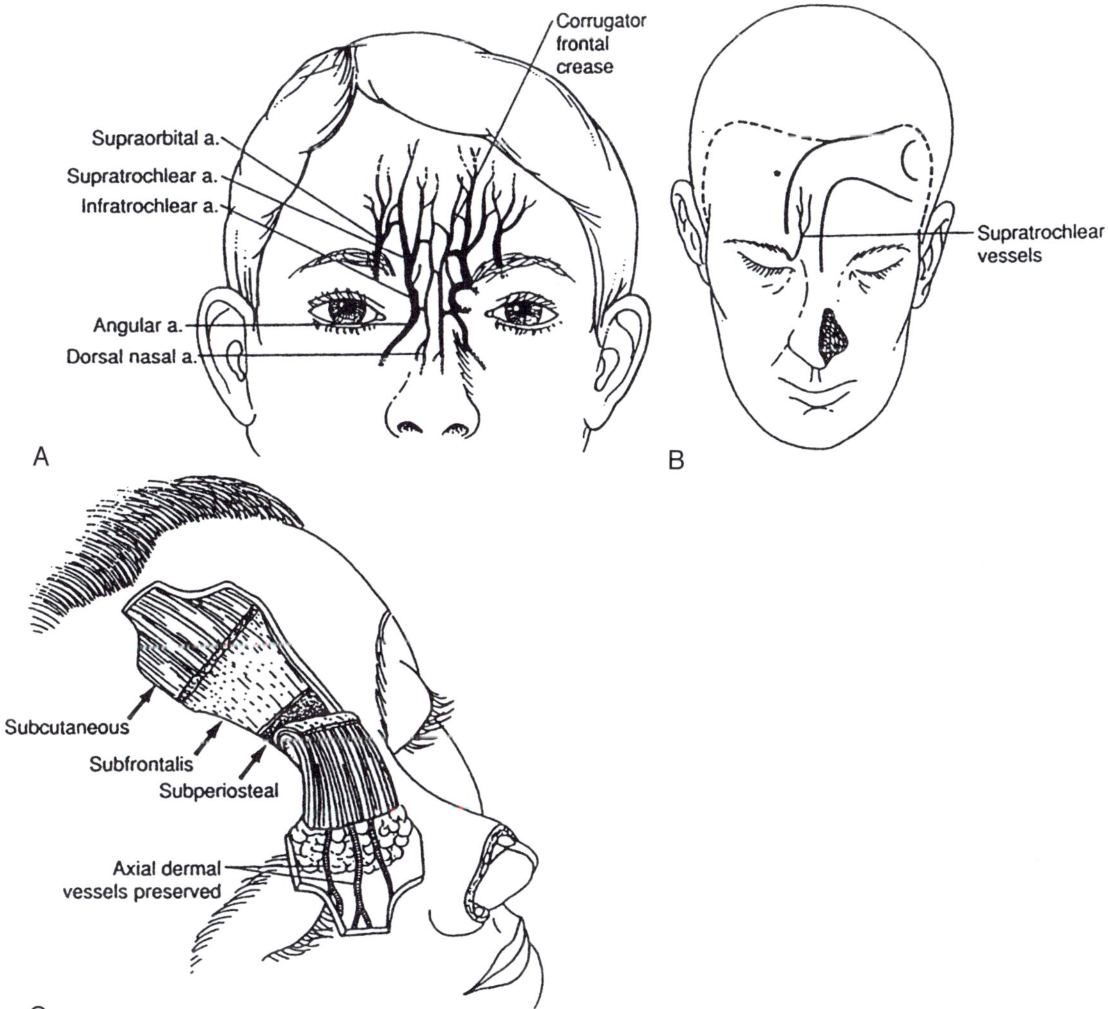

Figure 6 Paramedian forehead flap: (A) forehead blood supply; (B) paramedian forehead flap design; (C) flap elevation and thinning. (From Aston SJ; Beasley RW; Thorne CHM: *Grabb and Smith's Plastic Surgery*. 5th ed. Philadelphia: Lippincott-Raven, 1997.)

4. The pedicle is cut at a second stage approximately 3 weeks later.
5. This flap is rarely used today as it has essentially no advantages over the paramedian forehead flap.

V. COLUMELLA

Columellar reconstruction can be exceedingly difficult.

A. Nasolabial flaps—Best results are achieved with a nasolabial flap, preferably bilateral, and transferred on a superior pedicle.
B. Upper lip forked flaps—Useful in partial columellar loss or in the elderly patient with a long upper lip.
C. Forehead flap—A distal extension to the paramedian forehead flap may be rolled inward or pinched and molded to form the columella and to line the vestibules.
D. Chondrocutaneous composite graft—Auricular composite grafts may be useful for isolated columellar losses.

VI. DISTANT TRANSFERS

Distant transfers are useful when the forehead is not available and the defect is too large to repair by a graft

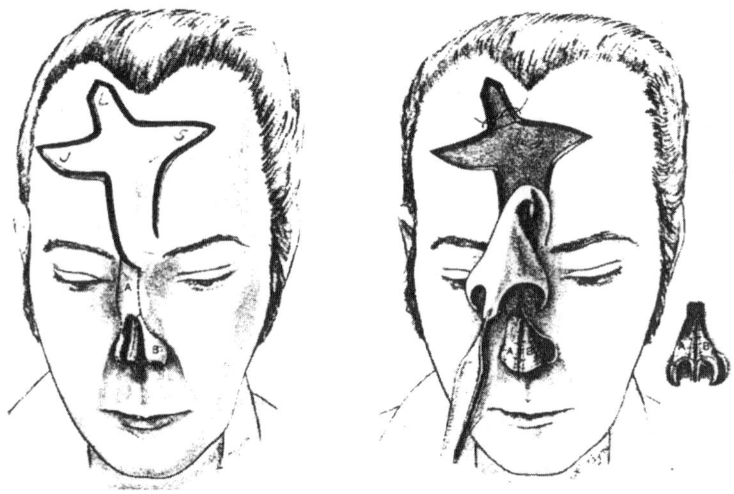

Figure 7 Gullwing flap. (From Millard DR Jr: Reconstructive rhinoplasty for the lower half of a nose. *Plast. Reconstr. Surg.* 53:135, 1974.)

or local flap. They frequently have the disadvantage of a poor color match. Flaps of primarily historical interest include brachial flaps (Tagliacozzi technique), cervical flaps, abdominal tube pedicle flaps, and deltopectoral flaps. Free flaps include:

1. Radial forearm free flap
   - First choice for free-tissue transfer total nasal reconstruction.
   - Thin, pliable tissue and easy to transfer.
   - Patients with normal Allen's test can provide an 8–10 cm vascular pedicle. Recipient vessels are usually the facial or superior labial arteries.
2. Dorsalis pedis free flap
   - Has large, thin skin paddle.
   - Like the radial forearm flap, can be harvested as an osseocutaneous transfer.

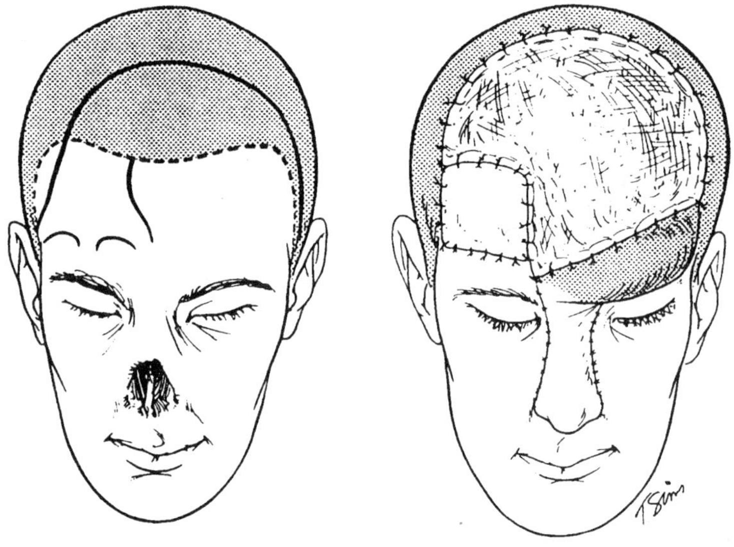

Figure 8 Design and transfer of scalping (converse) flap. (From Aston SJ; Beasley RW; Thorne CHM: *Grabb and Smith's Plastic Surgery*. 5th ed. Philadelphia: Lippincott-Raven, 1997.)

3. Postauricular free flap
   - A microvascular modification of the Washio technique.
   - The dermis of the flap, which is smooth and thin, may not resemble the thick, sebaceous nasal skin, but the donor site is very inconspicuous.
4. Helical free flap
   - Particularly suited to nostril restoration.
   - Auricular tissue is carried on the anterior branch of the temporal artery to bring the root of the helix to the nose as a composite helical free flap.
   - Limited to 3 × 3 cm surface area without distortion of the anterior ear.

VII. LINING

A. Indications and Timing

1. One should provide for nasal lining, skeletal elements, and external cover in a single operation. This ensures uniform healing and maximum flexibility of tissues for shaping.
2. For very large lining defects, staged reconstruction may be indicated. The proposed lining replacement is attached to the flap used for skin coverage at a preliminary procedure. Once the lining graft has taken, the flap is transferred. Although safer, this technique may result in cicatricial stiffening of the flap, which may limit shaping of the reconstruction.

B. Lining Techniques

1. Turn-in nasal flaps
   - Flap is hinged on the outer cicatricial edge and flipped over to span the defect.
   - Useful only in defects that have been present long enough to heal the margins. This technique is not appropriate for acute wounds.
2. Folded extranasal flaps
   - Forehead flap may be folded to resurface the interior of the nose. Five to seven mm can be reliably folded inward in a nonsmoker. This may result in a slightly thick reconstruction.
   - Nasolabial flaps can be burrowed under the alar base and inverted to provide nasal lining, or turned over on its subcutaneous pedicle with the skin of the flap facing intranasally to replace vestibular skin. The latter is frequently the lining flap of choice.
3. Skin graft to forehead flap
   - Preliminary skin graft may be used for the undersurface of a forehead flap to provide nasal lining.
   - A composite graft from the ear to the underside of the forehead flap may be used for simultaneous replacement of skin cover, lining, and skeletal support. It is helpful to fenestrate the cartilage of the graft to improve the take.
4. Septal hinge flap (Fig. 9)
   - Septal mucosa is removed ipsilateral to the defect, and an appropriately sized flap of septal cartilage is dissected. The septal trapdoor is made to open on a dorsal hinge toward the reconstructed side, so that the septal mucosa on its far side bridges the wound and lines the airway.
   - Caudally, flap reach is limited to the border of the upper lateral cartilages, because a sufficient amount of septum has to be left in place along the dorsum (approximately 1 cm wide) to support the midline, prevent collapse, and help with nasal projection.
5. Septal pivot flap (Fig. 10)
   - An anteriorly based septal mucoperichondrial flap may be used to serve as nasal lining.

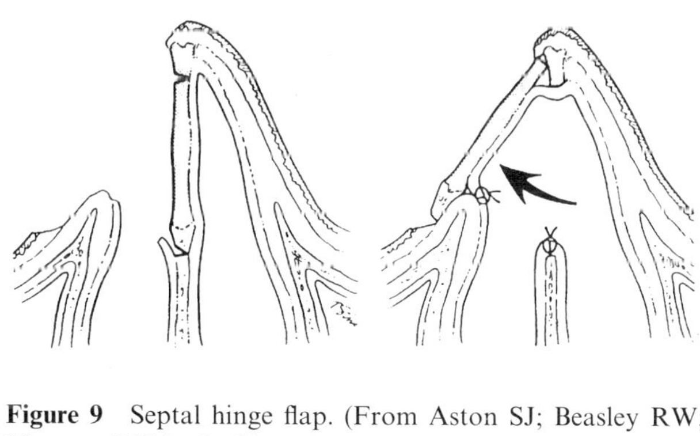

Figure 9 Septal hinge flap. (From Aston SJ; Beasley RW; Thorne CHM: *Grabb and Smith's Plastic Surgery*. 5th ed. Philadelphia: Lippincott-Raven, 1997.)

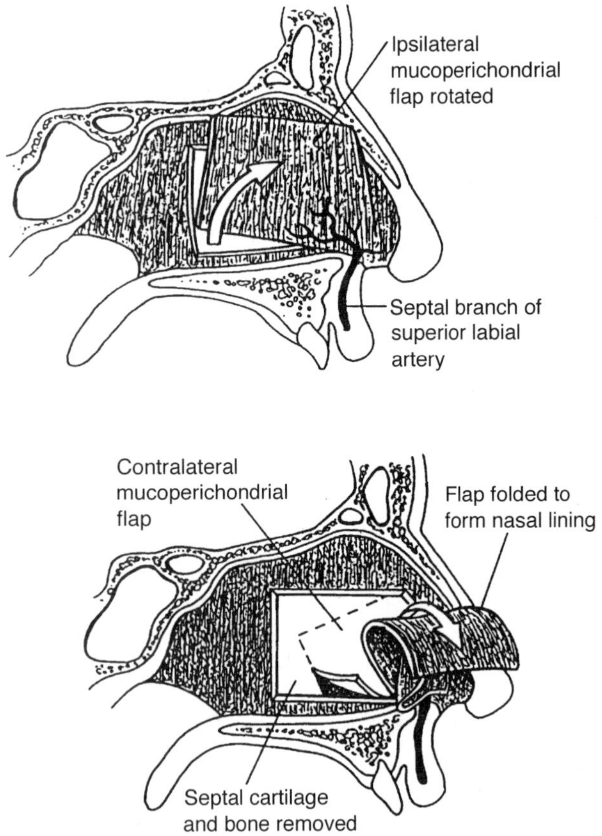

Figure 10 Septal pivot flap. (From Aston SJ; Beasley RW; Thorne CHM: *Grabb and Smith's Plastic Surgery*. 5th ed. Philadelphia: Lippincott-Raven, 1997.)

- A large rectangle of mucosa or a composite of mucosa and perichondrium is elevated from the septum, based on the septal branch of the superior labial artery.
- The flap pivots on an anterior-inferior point near the nasal spine and folds outward to provide lining for the nasal domes.

6. Mucosal advancement flap (Fig. 11)

- A bipedicled mucosal advancement flap is based medially on the remaining septum and laterally at the piriform aperture. The flap is advanced inferiorly to cover defects of lining along the alar rim.
- The vascularized mucosa can immediately support an auricular cartilage graft to give rigidity to the alar rim.

VIII. SKELETAL SUPPORT

A. Skeletal elements are an integral part of the initial nasal reconstructive plan in order to maintain normal soft tissue dimensions and prevent cicatricial collapse. Once soft tissues collapse and become fixed by scar, secondary elevation is disappointing.

B. Skeletally, the nose is composed of a rigid central scaffold and the more flexible lateral walls. The lateral walls serve in projecting the nose and maintaining tip elevation.

C. The alar cartilages tent the vestibule and keep the nostril wings open to allow airflow. Midline support of the reconstructed nose is needed to prevent tip collapse.

D. L strut

- A longitudinal piece of bone or cartilage is seated on the nasal radix and extended along the dorsum to the tip, where it is bent sharply to rest on the anterior nasal spine.
- A costal osteochondral graft from the fifth rib can be carved into appropriate hockey-stick configuration to project the tip and substitute for the medial crura. Its disadvantage is side-to-side instability and an excessively wide columella.

E. Hinged septal flap—An L-shaped flap of septum is hinged superiorly to provide nasal support.

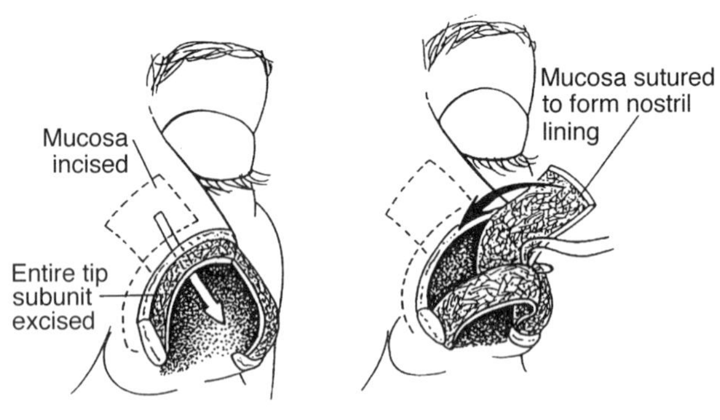

Figure 11 Mucosal advancement flap. (From Aston SJ; Beasley RW; Thorne CHM: *Grabb and Smith's Plastic Surgery*. 5th ed. Philadelphia: Lippincott-Raven, 1997.)

F. Septal pivot flap—Simultaneous lining and some dorsal skeletal support is provided with a composite flap of septum pivoting anteriorly.

G. Cantilever graft

- Perhaps the most widely used method for restoring skeletal support.
- A strong strut of bone is fixed to the nasal radix with screws or wires and extends along the dorsum down to the tip. Absolute rigid stability of the graft is important to prevent resorption.
- The remaining nasal bones often need to be lowered to accommodate the bone graft and to prevent an excessively high radix.
- Cranium, ilium, and rib are acceptable sources for these grafts.

H. Lateral support

- Nonanatomically placed cartilage grafts are necessary when reconstructing the ala to prevent collapse. This is particularly important close to the alar rim.
- Auricular cartilage is a good source for these grafts.

38

Lip Reconstruction

Babak J. Mehrara, M.D.,* **and Barry M. Zide, M.D., D.M.D.**
New York University Medical Center, New York, New York, U.S.A.

I. INTRODUCTION

1. Lip reconstruction is challenging for functional and aesthetic reasons. In addition, minor lip defects are noticeable at conversational distances.
2. Thus, important goals in lip reconstruction include maintenance of oral competence as well as aesthetic reconstruction of the lips and vermilion.

II. ANATOMY

The topography of the lips is an important consideration in reconstructive planning (Fig. 1). The area corresponding to the upper lip extends from one nasolabial fold to the other, including the philtral columns, vermilion, and intraoral mucosa. The lower lip includes the intraoral mucosa, vermilion, as well as the skin and soft tissues extending to the labiomental fold.

A. Musculature

1. Orbicularis oris
   - Primary muscle responsible for maintenance of oral competence, hence known as the oral sphincter.
   - Muscle fibers originate at the modiolus laterally and decussate in the midline and at the commissures.
   - Orbicularis oris muscle consists of two anatomically distinct muscle groups: the outer pars peripheralis and the pars marginalis (toward the vermilion).
2. Levator labii superioris
   - Acts as the primary lip elevator in conjunction with levator labii superioris alaque nasi.
   - Originates from the anterior portion of the maxilla and inserts into the lower two-thirds of the philtral columns superficial to the orbicularis oris muscle.
   - This muscle, along with the orbicularis oris, provides the bulk of the lower philtral columns.
3. Levator anguli oris: originates from the anterior portion of the maxilla and inserts on the upper lateral lip and modiolus, thereby acting in conjunction with zygomaticus major/minor muscles to elevate the commissures.
4. Zygomaticus major and minor
   - Act to draw upper lips up and back.
   - Originate from the zygoma and insert on the upper lateral lip and modiolus.
5. Mentalis
   - Is the central lower lip elevator.
   - Originates from the mandibular periosteum below the attached gingiva between the

**Current affiliation*: Memorial Sloan-Kettering Cancer Center, New York, New York, U.S.A.

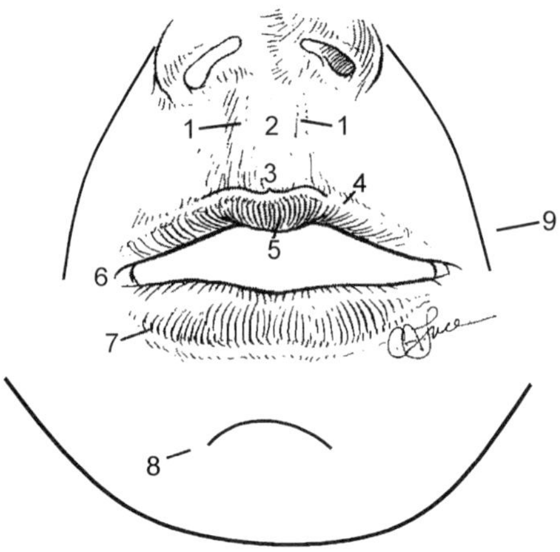

Figure 1 Topographic anatomy of the lips: (1) philtral columns; (2) philtral groove or dimple; (3) cupid's bow; (4) white roll; (5) tubercle; (6) commissure; (7) vermilion; (8) labiomental fold; (9) nasolabial fold. (Adapted from Zide BM: Deformities of the lips and cheek. In: McCarthy JG, ed. *Plastic Surgery*. Philadelphia: W.B. Saunders, 1990.)

lower lateral incisors and inserts into the entire chin pad.

- Contraction of this muscle elevates the chin pad and compresses it against the mandible, thus forcing the central lip upward. It is the muscle that allows "pouting."
- The upper fibers maintain lip position.

6. Depressor anguli oris, depressor labii inferioris: represent the primary lower lip depressors that originate from the mandibular border and insert into the lower orbicularis of the lower lip.

B. Innervation

1. Motor
   - Motor innervation of the lips is via the seventh cranial nerve (buccal and mandibular branches).
   - Orbicularis oris is innervated by the buccal branch only.
2. Sensory
   - Sensory innervation of the upper lip is via the infraorbital branch of the fifth cranial nerve (V2).
   - Sensory innervation of the lower lip is via the mental branch of the fifth cranial nerve (V3).

C. Blood Supply

1. The blood supply of the lips is derived from the paired labial arteries arising from the facial arteries.
2. A rich anastomotic network surrounds the lips, thus enabling extensive dissections.
3. Local flaps based on the labial arteries represent the basis for many reconstructive options.

D. Lymphatic Drainage

1. Lymphatic drainage of the lips occurs via the submandibular and submental lymph nodes.

III. PATHOPHYSIOLOGY

The vast majority of lip defects are secondary to cancer ablation. In addition, lip defects resulting from vascular malformations, trauma, and infectious complications are also commonly encountered.

A. Characteristics

1. Neoplasms of the lip are primarily related to actinic damage. Most lip neoplasms (approximately 95%) involve the lower lip since the upper lip is at least partially shielded from sun exposure by the nose.
2. Lip cancers demonstrate strong sex bias, with males affected approximately 9 times more frequently than females.
3. Upper and lower lips also differ in the incidence of different types of skin cancers. Upper lip carcinomas are usually basal cell types, while lower lip carcinomas are usually squamous cell carcinomas.
4. Fortunately, only a small minority (approximately 2–3%) of lower lip squamous cell carcinomas tend to involve the commissures. These tumors tend to behave more aggressively (up to 16% have evidence of metastasis on presentation) and are more difficult to reconstruct.

B. Squamous Cell Carcinomas of the Lips

These tend to behave less aggressively than those involving oral mucous membranes.

1. Primary lip squamous cell carcinomas less than 1.5 cm in diameter should be excised with a margin of 1.0 cm (unless Mohs' chemosurgery is

used). In addition, many authors recommend evaluation of the remaining lip vermilion with lip shave and histologic sampling to rule out premalignant or superficial malignancy.

2. Staging of squamous cell carcinomas is also important since the surgical stage has been directly correlated with survival. In surgical staging of squamous cell carcinomas, T1 represents a tumor <2 cm in greatest diameter, T2 = 2–4 cm, T3 >4 cm, and T4 = local tissue invasion.

IV. RECONSTRUCTION

A. Basic Tenets

Reconstruction of lip defects is preferentially performed using:

1. Same lip
2. Opposite lip
3. Local skin (cheek, nasolabial fold, etc.)
4. Free flap

B. Upper Lip Reconstruction

Aesthetic reconstruction of the upper lip is more challenging than that of lower lip defects, since care must be given to the reconstruction of the Cupid's bow and philtral columns. In addition, care must be taken to restore the shape and contour of the vermilion with accurate alignment of the white roll. Functionally, however, upper lip defects are less challenging than lower lip defects, since the lower lip primarily controls oral competence. Techniques used for upper lip reconstruction are summarized in Figure 2.

1. Partial-Thickness Defects

a. Partial-thickness defects can usually be closed by primary closure in the direction of relaxed skin tension lines (i.e., vertically).

b. Larger defects may occasionally require full-thickness skin grafting, and results in aesthetically pleasing results (for example, reconstruction of the entire philtral skin).

c. Conversion to full-thickness defects and coverage with lower lip flaps (e.g., Abbe flaps).

d. Local tissue flaps are commonly used. Examples include nasolabial flaps and cheek flaps. The use of local flaps may be problematic, however, since these flaps often result in the obliteration of aesthetic units, especially with facial animation (e.g., during smiling). In addition, movement of hair-bearing skin in male patients can result in noticeable scars.

2. Full-Thickness Defects

a. Defects <35% of Total Width:

- Usually can be closed primarily with good aesthetic results. Maximum defect size that can be closed primarily depends on skin laxity. Care must be given to precise alignment of white roll and muscle for optimum aesthetic and functional reconstruction. Closure of medial defects may cause distortion of the philtral columns.
- Abbe flaps (lip switch) and occasionally full-thickness grafts may be used for philtral column reconstruction in central lip defects. This technique may improve aesthetic outcome, especially in females, since the absence of philtral columns secondary to primary closure cannot be hidden by facial hair.

b. Defects >30% of Total Width:

- Local tissue flaps: large upper lip defects may be reconstructed with bilateral flaps.

  Abbe flaps (lip switch) may be used to reconstruct defects measuring up to 50% of the total width. These flaps may be combined with local tissue flaps, especially for reconstruction of philtral columns.

  Nasolabial flaps/cheek advancement flaps rely on perialar tissue with or without skin/soft tissue excisions to aid in tissue advancement. All flaps usually require revisions, and patients should be so advised. If excisions are limited to skin and limited subcutaneous tissues, these procedures have the potential to preserve innervated muscle tissue to close lip defects while maintaining sphincter function. However, original descriptions of some of these procedures called for full-thickness excisions that would denervate the lips. Examples of nasolabial/cheek advancement flaps include:

  - Bernard Von Burrow chelioplasty
  - Webster modification
  - Schuchardt flap

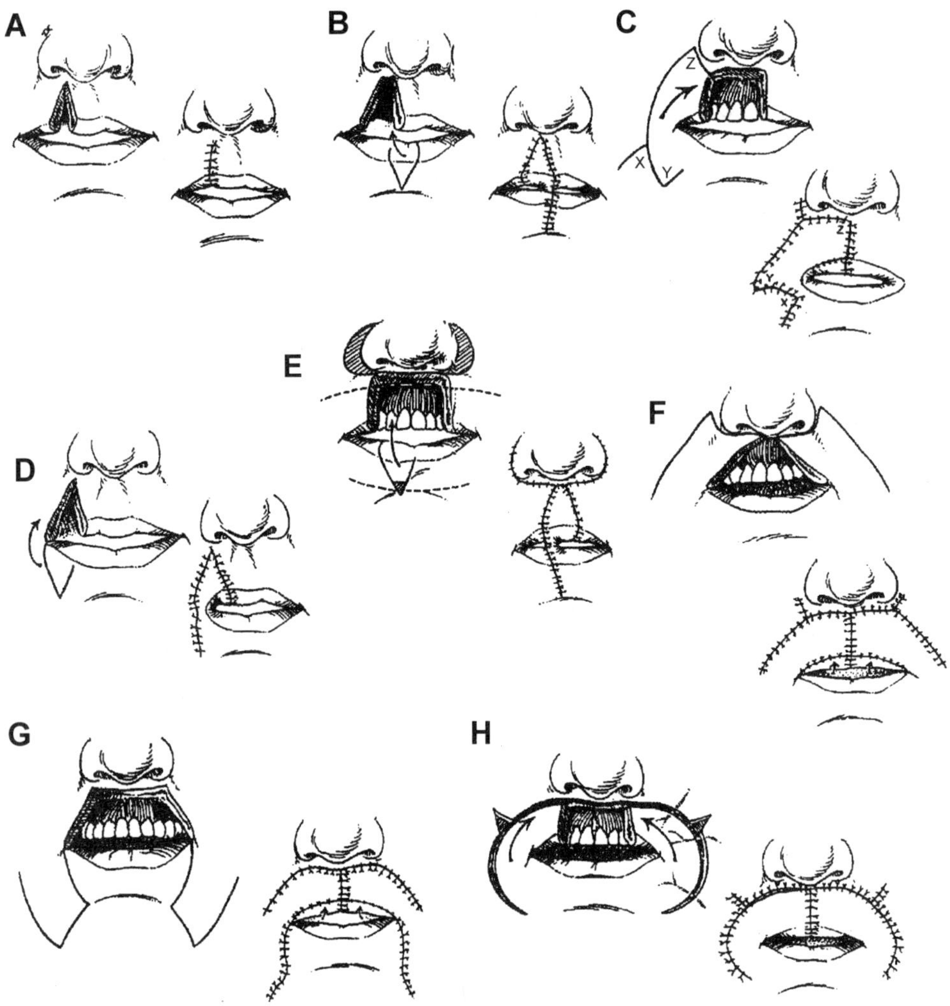

Figure 2 Techniques of upper lip repair: (A) wedge excision with direct closure; (B) Abbe (lip switch) flap; (C) reverse Gillies fan flap; (D) reverse Estlander flap; (E) Webster's combination procedure; (F) nasolabial flaps; (G) Kasanjian/converse lower cheek flaps; (H) reverse Karapandzic flap. (Adapted from selected readings in plastic surgery.) *Notes*: (A) cuts must be perpendicular to vermilion border; (B) switch flaps best put in center only. This size defect can be closed primarily with release as drawn; (C) rarely used-see Yotsuyanagi; (D) rarely done due to commissure distortion. (From Yotsuyanagi T, et al.: Functional and aesthetic reconstruction using a naso labial orbicularis oris myocutaneous flap for large defects of the upper lip. *Plast. Reconstr. Surg.* 101:1624, 1998.)

Oral circumference flaps

- Gillies fan flap is a rotation advancement flap that moves lateral lip and commissure medially. Results in distortion of commissure, often requiring a difficult commissure revision. In addition, this flap is associated with microstomia when used as bilateral flaps for the closure of large defects.
- McGregor flap is a modification of the Estlander flap (see below) and adds complete vermilionectomy with rotation around the commissure. Maintains commissure in position, but changes direction of muscle fibers with reosultant decreased sphinteric action.
- Innervated composite flaps (e.g., Karapandzic flap, Nakajima flap) are best dissected with loupe magnification to

preserve facial nerve branches and vessels. Thus, motor and sensory innervation of the orbicularis oris muscle are preserved, resulting in improved sphincteric function. The use of these flaps in larger defects may result in microstomia, thus complicating denture insertion and dental work. Microstomia is, to some extent, responsive to stretching exercise or devices. In addition, the scars associated with these flaps tend to be noticeable.

Combination flaps utilize combinations of above flaps to close larger defects.

Distant flaps are used only if local tissues are not available. Distant flaps are problematic because they are insensate and have no muscle function. The most commonly described flap is the radial forearm flap. A radial forearm flap may be suspended with palmaris longus tendon to aid in oral competence.

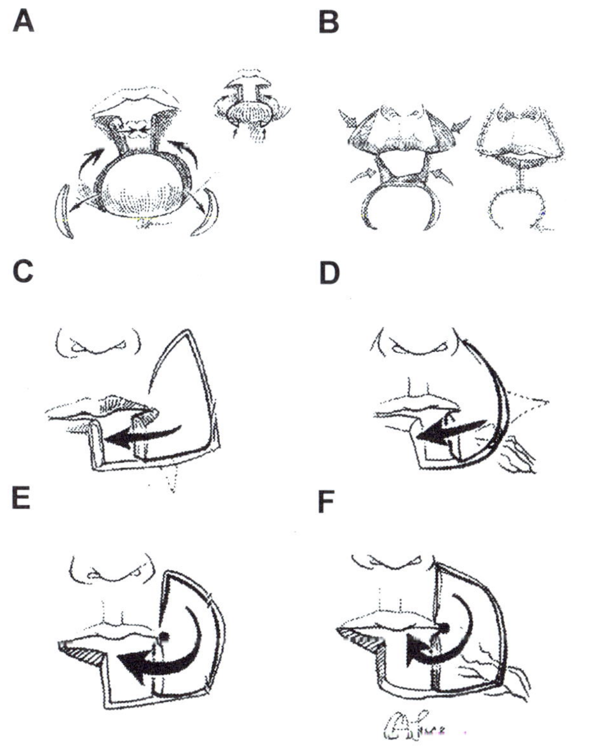

Figure 4 Techniques for closure of large (>33% total width) lower lip defects: (A) Schuchardt procedure; (B) Webster modification of the Bernard operation; (C) Gillies fan flap; (D) Karapandzic flap (innervated); (E) McGregor flap; (F) Nakajima flap. (Adapted from Zide BM: Deformities of the lips and cheek. In: McCarthy JG, ed. *Plastic Surgery*. Philadelphia: W.B. Saunders, 1990.)

C. Lower Lip Defects

These are encountered much more frequently than upper lip defects (due to increased actinic damage—see above). In addition, when lower lip reconstruction is performed, every effort should be made to maintain oral competence. Techniques used for lower lip reconstruction are summarized in Figures 3 and 4.

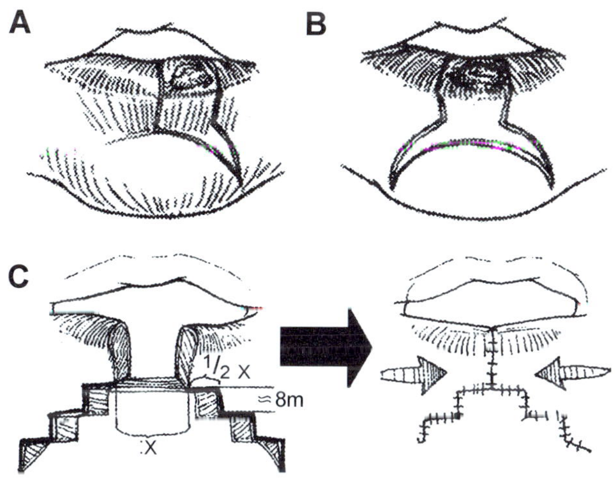

Figure 3 Techniques for primary closure of lower lip defects: (A) single barrel excision; (B) double barrel excision; (C) staircase/stepladder method: Not a great result as steps are often visible. (Adapted from Zide BM: Deformities of the lips and cheek. In: McCarthy JG, ed. *Plastic Surgery*. Philadelphia: W.B. Saunders, 1990.)

1. Defects less than 33% of total lower lip width can usually be closed primarily.
    - Techniques such as single barrel, double barrel, or stair-step excisions can be used successfully (Fig. 3).
    - V-shaped excisions are not recommended for tumor excision since tumor invasion can occur laterally or downward.
    - Flared W-plasty and barrel-shaped excisions avoid incisions across the labiomental fold, thus resulting in more cosmetic appearance by avoiding hypertrophic scarring.

2. Defects measuring 33–65% of total width
   - Local advancement flaps:

     Cheek advancement.

     Oral circumference advancement flaps (e.g., Schuchardt advancement flaps, Webster-Bernard flaps, gate flaps).

     Composite flaps (e.g., Gillies fan flap, McGregor flap, Karapandzic flap).

     Lip switch procedures (e.g., Abbe flap).
3. Defects measuring greater than 65% of total width are considered near-complete reconstruction (>80% is considered total reconstruction).
   - Bilateral Karapandzic flaps (approximately 80%)
   - Bilateral McGregor/Nakajima flaps (approximately 90%)
   - Webster-Bernard technique (approximately 100%)
   - Combination procedures
   - Distant flaps
   - Microvascular tissue transfers

D. Defects Involving the Commissures

1. Can be treated similar to upper/lower defects.
2. Commissure reconstruction can be provided with Estlander or McGregor flaps.
3. Larger defects may be combined with other procedures.

E. Vermilion Defects

1. Key Points for Reconstruction

a. Always mark the white roll with blue dots into the dermis.

b. Always cross white roll at 90° angles.

c. Do not suture the white roll (results in prolonged erythema and resultant obliteration).

d. If possible, maintain incisions within the vermilion.

2. Order or Preference for Vermilion Reconstruction

1. Advancement of same lip (V-Y advancement flaps or primary closure). Care must be taken to reapproximate muscle fibers to prevent future scar contraction and dimpling.
2. Other lip vermilion (unipedicled or bipedicle flaps).
3. Mucosal advancement flap.
4. Tongue flaps.
5. FAMM flaps (facial artery musculomucosal flap).

39

Mandible Reconstruction: Principles and Techniques

Michael Klebuc, M.D.
Baylor College of Medicine, Houston, Texas, U.S.A.
Larry H. Hollier, M.D.
Texas Children's Hospital and Baylor College of Medicine, Houston, Texas, U.S.A.

I. ETIOLOGY AND CLASSIFICATION OF MANDIBULAR LESIONS

A. Causes

1. Malignant and benign tumors
2. Penetrating and blunt trauma
3. Congenital abnormalities

B. Classification—Boyd (HCL) System (Fig. 1)

1. H (hemimandible)—condyle and lateral segment that does not cross the symphysis (midline).
2. L (lateral)—lateral segment without a condylar component; not crossing the symphysis.
3. C (central)—bony region between the mental foramina.

C. Tissue Classification

1. O—bone only
2. M—mucosa
3. S—skin
4. MS—mucosa and skin

II. RECONSTRUCTIVE GOALS

A. Achieve primary wound healing in a hostile environment (saliva, irradiated tissue).

B. Avoid fistula formation and exposure of bone grafts, hardware, and vascular structures.

C. Facilitate a complete oral rehabilitation:

- Oral competence (preserve lingual sulcus)
- Unencumbered mastication and swallowing without aspiration
- Dental occlusion (i.e., osseointegrated implants)
- Intelligible speech (mobile tongue)
- Intraoral sensation

D. Reestablish the aesthetic harmony to the lower third of the face (height, width, and projection) and avoid the "Andy Gump" deformity.

III. REGIONAL CHALLENGES

A. Anterior arch defects—altered relationships between the soft tissue-muscle complex of the oropharynx results in increased dysphagia, aspiration, and oral incompetence (greatest reconstructive challenge).

B. Lateral defects—masticatory muscles create upward/lateral displacement of residual fragments with resultant hollow deformity, malocclusion, and deviation with opening (most problematic when good dentition remains).

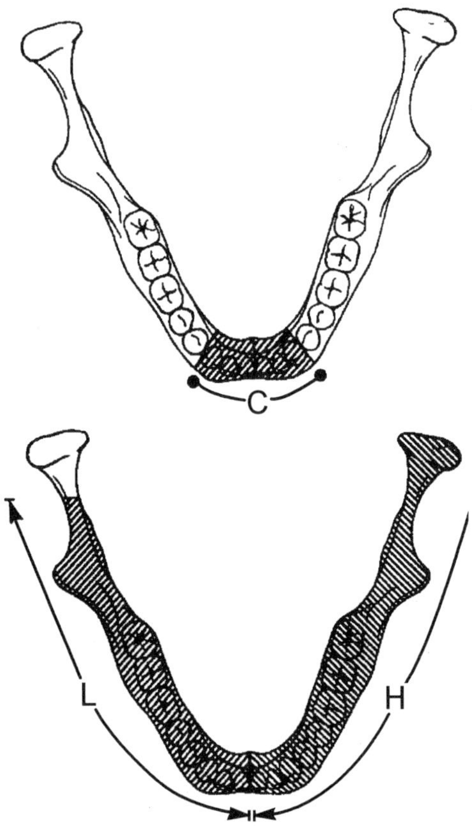

Figure 1 Boyd (HCL) classification of mandibular defects: C, central; L, lateral; H, hemimandible. (From Boyd B, Gullane P, Brown D: Classification of mandibular defects. *Plast. Reconstr. Surg*. 92(7):1266, 1993.)

C. Posterior defects—limited morbidity treating posterior defects that involve the condyle, without bony reconstruction, utilizing soft tissue free flaps.

IV. NONVASCULARIZED RECONSTRUCTIVE TECHNIQUES

A. Options include:

- Autogenous and alloplastic bone grafts
- Reconstruction plates
- Alloplastic trays with cancellous autograft bone

B. Requirements for successful nonvascularized reconstruction:

- Well-perfused soft tissue envelope without intraoral communication
- Contraindicated if pre- or postoperative radiation therapy is required

C. High failure rate in fibrosed or scarred recipient beds (multiple surgeries, gunshot wound).

D. Hyperbaric oxygen therapy: multiple pre- and postoperative treatment sessions may reduce complications and improve survival. Theoretic risk of stimulating growth of residual microscopic tumor rests.

E. High failure rate for segments >5 cm in length and in anterior (symphyseal) defects.

F. Autogenous and alloplastic bone grafts:

- Autogenous—inner or outer cortex of the iliac crest, split calvarial, rib.
- Alloplastic—freeze-dried mandible allograft filled with cancellous autograft, split rib allograft to create a biologic tray for cancellous autograft (allograft perforated with multiple drill holes).
- Indications—small (<5 cm) lateral bone–only defects approached extra orally in nonradiated tissue (i.e., fracture nonunions, benign tumors, supplementing previous vascularized bone flaps).

G. Rigid fixation—stabilization with reconstruction plates (2.4–3.5 mm diameter screws) limits resorption and infection. Three or more bicortical screws should be placed in the segments of residual native mandible.

H. Reconstruction plates:

- Utilized without bony reconstruction after palliative surgery in patients with limited life expectancy.
- Frequent failures due to screw loosening and plate fracture.
- High extrusion rate when combined with radiation therapy.
- Failure rates 48% in anterior defects and 17% in lateral defects.
- Very limited indications—palliation for poor prognosis patients with small, lateral defects, no history of radiation therapy, and robust local soft tissue or flap coverage.

I. Alloplastic trays and bone autograft:

- Metallic mesh and Dacron trays packed with cancellous bone graft.
- Utilized for limited, lateral defects.

- Tray frequently removed after bony integration.
- Failure rates approximately 48% in radiated and 30% in nonradiated reconstructions.

V. VASCULARIZED BONE FLAPS

A. Pedicle Flaps

1. Pectoralis + rib and trapeziu + scapula combinations are largely of historical interest.
2. Short bone segments with pedicle restricting mobility and insetting of flap.
3. Most tenuous perfusion in zone of interest.
4. Often-staged procedures.
5. Limited amount of cortical bone complicates plate fixation.

B. Microvascular Bone Flaps

1. Fibula Free Flap

1. Most frequently utilized microvascular reconstructive technique (Fig. 2).
2. Pedicle-peroneal artery and vein (up to 12 cm in length).
3. Bone length (22–27 cm)—6–8 cm preserved proximal and distal for knee and ankle stability.
4. Segmental blood supply enables multiple osteotomies.
5. Skin island—maximum 15 × 27 cm (donor defect < 4 cm wide can be closed primarily).
6. Preoperative planning:
   - Thorough peripheral vascular exam (pulses, skin and hair changes).
   - Imaging studies have a low yield if the physical exam is normal, but they are the only means to rule out peronea magna (dominant peroneal vessels) or congenital absence (incidence = 2–5%).
   - Color flow Doppler and magnetic resonance angiography are noninvasive and provide similar information as arteriograms and can map septocutaneous perforators.

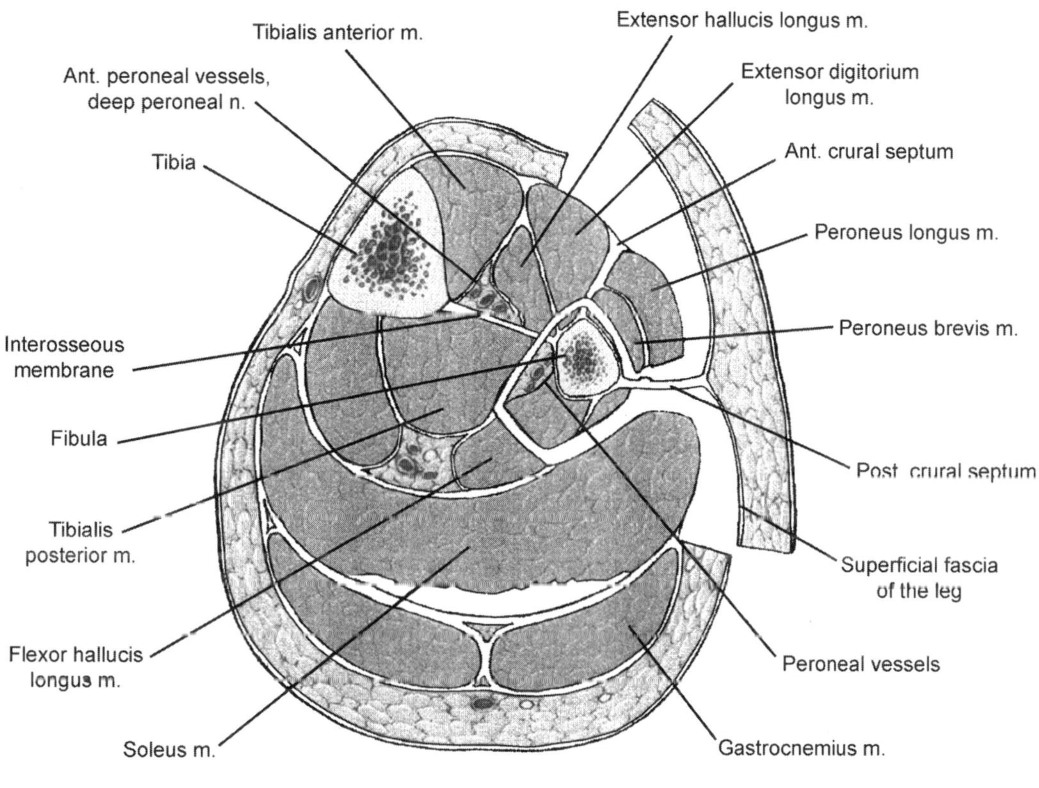

Figure 2 Cross-sectional anatomy of the fibular flap. (From Anthony J, Foster R: Mandible reconstruction with the fibula osteocutaneous free flap. *Operative Tech. Plastic Surg.* 3(4):233, 1996.)

7. Surgical suggestions:
   - Utilize contralateral leg if an intra-oral skin paddle is required (Fig. 3).
   - Design the skin island over the lower two thirds of the fibula to take advantage of the higher perforator density.
   - Plantar flexing the ankle intensifies the surface definition of the lateral soleus muscle and posterior crural septum facilitating perforator identification via Doppler.
   - Longer skin islands incorporate more septocutaneous perforators and are more reliable. Vascularity is preserved by deepithelializing the skin island if a smaller cutaneous paddle is required.
   - Dissection under tourniquet control.
   - Avoid the superficial branch of the peroneal nerve as it emerges between the peroneus muscles.
8. Dissection (Fig. 2):
   - Elevate fasciocutaneous skin island perfused by posterior crural septal perforators.
   - Lateral compartment—elevate peroneus muscles from fibula with 2 mm muscle cuff.
   - Vessels protected and proximal and distal osteotomies are created, which greatly facilitates exposure.
   - Anterior compartment—anterior crural septum and extensor digitorum longus elevated from bone (2 mm muscle cuff).
   - *Caution*—the anterior tibial vessels are frequently closer to the fibula than depicted in

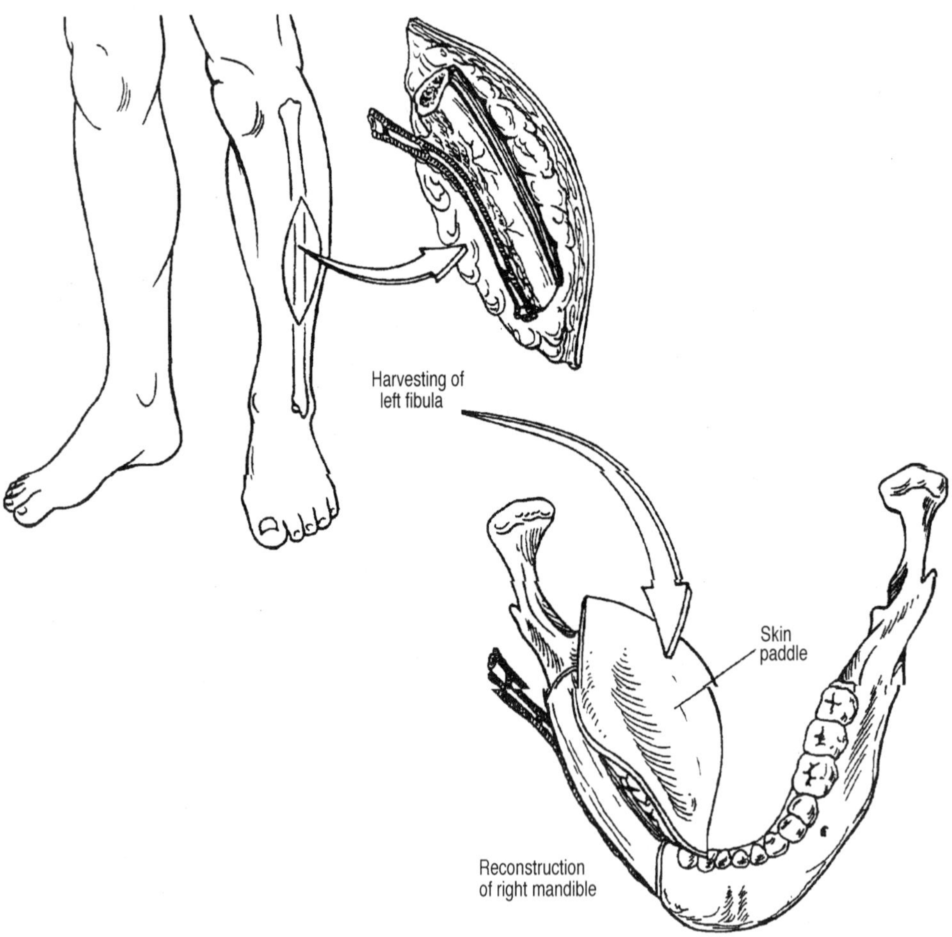

Figure 3 The contralateral leg is used preferentially if an intraoral skin island is required. This allows for intraoral skin paddle placement. If no skin paddle is needed, the ipsilateral leg is selected. (From Schusterman M: Free flap reconstruction of the mandible. In: Schusterman M, ed. *Microsurgical Reconstruction of the Cancer Patient*. Philadelphia, Lippincott-Raven, 1997, p. 43).

standard anatomy texts. Identify the peroneal vessels at the distal osteotomy if in doubt.

- Deep posterior compartment—divide interosseus membrane to expose the pedicle. Incorporate a liberal segment of flexor hallicus longus muscle with the flap to protect the perforators.
- Superficial posterior compartment—1 cm cuff of soleus muscle is harvested to preserve perforators (optional).
- Key point—bending the reconstruction plate to the native mandible prior to its division greatly facilitates contouring.
- Osteotomies proceed from distal to proximal as each cut reduces bony length up to 1 cm.
- Fixation to the reconstruction plate before peroneal vessel division reduces ischemia time.
- Elongate pedicle by proximal subperiosteal dissection and removal of unnecessary bone.

9. Postoperative care:
   - Closed suction drains are utilized.
   - Skin-grafted donor sites are placed in below-knee splints for 1 week, then progressive physical therapy and walking program to prevent contracture deformity of the deep posterior compartment musculature begun.
   - Usually fully ambulatory in 3 weeks.
   - Patients with primarily closed donor sites are splinted for 3–5 days and mobilized early.

2. Deep Circumflex Iliac Artery (Iliac Crest Composite) Free Flap

1. Pedicle—deep circumflex iliac artery (DCIA) and vein (length, 8–10 cm; diameter, 1.5–2.5 mm)
2. Tripartite composite flap:
   - Curved bone segment (14–16 cm)
   - Skin—soft tissue island can be as large as 10 × 15 cm over the iliac crest
   - Internal oblique muscle paddle
   - Capable of closing through-and-through defects
3. Surgical suggestions:
   - Approach femoral vessels and DCIA via inverted L incision over inguinal region.
   - DCIA originates from the external iliac artery above the inguinal ligament, lateral to the spermatic cord (Fig. 4).
   - Vessels run deep to the transversalis fascia toward the ASIS and cross the lateral femoral circumflex cutaneous and ilioinguinal nerves (division causes thigh paresthesia).
   - Eighty percent have ascending branch to internal oblique muscle 1 cm before ASIS (number of branches and takeoff are variable).
   - Musculocutaneous perforators start at the ASIS and run posteriorly for 10 cm.
   - Perforate abdominal wall muscles 1–1.5 cm above the iliac crest.
   - Traditionally, harvest the skin island with a 2.5 cm muscle cuff to protect perforators.
   - Periosteal arteries enter via the medial cortex permitting "split cortex modification" and osteotomies.
   - Split cortex modification—harvesting inner cortex alone provides bone segment of similar thickness to the mandible amiable to dental implants and decreased rates of hernia formation, gait disturbance, and contour deformity (Fig. 5).
   - Skin island is often bulky with limited independent motion in relation to the bone, which complicates flap insetting and often obliterates the lingual sulcus with intraoral use.
   - In 30% of cases, the skin island is harvested as an axial pattern flap on a dominant perforator "piercing vessel" to enhance mobility of the skin island.
   - Bone segment with ASIS incorporated resembles the mandibular angle and ramus when inverted.
   - Careful layered closure with heavy, nonabsorbable sutures (no drill holes in bone).
   - Always prebend reconstruction plate to native mandible.
4. Postoperative care:
   - Liberal use of closed-suction drains.
   - Start ambulation on postoperative day 3, with subsequent progressive rehabilitation program.

3. Scapular Free Flap

1. Pedicle:
   - Major pedicle is circumflex scapular artery and vein to skin island and bone (length, 5–6 cm; diameter, ~2.5 mm).

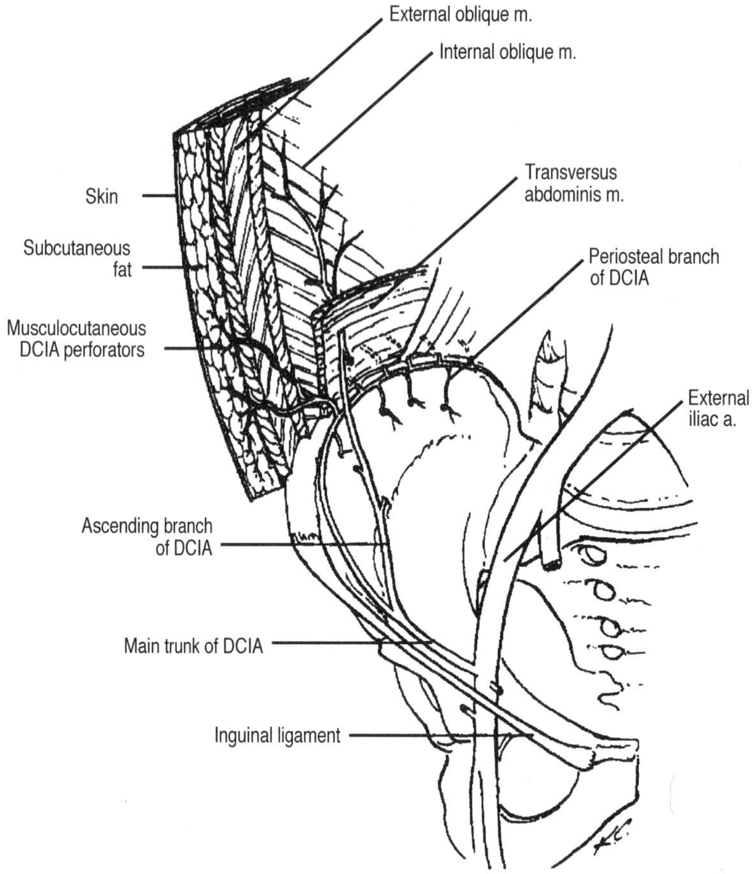

Figure 4 Vascular anatomy of the deep circumflex iliac artery system and the iliac crest free flap. (From Shenaq S, Klebuc M, Safak T, et al.: Mandibular reconstruction with the iliac crest composite microsurgical free flap. *Operative Tech. Plastic Surg.* 3(4):289, 1996.)

- Minor pedicle is thoracodorsal system-angular branch to bone (Fig. 6).

2. Bone: lateral scapular border; 1.5–2.5 cm thick and 12–16 cm long
3. Skin island: 7 × 20 cm (> 7 cm wide can be difficult to close primarily)
4. Preoperative planning:
   - Doppler the circumflex scapular artery in the triangular fossa approximately 2 cm superolateral to the apex of the posterior axillary fold.
   - Scapular flap skin island follows the transverse branch with medial border halfway between the medial scapular border and spine.
   - Parascapular skin island—from triangular fossa following the descending branch on an oblique course to the posterior iliac spine (Fig. 7).
5. Scapular bone, skin island, latissimus dorsi, and serratus anterior muscle can be transferred with a single anastomosis.
6. Surgical sequence:
   - Elevate the skin island and identify the circumflex scapular vessels exiting the triangular space. The margins of the triangular space are:

     Superior—teres minor

     Inferior—teres major

     Lateral—long head of triceps
   - Release teres major to improve exposure and suture to teres minor during closure.
   - Bone with dual blood supply:

     Proximally—branch of circumflex scapular vessels

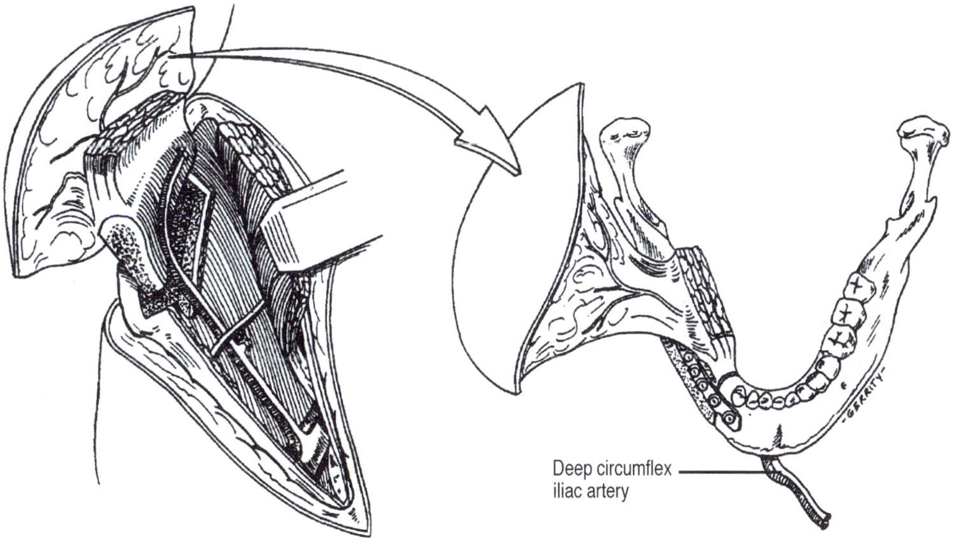

Figure 5 Split inner cortex DCIA flap. Note the 2.5 cm muscle cuff to protect the flap perforators. (From Schusterman M: Free flap reconstruction of the mandible. In: Schusterman M, ed. *Microsurgical Reconstruction of the Cancer Patient* Philadelphia: Lippincott-Raven, 1997, p. 57.)

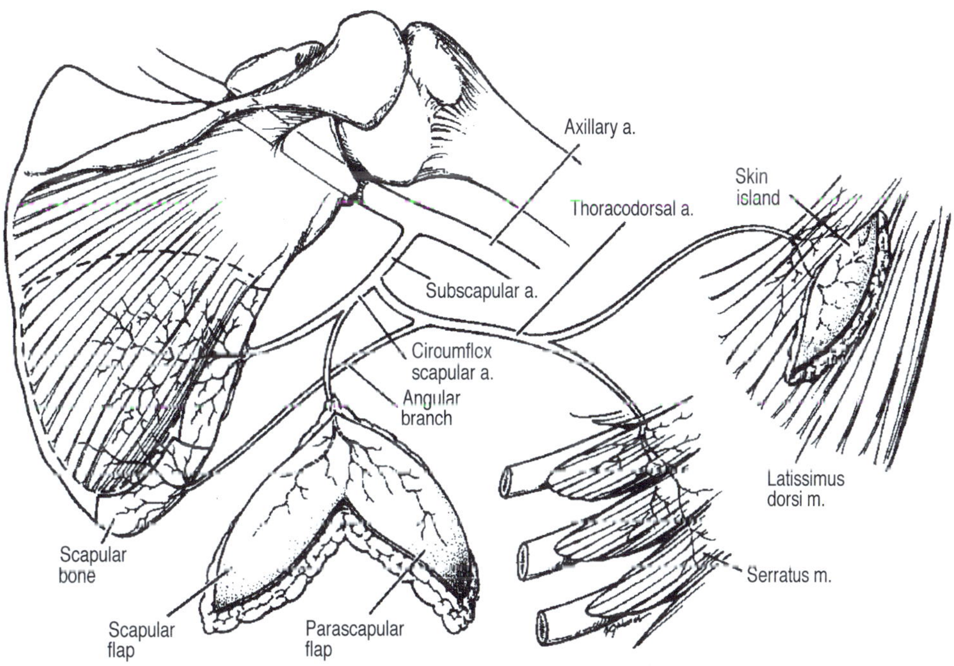

Figure 6 Vascular anatomy of the subscapular system. (From Sultan M: Mandible reconstruction with the scapula osteocutaneous flap. *Operative Tech. Plastic Surg*. 3(4):248, 1996.)

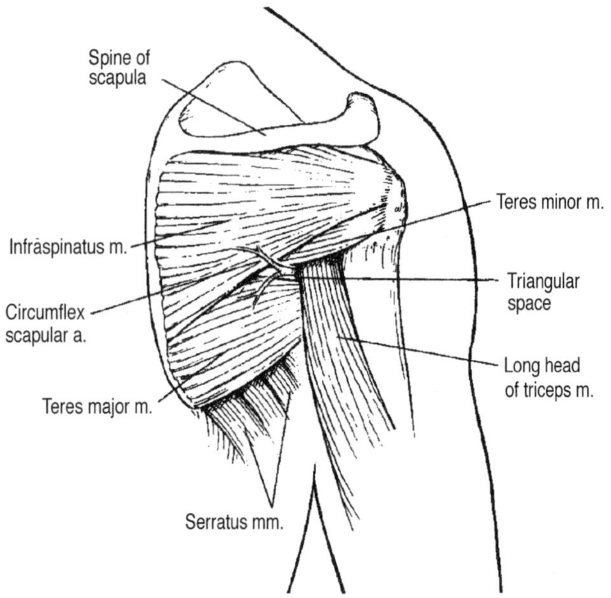

Figure 7 Borders of the triangular space. (From Sultan M: Mandible reconstruction with the scapula osteocutaneous flap. *Operative Tech. Plastic Surg.* 3(4):248, 1996.)

Distally—angular branch from the thoracodorsal vessels

- Elevating bone on the angular branch and skin island on the circumflex scapular vessels increases bone–soft tissue independence.

7. Pedicle length increased from 4–5 cm (circumflex scapular) to 13–15 cm by extending dissection to include the thoracodorsal vessels.
8. Bone—segment of cortico-cancellous bone 1.5–2.5 cm thick and 12–16 cm long from the lateral scapular border. Bony territory starts at the inferior angle and ends 2 cm before articular capsule.
9. Indication—large, spatially complicated soft tissue defect with limited bone requirements.
10. Drawbacks
    - Limited to hemimandible reconstruction (short bone segment).
    - Requires lateral decubitus positioning.
    - Proximity to head and neck negates a two-team approach.
    - Skin paddle is bulky in obese patients and lacks cutaneous nerve for neurotization.
11. Postoperative care: use of a sling to support the shoulder for 1 week, then begin graduated range of motion exercises.

4. Radial Forearm Free Flap

1. Pedicle—radial artery and venae comitantes (length is up to 20 cm; diameter approximately 2.5 mm) and cephalic vein (preferred for venous anastomosis) (Fig. 8).

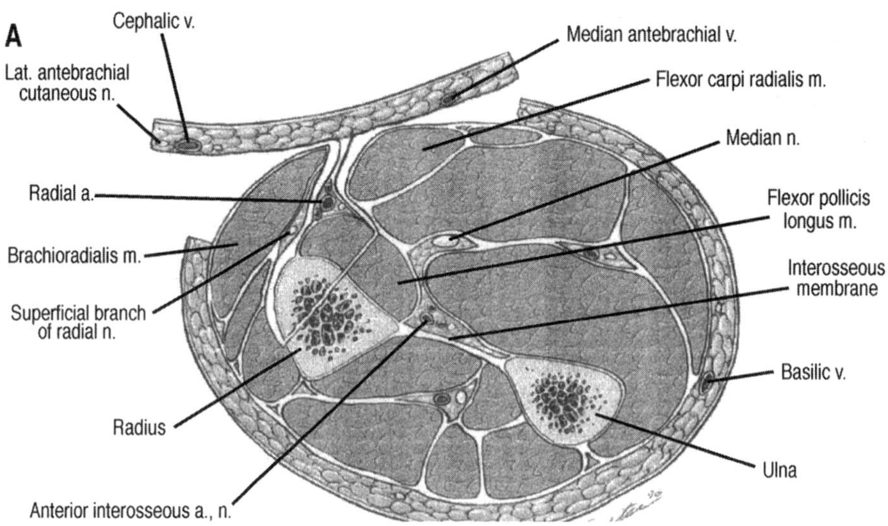

Figure 8 Cross-sectional anatomy of the radial forearm flap. (From Boyd B: Mandible reconstruction with the radial forearm flap. *Operative Tech. Plastic Surg.* 3(4):241, 1996.)

2. Bone—10 cm segment of the distal-lateral radius.
3. Skin island—thin; pliable; maximum dimension is 10 × 40 cm; skin island < 4 cm wide can be closed primarily.
4. Sensory nerve—lateal antebrachial cutaneous (C5–6).
5. Preoperative planning:
   - Use nondominant forearm as donor site.
   - Allen's test—special attention to blood flow to the thumb during the test.
   - *Key point*: Plan the flap with radial-dorsal orientation to include the cephalic vein.
   - Mark the upper extremity with a sign instructing the nursing staff to avoid IV catheters and blood draws.
6. Radial artery is located between the brachioradialis muscle (lateral) and flexor carpi radialis (medial).
7. Increased number of skin perforators in the distal half of the radial artery.
8. Surgical suggestions:
   - Skin island can be folded to provide external coverage and lining.
   - Avoid sacrificing the superficial branches of the radial nerve (neuroma formation and pain syndromes)
   - Leave paratenon of flexor tendons intact to facilitate skin graft closure.
   - Maximum bone segment is 12 cm long and less than one-third of the diameter of the radius (approximately 1 cm wide) (Fig. 9).
   - Insertion of the brachioradialis tendon is the distal limit of the bony component and pronator teres the proximal limit of the bony component.
   - Perforators to the bone pass through the flexor pollicis longus (must harvest a protective muscle cuff to protect the blood supply).
   - Beveled osteotomies are associated with a lower radius fracture rate than ones performed at right angles.
   - Reconstruction plates and iliac crest bone grafts are utilized primarily if any concern over radial stability arises.
9. Indications: useful for defects with extensive loss of lining and limited bone requirements.

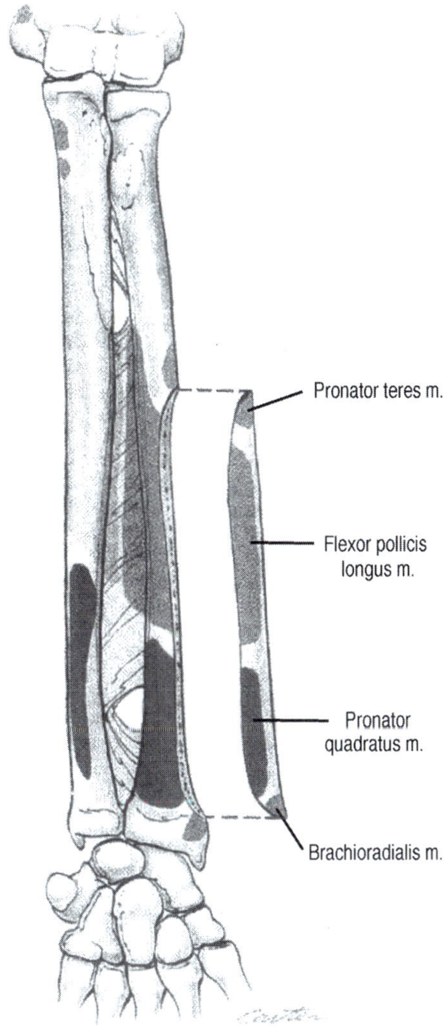

Figure 9 Osseous component of the radial forearm with corresponding muscle insertions. (From Boyd B: Mandible reconstruction with the radial forearm flap. *Operative Tech. Plastic Surg*. 3(4):241, 1996.)

10. Drawbacks:
    - Conspicuous donor site and complicated skin graft healing over tendon.
    - Postoperative radius fractures.
    - Insufficient bone height for use in central defects (unacceptable cosmetic deformity)
    - Intraoral hair on skin island.
11. Postoperative care:
    - Wrist and thumb in volar splint for 1 week, then above-elbow cast with the thumb free for

2 months, followed by a below-elbow cast for an additional month.

VI. TEMPOROMANDIBULAR JOINT RECONSTRUCTION

A. The temporomandibular joint is a ginglymoarthrodial joint—allows for hinge and gliding movements.

B. Reconstruction methods:

- Reconstruction plate with condylar head—useful in elderly patients where weak masticatory forces are unlikely to produce skull base erosion and perforation.
- Costochondral grafts—remodel in response to functional stresses. Will function in the absence of an articular disc and have growth potential for pediatric cases (unpredictable).
- Extended bone flap in conjunction with soft tissue arthroplasty (temporalis myofascial flap)—preserving a periosteal sleeve after excision of excess fibula improves the reconstruction.
- Replanting the condylar head from the resected specimen after frozen-section evaluation and processing (i.e., autoclave, freeze-drying).

VII. HARDWARE AND MAINTAINING BIMAXILLARY RELATIONSHIPS

A. Nonlocking titanium plates ($\geq$2.4 mm diameter screws), locking reconstruction plates, THORP hollow screw plating systems, and miniplates all provide adequate internal fixation.

B. *Key point*: Bend the reconstruction plate to the native mandible prior to mandibulotomy:

- Obviates the need for intermaxillary or external fixation
- Maintains dental relationships
- Reduces operative time
- Improves accuracy

C. Bimaxillary dental relationship can be maintained by:

- Arch bars—in dentulous patients
- Acrylic dental splints and circumandibular wires—in patients with poor or absent dentition
- Miniplates for temporary intermaxillary fixation

40

Complex Facial Reconstruction

Aldona Jedrysiak, M.D.
Baylor College of Medicine, Houston, Texas, U.S.A.
Larry H. Hollier, M.D.
Texas Children's Hospital and Baylor College of Medicine, Houston, Texas, U.S.A.

I. PRINCIPLES

A. Best results are obtained when the reconstruction is performed immediately to maintain function and prevent distortion secondary to scarring.

B. The ideal is a one-stage reconstruction with well-vascularized, thin, and pliable tissue containing all components to reconstitute the defect.

C. Preoperative evaluation should often be performed by a prosthetist to determine the need for a maxillofacial prosthesis.

D. Combination of alloplastic and autogenous techniques can been used to optimize the reconstructive result.

E. Microvascular tissue transfer is often useful in complex defects:

- Recipient vessels are the superficial temporal, facial, or cervical vessels.
- The team approach is preferred with simultaneous ablation and flap harvest.

II. MIDFACE RECONSTRUCTION

Includes the cheek, nose, orbital floor, maxilla, and palate.

A. Goals of Reconstruction

1. Restore the bony and soft tissue contour of the face
2. Rigid support for the soft palate
3. Oronasal separation
4. Support the globe
5. Obliterate the maxillary sinus
6. Restore or maintain function including respiration, speech, deglutition, and mastication

B. Skeletal Support

Skeletal support must often be incorporated within the reconstruction. Bone grafts/vascularized bone can be utilized.

C. Soft Tissue

1. Skin
   - Cervicofacial and cervicopectoral flaps are useful for large defects. The entire cheek can be reconstructed as an aesthetic unit, but frequently requires flap delay.
   - Fasciocutanous free tissue transfer (i.e., radial forearm) can provide reliable coverage.
2. Volume—free flaps are capable of transferring a large volume of tissue. Some surgeons prefer to utilize the soft tissue volume of flaps as a replacement for loss of skeletal support. Rectus abdominus flap is a popular option.

- Intraoral placement obliterates the maxillary sinus.
- Intraoral skin paddles tend to sag with time. Muscle should be left to re-epithelialize.

III. ORBITAL RECONSTRUCTION

Quality of outcome is determined by the eyelids. When the eyelids are absent, a good result is difficult to obtain.

A. Globe Present

1. Restoration of normal orbital volume is important to prevent enophthalmos.
2. Floor reconstruction:
   - Rib/cranial bone grafts or alloplast (titanium mesh/Medpor) are acceptable.
   - Anatomic restoration of the normal floor shape is important to prevent postoperative globe malposition.

B. Globe Absent

1. Adequate orbital volume must be preserved to allow for retention of prosthetic globe.
2. Orbital lining:
   - Skin grafts are most commonly used. Temporoparietal fascia flap may be used as a vascularized bed for graft, if necessary.
   - Temporary prosthesis should be maintained postoperatively to minimize contraction of the skin graft.
3. Prosthetic reconstruction—when lids are also absent, consideration should be given to complete prosthetic reconstruction of the defect.

IV. TOTAL NASAL RECONSTRUCTION (SEE CHAPTER 37)

Must reconstitute skin, lining, and support.

A. Skin

1. Forehead flap—most commonly used.
   - Based on supratrochlear vessels, with collateral blood supply from angular arteries.
   - A 3-cm forehead defect can be closed primarily; otherwise, donor site can be left to heal by secondary intention.
   - For patients with low hairlines, an extension into the hair can be made or the flap can be taken obliquely across the forehead to increase the flap length.
2. Scalping flap
   - Rarely indicated.
   - Most reliable way to provide tissue for total nasal reconstruction.
3. Radial forearm free flap
   - Provides large volume of thin pliable coverage, but color mismatch is a problem.
   - Should only be considered if a forehead flap is not an option.
   - Donor site scar is less than optimal.

B. Lining

1. Septal mucosal flaps—can be based anteriorly or dorsally.
2. Nasolabial turnover flaps.
3. Skin grafts—the underside of the forehead flap can be skin grafted while still on the forehead to provide lining as a preliminary procedure.

C. Skeletal Support

1. Cantilever bone grafts must be rigidly fixed to radix area with screws or plates.
2. Septum can be hinged or rotated to provide support, provided sufficient septum remains.

D. Prosthetic Reconstruction (See Chapter 43)

V. LIP RECONSTRUCTION (SEE CHAPTER 38)

A. Goals

1. Maintain competence of the oral sphincter
2. Maintain adequate stomal aperture
3. Restoration of skin and vermilion in a proper relationship
4. Provide sensation

B. Options

1. Remaining lip—defects <25–30% can often be closed primarily

2. Opposite lip:
   - Abbe flap—particularly good for central upper lip defects. Pedicle is divided at 10–14 days.
   - Estlander flap—good for lateral defects. Causes distortion of the commissure.
   - Gillies fan flap.
3. Adjacent tissue:
   - Cheek—Bernard Webster flap is capable of reconstructing 100% lower lip defects, but is a nonfunctional flap that acts essentially as a dam for oral secretions.
   - Karapandzic flap:

     Defects up to 80% are reliably closed. Microstomia may be a problem. The microstomia can be addressed at a second stage by an Abbe flap.

     Functional oral sphincter is maintained by preserved innervation to the flap during dissection.
4. Free flaps:
   - Best option is the radial forearm free flap.
   - Indication—defect of entire lip and adjacent cheek.
   - Oral competence is problematic. Flap should be suspended cephalad to zygomatic arch in sling-like fashion.

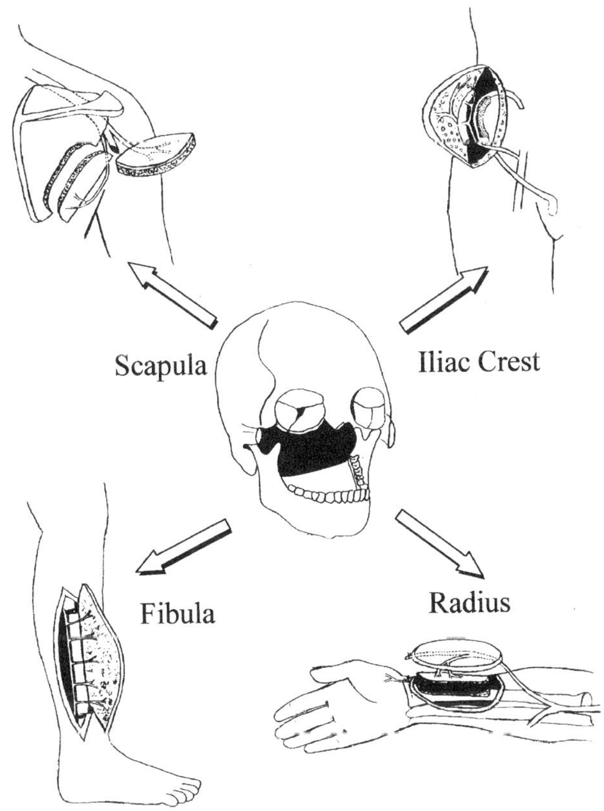

Figure 1 Osteofasciocutaneous flap options for reconstruction of facial defects.

VI. OSSEOUS RECONSTRUCTION OF COMPLEX FACIAL DEFECTS (FIG. 1)

A. Nonvascularized Bone Grafts

1. Necessitate a well-vascularized bed.
2. Large grafts (>6 cm), radiation, and significant scarring are relative contraindications.
3. May require adjuvant soft-tissue reconstruction at the time of their placement.

B. Vascularized Bone Grafts

1. Useful in reconstruction of maxillofacial defects with avascular recipient beds.
2. More difficult to contour than free grafts, due to limitations imposed by the pedicle.
3. Fibula osteocutaneous free flap is the flap of choice due to volume/length of bone and large skin island available.
4. Iliac crest, scapula, and radial forearm flaps are other microvascular options.

C. Osseointegrated Implants (See Chapters 12, 43, 114)

1. Concept—"anchor" placed in bone is integrated into new bone growth. Prostheses are then secured by screws into these anchors.
2. Thin skin covering of bone is preferred at the implant site. Bulky soft tissue interferes with interface of bone/prosthesis.
3. Dental implants, eyes, nose, and ears are the prostheses commonly utilized.

VII. FLAPS

A. Cervicofacial Flap

1. For reconstruction of complex cheek defects <6 cm in size.

2. Blood supply is based on the facial vessels.
3. Reliability is increased by elevating the flap in the sub-SMAS plane.
4. Flap must be back cut at the inferior limit of the dissection to increase reach.
5. Defects greater than 6 cm diameter can be covered by extending dissection onto the chest (cervicopectoral flap)

B. Temporoparietal Fascial Flap

1. Can be transferred as a pedicled or free flap.
2. Useful to cover exposed bone grafts to improve survival or as a vascularized bed for skin grafting over exposed cranium.
3. Plane of dissection is just deep to the hair follicles.
4. Before transfer as a free flap, explore the pedicle to detect possible venous anomalies, which can be present in up to one-third of the cases.

C. Galea-Frontalis Flap

1. Based anteriorly on supratrochlear/supraorbital system of vessels.
2. Plane of elevation is just above the galea in the subcutaneous tissue to incorporate the axial blood supply.
3. Excellent flap for coverage or fill of frontal sinus or cranial base defects.

D. Forehead Flap

1. For reconstructions of the midface, including cheek and nose.
2. Base of the flap should be kept narrow to increase its mobility.
3. Delay procedure can be used to increase the reliability of the flap in smokers.
4. Flaps larger than 3 cm leave donor defects that most often cannot be closed primarily. This should be left to heal by secondary intention for the best result.
5. Preoperative skin expansion can be used to allow donor site closure, but rebound contraction of the flap may be a problem.

VIII. FREE FLAPS (SEE CHAPTER 2)

A. Radial Forearm Flap

1. Based on radial artery; drained by venae comitantes and cephalic vein.
2. May carry vascularized bone between the insertions of the pronator teres and the brachioradialis. A cuff of flexor pollicis longus must be taken with the flap to maintain the perforators to the bone.
3. Skin is available from wrist flexion crease to upper third of the forearm.
4. Nerve (lateral antebrachial cutaneous nerve) may also be included to innervate the flap.
5. May be elevated as a fascia-only flap to allow primary closure of the donor site incision.
6. Normal Allen's test should be confirmed prior to flap harvest.
7. Disadvantage—unsightly donor site that must be skin grafted.

B. Scapular/Parascapular Free Flap

1. Highly versatile flap that provides a combination of skin, muscle, and bone for a spectrum of reconstructive problems.
2. Based on the circumflex scapular artery.
3. When used as an osteocutaneous flap, it can provide up to 15 cm of corticocancellous bone.
4. Flap can be deepithelialized to provide tissue for filling defects.
5. Disadvantages—thick cutaneous paddle and the intraoperative position change required for flap harvesting.

C. Fibula Free Flap (Flap of Choice for Mandibular Reconstruction)

1. Based on the peroneal artery and vein.
2. Thin, soft, and pliable skin paddle.
3. Can be used for both external skin coverage and intraoral lining.
4. Bone can be segmented by multiple osteotomies to conform to complex defects due to segmented reliable bone blood supply.

5. Preoperative angiography is indicated when preoperative vascular exam is abnormal to rule out peronea magna (dominant peroneal artery).
6. Skin blood supply is from the posterolateral intermuscular septum—septocutaneous and musculocutaneous branches from the peroneal artery through the flexor hallucis longus and soleus.

D. Rectus Abdominus Flap

1. Best for filling deep and large defects.
2. Provides large amount of tissue with long vascular pedicle (10 cm) and large vessels (2.5 mm).
3. No need for changing patient position intraoperatively, so simultaneous flap harvest is possible.
4. Skin paddle may be oriented vertically, horizontally, or obliquely. Oblique orientation allows harvest of a very large skin island.

E. Latissimus Dorsi Muscle Flap

1. Based on the thoracodorsal artery, which subdivides into lateral and medial branches within the muscle.
2. Large skin/muscle flap is possible. Can be combined with serratus anterior or scapular flap using the common subscapular pedicle.
3. Utilized because of its bulk, reliable anatomy, ample pedicle length and diameter, and minimal donor site morbidity.

F. Serratus Anterior Free Flap

1. Based on the serratus branch of the thoracodorsal artery and vein.
2. May include bone in the form of vascularized rib.
3. Scapular winging may occur if more than the lowest 3–4 slips of muscle are used.
4. May be harvested with latissimus muscle on same pedicle for coverage of the largest defects.

G. Deep Circumflex Iliac Artery Free Flap

1. Can be harvested with internal oblique muscle to increase volume.
2. Provides a large volume of high quality bone, but cannot be osteotomized as aggressively as fibula due to lack of segmental blood supply.
3. Useful for hemimandibular defects.

41

Principles of Orthognathic Surgery

Peter J. Taub, M.D., and H. Peter Lorenz, M.D.
Stanford University Medical Center, Stanford, California, U.S.A.

I. NORMAL ANATOMIC RELATIONSHIPS

Classic canons used as a point of reference and all relationships are approximate.

A. On frontal view of the face:

1. Eyebrows are usually arched laterally (highest peak is at the lateral limbus).
2. Eye fissure follows the pattern of the eyebrow (desirable angle off the horizontal is 2° lateral elevation).
3. Intercanthal distance is 28–32 mm (roughly equals distance from medial to lateral canthus).
4. Upper eyelids overlap the iris by 1–2 mm.
5. Midface width—from zygoma to zygoma—is divided into quarters, with each quarter the distance between the nasal alae.
6. Helix of the ear is on parallel with the hairline and slightly visible, protruding 1–1.5 cm from the mastoid process.
7. Length of the ear approximates the length of the nose.
8. Lower border of the earlobe is at the level of the subnasale.
9. Length of the upper lip is one-half the distance from the stomion to the menton.
10. Oral fissure is the length between one medial limbus to the other.

B. On profile view of the face:

1. Hairline to supraorbital rim is one-third of facial height.
2. Supraorbital rim to subnasale is one-third of facial height.
3. Subnasale to menton is one-third of facial height.
4. Anterior surface of the cornea projects 12–16 mm anterior to the lateral orbital rim and sits 8–10 mm posterior to the supraorbital ridge.
5. Nasofrontal angle is 130° in males and 134° in females.
6. Nasolabial angle is 100° in males and 105–108° in females.
7. Columella projects 4 mm caudal to the alar rim.
8. Long axis of the ear is 30° posterior to the vertical axis of the head.
9. Lower third of the face may be further divided into thirds with the subnasale to stomion representing one-third and the remainder representing two-thirds.
10. Upper lip usually rests slightly anterior to the lower lip.
11. In repose, the lips should contact one another.
12. Labiomental groove is 6 mm deep in males and 4 mm deep in females.

C. During puberty, the mandible grows more than the maxilla.

II. DEFINITIONS

- Buccal—toward the cheek.
- Lingual—toward the tongue.
- Distal—away from the midline.
- Mesial—toward the midline.

III. OCCLUSION

A. Described by the Angle classification of dental occlusion:

1. Class I occlusion—neutral occlusion where the mesiobuccal cusp of the maxillary 1st molar articulates with the buccal groove of the lower 1st molar.
2. Class II malocclusion—mandibular arch lies posterior to the maxillary arch ("overbite"). The mandibular 1st molar is distal to the class I relation. The mesiobuccal cusp of the maxillary 1st molar articulates anterior to the buccal groove of the 1st molar.
3. Class III malocclusion—mandibular arch lies anterior to the maxillary arch ("underbite"). The mandibular 1st molar is anterior to the class I relation. The mesiobuccal cusp of the maxillary 1st molar articulates posterior to the buccal groove of the mandibular 1st molar.

B. Centric occlusion is the position of maximal, bilateral, balanced contact between the maxillary and mandibular teeth.

C. Centric relation is the most retruded, unstrained position of the mandibular condyles within the glenoid fossa. Ideally, the jaws should be in centric occlusion and centric relation simultaneously.

D. Overjet and overbite:

1. Overjet describes the horizontal overlap of the incisors, which has a normal distance of approximately 2 mm. With excess overjet, the upper incisors are anterior to their normal position.
2. Overbite describes the vertical overlap of the incisors, which has a normal distance of approximately 2 mm. With excess overbite ("deep bite"), the upper incisors are lower than their normal position.

E. Occlusal cant:

1. Describes asymmetric growth or rotation of the maxilla or mandible.
2. Evaluated by examining the face from above the head as well as asking the patient to bite on a horizontally placed tongue blade.

IV. CEPHALOMETRIC ANALYSIS

A. Points to identify on the lateral cephalogram:

1. Sella—center of the sella turcica.
2. Nasion—bony nasofrontal junction.
3. Orbitale—most inferior point of the orbital cavity.
4. Point A—most posterior point on the maxillary alveolar process.
5. Point B—most posterior point on the mandibular alveolar process.
6. Pg (pogonion)—most anterior point on the mandibular symphysis.
7. Genion—point at the tip of the mandibular symphysis.
8. Menton—most inferior point on the mandibular symphysis.
9. Gonion—most inferoposterior point of the mandibular angle.
10. Porion—most superior point of the external auditory meatus.
11. Frankfurt horizontal plane—line between the porion and the orbitale.
12. Mandibular plane—line between gonion and menton.

B. Angles to calculate

1. SNA—relates the maxilla to the cranial base. Normal SNA angle is approximately 82°.
2. SNB—relates the mandible to the cranial base. Normal SNB angle is approximately 80°.
3. Mandibular plane angle—angle between the Frankfort horizontal plane and the mandibular plane.

It relates posterior facial height to anterior facial height.

Normal angle is approximately 21°.

The angle is more acute in patients with short-face syndrome and anterior open bite.

The angle is more obtuse in patients with long-face syndrome and a posterior open bite.

V. ORTHOGNATHIC SURGERY

A. Presurgical orthognathia aligns the teeth so that they are positioned directly above the mandible and below the maxilla.

B. Orthodontia is frequently required to eliminate the compensatory changes in the teeth. It aligns the occlusal surfaces of the teeth, removing the dental compensations. This initially worsens the malocclusion, but makes a stable class I occlusion possible after surgery.

C. The teeth frequently move in response to the malocclusion. For example, flaring of the lower incisors is seen with a class II malocclusion and retroclined lower incisors occur with a class III malocclusion.

D. Work-up includes photographs, radiographs (including lateral cephalogram and panorex views), and dental models.

E. Surgery is performed after cessation of mandibular growth, which occurs around the age of 17–18 years in males and slightly younger in females.

F. The radiographs should be performed over 6 months to ensure cessation of mandibular growth.

G. Presurgical manipulation of stone models is performed both to judge the amount of movement necessary and to ensure that the occlusal surfaces will be properly aligned. An acrylic splint with the occlusal surfaces in the planned postoperative relation is then created.

VI. COMMON OSTEOTOMIES USED IN ORTHOGNATHIC SURGERY

A. Le Fort I Osteotomy

1. Most commonly used osteotomy of the maxilla.
2. First performed for malocclusion by Wassmund.
3. The osteotomy is performed across the anterior maxilla 4–5 mm above the roots of the maxillary teeth and below the infraorbital foramen. The osteotomy is then continued through the lateral and medial maxillary walls below the nasolacrimal duct. The septum is separated from the vomer, and an osteotomy is performed between the maxillary tuberosity and pterygoid plate of the sphenoid.
4. Segmental osteotomies can be made in the alveolus and palate in order to widen or narrow the transverse width of the maxilla.
5. Complications:
   - Traction on the infraorbital nerve with resultant cheek and upper lip sensory loss.
   - Injury to the greater palatine neurovascular bundle.
   - Nasopalatine nerve injury—occurs during down-fracture and results in sensory loss to the premaxillary palatal mucosa.
   - Velopharyngeal insufficiency—usually only occurs in cleft palate patients who undergo moderate to severe advancement.

B. Le Fort II Osteotomy

1. First performed for nontrauma cases by Tessier in the 1960s.
2. True total maxillary osteotomy.
3. Performed through the nasofrontal junction and across the anterior maxilla. It may be anterior or posterior to the nasolacrimal apparatus.
4. Commonly used for the following conditions:
   - Binder's syndrome.
   - Crouzon's syndrome.
   - Hemifacial microsmia.
   - Severe maxillary hypoplasia involving the nose and infraorbital rims.

C. Le Fort III Osteotomy

1. Designed to enlarge the orbital cavity and advance the maxilla.
2. Performed through the zygomaticofrontal suture, the nasofrontal junction, medial orbital wall, orbital floor, and the zygomatic arch.

D. Sagittal-Split Osteotomy

1. Originally described by Trauner and Obwegeser in 1955.

2. Procedure of choice for advancement of the mandible, but may also be applied for setback in the case of prognathism.
3. Technique involves:
   - Buccal and anterior lingual subperiosteal dissection of the soft tissues off the ramus of the mandible.
   - A horizontal cut in the lingual cortex above the lingula.
   - A vertical cut on the buccal cortex at the level of the second molar to the antegonial notch.
   - A sagittal connection of the two osteotomies along the external oblique line.
4. Alveolar nerve remains with the distal bony segment.
5. In the case of a setback, a portion of the proximal segment is removed, equal in width to the amount of desired movement.
6. Following osteotomy, the condyles must be seated properly in the glenoid fossae to obtain the planned centric occlusion. Too low a placement will result in an anterior open-bite deformity because of premature molar contact. Too high a placement will result in compression of the condylar head and TMJ arthropathy.
7. Segments are held in wire fixation intraoperatively with a variable duration of postoperative elastic therapy.
8. There is a 1:1 relationship between the soft tissue and bone correction at the chin.
9. Complications:
   - Inferior alveolar nerve disturbance—occurs in the vast majority and results in some degree of sensory loss to the lower lip.
   - Lingual sensory nerve disturbance—occurs less commonly and results in loss of sensation of the tongue, floor of the mouth, and gingiva.
   - Mandibular branch of the facial nerve disturbance—rare.
   - Open bite deformity and/or TMJ arthropathy—results from poor placement of the condyles during centric occlusion.
   - Avascular necrosis of the proximal bony segment, secondary to over-aggressive stripping of soft tissue.
   - Relapse—may occur if the mandibular body is brought too far forward resulting in stretch of the suprahyoid muscles.

E. Vertical and Oblique Subcondylar Osteotomy

1. Used for mandibular setback—preferred approach in certain instances:
   - Distances greater than 10 mm.
   - Asymmetric mandibles.
   - Reoperative cases.
2. Vertical osteotomy was described by Caldwell and Letterman in 1954.
3. Oblique modification was described by Robinson in 1956.
4. May be performed:
   - Via an external approach, through an incision 1 cm below the angle of the mandible.
   - Via an internal approach, with a mucosal incision along the anterior border of the ramus from the coronoid process into the buccal sulcus to the second mandibular bicuspid.
5. Low incidence of inferior alveolar or lingual nerve injury.

F. Genioplasty

1. May be performed independently or in conjunction with orthognathic procedures.
2. Types of osteotomies include:
   - Sliding horizontal osteotomy (either anterior or posterior).
   - Transverse sliding osteotomy.
   - Horizontal osteotomy and replacement as a graft.
   - Wedge osteotomy for lateral shift of the midline.
3. Alloplastic implants are an alternative to genioplasty achieved by osteotomy.
4. Types of chin deformities treatable with genioplasty include:
   - Macrogenia.
   - Microgenia.

- Combined macrogenia and microgenia.
- Asymmetry.
- Pseudomacrogenia—excessive soft tissue.
- Pseudomicrogenia—retrogenia secondary to excessive maxillary growth and mandibular clockwise rotation.
- Witch's chin deformity—ptotic soft tissue.

G. Other

Long-term dysfunction of the distal inferior alveolar nerve (mental nerve) is rare.

VII. CLINICAL DENTAL-FACIAL SKELETAL ABNORMALITIES

A. Vertical Maxillary Excess—"Long Face Syndrome"

1. Clinical examination may reveal:
   - Increased lower-third facial height.
   - Narrowed nasal alar base.
   - Obtuse nasolabial angle.
   - Anterior open bite with associated mentalis strain or lip incompetence.
   - Excessive upper incisor and gingival show.
   - Retrognathia with clockwise autorotation of the mandible causing a more obtuse mandibular plane angle.
2. Cephalometric analysis shows an increased SNA angle and a decreased SNB angle.
3. Correction requires LeFort I osteotomy and posterior movement of the maxilla.
4. Mandibular advancement may be a necessary adjunctive procedure.
5. If true microgenia is present (rather than a normal mandible that appears deficient due to clockwise autorotation), osseous genioplasty may also be indicated.

B. Vertical Maxillary Deficiency—"Short Face Syndrome"

1. Clinical examination may reveal:
   - Diminished lower-third facial height.
   - Widened nasal alar base.
   - Acute nasolabial angle.
   - Deep bite with a protruding chin.
   - Deficient upper incisor and gingival show, producing an edentulous appearance.
   - Acute mandibular angle.
2. Correction often requires LeFort I osteotomy, horizontal advancement, and interpositional bone graft.
3. Genioplasty with posterior movement of the chin or wedge resection may also be needed to correct the diminished lower-third facial height.

C. Transverse Maxillary Deficiency

1. Long-term stability associated with maxillary transverse expansion and/or intrusion/extrusion is far superior to orthodontic tooth movement in the same direction.
2. Significant orthodontic expansion of the adult maxillary dentition is unstable and risks fenestration of the buccal cortical plate of the maxilla by tooth roots. The stability of orthodontic extrusion of the anterior teeth or intrusion of the posterior teeth to close an anterior open bite is unreliable.
3. If the deficiency is primarily posterior, a two-piece LeFort I osteotomy is indicated. This is usually done between the central incisors anteriorly and parasagitally through the hard palate while the maxilla is in the down-fractured position. This procedure is able to widen the maxilla 6–8 mm.
4. If the deficiency is primarily anterior in the region of the canine teeth, four-piece LeFort I osteotomy is indicated.
5. These procedures can also be done to narrow the maxilla in cases of transverse excess.

D. Mandibular Prognathism

1. Clinical exam may reveal dental changes that serve to compensate for the abnormal position of the mandible and class III malocclusion.
2. Protrusion of the maxillary teeth.
3. Lingual inclination of the mandibular teeth.

4. Treated with surgical procedures designed to setback the mandible. These include:
   - Sagittal split osteotomy.
   - Vertical subcondylar osteotomy.

E. Retrognathism

1. Small or retropositioned mandible.
2. Associated with a Class II malocclusion: mesiobuccal groove of the mandibular first molar is distal to the mesiobuccal cusp of the maxillary first molar.
3. Diagnosed on physical exam, cephalogram, dental casts, and photographs.
4. Syndromic patients may have coexisting condylar and coronoid process problems.
5. Associated etiologies include:
   - Hereditary (Treacher-Collins)—majority of cases in the United States.
   - Hemifacial microsomia.
   - Trauma.
   - Obligatory mouth breathing.
   - Thumb sucking.

F. Temporomandibular Joint (TMJ) Dysfunction

1. The mandible opens at the TMJ at an average interincisal distance of 40–50 mm.
2. The first 20–25 mm of opening is the result of hinge action at the TMJ.
3. The final 15–20 mm of opening is the result of anteroinferior translation of the mandibular condyles.
4. Patients with interincisal opening of less than 15 mm are severely disabled and may be candidates for TMJ therapeutic procedures:
   - Arthroscopy (with biopsy, debridement, and/or lavage).
   - Disk repositioning.
   - Removal of osteophytes.
   - Condylar replacement with an autogenous costochondral graft.
   - Alloplastic implantation (for severe cases only).

42

Facial Fractures

Michael C. Edwards, M.D.
Baylor College of Medicine, Houston, Texas, U.S.A.
Larry H. Hollier, M.D.
Texas Children's Hospital and Baylor College of Medicine, Houston, Texas, U.S.A.

I. FRONTAL SINUS FRACTURES

A. Anatomy and Mechanism

1. The frontal sinus consists of two paired irregular cavities.
2. The cavities are divided by septa that drain via the nasofrontal duct (NFD) through the ethmoidal air cells into the nasal cavity via the middle meatus.
3. The frontal sinus first appears radiographically at about 8 years of age:
   - May develop unilaterally in 10% of people.
   - Rudimentary development in 5%.
   - Absent in 4%.
4. The frontal bone is the strongest bone of the face:
   - Because of the high energy required, isolated fractures of the frontal bone are the least frequently encountered facial fracture.
   - The most common mechanisms of frontal sinus injury are direct blows to the glabella or supraorbital rims.
   - Less frequently, indirect fractures can be produced by transmission of forces from the lower facial skeleton.
5. Polytrauma, including intracranial hematoma, often accompanies frontal bone fractures.
6. Of the associated maxillofacial injuries, naso-orbito-ethmoidal (NOE) fractures are the most common.

B. Signs on Physical Exam

1. Most common signs:
   - Contusions
   - Lacerations
   - Hematomas in the area of the forehead or orbit, such as the classic spectacle hematoma
2. In the acute setting, swelling and bruising may obscure a visible or palpable step deformity secondary to an underlying fracture.
3. Larger supraorbital fractures are associated with hypesthesia in the distribution of the supraorbital nerve and orbital emphysema.
4. Swelling in the roof of the orbit produced by a displaced roof fracture will produce a characteristic downward and forward positioning of the globe.
5. Extension of the fracture posteriorly into the superior orbital fissure (SOF) and optic foramen

will produce superior orbital fissure syndrome or orbital apex syndrome (see Sec. II.B).

6. Due to frequently associated ocular injuries, evaluation of the visual system is essential. This must include inspection of the globe and examination of light perception, pupillary light reflex, and visual acuity.
7. Mental status changes may reflect associated brain injury and documentation of the patient's neurological status, including a Glasgow Coma Scale rating, is essential.
8. Fractures through the orbital frontal bone and anterior cranial fossa may have associated dural lacerations that may produce either otorrhea or rhinorrhea. This may be evidenced by the double ring sign (halo sign) when this fluid is absorbed onto a paper towel.

C. Radiographic Diagnosis

1. Plain films may detect displaced fractures. They may also demonstrate an air-fluid level in the frontal sinus or pneumocephalus.
2. The appropriate plain films consist of anteroposterior (AP) and lateral skull films, and Water's, submentovertex, and Caldwell views (Fig. 1).
3. CT scanning with 3-mm axial cuts is the most sensitive modality for diagnosing frontal sinus fractures. Displacement of the fracture fragments is easy to appreciate with this study.
4. The suspicion for a NFD duct injury or obstruction should be raised by fractures that are located inferior and medial in the frontal sinus.

D. Treatment

1. Operative approach is via a coronal incision.
2. The sinus is inspected after removing anterior table fragments.
3. Any blockage of the NFD preventing adequate drainage of mucosal secretions predisposes to mucocele formation. This generally presents years following the injury, but can be life-threatening.
4. Blockage of the NFD may be confirmed by instilling methylene blue in the sinus and failing to detect staining of pledgets placed in the nose at the level of the middle meatus.

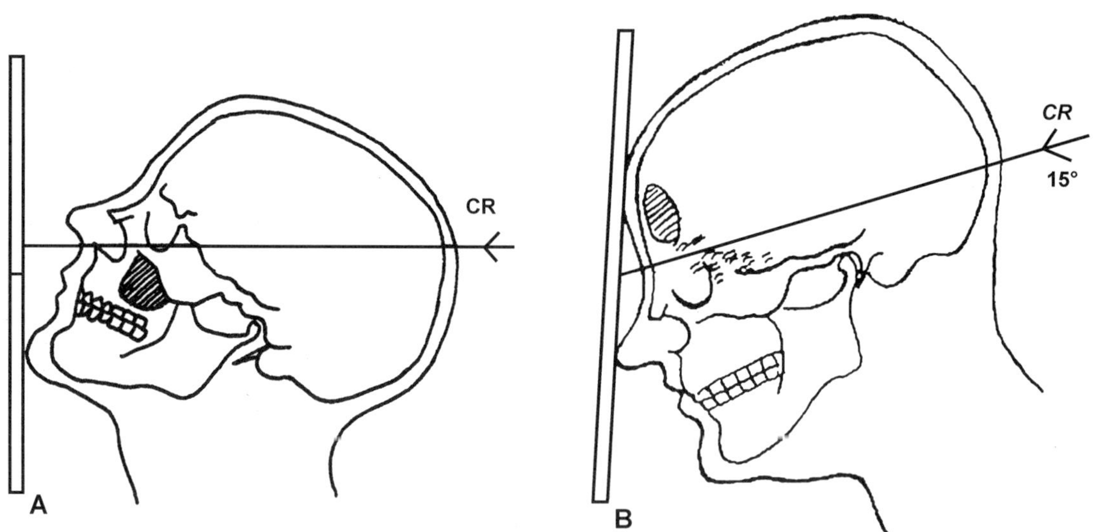

Figure 1 (A) Water's view. Position of the patient in relation to the film and the central ray (CR). Posteroanterior view for visualization of the maxillary sinuses, maxilla, orbits, and zygomatic arches. In this view, the petrous ridges are projected just below the floor of the maxillary sinuses. (B) Caldwell position. Posteroanterior view of the skull. This position is used to study fractures of the frontal bone, orbital margins, zygomaticofrontal sutures, and lateral walls of the maxillary sinuses. The paranasal sinuses are shown in this projection. The petrous ridges are shown at a level between the lower and middle thirds of the orbits (From Manson P: Facial injuries. In: McCarthy JG, ed. *Plastic Surgery*. Philadelphia: WB Saunders Company, 1990.)

5. Fractures of the NFD are treated by obliteration. This involves removing the sinus mucosa, burring the bone (eradicates mucosa in vascular pits of the sinus), and filling the sinus cavity with bone, muscle, or fat. Alternatively, the sinus may be simply left alone to be filled naturally by the process of osteoneogenesis.
6. The NFD must also be plugged with graft material to prevent repopulation of the sinus by migratory respiratory epithelium from the nose.
7. Displaced anterior table fractures should be repaired by repositioning and fixation with microplates (Fig. 2A).
8. Displaced fractures of the posterior table with a CSF leak require cranialization that entails removal of the posterior wall and sinus and NFD obliteration (Fig. 2B). This allows the brain to expand into the frontal sinus cavity.
9. Observation is indicated in nondisplaced anterior table fractures and posterior table fractures without CSF leakage.

E. Postoperative Care

1. Patient should be prohibited from nose blowing and sneezing.
2. Broad-spectrum antibiotics should be continued.
3. The head of the bed should be elevated to minimize edema.
4. Nasal decongestant sprays may be helpful.

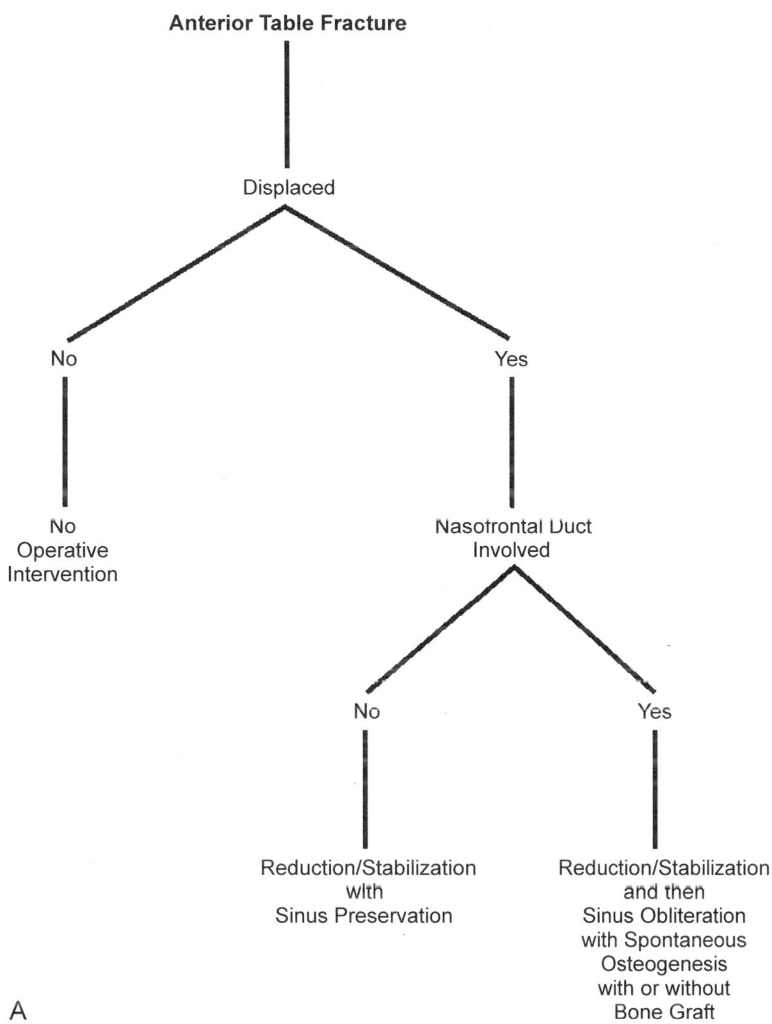

Figure 2 (A) Anterior table fracture management algorithm. (B) (see next page) Combined anterior/posterior table fracture management algorithm (From Rohrich RJ; Hollier LH; Management of frontal sinus fractures. *Clin. Plast. Surg*. 1992; 19:219.)

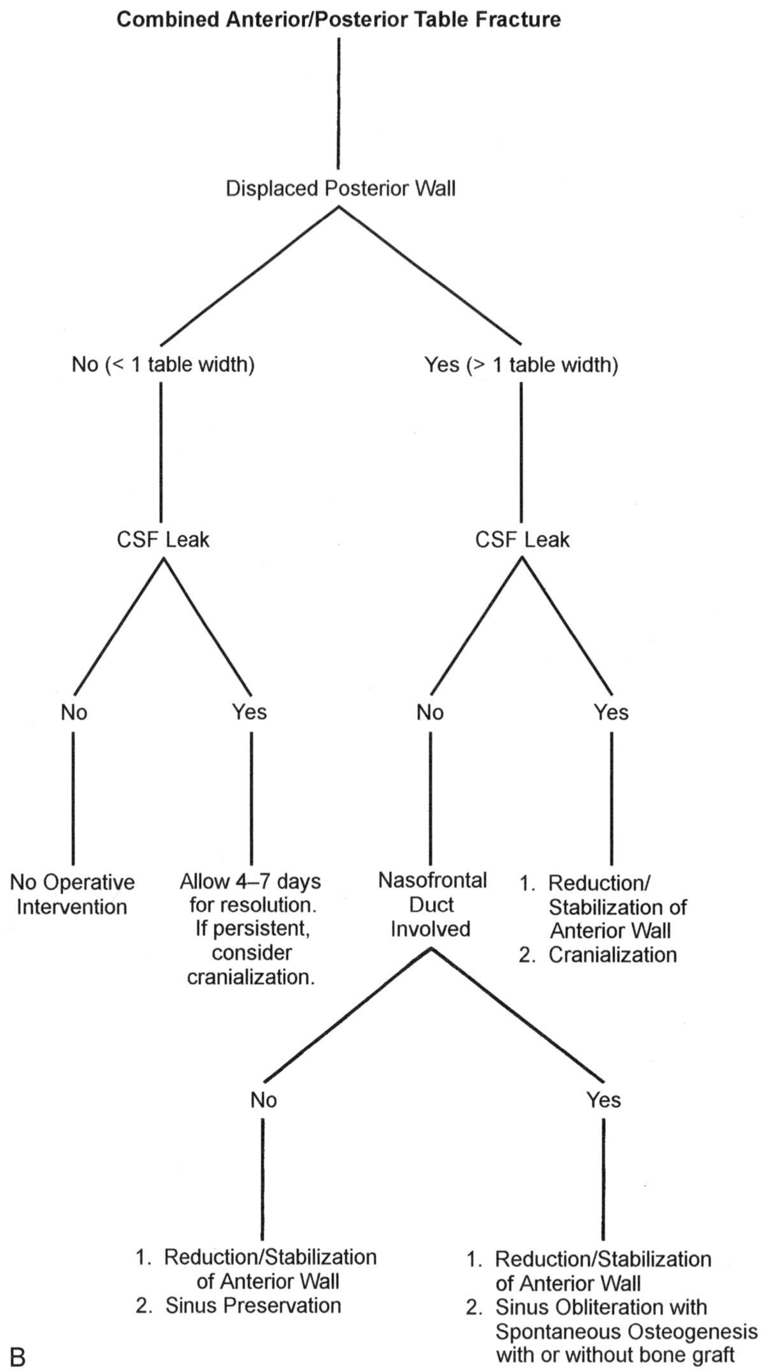

Figure 2 Continued.

II. FRACTURES OF THE ORBIT

A. Anatomy and Mechanism

1. The orbit is composed of seven bones:
   - Zygoma
   - Lesser and greater wings of the sphenoid bone
   - Frontal bone
   - Ethmoid bone
   - Lacrimal bone
   - Palatine bone
   - Maxilla
2. The superior orbital fissure (SOF) is a cleft that runs superior and lateral to the apex of the orbit, separating the greater and lesser wings of the sphenoid. Provides a path for the oculomotor nerve (CN III), trochlear nerve (CN IV), abducens nerve (CN VI), and the ophthalmic division of the trigeminal nerve (CN V1).
3. The inferior orbital fissure provides passage of the maxillary division of the trigeminal nerve (CN V2), branches of the sphenopalatine ganglion, and branches of the inferior ophthalmic vein.
4. The optic nerve enters the orbit superiomedially within the orbital cone approximately 45 mm posterior to the orbital rim.
5. Orbital blowout fractures are most often caused by a force applied to the orbital rim with resultant fracture of the orbital floor and sometimes the medial wall of the orbit.

B. Signs on Physical Exam

1. Orbital fractures are usually associated with periorbital edema, ecchymosis, and subconjunctival hemorrhage. Palpable bony step-offs may be appreciated along the orbital rim.
2. Oculomotor disturbances resulting in diplopia may be present. The most common cause of diplopia is extraocular muscle contusion, although the periorbita may be entrapped in the fracture.
   - If diplopia occurs and extraocular muscle entrapment is suspected, a forced duction test should be performed to rule out mechanical entrapment of the periorbital musculature. In the forced duction test, after the conjunctiva has been topically anesthetized, forceps are used to grasp the conjunctiva near the inferior oblique muscle. The globe is gently rotated, feeling for any restriction of motion.
   - Ophthalmologic consultation should be obtained in all cases of orbital fracture.
3. Enlargement of the orbital cavity may result in enophthalmos. Enophthalmos in excess of 2 mm results in a noticeable deformity, but this is not usually appreciated in the early postinjury period due to swelling.
4. Injury to the levator muscle or CN III will result in ptosis.
5. Fractures involving the SOF may produce superior orbital fissure syndrome, consisting of:
   - Ophthalmoplegia
   - A fixed and dilated pupil
   - Upper eyelid ptosis
   - Loss of the corneal reflex
6. Orbital apex syndrome is SOF with associated involvement of the optic nerve that impairs vision.
7. Fractures injuring the retina or optic nerve may result in a Marcus-Gunn pupil or afferent pupillary defect, in which a light shone in the affected eye will produce no pupillary constriction, but a light shone in the contralateral eye will constrict the affected pupil.

C. Radiographic Diagnosis

1. Thin section, axial, and coronal CT scanning is required for diagnosis.
2. Axial CT scans display the medial and lateral orbital walls well.
3. Coronal scans demonstrate abnormalities of the orbital floor, roof, and interorbital area.
   - Fractures of the floor are difficult to diagnose without coronal images. If the patient's neck cannot be hyperextended to obtain these views, they should be reconstructed from the axial images.
   - An oblique parasagittal reconstruction along

the long axis of the globe gives the best view of the orbital floor.

- Plain films are rarely useful. A Water's view may sometimes demonstrate the fractures.

D. Treatment

1. Treatment goals for orbital fractures include reduction of herniated orbital contents and reestablishment of normal orbital contour, volume, and function.
2. The indications for surgery include large floor defects (>1 cm^2), mechanical entrapment, and enophthalmos.
3. Reconstruction is achieved using open reduction and plating of fractures of the rim.
   - The orbital floor and medial wall may be reconstructed with autogenous bone grafts or alloplastic implants such as titanium mesh, porous polyethylene (Medpor), or silicone.
   - In floor reconstruction, it is important to recreate the normal anatomy of the floor to prevent enlarging the orbital volume that would result in enophthalmos (Fig. 3).

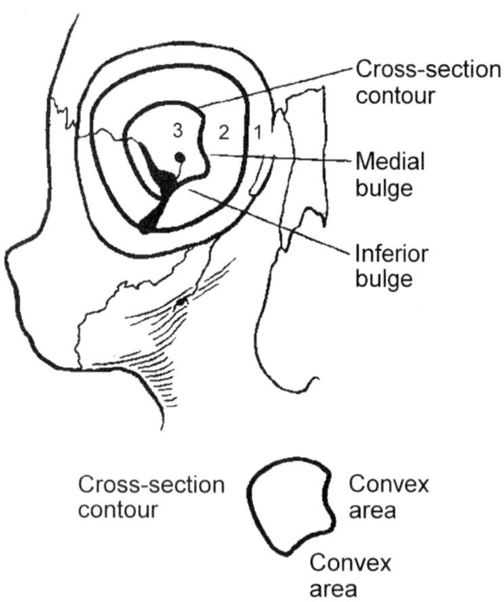

Figure 3 Anatomy of the orbit. Note the inferomedial bulge that arises in the posterior aspect of the orbit. This bulge is an important anatomic consideration to prevent enophthalmos after orbital reconstruction. (From Smith ML; Williams K; Gruss JS: Management of orbital fractures. *Oper. Tech. Plast. Surg*. 1998; 5:318.)

4. Infraorbital rim and floor fractures may be approached by subciliary, subtarsal, or transconjunctival incisions, with or without a lateral canthotomy to improve visualization. Medial wall fractures can be accessed via the above incisions, but a coronal incision greatly improves access.
5. At the end of the procedure, if lower lid tone is not felt to be sufficient, a lateral canthopexy and/or a Frost suture between the upper and lower eyelids should be placed to prevent ectropion.

E. Postoperative Care

1. The head of the bed should be elevated to minimize edema.
2. Eye lubrication with drops or ointment.
3. Frost suture should be removed in 24–48 h.
4. Instructions in massage of the lower lid to soften scar and decrease ectropion risk.

III. FRACTURES OF THE NASO-ORBITO-ETHMOID (NOE) COMPLEX

A. Anatomy and Mechanism

1. The NOE complex consists of:
   - Paired nasal bones
   - Nasal septum
   - Nasal cartilage
   - Nasal processes of the frontal bones
   - Frontal processes of the maxilla
   - Lacrimal bones
   - Ethmoid bone
   - Sphenoid bones
2. The NOE complex also contains the attachment of the medial canthal ligament, a tendinous insertion of the orbicularis oculi. The medial canthal ligament consists of anterior and posterior attachments to the lacrimal crests (which surround the lacrimal sac) and a superior attachment to the nasofrontal region (Fig. 4).
3. When a blunt force is directed over the bridge of the nose, the skeletal support of the nose is projected backward between the orbits, resulting in a NOE-type fracture.
4. Fractures may be unilateral (36%) or more commonly bilateral (64%).

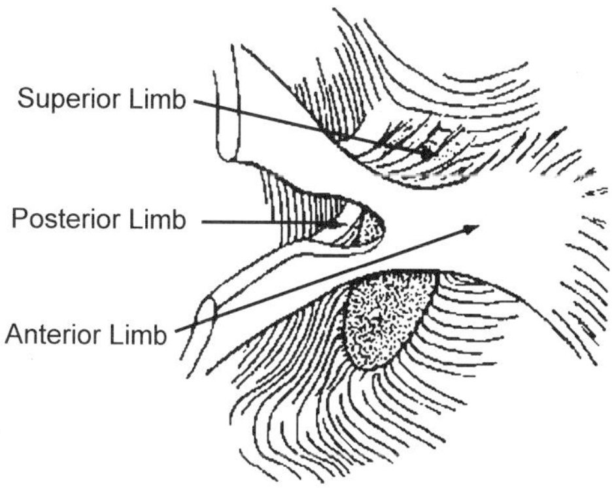

Figure 4 Diagrammatic insertion of the medial canthal ligament. There are three limbs: superior, anterior, and posterior. The anterior limb fans out onto the lateral surface of the nasal bone. The posterior limb is thin, attaching to the posterior aspect of the lacrimal fossa. The superior limb hoods the lacrimal sac and joins the junction of the frontal process of maxilla with the internal angular process of the frontal bone. (From Leipziger LS, Manson P. Nasoethmoid orbital fractures. Current concepts. *Clin. Plast. Surg.* 1992; 19:167.)

5. NOE fractures are often accompanied by orbital blowout fractures.

B. Signs on Physical Exam

1. Clinical presentation of NOE fractures usually consists of glabellar, periorbital, and nasal ecchymosis. Characteristically, patients present with a loss of dorsal nasal prominence.
2. Bimanual examination over the canthal region may detect bony crepitus.
3. The lower eyelid should be placed on lateral traction and the canthal ligament palpated to detect if its attachments are intact (bowstring test). Disruption of these ligaments results in traumatic telecanthus with an increase in the distance between the medial canthi.
4. Epiphora may be seen with disruption of the lacrimal system.
   - The system's continuity may be tested by placing fluorescein dye in the fornix and observing for uptake on a cotton-tip applicator placed in the inferior meatus.
   - Approximately 15% of NOE fractures will ultimately need a procedure to allow for lacrimal drainage, but this is not performed at the time of fracture fixation.
   - CSF rhinorrhea may be found due to fracture of the cribiform plate.

C. Radiographic Diagnosis

1. Thin-section axial CT scan is the imaging modality of choice.
2. Plain radiographs are generally not useful.
3. NOE fracture classification:
   - Type I = single-segment central fragment with medial canthal tendon attached.
   - Type II = comminuted central fragment fractures with medial canthal tendon still attached to a bone fragment.
   - Type III = comminuted fracture with canthal tendon avulsion.

D. Treatment

1. Treatment goals for NOE fractures include the reduction and stabilization of fractures, reestablishment of intercanthal distance, and reestablishment of dorsal nasal height and projection.
2. All fracture sites must be thoroughly explored through a coronal incision. A lower lid incision may improve visualization.
3. The canthal tendon should be identified and looped with wire suture. This should then be passed transnasally with a posterior and superior vector of pull to establish medial canthal position.
4. All fracture fragments should be reduced and plated.
5. Frequently, dorsal nasal support must be restored using a cantilever bone graft.

E. Postoperative Care

1. The head of bed should be elevated to minimize edema.
2. The patient should not blow his/her nose for several weeks.
3. Epiphora should resolve as edema resolves. Persistence requires reassessment.
4. Antibiotics should be initiated to prevent meningitis.

5. CSF leakage is not uncommon and should resolve within 7–14 days. If not, consideration should be given to a lumbar drain.

IV. NASAL FRACTURES

A. Anatomy and Mechanism

1. The nose consists of the paired nasal bones and the paired upper and lower lateral cartilages (Fig. 5).
2. The midline septum consists of the vomer, the perpendicular plate of the ethmoid, the quadrangular cartilage, and the nasal crest of the maxilla.
3. Blood supply:
   - Ophthalmic artery.
   - Anterior and posterior ethmoidal branches of the internal carotid artery.
   - The facial (superior labial branch) and internal maxillary branches (sphenopalatine, greater palatine, and infraorbital branches) of the external carotid artery also supply the nose.
   - The internal carotid branches supply the nose primarily superior to the middle turbinate; the external carotid branches supply the area inferior to this.
4. The external nose is innervated primarily by:
   - Infraorbital nerve.
   - Anterior ethmoid nerve.
   - Supratrochlear nerve.
5. The internal nose is innervated primarily by the ethmoidal, sphenoidal, and nasopalatine nerves.
6. The nasal bone is the weakest part of the facial skeleton and constitutes approximately 40% of all facial fractures.
7. Frontal trauma to the nasal dorsum often fractures the thin lower half of nasal bones and the septum.
8. Lateral forces in younger patients tend to result in fracture-dislocations of large segments, whereas older patients tend to have comminution.
9. Higher forces may result in extension of the fracture into the NOE region.

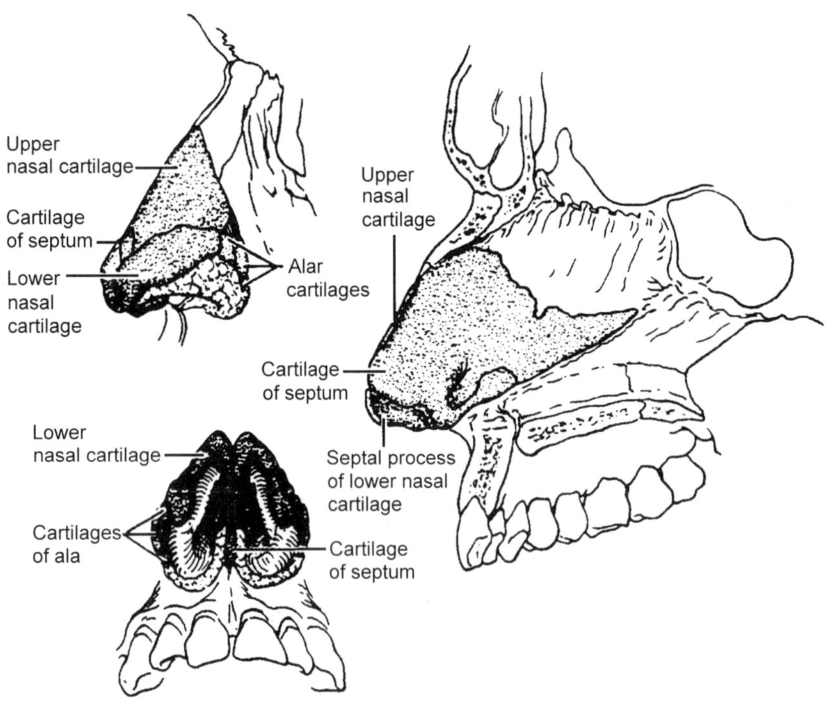

Figure 5 The external and internal cartilaginous framework of the nose. (From Rowe NL; Williams JL; eds: *Maxillofacial Injuries*. New York: Churchill Livingstone, 1985.)

B. Signs on Physical Exam

1. Nasal fractures are readily diagnosed by physical exam with the palpation of tenderness, mobility, and bony crepitus.
2. Nasal deviation may be apparent.
3. Intranasal examination may reveal deviation of the septum or septal hematomas.
4. Epistaxis may be present.

C. Radiographic Diagnosis

1. Radiographs are not necessary to make the diagnosis.
2. Plain films may be obtained for legal documentation.
3. CT exam is warranted when there is suspicion of other facial fractures. This is especially important in the evaluation of NOE fractures.

D. Treatment

1. Epistaxis can usually be stopped by direct pressure.
   - Correcting hypertension and the use of vasoconstrictive sprays may also be helpful.
   - In severe cases with ongoing hemorrhage, placement of a Foley catheter with the balloon position posteriorly may tamponade the bleeding.
   - Blood clots should be extracted and any septal hematoma should be evacuated by incision of the mucoperichondrium to prevent septal necrosis.
2. Goals of treatment include reelevation and alignment of the nasal bones, and return of the nasal septum to the midline.
3. Fractures should be treated at the time of initial evaluation by closed reduction.
4. After 24 h, edema obscures the visible deformity and reduction is best deferred for approximately 7 days when swelling has decreased.
5. Fractures treated later than 1–2 weeks may not be amenable to closed reduction.
6. For reduction, the nose is packed with cotton pledgets soaked in 4% cocaine or 1:100,000 epinephrine. The infraorbital, supratrochlear, and intranasal nerves may be infiltrated with 1–2% lidocaine with 1:100,000 epinephrine.
7. The surgeon should wear a fiberoptic headlight.
8. A nasal speculum should be used. Asch or Walsham forceps facilitate manipulation of the nasal bones.
9. After reduction, silicone nasal splints are placed and sutured to the membranous septum to prevent the formation of synechiae. An external splint is then applied on the dorsum.
10. Delayed treatment of severe nasal fractures often requires formal rhinoplasty.

E. Postoperative Care

1. Nasal splints are kept in place for 7–10 days.
2. The head of the bed should be elevated.
3. No nose blowing for several weeks.
4. No glasses should rest on the nasal dorsum.

V. FRACTURES OF THE MALAR COMPLEX AND ZYGOMATIC ARCH

A. Anatomy and Mechanism

1. The zygoma is also known as the malar bone or tripod.
   - It articulates with the frontal bone, maxilla, temporal bone, and greater wing of the sphenoid along the lateral orbital wall.
   - The zygomaticotemporal and zygomaticofacial nerves exit through small foramina in the zygoma to supply sensation to the soft tissues of the malar eminence.
2. Zygomatic arch fractures can occur as isolated fractures secondary to direct blows with the remaining articulations of the zygoma remaining intact.
3. The zygoma fractures at all of its articulations, most often secondary to a direct blow. Displacement may be increased by the pull of the masseter muscle as it attaches to the arch.

B. Signs on Physical Exam

1. For isolated arch fractures, depression of the arch may be appreciated.
2. Trismus from impingement of the arch on the coronoid process is possible.

3. Zygoma fractures, by definition, involve the orbit with resulting periorbital and subconjunctival hemorrhage frequently seen.
4. Loss of malar prominence may be apparent, especially when examined from the basilar view.
5. Inferior displacement of the zygoma results in a corresponding inferior displacement of the lateral canthal mechanism that is attached to Whitnall's tubercle, located approximately 10 mm below the zygomaticofrontal suture. This produces a characteristic antimongoloid slant to the palpebral fissure.
6. The infraorbital nerve is often lacerated or contused, resulting in anesthesia of the anterior cheek, upper lip, and lateral aspect of the nose.
7. Enophthalmos may result from increased orbital volume as the zygoma comprises a large portion of the lateral orbital wall.

C. Radiographic Diagnosis

1. Water's view provides information regarding the fracture and is the best plain film for zygomaticomaxillary complex (ZMC) fractures.
2. Submentovertex view provides detail of the zygomatic arch.
3. Thin-section axial CT scanning is essential to accurately detail the anatomy of the fracture, particularly with respect to displacement.
4. Orbital floor blowout fractures often accompany zygomatic fractures and are best appreciated on coronal images.

D. Treatment

1. The goals of treatment include restoration of skeletal buttresses and restoration of orbital volume.
2. For malar complex fractures, the indications for surgery include fractures that display significant displacement. This is best appreciated on the axial CT at the level of the articulation of the zygoma with the greater wing of the sphenoid (lateral orbital wall).
3. The standard of treatment for any displaced fracture is open reduction and internal rigid fixation.
4. Incisions employed:
   - Intraoral (gingivobuccal sulcus)
   - Lower eyelid (similar to orbital floor fractures)
   - Upper eyelid (lateral portion of blepharoplasty incision)
   - With these incisions, three buttresses may be plated: zygomaticofrontal, zygomaticomaxillary, and infraorbital rim.
5. Severe fractures with comminution may require a coronal incision to allow visualization and plating of the arch.
6. The lateral orbital wall forms a broad articulation with the zygoma and is a good location to check reduction.
7. At the end of the procedure, the facial soft tissues should be resuspended using a suture placed through the periosteum of the cheek and securing this cephalad through drill holes to the orbital rim laterally.
8. As with orbital fractures, lateral canthopexy and/or Frost suture should be used to prevent ectropion if lower lid tone is diminished.
9. The indication for operative management of isolated arch fractures includes visible displacement (contour deformity) or trismus.
   - The approach is a Gillies incision (temporal scalp) with an elevator slid down to the posterior surface of the arch traveling along the surface of the temporalis.
   - An intraoral approach may be used.
   - The fracture is elevated and, if unstable, can be secured with a suture passed under bone and tied over a metal eye patch placed over the arch as a stent.

E. Postoperative Care

1. Frost sutures must be removed in 24–48 h.
2. Eye lubrication should be used.
3. Intraoral hygiene is important if an incision was made here. Half-strength hydrogen peroxide, Peridex, or normal saline rinses are adequate.

VI. FRACTURES OF THE MAXILLA AND MIDFACE

A. Anatomy and Mechanism

1. The midface is composed of a system of vertical and horizontal buttresses, which are areas of thicker bone that provide resistance against forces applied to the face.

2. The strong vertical buttresses maintain the vertical dimensions of the face. These include.

   - Nasomaxillary (NM) buttress—extends along the pyriform aperture and medial orbital rim.
   - Zygomaticomaxillary (ZM) buttress—extends from the maxillary alveolus up through the zygoma to the zygomaticofrontal suture.
   - Pterygomaxillary (PM) buttress—extends to the cranial base from the posterior portion of the maxilla.

3. Fractures of the maxilla vary from simple dento-alveolar fractures to comminuted fractures of the entire midface, depending on the magnitude and direction of applied force.
4. In a complete maxillary fracture, all vertical buttresses are interrupted.

   - Le Fort I fractures go through the maxilla at about the level of the piriform rim, including the entire alveolar process, the palate, and the pterygoid processes.
   - Le Fort II fractures include the Le Fort I fragment but extend cephalad to involve part of the inferomedial orbit and extend across the nose to isolate a pyramidal-shaped maxillary segment.
   - Le Fort III fractures result in craniofacial dysjunction with the fracture extending through the frontozygomatic suture, nasofrontal suture, across the floor of the orbits, and the zygomatic arches.

5. Fractures of the maxilla may also occur in a sagittal direction, usually beginning adjacent to the cuspid tooth.
6. Pure Le Fort I, II, or III fractures are less common than mixed fractures involving one Le Fort level on one side and a different Le Fort level on the other side.

B. Signs on Physical Exam

1. The midface may have an elongated, retruded appearance (dishface).
2. Intraoral examination may reveal lacerations in the gingiva or mucosa.
3. Examination of occlusion is important.
4. Malocclusion is possible, especially an anterior open bite.
5. Grasping the anterior maxilla between the thumb and index finger while stabilizing the head may demonstrate mobility of the midface.
6. Lip or palatal lacerations often accompany palatal fractures.

C. Radiographic Diagnosis

1. Plain films including Water's and Caldwell views may demonstrate fracture lines and maxillary sinus opacification.
2. Axial CT scanning is essential for the diagnosis of maxillary fractures.
3. Fractures must extend through the pterygoid plates to be properly termed a Le Fort fracture.

D. Treatment

1. If the airway is compromised by bleeding or swelling, particularly when a mandible fracture is present, one must consider intubation or tracheostomy at the time of initial evaluation.
2. It is most important to reestablish normal dental occlusion.
3. Arch bars and intermaxillary fixation (IMF) are performed initially.
4. Exposure and plating is determined by the level of injury.

   - For LeFort I fractures, an intraoral incision is used and the ZM/NM buttresses are plated.
   - For LeFort II fractures, intraoral and lower lid incisions are used and the ZM buttress is plated. The medial fracture is usually plated along the orbital rim.
   - For LeFort III fractures, intraoral and coronal incisions are used to access all fracture sites. The zygomatic arch, ZF suture, and nasofrontal regions are plated.
   - Usually, IMF can be removed at the end of case, but the arch bars should be maintained for possible postoperative elastic traction to adjust minor occlusal discrepancies.

E. Postoperative Care

1. If in IMF, nasagastric suction should be continued until the patient is awake and alert with normal gastrointestinal function.

2. Nasal vasoconstrictors may be utilized to help maintain a patent nasal airway.
3. Head of bed elevation should be maintained to lessen postoperative edema.
4. Maintenance of oral hygiene is essential, including oral rinses.
5. The patient should be maintained on a soft diet.
6. After 6–8 weeks, the arch bars can be removed in the office.

VII. FRACTURES OF THE MANDIBLE

A. Anatomy and Mechanism

1. The U-shaped mandible is composed of the body, symphysis, rami, condyles, and the coronoid processes (Fig. 6A).
2. The mandible is thin at the angles where the body joins with the ramus. This is further weakened by an unerupted third molar.
3. The mandible is also weak at the neck of the condyle (subcondylar area).
4. The anterior body and parasymphyseal area are weakened by the long root of the cuspid tooth and the mental foramen.
5. The inferior alveolar nerve and artery enter through the lingula on the medial border of the ramus and travel in a canal to exit at the mental foramen at the level of the 1st and 2nd bicuspid.
6. The mandible is the strongest facial bone, but is one of the most frequently fractured. Greater than 50% of mandible fractures are multiple.
7. In order of decreasing frequency, the most common sites for fracture are (Fig. 6B):
   - Condyle—36%
   - Body—21%
   - Angle—20%
   - Parasymphysis—14%
   - Ramus—3%
   - Alveolar process—3%
   - Coronoid process—2%
   - Symphysis—1%
8. Muscle attachments strongly influence the degree and direction of displacement.
   - The temporalis muscle attaches to the coronoid process
   - The masseter and medial pterygoid muscles attach to the angle of the mandible
   - The lateral pterygoid muscle attaches to the temporomandibular joint (TMJ) and condylar neck.
9. Direction of muscle pull:
   - The posterior group of mandibular muscles consists of the masseter, temporalis, medial pterygoid, and lateral pterygoid. These exert strong upward, forward, and medial force.
   - The anterior or depressor group of muscles consists of the geniohyoid, genioglossus, mylohyoid, and digastric muscles. They displace the fracture fragments downward, posteriorly, and medially.
   - The direction and angulation of fracture lines may accordingly be favorable or unfavorable for displacement of the fracture.

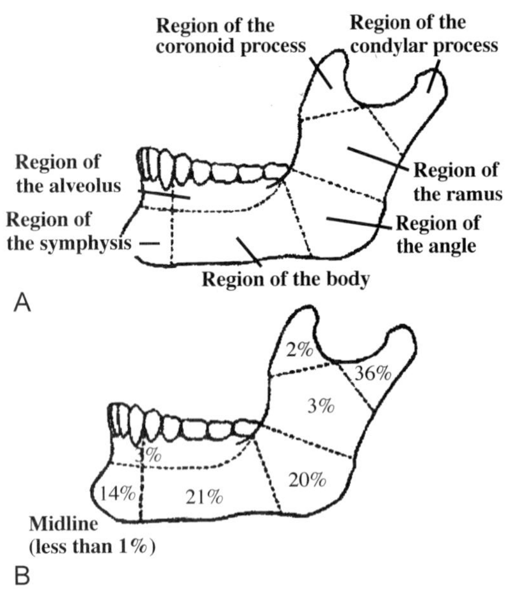

Figure 6 Anatomic regions and frequency of fractures. (A) Anatomic regions of the mandible. (B) Frequency of fractures in those regions. (From Manson P. Facial fractures. In: Aston S; Beasley R; Thorne C; eds: *Grabb and Smith's Plastic Surgery*. Philadelphia: Lippincott-Raven Publishers, 1997.)

B. Signs on Physical Exam

1. Pain is present on motion and palpation.
2. Malocclusion may be present.

3. Disruption of the inferior alveolar nerve may produce numbness in the distribution of the mental nerve and ipsilateral teeth.
4. The patient may have difficulty opening the mouth (trismus).
5. Intraoral inspection may show a gap in dentition, loose teeth, or a laceration.
6. Subcondylar fractures are associated with deviation of the chin to the ipsilateral side.

C. Radiographic Diagnosis

1. A mandibular series of plain x-rays includes lateral, posterior-anterior skull, right and left lateral obliques, a Towne projection, and submental vertex (SMV) projection.
2. A panoramic radiogram (Panorex) is the most useful x-ray, providing a view of entire mandible on one film. This allows assessment of all fractures, the status of the teeth, and the location of inferior alveolar canal. Because of distortion inherent in this radiograph, it may be supplemented by a PA x-ray of the mandible for most accurate diagnosis.
3. CT scan is generally not necessary, but may be used in cases with extreme comminution and in assessing whether an intraarticular condylar fracture is present.

D. Treatment

1. Initially, airway maintenance is paramount, as with maxillary fracture.
2. At surgery, the most important goal is to establish preinjury dental occlusion.
3. The operation performed depends on displacement and fracture location
   - A nondisplaced fracture may usually be treated by IMF for 4–6 weeks.
   - For displaced subcondylar fractures:

     IMF for 2–6 weeks *or*

     ORIF if bilateral and associated with midface fracture, foreign body in the joint capsule, lateral extracapsular displacement, displacement into the middle cranial fossa or temporal fossa with clinical disability, open fractures such as shotgun blasts, or fracture preventing reduction. Submandibular (Risdon), retromandibular (Hines), or preauricular incisions are used. The facial nerve is at risk in this exposure.
   - For displaced parasymphysis fractures, usually perform ORIF with a tension band (2.0 mm diameter plate + screws) or arch bar superiorly and a lower border plate (2.0 mm or 2.4 mm diameter plate + screws). An intraoral incision may be used.
   - For displaced body fractures, usually perform ORIF with a tension band (2.0 mm) or arch bar superiorly and lower border plate (2.0 or 2.4 mm). Intraoral or external incisions may be used.
   - Displaced angle fractures usually require ORIF with a tension band superiorly and lower border plate.
4. After fixation, IMF is removed and occlusion is checked. If malocclusion is present, remove fixation and repeat ORIF.
5. Decision to replace IMF at end of procedure is contingent upon stability of the fixation. If rigid stabilization has been achieved, IMF generally is not necessary.
6. For teeth in the line of the fracture, remove the teeth if they prevent reduction or are diseased/damaged.
7. Fractures involving significant bone loss or severe infections may require external fixation (Joe-Hall-Morris technique).

E. Postoperative Care

1. IMF places the patient at increased risk for aspiration. Nasogastric suction should be utilized at the time of surgery and postoperatively until the patient is extubated, alert, and GI function is normal.
2. Antibiotics are given perioperatively, usually penicillin or clindamycin.
3. A soft diet is continued for 6–8 weeks.
4. Frequent checks of occlusion are performed. Elastics may be used to compensate for only very minor discrepancies.
5. Radiographic evidence of consolidation at the fracture site lags behind clinical healing.
6. Arch bars are removed in the office after the fracture has fully healed (6–8 weeks).

43

Maxillofacial and Craniofacial Prosthetics

Lawrence E. Brecht, D.D.S.
New York University School of Medicine and New York University College of Dentistry, New York, New York, U.S.A.

The restoration of craniomaxillofacial defects may not always be possible through the use of autogenous tissues and reconstructive plastic surgery. In such instances, a prosthesis may be required to restore the patient's facial form and function. Many of these prostheses are made as a direct result of earlier medically necessary care, and generally none are considered cosmetic.

I. TERMINOLOGY

A. Prosthesis—an artificial replacement for an absent human body structure or a therapeutic device to improve or alter function or to accomplish a desired reconstructive result.

B. Prosthodontics—that branch of dentistry pertaining to the restoration and maintenance of oral function, comfort, appearance, and health of the patient. This involves restoration of natural teeth and/or the replacement of missing teeth and contiguous oral and maxillofacial tissues with artificial substitutes.

C. Maxillofacial prosthetics—that branch of prosthodontics concerned with the restoration or replacement of the stomatognathic structures with prostheses that may or may not be removed on a regular or elective basis.

D. Craniofacial prosthesis—that branch of maxillofacial prosthetics concerned with the replacement of hard and/or soft tissues of the craniofacial region with prostheses that may or may not be removed on a regular or elective basis.

E. Osseointegration—the direct attachment of living osseous tissue to an inert, alloplastic material (e.g., titanium) without an intervening connective tissue.

F. Splint—a rigid or flexible device that maintains a displaced, injured, or movable part in position in order to restrict motion.

G. Stent—eponym (Dr. Charles Stent—English dentist) for a device used in conjunction with a surgical procedure to keep a skin graft in place or to provide support for anastomosed structures. The stent is often modified with acrylic resin or dental modeling compound intraoperatively.

H. Appliance—something developed by the application of ideas or principles that is designed to serve a special function.

I. Moulage—the impression of a body structure that can produce a model of the structure when converted to a positive replica (such as when poured with dental stone).

II. ETIOLOGY OF DEFECTS

A. Congenital

1. Cleft lip, cleft alveolus, and cleft palate
2. Treacher-Collins syndrome

3. Hemifacial microsomia
4. Other congenital syndromes
5. All of the above may include anomalies that require a prosthesis as part of their short- or long-term management.

B. Acquired

1. Surgical ablation of tumors constitutes a major source for both intraoral and extraoral defects that require management through the use of prostheses.
2. Trauma, such as motor vehicle accidents (MVAs), gunshot wounds, burns (thermal, electrical and chemical), and human and animal bites also result in craniomaxillofacial defects.

C. Developmental

1. Cerebrovascular accidents
2. Amyotrophic lateral sclerosis
3. Oro-facial dyskinesia
4. Other conditions with a neurogenic etiology
5. All of the above may lead to orofacial deficits that may be ameliorated with various maxillofacial prostheses.

III. CLASSES OF PROSTHESES

A. Intraoral Prostheses

1. Surgical Obturator Prosthesis

a. When a maxillary tumor is resected, a surgical obturator prosthesis is inserted intraorally intraoperatively or immediately following the surgical procedure.

b. It serves to separate the oral and nasal cavities, allowing the patient to speak and swallow fairly normally without fluid or air leaking into the nasal passage. The prosthesis also supports surgical packing and a skin graft if one is used to line the defect.

c. This prosthesis usually is replaced by an interim or definitive obturator prosthesis after appropriate healing.

d. It is fashioned from heat-processed acrylic and usually retained by wire clasps that engage undercuts on adjacent teeth. When there are no teeth or insufficient teeth for retention, the surgical obturator may be retained using transalveolar, circumzygomatic, or other suspensory wiring.

e. The surgical obturator is first removed 7–10 days after surgery and is modified on a weekly or biweekly basis by the prosthodontist to ensure its proper fit.

2. Interim Obturator Prosthesis

a. Fabricated when the initial healing of maxillectomy has been completed.

b. May require frequent modifications.

c. Used for 6–9 months postresection.

3. Definitive Obturator Prosthesis

a. Fabricated following complete healing at 6–9 months postresection.

b. It artificially replaces part or all of the maxilla and associated teeth.

c. Fabricated from cast chromium-cobalt, titanium, or gold along with acrylic polymers.

d. Retained by metal clasps around teeth

e. Tissue undercuts adhesives or osseointegrated implants.

4. Surgical Stent

a. Prosthesis that gives support to a split- or full-thickness skin graft to improve adaptation of the graft, facilitate healing, and minimize scarring.

b. Fabricated from acrylic or composite resins, dental molding compound, or gutta percha.

c. Retained by clasps, screws placed into adjacent bone, sutures, or surgical wiring (i.e., circummandibular wiring).

d. Usually in place less than 4 weeks.

5. Palatal Lift Prosthesis

a. Prosthesis serves to elevate the intact soft palate superiorly to affect velopharyngeal closure.

b. Improves speech projection and reduces hypernasality.

c. Fabricated from acrylic and chromium-cobalt, titanium, or gold alloys.

d. Worn on the palate and retained by clasps to teeth.

e. Contraindicated in edentulous patients.

6. Trismus Appliance

a. This is an occlusal device that serves as a dynamic bite opener to reduce mandibular trismus, it provides a constant and gradual force that increases opening. The device is fabricated from acrylic and stainless steel wires.

7. Commissure Splint

a. Also known as a "lip splint," it is a device placed between the lips to assist in increasing the opening between the lips.
b. Its purpose is to stretch the commissures of the lips following chemical or electrical burns to the lips.

8. Nasoalveolar Molding Appliance

a. A combined intraoral and extraoral device that is indicated for infants with cleft lip, alveolus, and palate.
b. Serves to mold the intraoral alveolar segments closer together, while a nasal stent molds the nasal cartilages into a more normalized form.
c. Fabricated from acrylic and a soft liner material.
d. Must be modified weekly to accommodate the changes in the alveolus.
e. The appliance improves the hard and soft tissue foundation for the surgeon prior to reconstruction.
f. The appliance is held in place only with surgical tape on the infant's cheeks.
g. The appliance is effective in treating both unilateral and bilateral cleft conditions.

9. Speech Aid Prosthesis

a. Also known as a speech bulb, this prosthesis serves to improve speech quality in both children and adults. It obturates or seals off the palatal cleft or fistula or may assist an incompetent soft palate.
b. Fabricated from acrylic, chromium-cobalt, titanium, or gold alloy.
c. When teeth are present, the prosthesis is retained by clasps. When teeth are absent, adhesive, magnetics, or clip interlocks attached to osseointegrated implants retain the appliance in position.

B. Extraoral Prostheses

1. Auricular Prosthesis

a. Removable prosthesis to replace all or part of the external ear.
b. Fabricated from custom-shaded, medical-grade, heat-processed silicone elastomer.
c. Retained by skin adhesives, magnets, or clip interlocks to osseointegrated implants placed in the parieto-temporal region.
d. The ideal method to replace adult ear lost to trauma or ablation. Congenital microtia is usually more suited to autogenous reconstruction.

2. Orbital Prosthesis

a. Artificially replaces the eye, eyelids, and adjacent hard and soft tissues lost due to trauma or surgery.
b. Serves to restore normal appearance, seals the defect from the external environment, and maintains normal humidity of the adjacent maxillary sinus, oral cavity, and nasal cavities.
c. Skin portion of the prosthesis is made from medical-grade, heat-processed silicone elastomer.
d. Retained by skin adhesives, tissue undercuts, mechanical attachment to eyeglasses, or magnetic or clip interlocks to osseointegrated implants placed into surrounding bones of orbit.
e. The portion of the orbital prosthesis that replaces the missing eye is termed an ocular prosthesis. Patients who have not lost the soft tissues surrounding the globe (i.e., eyelids) usually only require an ocular prosthesis.

3. Nasal Prosthesis

a. Removable prosthesis that restores normal appearance to all or part of the nose.
b. Maintains normal moisture in the nasal cavity and sinuses.
c. Provides support for eyeglasses.
d. Fabricated from medical-grade, heat-processed silicone elastomer.
e. Retained in position by skin adhesives or magnets or clip interlocks to osseointegrated implants placed in surrounding nasomaxillary bones. Adhesive-retained prosthesis an excellent interim restoration while patient awaits nasal reconstruction.

4. Facial Prosthesis

   a. Removable prosthesis that serves to restore, as much as possible, facial appearance to the portion of the face that was lost to surgery, trauma, or congenital absence.
   b. Fabricated from medical-grade, heat-processed silicone elastomer.
   c. Retained in position by skin adhesives, eyeglasses, magnets, or clip interlocks to osseointegrated implants.

5. Cranial Prosthesis

   a. Also termed cranioplasty prosthesis, the cranial prosthesis is a biocompatible permanent prosthesis that serves to separate dura from skin and to protect exposed brain from trauma when calvarial grafts are not possible.
   b. Reestablishes contours of the skull.
   c. Fabricated from heat-processed acrylic, tantalum, or titanium.
   d. May be fashioned with CAD/CAM and CT scan data.

IV. PATIENT MANAGEMENT

A. Ideally, the patient requiring maxillofacial or craniofacial prosthetic care will be evaluated by the maxillofacial prosthodontist in conjunction with the surgeon prior to any surgical intervention, either ablative or reconstructive. Presurgical records of the patient should be obtained.

B. The fabrication of a surgical prosthesis will require lead time as well. The team approach to the management of the maxillofacial or craniofacial prosthetic patient will invariably yield a superior surgical and prosthetic result when compared to an independent management style.

44

Embryology of the Head and Neck

James P. Bradley, M.D., and Henry K. Kawamoto, D.D.S., M.D.
David Geffen School of Medicine at UCLA, Los Angeles, California, U.S.A.

An understanding of the development of the head and neck in the embryo gives the plastic surgeon insight into the basis of craniofacial form, the function of cranial nerves, and anomalies of the head and neck that occur because of alterations in development.

I. EARLY DEVELOPMENT

A. The cranial portion of the embryo begins development in the middle of the third week with differentiation of three germ layers (ectoderm, endoderm, and mesoderm).

B. Neural crest cells are of ectodermal origin but consist of pluripotent ectomesenchymal tissue comparable to the three primary germ layers. Neural crest cells migrate along cleavage planes between germ layers and differentiate into connective tissue, muscle, nervous tissue, endocrine tissue, and pigment cells.

II. THE PHARYNGEAL (BRANCHIAL) APPARATUS*

A. Pharyngeal Arches

1. Formation

a. Neural crest cells migrate and contact with endodermal cells, causing mesenchymal swellings and differentiation (fourth week). Mesenchymal cells become myoblasts, and neural crest cells give rise to skeletal and connective tissue.

b. Paired pharyngeal arches develop cranially to caudally (Fig. 1).

2. Four Essential Elements (Table 1)

a. Cartilage: central skeleton of arch that gives rise to cartilage, bone and ligamentous structures

- First arch cartilage (Meckel's and Quadrate cartilage):

  Skeletal

  Endochondral ossification of cartilage precursor leads to formation of (1) malleus and mandibular condyles (Meckel's) and (2) incus and greater wing of the sphenoid bone (quadrate).

  Membranous ossification of arch dermal mesenchyme leads to formation of (1) mandibular body and ramus (mandibular prominence) and (2) maxilla, zygoma, and squamous portion of the temporal bone (maxillary prominence).

  Ligamentous = anterior ligament of malleus.

- Second arch cartilage (Reichert's cartilage):

* From *branchia*, Greek for "gill."

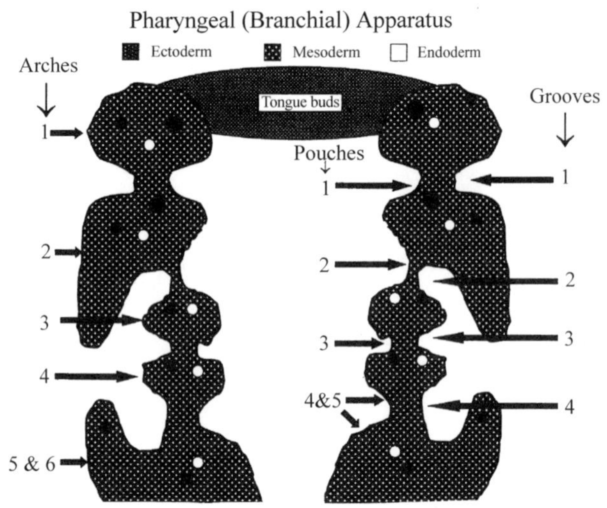

Figure 1 Coronal section of head, neck, and upper thorax of embryo at 5 weeks gestation, demonstrating the pharyngeal apparatus. From cranial (top) to caudal (bottom): mesenchymal tissue that will become tongue buds are seen, followed sequentially by the pharyngeal arches, grooves and pouches one through six, and then tissue that will become the esophagus. (Modified from Moore KL, ed. *The Developing Human*. 4th ed. Philadelphia: Saunders, 1988, p. 174.)

Skeletal = stapes, styloid process of temporal bone, lesser cornu, and superior part of the hyoid bone.

Ligamentous = stylohyoid ligament.

- Third arch cartilage: greater cornu and inferior part of body of the hyoid bone.
- Fourth arch cartilage: laryngeal cartilages.

3. Aortic Arch Artery

Joins the ventral heart and dorsal aorta.

4. Cranial Nerves—Sensory and Motor

a. First arch (mandibular arch): trigeminal nerve (CN V)

- Maxillary division (V2)—sensory
- Mandibular division (V3)—sensory and motor that includes the muscles of mastication (temporalis, medial and lateral pterygoids, masseter), mylohyoid, anterior belly of digastric, tensor tympani, and tensor veli palatini.

b. Second arch (hyoid arch)—facial nerve (CN VII).

c. Third arch—glossopharyngeal nerve (CN IX).

d. Fourth arch—superior laryngeal branch of the vagus nerve (CN X).

e. Fifth and sixth arches—recurrent laryngeal branch of the vagus nerve (CN X).

5. Muscles

Arch derivatives correspond to innervation (see cranial nerves above). Also, muscle development depends on innervation (e.g., Möbius' syndrome is a failure of facial nerve development and ineffective facial expression musculature).

B. Pharyngeal Grooves

External clefts between pharyngeal arches (Fig. 1).

1. The first pharyngeal groove becomes the external auditory canal.
2. Other pharyngeal grooves (2–4) are obliterated as the cervical sinus.
3. Failure of a groove to be obliterated by the sixth week of gestation can result in branchial fistulas, sinus tracts, or cysts (depending on the remaining remnant).
    - These anomalies are identified along the anterior border of the sternocleidomastoid (SCM) muscle, at any point from the external auditory canal to the clavicle.
    - Second branchial cleft remnant: most common, found externally in area of the middle to lower third of the SCM. Tract passes over the glossopharyngeal nerve and between external and internal carotid arteries to the tonsillar fossa.
    - Third branchial cleft remnant: passes beneath the internal carotid artery.
    - First branchial cleft remnant: rare; above the hyoid; may involve the facial nerve.

C. Pharyngeal Pouches

Internal cleft between pharyngeal arches (Fig. 1).

III. DEVELOPMENT OF THE FACE: 4–8 WEEKS (Fig. 2)

A. The primitive mouth or the stomodeum is formed from five facial prominences, which

Table 1 Branchial Arch Derivatives

Arch	First arch (mandibular)	Second arch (hyoid)	Third arch	Fourth arch	Fifth and sixth arches
Arch artery	Maxillary artery, terminal branch Portion of external carotid artery	Stapedial artery	Proximal internal carotid artery Part of common carotid artery	Aortic arch (Left) = Innominate and right subclavian artery (Right) = distal pulmonary artery	Proximal pulmonary arteries Ductus arteriosus (left arch)
Nerves	Trigeminal (CN V)	Facial (CN VII)	Glossopharyngeal (CN IX)	Superior laryngeal branch of vagus (CN X)	Recurrent laryngeal branch of vagus (CN X)
Muscles	Muscles of mastication[a] Anterior belly of digastric Myohyoid Tensor tympani palatini Tensor veli palatini	Muscles of facial, expression[b] Posterior belly of digastric Stylohyoid Stapedius	Stylopharyngeus	Constrictors of pharynx Cricothyroid Levator veli palatini Palatopharyngeus Palatoglossus	Intrinsic muscles of larynx (except cricothyroid)
Cartilage precursors	Maxillary[c] (quadrate) → Cartilage — Greater wing of sphenoid, incus	Reichert's cartilage	Third arch cartilage	Fourth arch cartilage	Sixth arch cartilage
Skeletal elements	Maxillary[d] prominence → Maxilla, zygoma, temporal bone (squamous portion) Mandibular[c] (Meckel's) → Cartilage — Malleus, mandibular condyles Mandibular[d] prominence → Body/ramus of mandible	Stapes Styloid process Lesser cornu of hyoid Upper hyoid bone	Greater cornu of hyoid Lower hyoid bone	Laryngeal cartilages[e]	Laryngeal cartilages[e]
Ligaments	Anterior ligament of malleolus Sphenomandibular ligament	Stylohyoid ligament			
Endodermal pouch[f]	D: Auditory tube and middle ear cavity form from tubotympanic recess V: Obliterated by tongue	D: Palatine tonsillar fossa V: Obliterated by tongue	Inferior parathyroid V: Thymus	D: Superior parathyroid V: Lateral thyroid, vestigial thymus	5th—Ultimobranchial body, calcitonin "C cells" 6th—None

[a] Temporalis, masseter, medial and lateral pterygoids.
[b] Buccinator, auricularis, fronto-occipitalis, platysma, orbicularis oculi, and orbicularis oris.
[c] Ossification of cartilaginous precursors forms endochondral bone.
[d] Direct ossification of arch dermal mesenchyme forms membranous bone.
[e] The cartilages of the larynx include thyroid, cuneiform, cricoid, arytenoids, and corniculate.
[f] D = dorsal and V = ventral endodermal pouch derivatives.

are separated by grooves. Although separate, mesenchymal migration occurs freely between the five prominences.

- Paired maxillary prominences (first pharyngeal arch)—lateral border of the stomodeum.
- Paired mandibular prominences (first pharyngeal arch)—caudal border of the stomodeum.
- Single frontonasal prominence—central process from mesenchymal tissue ventral to the forebrain. Not from a branchial arch. Forms the cranial boundary of the stomodeum.

B. Midface: quadrate cartilage within the maxillary prominence forms the incus and greater wing of the sphenoid bone. The maxilla, zygoma, and the squamous portion of the temporal bone are formed through membranous ossification of the maxillary prominences (cartilage serves only as a template, not a precursor, for ossification and is then obliterated).

C. Lower face: Meckel's cartilage within the mandibular prominences forms the malleus and the mandibular condyles. The body and ramus of the mandible form through membranous ossification of the mandibular prominences.

D. Nose: "nasal placodes" form in the inferior lateral aspect of the frontonasal prominence because of ectodermal thickening. As bordering medial and lateral nasal prominences continue to grow, deepening results in "nasal pits." Maxillary prominences and the medial and lateral nasal prominences migrate medially and fuse to produce continuity of the nose, upper lip, and palate, and separation of the oral and nasal cavities.

- Cupid's bow region of the upper lip, the nasal tip, the premaxilla, primary palate, and nasal septum all develop from the merger of the medial nasal prominences.
- The nasal alae develop from the lateral nasal prominences.
- The nasolacrimal groove develops from a furrow separating the lateral nasal prominence from the maxillary prominence. Epithelial cells line this groove to form the nasolacrimal duct, which becomes patent sometime after birth. Lack of fusion in this area results in an oblique facial cleft (Tessier #3 facial cleft).

E. Maldevelopments of the face:

- Unilateral cleft lip = failure of fusion of the medial nasal prominences and maxillary prominence on one side.
- Bilateral cleft lip = maxillary prominences failed migration and did not fuse to the medial nasal prominences. Maxillary prominences remain lateral to the merged medial nasal prominences, which manifest as prominent, overprojected premaxilla and prolabium.

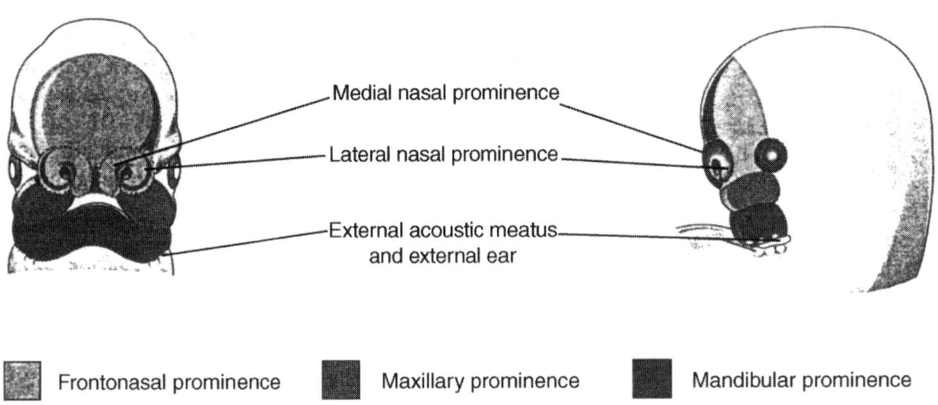

Figure 2 Anterior and lateral diagrams illustrating the developing human face at about 5 weeks gestation. Frontonasal prominence, maxillary prominences, and mandibular prominences are shaded. The medial and lateral nasal prominences and external auditory canal are identified. (From Moore KL, ed. *The Developing Human*. 4th ed. Philadelphia: Saunders, 1988, p. 190.)

- Macrostomia (Tessier #7 facial cleft) = failure of union of the maxillary and mandibular prominences at the lateral oral commissure.
- Median cleft of the upper lip (Tessier #0 facial cleft) = failure of fusion of the median nasal prominences.
- Central defect of the lower lip and chin (Tessier #30 facial cleft) = failure of fusion of the mandibular prominences.

F. Eyes: similar to nasal development, "lens placodes" form at the lateral aspect of the frontonasal prominence. Neural connections to the forebrain ("optic stalks") stimulate differentiation. Invaginations of placodes form "optic vesicles."

- Optic nerves develop from the optic stalks.
- Lenses develop from the lens placodes.
- Optic cups develop from the optic vesicles. Neural crest cell migration surrounds the optic cups to form the sclera, choroids, and the ciliary bodies. Neural crest cell migration over the lens forms the cornea.
- Eyelids form from folds of surface ectoderm that overgrow the eyes.

IV. PALATE DEVELOPMENT

A. Frontonasal prominence → becomes the merged median nasal prominences → become the median palatine process → becomes the primary palate (premaxillary portion of maxilla).

B. Maxillary prominences → become the lateral palatine processes → become the secondary palate. The posterior half of the secondary palate remains unossified as the soft palate.

C. Lateral palatine processes move from a vertical orientation to a horizontal orientation as the tongue descends. Then, fusion between opposing lateral palatine processes and the anterior median palatine process forms an intact palate. Fusion occurs with apoptosis (programmed cell death) of the medial edges.

D. The nasal septum (also formed from the merged median nasal prominences) then fuses with the nasal side of the palate.

E. Cleft palate results from a failure of fusion of the mesenchymal masses of the median palatine process to the lateral palatine process (cleft of primary palate) or failure of fusion of the mesenchymal cells between the two lateral palatine processes (cleft of the secondary palate).

F. Pierre Robin sequence—"sequence" of events resulting in micrognathia, glossoptosis, and cleft palate. Events include a large tongue pushed up into the oropharynx by the small mandible, causing continue vertical orientation of the lateral palatine processes (shelves) and a wide "U-shaped" cleft palate.

V. NASAL CAVITIES DEVELOPMENT

A. Nasal placodes → become nasal pits → become nasal sacs (deepening is a result of continuous growth of median and lateral nasal prominences).

B. An oronasal membrane separates the nasal sacs from the oral cavity. The choanae foraminae forms when this membrane ruptures.

C. The choanae is initially located behind the primary palate but shifts posteriorly with formation of the secondary palate and fusion of the lateral palatine processes and nasal septum.

D. The superior, middle, and inferior conchae are formed from elevations of the lateral nasal walls.

E. Paranasal sinuses are formed from diverticuli of the lateral nasal walls that extend into the maxillary (third month), sphenoid (fifth month), ethmoid (fifth month), and frontal (6 years) bones.

VI. EXTERNAL EAR (AURICLE) DEVELOPMENT

A. Six hillocks (swellings) develop into the characteristic shape of the ear by 8 weeks.

- Anterior three hillocks and posterior three hillocks are separated by the first branchial groove.
- Anterior three hillocks from the first branchial (mandibular) arch.
- Posterior three hillocks from the second branchial (hyoid) arch.

B. External auditory meatus develops from the first branchial groove (dorsal aspect of the cleft between the first and second branchial arches).

C. Ear development begins while it is still located in the cervical region, with subsequent cranial migration of the ear. Microtia patients with partial arrest of development have caudally placed maldeveloped ears.

VII. TONGUE DEVELOPMENT

A. Anterior two thirds of the tongue:

- Median tongue buds (tuberculum impar) elevate from the floor of the pharynx.
- Distal tongue buds (lateral lingual swellings) grow over the tuberculum impar and fuse in the midline at the medium septum of the tongue.
- Origin is from the first branchial arch and innervation is supplied by the lingual nerve, a branch of the mandibular division of the trigeminal nerve (V3).

B. Posterior one third of the tongue:

- The hypobranchial eminence (derived from the third and fourth arches) grows over the copula (derived from the second arch) and completely covers it.
- The glossopharyngeal nerve (third branchial arch) and the superior laryngeal branch of the vagus nerve (third branchial arch) supply sensory innervation. Since the facial nerve (second branchial arch) is completely covered (the copula), it does not provide sensation.

C. The terminal sulcus is a V-shaped groove that separates the anterior and posterior tongue.

D. The hypoglossal nerve innervates all muscles of the tongue except the palatoglossus (vagus nerve).

E. Congenital malformations:

- Cyst (thyroglossal duct remnant) or fistula (thyroglossal duct opening through the foramen cecum).
- Macroglossia/microglossia.
- Bifid tongue or cleft: failure of union of tongue buds.
- Ankyloglossis or tongue-tie: the frenulum extends to the tip of the tongue and prevents unrestricted movement.

VIII. THYROID DEVELOPMENT

A. Thyroid diverticulum develops from endodermal proliferation of the foramen cecum of the tongue and descends into the neck in front of the hyoid bone and laryngeal cartilages.

B. The thyroglossal duct is formed in the tract of the descent, but usually degenerates by the seventh week. A thyroglossal duct cyst may occur anywhere along the midline descent.

C. When its final position is reached in front of the trachea at the level of the first and second tracheal rings, two lobes are formed connected by an isthmus. The gland plays an important role in metabolism.

45

Birth Defect Syndromes with Craniofacial Components

Lisa A. Schimmenti, M.D.
David Geffen School of Medicine at UCLA, Los Angeles, California, U.S.A.

Birth defects represent a major pediatric health issue. One in every 30 infants is born with some form of birth defect, and half of all pediatric hospital admissions are related to medical management and treatment of birth defects. Many of the known birth defect syndromes present serious craniofacial malformations requiring surgical intervention to restore normal function to the facial and oral structures. The aim of this chapter is to introduce the reader to some of the common birth defects and syndromes encountered in the craniofacial clinic population. Many birth defects have a hereditary component; thus, referral to genetic services for medical management and genetic counseling remains part of the standard of care for the patient and family.

I. OROFACIAL CLEFTS

A. Nonsyndromic Cleft Lip and Palate and Isolated Cleft Palate

Nonsyndromic cleft lip and isolated cleft palate are common and the incidence varies by race. The incidence is 1.34/1000 (1/750) in whites, 2.6/1000 (1/375) in Asians, and 0.41/100 (1/2450) in African Americans. Nonsyndromic clefting implies that the affected individual does not have other major malformations or developmental delay.

B. Non-Syndromic Clefts

1. Cleft-lip and palate (CLP): Patients with non-syndromic CLP represent the largest group in craniofacial clinics. CLP is considered a separate entity from isolated cleft palate (CPO) in that the prevalence, sex ratios, ethnic distribution, and embryology are different.

- Prevalence: The birth prevalence of non-syndromic CLP is about 0.8 per 1000 live births.
- Heredity and genetic issues: The pattern of heredity of CLP is complex and may have environmental and genetic components.

  The probability of having a child with CLP for individuals who are affected is 3–5%, assuming that there are no other first-degree relatives who are affected.

  For the parents of a child with a cleft, the recurrence probability is also 3–5%.

  The risk for recurrence goes up to 7% if the proband has a bilateral cleft.

  If there are two affected first-degree relatives, the risk is 10–20%.
- Sex ratios: Males are affected twice as often as females.
- Clinical manifestations: Children with CLP need to be examined carefully for other birth abnormalities including cardiac defects, genital defects, other structural birth anomalies, and growth and developmental delays.

2. Cleft palate only (CPO) or isolated cleft palate:
   - Prevalence: The prevalence of CPO is 0.3 in 1000 live births.
   - Heredity and genetic: Heredity for CPO is similar to that of CLP with a recurrence rate of 4% in families with no other affected members.
   - Sex ratios: Females tend to be affected twice as often as males.
   - Clinical manifestation: Children with CPO need to be examined carefully for other birth defects. The typical palatal cleft has a V-shaped appearance. The mandible is usually normal in size (decreased in size in Pierre-Robin sequence). Patients with CPO have a higher risk of having a syndrome.
3. Prevention of nonsyndromic clefts:
   - A number of studies have suggested that folic acid may prevent clefting. It is recommended that women of childbearing years have a diet enriched with folic acid and begin to take prenatal formulated vitamin preparations 3 months prior to conception to reduce the risk of neural tube defects and clefting.
   - Significant cigarette smoking may increase the risk of clefting in genetically susceptible individuals.

II. SYNDROMIC CLEFTS

Of the children with CLP or CPO, 30–35% may have a genetic syndrome. Genetic evaluation is warranted in children with oral clefts and other malformations or developmental disabilities.

A. 22q Deletion Syndrome

22q deletion syndrome has been called velocardiofacial syndrome and DiGeorge syndrome. With the advent of fluorescent in situ hybridization (FISH) probes for the critical region, 22q11, the preferred method of diagnosis is by FISH. Ninety-five percent of the patients have a demonstrable deletion by FISH.

1. Incidence: The syndrome occurs in 1 in 4000 live births.
2. Genetics: In about 94% of individuals, a demonstrable deletion of 22q11 by FISH occurs de novo. In about 6% of probands, the parents harbor the deletion.
3. Clinical manifestations:
   - In the craniofacial clinic, the majority of the patients present with cleft palate, velopalatal insufficiency, and developmental or behavioral difficulty.
   - Seventy-four percent of patients with 22q deletion syndrome have cardiac defects, particularly conotruncal and ventricular septal defects.
   - Other clinical manifestations of the syndrome include:

     T-cell deficiencies.

     Hypocalcemia in the newborn period.

     Learning and behavioral difficulties.

     Unusual facial appearance, including long noses with narrow alae nasae, abnormal pinnae, short stature, and long tapering fingers.
4. Management issues: Patients with 22q deletion syndrome require evaluation for cardiac defects, immunodeficiency, and hypocalcemia. Of particular concern for surgeons performing pharyngoplasty is medial displacement of the carotid arteries.

B. Van der Woude Syndrome (VWS)

1. VWS represents a familial clefting syndrome characterized by paramedian lower lip pits, missing teeth (particularly the lateral maxillary incisors), and CLP or CPO.
2. Penetrance is nearly complete with variable expression. It is estimated that 2% of the cleft population may have VWS.
3. Careful examination of the probands and family members for the presence of lip pits and missing teeth should be part of a craniofacial examination.
4. Recurrence risk for clefting is higher in VWS than for nonsyndromic clefting.
5. The risk for clefting may vary by family and may have a molecular basis. Estimated risk of clefting in subsequent offspring to a parent with lip pits varies from 11 to 23%.

6. VWS has been mapped to chromosome 1q32-42. The causative gene has not been isolated.

C. Pierre Robin Sequence

Pierre Robin sequence represents a triad of mandibular hypoplasia, glossoptosis, and cleft palate.

1. The palatal cleft is typically U-shaped.
2. The clefting has been suggested to occur as a result of the tongue obstructing the fusion of the palatine shelves.
3. Underlying causes: A number of genetic syndromes have been associated with Robin sequence. Thirty percent of children with Pierre Robin sequence may have Stickler syndrome. Stickler syndrome is caused by mutations in COL2A and COL11 genes. Patients may present with cleft palate, high myopia, flat midface, and hearing loss. Arthropathy may develop by the fourth decade. Mitral valve prolapse occurs in over half of the patients and must be considered for antibiotic prophylaxis during dental treatments.
4. Management issues: All children with Pierre Robin sequence should be evaluated by genetics and ophthalmology to rule out Stickler syndrome, as this disorder is associated with high myopia, retinal detachment, and loss of vision. Vision loss can be prevented by regular ophthalmologic follow-up.

D. Holoprosencephaly

1. This is a relatively rare syndrome, with an incidence of 1 in 16,000.
2. Patients may present with midline cleft lip and palate (Tessier #0 cleft), but will frequently have unusual manifestations such as panhypopituitarism, microcephaly, and severe developmental delay.
3. Mutations in genes expressed in early forebrain development, including sonic hedgehog, SIX3, and ZIC2, have been identified in individuals with holoprosencephaly. Many cases are sporadic. However, parents should be evaluated for subtle signs of holoprosencephaly such as learning disability and single central incisor. Genetic evaluation should be undertaken for counseling and diagnostic purposes.

E. Trisomy 13

1. This is a rare syndrome that occurs in 1 in 25,000 live births.
2. The majority of infants do not live more than 1–2 months. However, a child with mosaic trisomy 13 or partial trisomy 13, due to an unbalanced chromosome translocation, can survive for longer periods.
3. Infants may present with CLP, polydactyly, punctate scalp defects, holoprosencephaly, iris colobomas, and severe developmental disability.
4. Diagnosis is by chromosome study.

F. Wolf-Hirschhorn Syndrome

1. This syndrome is caused by deletion of part of the short arm of chromosome 4. This is also called 4p-syndrome and occurs in 50,000 live births.
2. Infants are severely delayed and may present with CLP.
3. Affected individuals have a striking wide nasal bridge with high-arched eyebrows.
4. At least half of affected infants have congenital heart disease.

III. TERATOGEN-INDUCED CLEFTS

An important part of history taking for new patients with clefting is medication/alcohol and drug exposure during pregnancy. There are a number of medications that, when taken early in pregnancy, have been known to induce clefts and other malformations. As in other birth defect syndromes, the malformation occurs early in gestation before 10 weeks. The timing of the exposure is, therefore, important.

A. Fetal hydantoin syndrome: Exposure of the fetus during the first 10 weeks of pregnancy to dilantin and related drugs for control of maternal seizures may cause a syndrome characterized by CLP and short tapered fingers with hypoplastic nails. The infants have normal intelligence and are not at increased risk for passing the clinical manifestations onto their offspring.

B. Fetal alcohol syndrome: Exposure of the fetus to alcohol during gestation may produce a clinical syndrome consisting of growth retardation, developmental delay, short palpebral fissures, long smooth philtrum, thin vermilion border, congenital heart disease (mostly ventricular septal defects), and occasionally cleft palate.

C. Other teratogens associated with clefting:

- Retinoic acid is commonly used for treatment of acne and wrinkles and has been associated with clefting. Other malformations associated with use of retinoic acid early in gestation include colobomas of the eye.
- Steroid usage and cigarette smoking are also associated with clefting.

IV. CRANIOSYNOSTOSIS

The craniosynostosis syndromes represent a group of disorders characterized by premature fusion of multiple cranial sutures.

1. These result in skull deformity, midface hypoplasia, exorbitisim, obstruction of the upper airway, and possible loss of vision and hearing.
2. Syndromes may or may not have involvement of the limbs.
3. Craniosynostosis affects 1 in 3000 newborns.

A. Molecular Basis

1. Fibroblast growth factor receptors (FGFRs): In humans, four fibroblast growth factor receptors have been identified:
   - The FGFRs are receptors for the FGF family of signaling molecules that affect growth and development.
   - The FGFRs are transmembrane molecules with an extracellular domain characterized by three IgG type lopps, a short membrane spanning region, and two tyrosine kinase domains.
   - Mutations in the genes for FGFR1, 2, and 3 have been associated with craniosynostosis syndromes. These mutations typically occur in the extracellular domain of the molecule for syndromes with craniosynostosis.
   - FGFR 1 maps to 8p, FGFR2 maps to 10q24, and FGFR3 maps to 4p.
2. TWIST: TWIST is a basic helix-loop-helix transcription factor and maps to chromosome 7q21. Individuals with Saethre-Chotzen syndrome have been identified with TWIST mutations or deletions.
3. MSX2: MSX2 is a homeobox transcription factor that maps to chromosome 5q. Mutations in the homeodomain of MSX2 have been identified in a family with Boston-type craniosynostosis.

B. Crouzon Syndrome

1. Persons with Crouzon syndrome have primarily premature fusion of the coronal sutures, although all sutures may be involved.
2. Midface hypoplasia, small nose, exorbitism, and upper airway difficulties may be observed.
3. The hands and feet in Crouzon syndrome are normal.
4. Mutations have been observed in FGFR2.
5. Patients with Crouzon syndrome and acanthosis nigricans have been identified with mutations in FGFR3.
6. Inheritance is autosomal dominant.

C. Pfeiffer Syndrome

1. The facial abnormalities observed in Pfeiffer syndrome are similar to those seen in patients with Crouzon syndrome.
2. In addition to craniofacial anomalies, individuals with Pfeiffer syndrome have hand and foot anomalies consisting of broad thumbs and great toes, brachydactyly, and sometimes syndactyly.
3. Mutations in FGFR1 and FGFR2 have been identified.
4. Inheritance is autosomal dominant.

D. Apert Syndrome

1. Apert syndrome, also known as acrocephalosyndactyly, results from mutation in FGFR2.
2. Most affected individuals have a new mutation that is not inherited.
3. Individuals with Apert syndrome have acrocephaly, high-arched palate, midface hypoplasia, and hand/foot anomalies.
4. The hand anomalies are characterized by broad thumbs and variable syndactyly of digits 2, 3, 4, and 5.

5. Feet have broad everted great toes with variable syndactyly and a common nail.
6. Many individuals with Apert syndrome exhibit developmental disabilities; however, this is not always the rule.
7. Inheritance is dominant.

E. Saethre-Chotzen Syndrome

1. Saethre-Chotzen syndrome is another autosomal dominant craniosynostosis syndrome characterized by brachycephaly with variable synostosis of coronal, metopic, and lambdoid sutures.
2. Limb findings include short digits, abnormal thumbs, clinodactyly, broad toes, and limited extension at the elbows.
3. Palpebral ptosis is observed in patients with the syndrome.
4. Mutations in TWIST and FGFR2 have been identified in affected individuals and their relatives.

F. Isolated Coronal Synostosis

Isolated coronal synostosis with variable hand and feet abnormalities has been associated with a recurrent autosomal dominant mutation in FGFR3, a proline-to-arginine substitution at amino acid 250. This also referred to as Muenke synostosis.

G. Other Craniosynostosis Syndromes

There are over 100 syndromes with craniosynostosis and abnormalities of limbs and other birth defects.

V. OCULOAURICULOVERTEBRAL SPECTRUM

Oculoauriculovertebral (OAV) spectrum has also been called hemifacial microsomia. Goldenhar syndrome refers to patients with the additional ocular findings listed below. The current accepted term is OAV spectrum. The prevalence has been estimated at 1 in 5600 live births.

A. Clinical Manifestations

The facial phenotype consists of unilateral and sometimes bilateral microtia with abnormal or absent helices and ear canals, mandibular hypoplasia with sometimes absent ramus or condyle, epibulbar dermoids, and vertebral anomalies. In many patients there is midface flattening on the affected side.

1. Facial findings:
   - The majority of individuals exhibit varying degrees of facial asymmetry resulting from maxillary or mandibular hypoplasia.
   - A soft tissue component may contribute to the facial hypoplasia.
   - The asymmetry may be plainly obvious to the observer or may be as mild as a slight occlusal cant that is only demonstrable when the patient holds a tongue blade between the teeth.
2. Ear findings:
   - Ear findings can range from preauricular tags to complete anotia.
   - Patients may present with unilateral microtia, stenotic ear canals, absent lobule, or caudally displaced pinnae.
   - As many as half of affected patients have hearing loss.
   - Bilateral ear abnormalities are common as well.
3. Eye findings (Goldenhar syndrome):
   - Eye findings include epibulbar dermoids. These soft tissue masses have a white or pinkish appearance and usually occur on the inferotemporal portion of the eye. The epibulbar dermoids do not have visual sequelae unless they encroach upon the cornea.
   - Other ocular findings include exotropia, colobomas of the globe or eyelids, microphthalmia, or cystic eyes.
   - Occasionally, shortening of the palpebral fissure on the affected side of the face will develop.
4. Oral and mandibular findings:
   - Patients may exhibit macrostomia or an overt lateral facial cleft on the affected side.
   - Cleft lip and palate have been reported in 7–15% of patients.
   - Velopharyngeal incompetence has also been reported.
   - There may be asymmetry of the tongue on the affected side.
   - The mandibular ramus and condyle may be hypoplastic or absent.

5. Skeletal findings:
   - Abnormalities of the cervical spine may be present in one-third of patients.
   - Limb anomalies including radial ray malformations have been reported.
6. Other organ systems:
   - The majority of patients have normal intelligence. If a patient exhibits developmental delay, a genetic evaluation is warranted to rule out a chromosome abnormality.
   - Cranial nerve palsies are not uncommon.
   - Cardiac abnormalities have also been reported.

B. Genetics

The genetic basis of OAV is unknown. Most cases are sporadic, with a recurrence risk of 3–4%. Autosomal dominant inheritance has been documented in a few reports. If the patient has learning disability, congenital heart disease or palatal malformations, chromosome studies with 22q FISH should be considered. A genitourinary history should be elicited, and search for renal anomalies should be considered.

C. Management Issues

C-spine films to rule out vertebral anomalies should be performed on OAV patients.

VI. TREACHER-COLLINS SYNDROME (MANDIBULOFACIAL DYSOSTOSIS)

Patients with mandibulofacial dysostosis, more commonly known as Treacher-Collins syndrome, present a relatively recognizable pattern of facial malformations.

A. Facial Findings

The most salient findings are:

1. Symmetric appearance of severe maxillary flattening with hypoplastic or incompletely formed zygomatic arches.
2. Down-slanting palpebral fissures.
3. Coloboma (notch) of the lower lid.
4. The ears may be small, inferiorly displaced, or completely absent. In the presence of absent ears, the middle ear structures may be malformed or absent.
5. The mandible is small with hypoplastic condyles.
6. In about 25% of patients, a wisp of hair grows on the face toward the cheek.
7. Cleft lip and palate have also been reported.
8. The limbs are spared, as are other organ systems.

B. Genetics

1. Mandibulofacial dysostosis is an autosomal dominant disorder.
2. The majority of patients come from families where there are other affected family members.
3. About 60% of affected individuals are "new mutations."
4. The gene for mandibulofacial dysostosis has been mapped to chromosome 5q32-33.1.
5. The gene, TCOF1, encodes a protein "treacle."

VII. FRONTONASAL DYSPLASIA

A. The descriptive term "frontonasal dysplasia" (also known as frontonasal malformation) was coined by Sedano et al. in 1970. The term describes a malformation of the midface that can be considered to result from a wide "splitting" of the frontonasal process during the early part of development (before 7 weeks).

B. The facial malformations include hypertelorism, a broad nasal root, a bifid or absent nasal tip, widow's peak, and defects of the anterior cranium including anterior encephalocoele.

C. The genetics of the disorder are uncertain.

D. Most patients have normal intelligence and no other malformations.

E. Occasionally, brain abnormalities have been reported, as have other defects including cardiac and limb anomalies.

VIII. ORAL-FACIAL-DIGITAL SYNDROME TYPE 1 (OFD1)

OFD1 is characterized by midline facial defects, including median cleft lip and palate.

A. Facial Features

1. Affected individuals are usually women, except for the rare reports of OFD1 in men with Klinefelter syndrome.

2. Affected individuals may have midline cleft lip and palate with thick frenulae along upper and lower alveolar/buccal surfaces, a bilobed, trilobed or multilobed tongue, and lingual hamartomas.
3. Affected patients may have dystopia canthorum, down-sloping palpebral fissures.
4. In young patients, milia may be present on the pinnae.

B. Limbs

The hands exhibit short digits and the thumb is short with ulnar deviation. Clinodactyly and syndactyly also have been reported. Feet may demonstrate similar abnormalities.

C. Renal Manifestations

There have been a number of reports of individuals who have developed cystic kidneys. Assessment of renal function and anatomy by ultrasound should be considered in affected individuals.

D. Genetics

1. This disorder generally affects only females.
2. Affected mothers may report a history of recurrent pregnancy loss.
3. OFD1 is an X-linked dominant disorder that is lethal in males.
4. Half of the female offspring of an affected woman will be affected. Half of her male fetuses will inherit the gene, but will not be born; they will present as early miscarriages.
5. The locus maps to Xp22. The causative gene has not been identified.

IX. INTERNET RESOURCES FOR GENETIC DISORDERS

A. Online Mendelian Inheritance in Man (OMIM): This is a database of known genetic diseases with current literature citations (http://www.ncbi.nlm.nih.gov/omim/). There are links to Genbank and the Alliance of Genetic Support Groups.

B. Gene Clinics: This database has outlines of clinical knowledge for genetic syndromes. It is a relatively new database, and the number of diseases listed on the database is growing. The website address is http://www.geneclinics.org. This database will also include a referral base for clinical genetic resources in the United States.

46

Rare Craniofacial Clefts

Wayne Ozaki, M.D., D.D.S.
Oregon Health and Science University, Portland, Oregon, U.S.A.
Henry K. Kawamoto, Jr., M.D., D.D.S.
David Geffen School of Medicine at UCLA, Los Angeles, California, U.S.A.

A craniofacial cleft is among the most disfiguring of all facial anomalies. Although they appear bizarre and seem to defy description, most craniofacial clefts occur along predictable embryologic lines.

I. EPIDEMIOLOGY

A. Incidence = approximately 1.4–4.9 per 100,000 live births.

B. Comparison of rare craniofacial clefts to common clefts has approximate incidence of 9.5–34 per 1000.

II. ETIOLOGY

A. In the majority of cases, etiology is unknown.

B. Treacher Collins syndrome—autosomal dominant with variable penetrance.

C. Goldenhar syndrome—autosomal dominant with variable penetrance.

D. Amniotic band syndrome.

E. Environmental factors—radiation, infection, maternal metabolic imbalances, and drugs (anticonvulsants, chemotherapeutic agents, steroids, and tranquilizers).

III. THEORIES OF FACIAL CLEFTING

A. Failure of fusion of the facial processes.

B. Failure of mesodermal migration and penetrance of neuroectoderm.

IV. CLASSIFICATIONS

A. American Association of Cleft Palate Rehabilitation Classification by Harkins et al. in 1962.

B. Karfik Classification in 1966.

C. Van der Meulen and Associates Classification in 1983.

D. Median Tissue Deficiency Classification by DeMyer in 1964.

E. Median Excess Tissue Classification by DeMyer in 1967.

F. Tessier Classification in 1976 (Figs. 1 and 2).

V. TESSIER CLASSIFICATION OF CLEFTS

A. General

1. The most enduring, complete, and clinically relevant classification, which links clinical observations to underlying skeletal deformity.

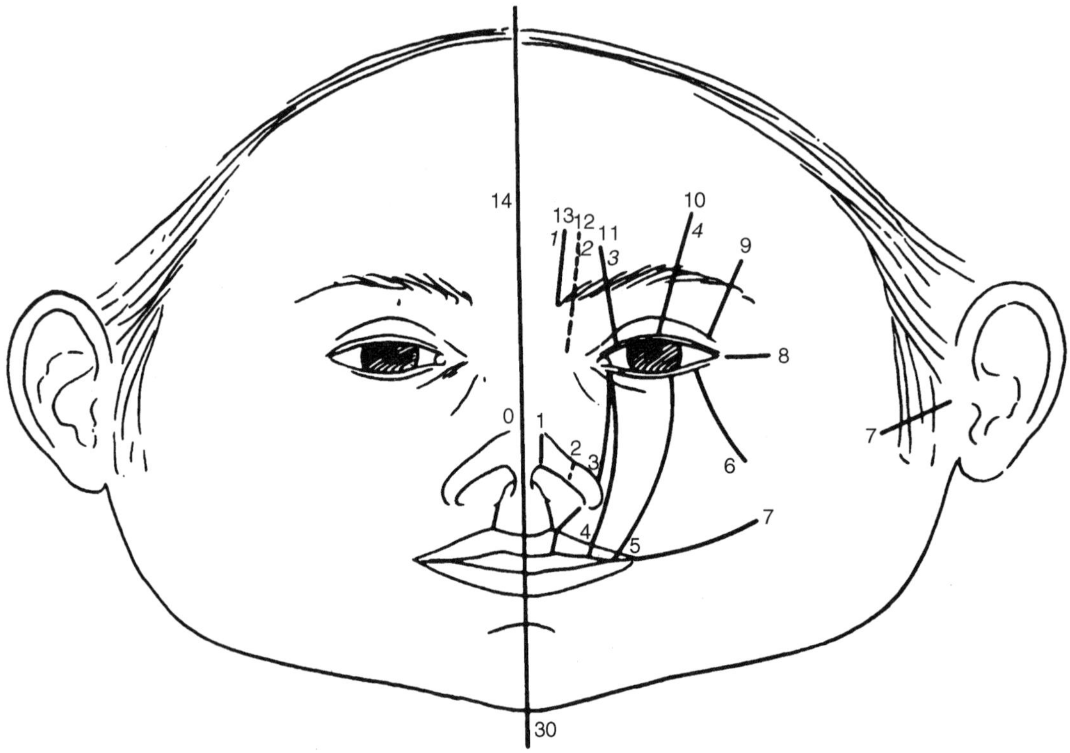

Figure 1 Tessier classification of craniofacial clefts. Lines represent soft tissue clefts. (Courtesy of Dr. P. Tessier.)

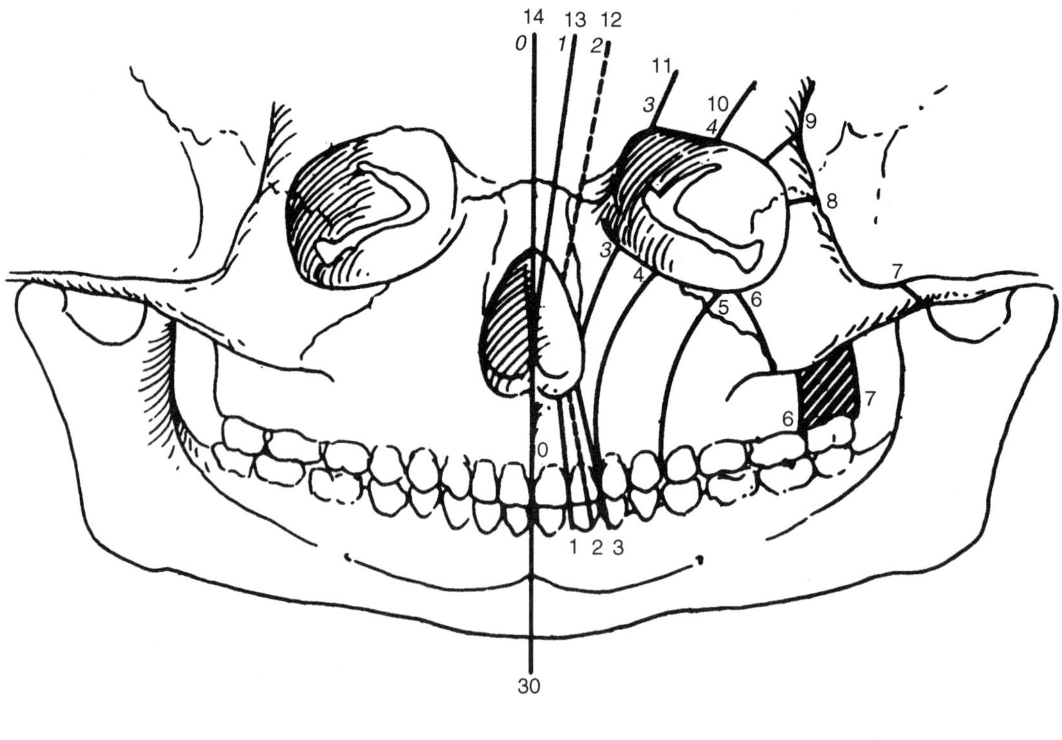

Figure 2 Tessier classification of craniofacial clefts. Lines represent skeletal clefts. (Courtesy of Dr. P. Tessier.)

2. Numbered from 0 to 14, these cleft types follow well-defined "time zones."
3. The eyelids and orbits define the classification axis and divide the face into upper and lower hemispheres.
4. Clinically observed combinations: 0 and 14, 1 and 13, 2 and 12, 3 and 11, 4 and 10, 5 and 9, and 6 and 8. Note that the combinations typically add up to the number 14.
5. Tessier cleft number 7 is the most lateral craniofacial cleft.

B. Number 0 Cleft

1. Soft tissue characteristics, in cases of widening or duplication:
   - True midline cleft
   - Diastema between the central incisors
   - Bifid labial frenulum
   - Broad philtral columns
   - Bifid nose
   - Duplicated nasal septum
2. Soft tissue characteristics, in cases of agenesis or hypoplasia, are associated with:
   - Holoprosencephaly
   - False midline cleft
   - Absent philtral column
   - Rudimentary or absent columella
   - Cleft of the primary and secondary palate
   - Nasal hypoplasia
   - Vestigial nasal septum
   - Nasal tip depression
3. Bony characteristics, in cases of widening or duplication:
   - Keel-shaped maxilla with anterior teeth angled medially
   - Anterior open bite
   - Cleft in the primary and secondary palate
   - Duplicated anterior nasal spine and bony septum
   - Vertical maxillary hypoplasia
   - Broad and flattened nasal bones
   - Enlargement of ethmoid and sphenoid sinuses
   - Orbital hypertelorism
4. Bony characteristics, in cases of agenesis or hypoplasia:
   - Absent nasal bone and bony septum
   - Hypoplastic ethmoid bones
   - Orbital hypotelorism
   - Eye deformities
   - Congenital forebrain deformities
5. Soft tissue and bony characteristics (lower face):
   - A number 30 cleft is the caudal extension of a number 0 cleft
   - Median cleft between the central incisors and mandibular symphysis
   - Neck deformities
   - Absent hyoid bone
   - Abnormal thyroid cartilage
   - Atrophic neck muscles
   - Bifid tongue
   - Ankyloglossia

C. Number 1 Cleft

1. Soft tissue characteristics:
   - Facial cleft is the same as for a common cleft
   - Notched alar dome
   - Broad columella
   - Nasal tip and septum are deviated away from the cleft
   - Furrows along the nasal dorsum
   - Cleft is medial to the malpositioned medial canthus
   - Vertical distopia
   - Telecanthus
2. Bony characteristics:
   - Keel-shaped maxilla with medially facing teeth
   - Anterior open bite
   - Cleft is between the central and lateral incisors and into the pyriform aperture, through the primary and secondary palate, and then between nasal bone and maxilla
   - Flattened nasal bones
   - Ethmoid hypertrophy
   - Orbital hypertelorism

D. Number 2 Cleft

1. Soft tissue characteristics:
    - Cleft lip lies in the region of common clefts
    - Hypoplasia of the mid-alar cartilage
    - Flattened lateral nose
    - Broad nasal dorsum
    - Cleft passes medial to the palpebral fissure
    - Normal lacrimal drainage
    - Laterally displaced medial canthus
2. Bony characteristics:
    - Cleft between the lateral incisor and canine into the pyriform sinus
    - Intact maxillary sinus
    - Complete cleft of the primary and secondary palate
    - Intact nasal septum, deviated away from the cleft
    - Passes between the nasal bones and maxilla
    - Hypoplastic ethmoid and frontal sinuses
    - Orbital hypertelorism

E. Number 3 Cleft

1. Soft tissue characteristics:
    - Most common Tessier cleft
    - Cleft is along philtral column into the nasal floor
    - Vertical shortening between the ala and lower lid
    - Short nose
    - Upward pull of the alar base
    - Disrupted lacrimal system and lower canaliculus
    - Lower lid colobomas.
2. Bony characteristics:
    - Cleft passes between the lateral incisor and canine
    - Flat maxillary arch
    - Communicates with the pyriform and maxillary sinuses
    - Passes lateral to the nasal bone, through the lacrimal groove, and into the orbit

F. Number 4 Cleft

1. Soft tissue characteristics:
    - Cleft is lateral to Cupid's bow and medial to the oral commissure
    - Ala are superiorly positioned
    - Passes into the lower eyelid
    - Severe soft tissue deficit between the lip and eyelid
    - Normal nasolacrimal system and medial canthus
2. Bony characteristics:
    - Cleft passes between the lateral incisor and canine, then lateral to the pyriform aperture, through the maxillary sinus, medial to infraorbital foramen, and through the inferior orbital rim

G. Number 5 Cleft

1. Soft tissue characteristics:
    - Cleft lip is just medial to the oral commissure
    - Passes lateral to the ala
    - Short nose
    - Superiorly rotated alar base
    - Into the lower eyelid at its superior extent
2. Bony characteristics:
    - Cleft is between the premolar teeth, then passes lateral to the infraorbital nerve and maxillary sinus, into the lateral orbital rim and floor
    - Hypoplastic maxillary sinus

H. Number 6 Cleft

1. Soft tissue characteristics:
    - Similar to Treacher Collins syndrome
    - Cheek furrow from the commissure to the lateral eyelid
    - Inferiorly displaced lateral palpebral fissure
    - Lateral colobomas
    - Ear deformities and hearing deficits are common
2. Bony characteristics:
    - No alveolar cleft
    - Tilted occlusal plane
    - Cleft is through the zygomatico-maxillary suture, into the lateral orbital rim
    - Hypoplastic zygoma

I. Number 7 Cleft

1. Soft tissue characteristics:
    - Same cleft as hemifacial microsomia and Goldenhar syndrome

- Soft tissue furrow from the oral commissure to the preauricular hairline
- Possible external and middle ear malformations
- Occasional parotid gland defects
- Occasional abnormalities of cranial nerves 5 and 7 and corresponding temporalis muscles

2. Bony characteristics:
   - Cleft is through the pterygomaxillary junction
   - Hypoplasia of the posterior maxilla and mandibular ramus
   - Canted occlusal plane
   - Hypoplastic coronoid process and condyle
   - Anterior open bite on the affected side
   - Severely malformed zygoma and arch
   - Asymmetric cranial base and glenoid fossa
   - Abnormal sphenoid

J. Number 8 Cleft

1. Soft tissue characteristics:
   - Seldom an isolated cleft; usually a part of Treacher Collins syndrome
   - Begins at the lateral palpebral fissure and extends onto the temporal area
   - True lateral coloboma (dermatocele)
   - Absent lateral canthus
2. Bony characteristics:
   - Cleft of the frontozygomatic suture
   - Absent or hypoplastic zygoma
   - Downward slanting lateral palpebral fissure (Treacher Collins)

K. Number 9 Cleft

1. Soft tissue characteristics:
   - Extremely rare
   - Cleft is through the lateral third of the upper eyelid and eyebrow
   - Distorted lateral canthus distorted
   - Cranial nerve palsy is common
2. Bony characteristics:
   - Cleft is through the superolateral angle of the orbit, through the greater wing of the sphenoid to the squamousal temporal bone
   - Cranial base abnormalities

L. Number 10 Cleft

1. Soft tissue characteristics:
   - Cleft of the middle eyelid and eyebrow
   - Elongated palpebral fissure
   - Possible amblyopia
   - Possible colobomas
   - Hair projection from the temporo-parietal region to the lateral brow
2. Bony characteristics:
   - Cleft is through the supraorbital rim, frontal bone, and orbital roof lateral to the supraorbital nerve
   - Encephalocele is common
   - Hypertelorism

M. Number 11 Cleft

1. Soft tissue characteristics:
   - Cleft traverses the medial eyelid and eyebrow
   - Frontal hair projection
2. Bony characteristics:
   - Cleft is either lateral to the ethmoids and through the supraorbital rim or through the ethmoid air cells to produce orbital hypertelorism
   - Normal cranial base

N. Number 12 Cleft

1. Soft tissue characteristics:
   - Cleft is medial to the medial canthus
   - Eyebrow colobomas
   - Lateral displacement of the medial canthus
   - No eyelid clefts
   - Paramedian frontal hair projection
2. Bony characteristics:
   - Cleft passes through the flattened, frontal process of the maxilla, through hypertrophy of the ethmoid air cells to produce orbital hypertelorism and telecanthus
   - Enlarged frontal and sphenoid sinuses
   - No encephalocele

O. Number 13 Cleft

1. Soft tissue characteristics:
   - Encephalocele

- Cleft is medial to eyelids and eyebrows
- V-shaped frontal hair projection

2. Bony characteristics:
   - Paramedian cleft traverses the frontal bone and courses across a widened olfactory groove
   - Widened cribiform plate
   - Hypertrophy of ethmoid sinus
   - Hypertelorism
   - Orbital distopia

P. Number 14 Cleft

1. Soft tissue characteristics, in cases of agenesis or hypoplasia:
   - Holoprosencephalic disorders
   - Microcephaly
   - Hypotelorism
   - Forebrain malformations
2. Bony characteristics, in cases of agenesis or hypoplasia:
   - Absence of midline cranial base
   - Flattened frontal bone
   - No pneumatization of the frontal sinus
3. Soft tissue characteristics, in cases of widening or duplication:
   - Frontonasal encephalocele
   - Lateral orbital displacement
   - Hypertelorism
   - Telecanthus
   - Midline hair projections
4. Bony characteristics, in cases of widening or duplication:
   - Bifid crista galli and perpendicular plate of the ethmoid
   - Ethmoid is pneumatized
   - Rotated greater and lesser wings of the sphenoid, causing a short middle cranial fossa

VI. TREATMENT

1. Treatment plans cannot be rigidly standardized.
2. Timing is governed by severity of the malformation. Surgery should be delayed if the malformation is mild; surgery should be performed early if the deformity is severe or if functional issues are present.
3. Soft tissue clefts and cranial defects are corrected during infancy. Midface bone grafting and reconstruction are performed in an older child, and orthognathic surgery is performed in adults.
4. Soft tissue clefts are closed with Z-plasties and local tissue flaps. When possible, place incisions along aesthetic lines.
5. Lip—align the vermilion as in common cleft lip and restore muscle continuity. If the cleft is lateral to the philtral column, excise the intervening tissue.
6. Oral commissure—restore the cleft laterally with straight-line repair and a Z-plasty medially. Place the scar along the nasolabial fold.
7. Nose—excise the cleft, repair the nasal cartilages, perform local rotation flaps and Z-plasties for the retracted ala, and place cartilage grafts or composite grafts as necessary. Nasal lining is obtained from the nasal septum. Nasal reconstruction is achieved with a cantilevered cranial bone graft.
8. Orbit—reconstruct with bone grafts to restore continuity and to correct distopia.
9. Eyelid—accurately position the medial canthus and secure with transnasal wiring. Lateral canthoplasties are performed as necessary. Transposition flaps are utilized for eyelid skin deficit; palatal grafts for conjunctiva deficit; and Z-plasty to correct a number 8 soft tissue cleft.
10. Eye—urgent surgical intervention is indicated if the eye is exposed from colobomas in order to prevent corneal ulceration.
11. Lacrimal apparatus—when the cleft disrupts the canalicular system, correct with silastic stents or dacryocystorhinostomy when necessary.
12. Severe hypotelorism is corrected with facial bipartition or subcranial Le Fort III osteotomy and bone grafts.
13. Forehead and orbital reconstruction is with cranial bone grafts, if available.
14. Alternatives to cranial bone are rib, iliac crest, or alloplastic materials.
15. Alloplastic material includes polymethylmethacrylate, hydroxyapatite, resorbable tricalcium

phosphate, silicon, and hard tissue replacement (Walter Lorenz®).

16. Contraindications to alloplasts include placing material near sinuses, history of craniofacial infection, and inadequate soft tissue coverage.
17. Disadvantages of alloplasts: increased infection rate, extrusion, and local tissue reaction.
18. Lower lip—V-excision of the cleft and closure in layers. A Z-plasty is performed to release the frenulum. A bifid tongue is excised and closed in layers.
19. Midline mandible—correct midline mandibular clefts when the child is older and bone graft as necessary.
20. Lateral mandible—correct severe deformity with a costochondral graft. Correct moderate deformity with distraction osteogenesis. Mild deformities can be observed until the patient becomes an adult, then correct with orthognathic surgery (maxillary Le Fort I osteotomy and mandibular sagittal split osteotomy).
21. Final correction of large and severe soft tissue deficit is usually accomplished with a fasciocutaneous free flap.

47

Craniosynostosis

Babak J. Mehrara, M.D.*
New York University Medical Center, New York, New York, U.S.A.

Michael T. Longaker, M.D.
Stanford University Medical Center, Stanford, California, U.S.A.

I. DEFINITION

Craniosynostosis is defined as a premature fusion of one or more cranial sutures with resultant abnormality in cranial shape. Calvarial growth normally occurs perpendicular to the sutures. Thus, growth restriction, secondary to suture fusion, results in redirection of calvarial growth parallel to the fused suture.

II. EPIDEMIOLOGY

A. Incidence

Craniosynostosis is a relatively common craniofacial disorder with an incidence of 1:1500 to 1:1900 live births.

B. Inheritance

1. Occurs as a syndromic or nonsyndromic disorder.
2. Nonsyndromic cases are usually sporadic, although inherited forms have been described.
3. Sporadic craniosynostoses (95%) far outnumber syndromic cases (5–6%).
4. Over 100 syndromes that have craniosynostosis as part of a constellation of abnormalities have been described, including Crouzon, Pfeiffer, and Apert syndromes. Syndromic craniosynostoses are usually transmitted via autosomal dominant or autosomal recessive mechanisms. Sporadic transmission has also been reported, however.

III. ETIOLOGY

Exact etiology is unknown and likely to be multifactorial with genetic, maternal, positional, and infectious contributions.

A. Numerous theories exist:

1. Virchow (1851) advocated the concept that abnormality is primarily localized to the cranial suture with resultant secondary defects in the cranial base.
2. Moss and others have hypothesized that abnormalities in the cranial base cause abnormal sutural development.
3. More recently, Mehrara, Longaker, Ogle, and Opperman have identified that the dura mater underlying a cranial suture is an important determinant of sutural fate in murine models of normal suture fusion.

B. Genetic link is important:

1. Numerous authors have demonstrated mutations in fibroblast growth factor receptors (FGFRs). Mutations were first identified in syndromic cases of craniosynostosis, although,

Current affiliation: Memorial Sloan-Kettering Cancer Center, New York, New York, U.S.A.

more recently, Mulliken et al. and others have identified similar mutations in sporadic cases. The majority of mutations are gain of function mutations with ligand-independent activation of the receptor, resulting in overactivity of fibroblast growth factor.

2. Gain of function mutations in the transcription factor *MSX-2* have been associated with Boston-type craniosynostosis.
3. Laboratory studies have also implicated an important role for fibroblast growth factors in the regulation of pathologic and programmed cranial suture fusion in murine models. In addition, these studies have identified a number of other osteogenic growth factors, including transforming growth factor beta and bone morphogenetic proteins.

IV. ANATOMY AND TERMINOLOGY

Normal major cranial sutures include metopic, sagittal, coronal, and lambdoidal sutures.

A. Common types of craniosynostosis:

1. Sagittal suture (scaphocephaly)—most common type of single suture synostosis.
2. Metopic suture (trigonocephaly).
3. Unilateral coronal suture (anterior plagiocephaly).
4. Bilateral coronal suture (brachycephaly).
5. Lambdoidal (posterior plagiocephaly)—least common type of single suture synostoses.
6. Positional (deformational) plagiocephaly—not considered to be a true craniosynostosis with fusion of cranial sutures, but rather represents an alteration in calvarial shape due to newborn supine positioning during sleep.

V. PHYSIOLOGY

Alterations in calvarial growth can result in a number of functional problems including increased intracranial pressure, mental retardation, seizures, hydrocephalus, and blindness.

A. Increased Intracranial Pressure (ICP)

Brain volume reaches approximately 50% of adult levels by 6 months of age and normally triples by the first year of life. Thus, restriction in calvarial growth, particularly due to the fusion of multiple sutures, may result in a decrease in calvarial size and increased ICP. Not all children with craniosynostosis have increased ICP, however.

1. Marchac and Reinier (1982) demonstrated that 42% of patients with fusion of multiple sutures had elevated ICP. In contrast, increased ICP was found in only 13% of patients with a single fused suture. Interestingly, the authors demonstrated that abnormal ICP normalized after surgical correction and cranial vault remodeling, although this result has been debated.
2. Apert syndrome represents a possible exception to the increased incidence of elevated ICP pressures in patients with multiple fused sutures. This is likely related to the large midline calvarial defect present in many of these patients.
3. Papilledema, visual disturbances, seizures, nausea, gait abnormalities, anorexia, developmental delay as well as "thumb printing" on radiographs are important clinical signs and symptoms of elevated ICP.

B. Mental Retardation

1. The true incidence of mental retardation with craniosynostosis is unknown.
2. Some patients with syndromic craniosynostoses display developmental delay (Apert syndrome), while others can have "normal" mentation (Crouzon syndrome).
3. The main problem with analyses of mental acuity in relation with craniosynostosis has been the use of IQ testing, since these tests are not thought to be sensitive enough to assess intellectual abilities of young children. Thus, IQ testing has not consistently shown improvements in mental function after surgery.
4. Children with single suture synostosis generally have normal mentation. In fact, it has been suggested that IQ < 70 in association with single suture synostosis is likely related to a primary brain malformation and not due to premature suture fusion.

C. Visual Abnormalities

Optic nerve atrophy and papilledema are relatively common with multiple suture synostosis. These changes are likely related to increased ICP and optic nerve compression. Crouzon syndrome is most commonly associated with optic nerve dysfunction.

D. Hydrocephalus

Hydrocephalus is an increase in ventricular size and represents a relatively infrequent finding in isolated craniosynostosis. Hydrocephalus is more commonly noted in syndromic craniosynostosis and is thought to represent, at least in part, dystrophic brain development since ventricular enlargement has not been shown to correlate with elevated ICP. Worsening hydrocephalus in a series of CT scans does correlate with elevated ICP and should be assessed.

VI. CLINICAL EVALUATION

History and physical examination are important in the diagnosis of craniosynostosis.

A. Evaluation of a patient with abnormal calvarial shape should include a thorough analysis of:
   1. Family history
   2. Onset of abnormal calvarial shape
   3. Prenatal/maternal factors
   4. Developmental milestones
   5. Symptoms of elevated ICP (lethargy, anorexia, seizures, visual disturbances)

B. Physical examination should include analysis of:
   1. Overall facial/calvarial shape and head circumference
   2. Sutural ridging
   3. Fontanelles—location, open vs. closed, soft vs. bulging
   4. Age-appropriate neurologic exam
   5. Funduscopic exam of the eyes

C. Radiologic analysis should include:
   1. AP, lateral, and Towne's view x-rays
   2. C-spine x-rays including lateral and flexion/extension views to rule out cervical spine abnormalities
   3. CT scan to analyze:
      - Bone
      - Soft tissues and brain
      - Possible 3-D reconstruction
      - Preoperative planning
   4. MRI is useful in Apert and Pfeiffer syndromes to analyze the posterior fossa and foramen magnum.

VII. SURGICAL MANAGEMENT

A. Goals of surgical treatment of craniosynostosis are to decrease ICP and achieve normal calvarial shape.

B. Timing of surgery is debated. Most centers recommend early treatment (less than 1 year of age). Treatment may be hastened by evidence of increased ICP or visual disturbances. Surgery prior to 1 year of age is advocated since calvarial bone is softer and easily molded. In addition, children younger than 1 year of age are capable of healing large calvarial defects spontaneously. In general, cranial vault remodeling, frontal bone advancement, and shunt surgery (if needed) are performed before the first birthday.

VIII. ISOLATED SYNOSTOSIS

A. Metopic Suture (Trigonocephaly)

1. Metopic suture is the first cranial suture to fuse (less than 2 years of age).
2. Premature fusion results in a "keel"-shaped head.
3. Trigonocephaly is relatively uncommon and is seen in less than 10% of isolated synostosis.
4. Associated findings include hypotelorism, upward slanting of lateral canthi, and a triangular shape of the supraorbital ridge.
5. Usually not associated with increased ICP (<4%).
6. Some children display evidence of mental retardation and frontal lobe maldevelopment.
7. Surgical treatment involves supraorbital and lateral orbital rim advancement with frontal bone remodeling.

B. Sagittal Suture (Scaphocephaly)

1. Scaphocephaly represents the most common form of isolated craniosynostosis and results in increased anterior-posterior length and decreased width ("boat-like" head).
2. Most commonly sporadic (<2% familial predisposition).
3. Males are more commonly affected than females (4:1).
4. May involve part or all of the suture. Partial involvement may result in calvarial deformity that is primarily posterior, anterior, or central.

5. Surgical treatment involves strip craniectomy, cranial vault remodeling, and frontal/parietal/occipital "barrel-stave" osteotomies to increase biparietal and bitemporal dimensions.

C. Unilateral Coronal Suture Synostosis (Anterior Plagiocephaly)

1. Uncommon with an approximate incidence of 1:10,0000 live births.
2. Fusion results in ipsilateral flattening of the fronto-parietal region, bulging of the ipsilateral squamous portion of the temporal bone with resultant effacement of the temporal fossa, and shortening of the lateral orbital wall.
3. "Harlequin" orbit is a radiographic finding that is pathognomonic for anterior plagiocephaly ipsilateral to the involved coronal suture. The radiologic appearance is caused by ipsilateral superior displacement of the lesser wing of the sphenoid.
4. Other physical findings include deviation of the nose toward the affected side and chin deviation to the contralateral side.
5. Surgical treatment involves strip craniectomy and unilateral or bilateral forehead remodeling with reshaping and repositioning of the supraorbital bandeau to improve forehead symmetry.

D. Unilateral Lambdoidal Synostosis (Posterior Plagiocephaly)

1. Extremely rare, but commonly confused with positional (deformational) plagiocephaly.
2. Unlike deformational plagiocephaly (see below), true lambdoidal synostosis does not respond to molding helmets and nonsurgical therapy.

E. Deformational Plagiocephaly

1. This abnormality in cranial shape is not due to premature cranial suture fusion, but is due to abnormal calvarial molding secondary to supine newborn positioning during sleep.
2. The increased incidence of this problem has been contributed to the "back-to-sleep" campaign that advocated placing infants on their backs when sleeping to reduce the rates of sudden infant death syndrome.
3. Results in a calvarium that has a distinctive "parallelogram" shape.
4. Can cause either frontal or posterior shape changes.
5. Also seen with torticollis or abnormal shortening of the sternocleidomastoid muscle.
6. Treatment involves the use of molding helmets worn 23 h per day and sleeping in the prone position. Close follow-up until normalization of calvarial contour is critical. Molding helmet therapy should be instituted prior to 9 months of age for best effects.

IX. CRANIOSYNOSTOSIS SYNDROMES

These are well-recognized craniofacial abnormalities that combine craniosynostosis with a constellation of pathologic findings. To date, over 100 such syndromes have been described.

A. Transmission is usually genetic with autosomal dominant, autosomal recessive, or X-linked patterns described.

B. Variable penetrance is common in involved families.

C. Common features include mid-face hypoplasia, premature cranial suture fusion, and cranial base abnormalities. Differentiating factors often include limb anomalies and mentation.

D. Etiology is not completely understood, although genetic abnormalities are thought to play a crucial role (see above). Most common genetic abnormalities involve mutations in fibroblast growth factor receptors (FGFRs). Exact mechanisms by which these mutations result in phenotypic abnormalities are unclear, since identical mutations have been shown to be associated with different syndromes.

X. COMMON SYNDROMES

A. Apert Syndrome (Acrocephalosyndactyly Type I)

1. First described by Apert in 1906.
2. Relatively rare, with an approximate incidence of 1:160,000 live births.
3. Most cases are sporadic, but autosomal dominant transmission has also been reported.

4. Affected children demonstrate exorbitism, midface hypoplasia, and class III malocclusion with resultant flat, elongated forehead, and bitemporal widening. Other features include occipital flattening, beaked nose, and downward slanting palpebral fissures.
5. Craniosynostosis and calvarial vault deformity are variable but most commonly result in bilateral coronal suture synostosis with shortened anterior-posterior calvarial length and increased cranial height (turribrachycephaly).
6. Hand/feet anomalies (syndactyly) are distinctive features. Syndactyly has varying degrees of involvement but usually involves the 2nd, 3rd and 4th digits.
7. Often associated with elevated incidence of increased intracranial pressure (ICP) and hydrocephalus.
8. Most children demonstrate developmental delay, but some have normal intelligence.

B. Crouzon Syndrome (Acrocephalosyndactyly Type II)

1. First described by Crouzon in 1912.
2. Autosomal dominant transmission with variable penetrance.
3. More common than Apert syndrome with an incidence of 1:25,000 live births.
4. Premature fusion of bilateral coronal sutures (brachycephaly) is the most common calvarial phenotype. Other abnormalities, including cloverleaf skull, scaphocephaly, and trigonocephaly, have been reported.
5. Timing of premature suture fusion is variable with fusion by 2–3 years of age most common. Fusion by birth also described, but less common.
6. Maxillary hypoplasia and exorbitism similar to Apert syndrome. In addition, normal mandibular growth together with maxillary hypoplasia results in class III malocclusion.
7. Ocular exorbitism can be severe and lead to corneal ulceration or herniation.
8. Conduction hearing deficits are common.
9. Mentation is usually normal.
10. No commonly reported limb anomalies.
11. Increased incidence of elevated intracranial pressures.

C. Saethre-Chotzen Syndrome (Acrocephalosyndactyly Type III)

1. First described by Saethre in 1931 and Chotzen in 1932.
2. Autosomal dominant transmission.
3. Phenotypic features include brachycephaly with low-set frontal hairline, facial asymmetry, eyelid ptosis, maxillary hypoplasia, and short stature.
4. Partial syndactyly is commonly seen and usually involves the 2nd and 3rd digits.
5. Usually normal intelligence.

D. Pfeiffer Syndrome (Acrocephalosyndactyly Type V)

1. First described in 1964.
2. Mode of transmission usually autosomal dominant with variable penetrance.
3. Craniofacial features are similar to Apert syndrome, with turribrachycephaly secondary to bilateral coronal suture and sagittal suture synostosis.
4. Midface growth disturbance is also similar to Apert syndrome, with maxillary hypoplasia, exorbitism, and class III malocclusion.
5. Hypertelorism and down-slanting palpebral fissures are also commonly seen.
6. Distinctive feature is broad thumbs and great toes.
7. Usually normal intelligence.

XI. SURGICAL MANAGEMENT OF SYNDROMIC CRANIOSYNOSTOSIS

Most modern surgical techniques used in the treatment of syndromic craniosynostoses are based on the work of Paul Tessier, an innovative French surgeon who pioneered craniofacial surgery in the 1950s–1960s. Initial surgical management of syndromic craniosynostosis is designed to improve calvarial shape, release synostosed sutures with resultant cranial vault decompression, and upper orbital repositioning to improve exorbitism. Secondary procedures are designed to address midface abnormalities and class III malocclusion.

A. Fronto-Orbital Advancement

1. Usually performed before the first birthday (6–12 months).
2. Operative strategy is designed to release the synostosed suture and achieve simultaneous

cranial vault decompression and remodeling with repositioning of the supraorbital bar.

3. Multidisciplinary, intracranial approach involving neurosurgical and plastic surgical teams.
4. Advancement of the supraorbital bar in a tongue-and-groove fashion with fixation using absorbable mini-plates.
5. Overcorrection is important.
6. Secondary fronto-orbital advancements and calvarial vault remodeling may be required later in life.

B. Correction of Midface Deformity

1. Midface advancement is usually performed with subcranial Le Fort III osteotomy, as popularized by Tessier.
2. Monoblock advancement was developed by Fernando Ortiz-Monastario and combines fronto-orbital advancement with Le Fort III osteotomy. This procedure is usually performed in older children (i.e., >8 years of age) since surgery may be associated with an increased incidence of infection due to the creation of a retroorbital dead space that possibly communicates with the nasal cavity.
3. Timing of surgical intervention is controversial:
   - Some surgeons advocate early (4–7 years of age) treatment to improve facial contour, thus contributing to more normal psychosocial development. Early treatment, however, may require a repeat Le Fort III advancement after skeletal maturity.
   - Others wait until skeletal maturity (14–18 years of age) unless early intervention is forced by mitigating circumstances such as airway obstruction or severe exorbitism despite fronto-orbital advancement.

C. Orthognathic Surgery

This surgery is performed to correct class III malocclusion. Correction is usually performed after skeletal maturity (14–18 years) using Le Fort I maxillary advancement with or without genioplasty.

48

Craniofacial Microsomia

J. Timothy Katzen, M.D.
Santa Monica, California, U.S.A.
Joseph G. McCarthy, M.D.
New York University School of Medicine, New York, New York, U.S.A.

I. SYNONYMS

1. Hemifacial microsomia
2. Oculoauricularvertebral spectrum
3. First and second branchial arch syndrome
4. Otomandibular dysostosis
5. Lateral facial dysplasia
6. The variety of names suggests the broad clinical spectrum and incomplete understanding of this syndrome.

II. CRANIOFACIAL MICROSOMIA

A. Unilateral and Bilateral

The nomenclature is somewhat vague and misleading. Most cases of "unilateral" craniofacial microsomia do indeed have bilateral manifestations. Clinical and radiographic examination of "unilateral" cases usually reveals additional abnormalities on the "normal" or "less affected" side.

B. Incidence

- Incidence is 1 in 4000–5642 births. There was a marked increase in the number of cases associated with thalidomide usage in the early 1960s.
- Ratio of male to female is 3:2.
- Ratio of right to left side of face being involved is 3:2.

C. Physical Examination

Physical examination shows regional hypoplasia or abnormalities of:

1. Mandible
2. Maxilla
3. Temporozygomatic arch complex
4. Temporomandibular joint
5. Other components of the craniofacial skeleton (orbit, cranium)
6. Auricular complex
7. Associated soft tissues (including muscles of mastication, subcutaneous tissue, and cranial nerves)

D. Etiopathogenesis

1. Unlike in Treacher Collins syndrome, the genetic component in craniofacial microsomia is ill defined, and there is no evidence of genetic transmission except in a few patients.
2. The recurrence rate in a first-degree relative is estimated to be 3%.
3. Current etiopathogenic theories favor an intrauterine event. Many believe that vascular defects in the stapedial artery (with resulting hemorrhage) may account for the abnormal development of the first and second branchial arches.

The stapedial artery is a temporary vascular supply for the primordia of the first and second branchial arches.

E. Embryology

The ear serves as a frame of reference in this syndrome because of its developmental relationship with the jaw.

1. The first branchial arch leads to the formation of:
   - The anterior part of the auricle
   - The maxilla, palatine bone, and zygoma—all develop from the maxillary process of the first branchial arch
   - The mandible—develops from the mandibular process
   - The muscles of mastication—temporalis, masseter, medial and lateral pterygoids
2. The second branchial arch leads to the formation of:
   - The remaining portions of the external ear
   - The muscles of facial expression, posterior belly of the digastric, stylohyoid, and stapedius muscles

F. Skeletal Deformities

1. Jaw deformity: the most conspicuous deformity of craniofacial microsomia is hypoplasia of the mandible on the affected side.
   - The ramus of the mandible is short or virtually absent.
   - The body of the mandible curves upward to join the short ramus. The body of the mandible on the "unaffected" side shows increased horizontal length and an increase in the gonial angle.
   - The condyle malformations vary from minimal hypoplasia to complete absence, in association with hypoplasia of the ramus. In all patients, condylar abnormalities can be demonstrated and this finding may be the pathognomonic finding for the syndrome.
   - The chin is deviated to the more affected side.
   - There is an occlusal cant in a cephalad direction on the affected side.
   - Pruzansky classified mandibular deformities as follows (Fig. 1):

     Grade I: minimal hypoplasia

     Grade II: small condyle and ramus; flattened condylar head; absent glenoid fossa; coronoid process may be absent

     Grade III: severely hypoplastic or absent ramus
   - Polley and Figueroa found that mandibular growth deficiency is usually closely related to the degree of hypoplasia of the condyle. The mandibular defects can cause:

     Occlusal cant, which becomes higher on the more affected side

     Restricted movement and development of the maxillary dentoalveolar process in the superoinferior dimension

     Delay of molar teeth development and eruption
2. Other skeletal deformities on the affected side include:
   - Maxilla: hypoplasia on the more affected side
   - Styloid process: smaller and shorter on the affected side
   - Mastoid process: flattened with reduced or absent pneumatization

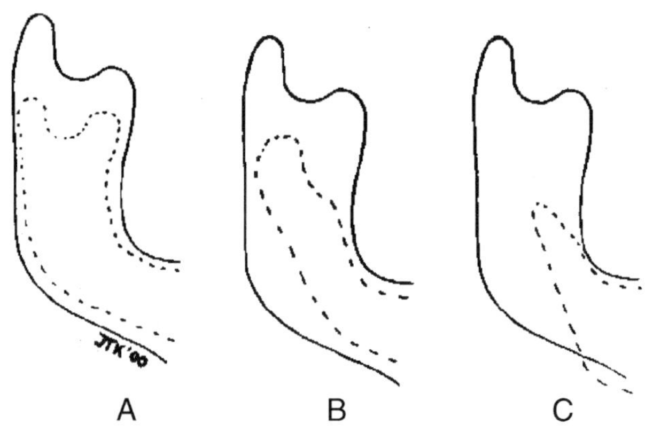

Figure 1 Pruzansky classification. Normal mandible is in solid outline, affected mandible is in dashed outline. (A) Grade I: minimal hypoplasia; (B) Grade II: small condyle and small ramus, flattened condylar head, absent glenoid fossa, and the coronoid process may be absent; (C) Grade III: severely hypoplastic or absent ramus.

- Zygoma: underdeveloped with a flattened eminence
- Frontal bone: flattening of the affected side, with an appearance similar to plagiocephaly without radiographic evidence of coronal synostosis
- Vertebrae: hemivertebrae, fused vertebrae, spina bifida, and scoliosis have been reported

G. Muscular Deformities

1. Lateral pterygoid muscle: results in limited protrusion and lateral movement. On testing for lateral pterygoid muscle function, patients will not be able to shift their mandible to the *unaffected* side.
2. Temporalis muscle: reduced in size.
3. Masseter muscle: reduced in size.
4. Soft palate musculature: abnormal contraction vector.

H. Nervous System Deformities

1. Cerebral: uncommon, but the following have been reported:
   - Ipsilateral cerebral hypoplasia, hypoplasia of the corpus collosum, hydrocephalus, lipomas, and unilateral hypoplasia of the brain stem and cerebellum
   - Mental retardation
   - Epilepsy
2. Cranial nerves:
   - Facial paralysis (most common): due to abnormal facial musculature, path of the facial nerve through temporal bone, and/or hypoplasia of the intracranial portion of the facial nerve and nucleus in brain stem.
   - Congenital hearing loss may be due to malformed inner ear, hypoplasia of cochlear nerve, and brain stem auditory nuclei. Hypoplasia of cranial nerves 9–12 may also be present.
   - Uncommon, but the following have been reported:

     Unilateral and bilateral arrhinencephaly

     Unilateral agenesis and hypoplasia of optic nerve

     Congenital ophthalmoplegia and Duane's retraction syndrome

     Hypoplasia of the trochlear nerve

     Hypoplasia of the abducens nerve

     Congenital trigeminal anesthesia

I. Soft Tissue Deformities

1. Auricular deformity: a typical feature of craniofacial microsomia:
   - Meurmann proposed the following classification:

     Grade I: smaller, malformed auricles

     Grade II: only a vertical remnant of cartilage and skin with a small anterior hook and complete atresia of canal

     Grade III: auricle almost entirely absent except for a small lobular remnant
   - The above degree of auricular deformity:

     Does not correlate with hearing function; computed tomography (CT), not auricular morphology, is the only indicator of middle ear structure

     Does correlate with the underlying ipsilateral mandibular deformity
2. Other soft tissue deficiencies have been noted in the:
   - Skin
   - Subcutaneous tissue
   - Tongue
   - Parotid gland
   - Eye and eyelid

J. Classification

The deformity in craniofacial microsomia varies in extent and degree, and there are many shades of expression, according to the degree of involvement of the first and second branchial arches and adjacent skeletal structures. In the severe form, all structures derived from the first and second branchial arches are hypoplastic. In other milder types, either the auricular or jaw dysplasias may predominate. Because of the heterogeneous nature of craniofacial microsomia, it is difficult to classify the individual deformity.

1. Harold, Vargervik, and Chierici proposed the following phenotypic classification:
   - Type I (A). The classic type characterized by unilateral facial underdevelopment without

microphthalmos or ocular dermoids. Patient may or may not possess vertebral, cardiac, or renal anomalies.

- Type I (B). Similar to Type I (A), except for the presence of microphthalmos.
- Type I (C). Bilateral asymmetric type; one side is involved more severely.
- Type I (D). Complex type that does not fit Types I (A-C). These patients do not display limb deficiencies, frontonasal phenotype, or ocular dermoids.
- Type II. Limb deficiency type. This may be unilateral or bilateral and with or without ocular abnormalities.
- Type III. Frontonasal phenotype. Relative unilateral underdevelopment of the face in the presence of hypertelorism. Patients may have ocular dermoids and/or vertebral, cardiac, or renal abnormalities.
- Type IV (A = unilateral or B = bilateral). Goldenhar type with facial underdevelopment in association with ocular dermoids, with or without coloboma.

2. Mulliken and Padwa proposed the OMENS phenotypic classification:
   - *O*rbital distortion
   - *M*andibular hypoplasia
   - *E*ar anomaly
   - *N*erve involvement
   - *S*oft tissue deficiency
3. "Formes frustes" or microforms are more frequent than generally acknowledged. These are usually subtle cases of deficient soft tissue or small degrees of macrostomia.

III. TREATMENT

A. Goals

1. Optimize occlusion
2. Improve craniofacial appearance:
   - Reconstruction of the craniofacial skeleton
   - Augmentation of soft tissues
3. Treatment of associated conditions such as auricular malformations and facial paralysis

B. Preoperative Evaluation

1. Airway evaluation (may need sleep study)
2. Baseline photography
3. Head CT
4. Hearing evaluation
5. Orthodontic evaluation

C. Surgical Treatment of Skeletal Deficiencies

1. Mandible

   In the past, the surgical treatment of craniofacial microsomia required multiple, invasive operations, often requiring bone grafts. Distraction osteogenesis has revolutionized the treatment of the mandible in craniofacial microsomia and has made surgical correction less invasive with reduced morbidity and more predictable results.

   - Most forms of craniofacial microsomia can be successfully treated with distraction osteogenesis.
   - Ancillary or subsequent orthodontic therapy may be needed to restore the occlusion.
   - More severe cases (Pruzansky III) may need to be treated with costochondral and/or iliac bone grafts with or without subsequent distraction osteogenesis.
2. Maxilla:
   - Often corrects with mandibular distraction in the younger patient. The older child may require postdistraction orthodontic therapy.
   - Surgical correction (Le Fort I osteotomy) should be undertaken when:

     The maxillary teeth have erupted

     Craniofacial growth is completed
   - Conditions that may require such correction include:

     Anterior open bite after mandibular distraction

     Vertical maxillary "excess" on the less affected side requiring impaction

     Narrow maxilla requiring widening
3. Nose:
   - Usually deviates to the side of involvement

- Should be corrected only after the maxilla is in adequate position
- Usually requires nasoseptal reconstruction

4. Chin:
   - Deformity usually prohibits correction with a chin implant
   - Treatment usually consists of an asymmetric, jumping (three-dimensional) genioplasty
   - Usually completed at the same time as a rhinoplasty

D. Typical Treatment Plan and Timing

1. Unilateral or bilateral mandibular distraction (usually done as early as 2 years of age; occasionally earlier for severe sleep apnea).
2. Cranial vault remodeling if necessary (usually done after the patient is 6 months old).
3. Mandibular distraction may need to be repeated (depending on growth).
4. Le Fort I osteotomy (occasionally done between ages 16 and 18 years); concomitant maxillary-mandibular distraction can also be considered.
5. Jumping or sliding genioplasty (usually done between ages 15 and 17 years).
6. Nasoseptal reconstruction (usually done between ages 15 and 17 years).
7. Microvascular free flap (typically parascapular donor site) to correct soft tissue deficiencies in the cheek area (usually done after 7 years of age).
8. Microtia repair (usually commenced after 8 years of age).

49

Distraction Osteogenesis

J. Timothy Katzen, M.D.
Santa Monica, California, U.S.A.

Joseph G. McCarthy, M.D.
New York University School of Medicine, New York, New York, U.S.A.

I. BASIC CONCEPTS

A. Distraction osteogenesis is defined as a surgical technique for reconstruction of skeletal deformities. It involves the gradual and controlled displacement of surgically created osteotomies. After creating an osteotomy, an external force is applied to the edges of the separated bony segments by a distraction device The device gradually separates the bone and associated soft tissue. Distraction stimulates bone generation and causes soft tissue elongation and hypertrophy. The process continues as long as the tissues are distracted or stretched. After the desired result is achieved, distraction is stopped and the callus is allowed to consolidate into bone.

B. The ability to reconstruct combined deficiencies in bone and soft tissue makes distraction osteogenesis a unique and invaluable technique.

C. There are six basic steps of distraction osteogenesis

- Osteotomy or corticotomy
- Application of a fixation/distraction device
- Latency period: time from surgery to activation of distraction force
- Activation of distraction force
- Consolidation period: time from cessation of activation to evidence of mineralization within the bone regenerate
- Removal of the distraction device

II. HISTORY

A. Codivilla (1905) was the first to describe the concept of bone lengthening in a human femur.

B. Abbott (1927) lengthened the tibia via a compressed spring.

C. Ilizarov (1951) is credited with describing the biologic basis and popularizing the clinical feasibility of distraction osteogenesis:

- He focused on the management of limb (long bone) deformities, especially difficult traumatic and developmental limb deformities often complicated by nonunions, malunions, and nonhealing wounds.
- He found that new bone and soft tissue could be formed by:

  Minimal soft tissue dissection with corticotomy
  Slow transport of skeletal fragments
  Rigid fixation
  Maintenance of skeletal loading

- He popularized the use of:

  Percutaneous wires to manipulate bone fragments

  Ring external fixators to stabilize the wires

  Threaded rods and hinges to stabilize the ring external fixators; these were adjustable and provided rigid fixation to healing bone fragments

D. Snyder (1973) reported on canine mandibular distraction.

E. McCarthy and colleagues at New York University reported on canine distraction of the mandible (1990), midface (1995), and zygoma (1994). They also performed the first craniofacial distractions (1989).

III. BIOLOGY

A. The distraction gap is divided into four zones:

- Fibrous central zone with collagen fibers arranged parallel to the axis of distraction
- Transition zone of early bone formation
- Bone remodeling zone with bone spicules
- Mature bone zone

B. Callotasis is the gradual stretching of the reparative callus that forms around bone segments interrupted by osteotomy or fracture. Callotasis consists of three sequential clinical periods:

- Latency: the period from bone division to the onset of distraction; this is the time required for adequate callus formation
- Distraction: the period when gradual traction is applied and new bone (the regenerate) is formed.
- Consolidation: the period of rigid fixation that allows maturation and corticalization of the regenerate after distraction forces are discontinued

C. Bone generated by distraction osteogenesis is indistinguishable from mature natural bone.

D. Associated soft tissue changes:

- Force of distraction:

  Is transmitted directly to overlying muscles

  Stimulates muscles to elongate and multiply (distraction histogenesis)

- Tissues that have been shown to undergo histogenesis include gingiva, skin, fascia, muscle, cartilage, blood vessels, and peripheral nerves.
- Traditional orthognathic surgical manipulation of the craniofacial skeleton has been associated with a high incidence of relapse, presumably from soft tissue memory causing muscle to pull bone fragments back to their original location. Muscle synthesis and the slow adaptive changes associated with distraction osteogenesis have allowed for larger skeletal movements. In addition, the manipulations have less potential for relapse.

IV. MANDIBULAR DISTRACTION

A. Objectives

1. Lengthen the ramus and/or body (unifocal distraction).
2. Reconstruct a mandibular defect (bifocal or transport distraction).
3. Reconstruct the temporodandibular joint (transport distraction after gap arthroplasty).
4. Achieve satisfactory occlusion.

B. Surgical Technique

1. Obtain preoperative clinical and dental examinations, cephalograms, and 3D CT scans to:
   - Evaluate tooth buds and bone morphology and density
   - Plan positioning of the osteotomy and vector of distraction
2. Expose the mandible via an intraoral incision.
3. Isolate the proposed osteotomy site.
4. Place the distraction pins and device.
5. Complete the osteotomy.
6. Close the soft tissue.

C. Types of Devices

1. External or extraoral: allows precise (multiplanar) postoperative manipulation of distraction vector.

2. Intraoral: avoids facial scarring, but is not applicable in the severely hypoplastic mandible.

D. Clinical Applications (Any Condition with a Mandibular Deficiency)

1. Congenital conditions and syndromes:
   - Craniofacial microsomia
   - Developmental micrognathias
   - Treacher Collins and Nager syndromes
   - Pierre Robin sequence
2. Posttraumatic deformities including temporomandibular joint (TMJ) ankylosis.
3. Postsurgical tumor resection with and without radiation history.
4. Patients who are tracheostomy dependent; distraction may eliminate soft tissue airway obstruction.

V. MAXILLARY OR MIDFACE DISTRACTION

A. Objectives

To correct midface deficiencies and associated malocclusions and to improve appearance.

B. Surgical Technique

1. Obtain preoperative clinical and dental examinations, cephalograms, and 3D CT scans to:
   - Evaluate tooth buds and bone morphology and density
   - Plan positioning of the osteotomy and vector of distraction
2. Expose the midface through an intraoral labiobuccal or coronal incision.
3. Complete the osteotomy; this may be a Le Fort I, II, or III (Le Fort I osteotomies must be placed cephalad in the growing child to avoid the tooth buds).
4. Mobilize the soft tissue.
5. Place the pins and distraction device.
6. Close the soft tissue.

C. Types of Devices

1. External: the "rigid external device"—stability relies on a neurosurgical halo, which is attached to the cranium and forces the maxilla to be distracted.
2. Internal: intraoral and extraoral.

D. Clinical Applications (Any Condition with a Maxillary or Midface Skeletal Deficiency)

1. Congenital:
   - Maxillary hypoplasia associated with cleft palate repair
   - Apert/Crouzon/Pfeiffer/craniosynostosis syndromes
2. Posttraumatic deformities.
3. Postsurgical tumor resection.
4. Obstructive airway disease (sleep apnea) associated with maxillary hypoplasia.

VI. ALVEOLAR RIDGE DISTRACTION

A. Objectives

To replace alveolar deficiencies in the mandible and maxilla:

1. Improve ridge aesthetics.
2. Create an alveolar ridge of sufficient volume for tooth implants.
3. Improve periodontal environment and adjacent teeth.
4. Expand alveolus for orthodontic tooth movement.

B. Surgical Technique

1. Obtain preoperative cephalograms and 3D CT dentascans to:
   - Evaluate tooth buds and bone topography/density
   - Plan positioning of the osteotomy and vector of distraction
2. Expose the defect through an intraoral buccal incision.
3. Complete the U-shaped osteotomy around the defect.
4. Place the pins and distraction device.
5. Close the soft tissue.

6. After the distraction phase, the lead screw is left in place until bone healing occurs.
7. The reconstructed site is suitable for osteointegrated implants or movement of a tooth with orthodontic therapy.

C. Types of Devices

Intraoral.

D. Clinical Application

1. Edentulous jaws.
2. Postsurgical resection.
3. Posttraumatic deformities.
4. Postreconstruction.
5. Congenital deficiencies.

VII. TEMPOROMANDIBULAR JOINT (TMJ) DISTRACTION

A. Objectives

To replace a deficient or nonfunctioning TMJ.

B. Surgical Technique

1. Obtain preoperative cephalograms and 3D CT scans to:
   - Evaluate tooth buds, bone topography and density, and extent of ankylosis
   - Plan positioning of the osteotomy and vector of distraction
2. Expose the TMJ through a preauricular incision.
3. Expose the mandible through an intraoral incision.
4. Perform a gap arthroplasty, if indicated.
5. Place pins and distraction device.
6. Cut a "reverse L" osteotomy: from the sigmoid notch, posterior to the path of the inferior alveolar nerve, to a position 1.5 cm above the gonial angle.
7. Contour a pseudo-glenoid fossa.
8. Close the soft tissue.
9. The distracted bone creates a new TMJ: constant movement, coupled with physical therapy, does not allow conversion of the regenerate into bone; rather, a fibrocartilaginous cap is created over the head of the pseudocondyle.

C. Types of Devices

External.

D. Clinical Application

Ankylosis due to:

1. Congenital defects.
   - Craniofacial microsomia
   - Degenerative joint disease
2. Traumatic defects.
3. Surgical resections.
4. Failed TMJ implants.

VIII. CRANIAL VAULT DISTRACTION (BASED ON LABORATORY STUDIES, NOT CLINICAL SERIES)

A. Objectives

To expand intracranial volume and improve morphology:

1. Separation of cranial bones following linear craniectomy.
2. Allows for normal growth of the brain.

B. Surgical Technique

1. Obtain preoperative clinical examinations, 3D CT scans, airway examination, and ocular examination.
2. Expose the cranial suture involved.
3. Resect the prematurely fused suture.
4. Place a spring-loaded device across the released suture.
5. Close the soft tissue.

C. Types of Devices

1. Internal springs.
2. Internal devices with transcutaneous distraction activation ports.

D. Clinical Applications

A. Congenital conditions and syndromes:
   - Isolated craniosynostosis
   - Apert/Crouzon/Pfeiffer/craniosynostosis syndromes

IX. SUCCESSFUL DISTRACTION OSTEOGENESIS

A. Surgical Technique

1. Preservation of osteogenic tissues and blood supply during osteotomy; minimize dissection of periosteum, nutrient artery, and bone marrow, as all are important in new bone formation.
2. Correct osteotomy placement.
3. Correct calculation of distraction vector. Distraction generates tension that stimulates new bone formation parallel to the vector of distraction. Osteotomy and vector projection must, therefore, be carefully planned.

B. Postoperative Course

1. Latency period:
   - Time from surgery to activation of distraction force
   - Allows for formation of fibro-vascular bridge
   - Usually 5–7 days (shorter in infants)
2. Rate of distraction:
   - Less than 0.5 mm per day can:

     Intensify the biosynthetic activity of cartilage cells

     Result in accelerated osteogenesis

     Lead to premature ossification
   - Greater than 1.5 mm per day can lead to:

     Local ischemia in the regenerative zone

     Delayed ossification

     Pseudoarthrosis/fibrous union
   - 1 mm per day recommended
3. Rhythm of distraction:
   - Is defined as the number of distraction events per day
   - 0.25 mm four times per day or 0.5 mm twice per day recommended
4. Stability of fixator
   - The distraction device must be stable enough to support the newly formed microcolumns of bone.
   - The bending or shearing of microcolumns results in fracture with local hemorrhage and the production of fibrocartilage. This leads to unsatisfactory distraction results (i.e., fibrous non-union).
5. Consolidation period:
   - The distraction device is left in place for maturation and remodeling of the new bone.
   - This period lasts approximately 8 weeks.
   - Radiographs are taken during the later part of this period to examine the quality of the regenerated bone; radiographic cortical outline is the best indicator as to when to remove the distraction device.

X. ADVANTAGES OF DISTRACTION OSTEOGENESIS

A. Utilizes natural healing process of bone.

B. Recreates native bone properties.

C. Lengthens associated soft tissue.

D. Decreases surgical trauma and is less invasive.

E. Avoids bone grafts and donor site pain and scarring.

F. Decreases blood loss and need for blood transfusions.

G. Decreases swelling.

H. Decreases operating time and hospital stay.

I. Intermaxillary fixation not usually necessary and patients can maintain an active lifestyle.

J. Decreases risk of infection.

K. Decreases morbidity.

L. Predictable surgical results.

M. Achieves corrections in three planes of space.

N. Decreases potential for relapse.

O. Can treat children at an early age, which leads to:
   - Improvement of neuromuscular function
   - Potential for subsequent growth of affected skeletal parts
   - Possible avoidance of secondary deformities
   - Decreased psychological impairment

P. Decreases costs.

XI. COMPLICATIONS OF DISTRACTION

A. External facial scar due to pin tract scar with the external device.

B. Pin tract infection:
   - Usually can be easily managed with local wound care alone
   - May need oral antibiotics if severe

C. Device pins may be placed accidentally in a tooth bud:
   - Typically occurs in young patients with tooth buds close to the mandibular border.
   - May lead to the loss of that tooth and the development of a dentigerous cyst during distraction phase.

D. Fracture of the bone.

E. Premature consolidation.

F. Undesirable transport vector.

G. Ankylosis.

H. Parotid fistula with mandibular distraction.

XII. DISTRACTION FAILURE

A. Failure due to:
   - Quality and volume of the host bone
   - Surgical technique
   - Lack of stabilization
   - Patient compliance

B. Treatment options depend on cause, but can include:
   - Repeat distraction
   - Costal or iliac bone graft, with or without subsequent distraction
   - Minor occlusal discrepancies after mandibular distraction, corrected with interdental elastic therapy

XIII. THE FUTURE

A. Ideal Distraction Device Characteristics

1. Miniaturized.
2. Internal to avoid cutaneous scarring.
3. Provide constant and equal distraction throughout the day since maximal osteogenesis is achieved with continuous distraction.
4. Allow for easy and multidimensional manipulation during activation phase.
5. Allow for easy removal or be biodegradable.

B. Applications

1. Orbital transport distraction to correct for hypertelorism/hypotelorism.
2. Cranial distraction to correct cranial vault abnormalities.

C. Biomolecular Manipulation

1. Addition of growth factors to distraction site to accelerate or shorten the consolidation phase.
2. Gene manipulation.

50

Presurgical Orthodontics and Orthopedics

Clarice Law, D.M.D., M.S., and Kang Ting, D.M.D., D.Med.Sc.
UCLA School of Dentistry, Los Angeles, California, U.S.A.

There are numerous approaches to the treatment of the cleft lip and palate patient. Orthodontic treatment protocols therefore vary with different teams. In general, presurgical orthodontics may take place at four different time periods—infancy, primary dentition, mixed dentition, and permanent dentition. Each of these periods of treatment serve to facilitate the three major surgical interventions common to the treatment of patients with cleft lip and palate, which include primary lip and palate closure, alveolar bone grafting to the cleft site, and orthognathic surgery.

In addition to skeletal and soft tissue defects, cleft lip and palate patients also commonly exhibit various dental anomalies, particularly in the cleft area. Patients may have hypodontia, microdontia, supernumerary teeth, or ectopic eruption. The lateral incisors and canines, being adjacent to the cleft site, are most often affected. Orthodontic treatment is part of the multidisciplinary dental care that can address these dental anomalies by properly positioning the teeth in the alveolus for dental restoration.

I. INFANCY

A. Rationale for Intervention

1. Pre-surgical orthopedic intervention within the first few weeks is a controversial subject since it is generally agreed that presurgical orthopedics at this stage will not improve the dental/orthodontic alignment. Its benefit on maxillary growth is also questionable.
2. On the other hand, many surgeons prefer to have displaced tissue repositioned with presurgical orthopedics prior to surgery in order to minimize the amount of repositioning necessary during the surgical procedure itself. Repositioning the cleft segments through presurgical orthopedics can reduce the need for lip adhesion and the size of the cleft palate and hence reduce the extent of scarring and tension from scarring that may inhibit normal maxillary growth and development (Fig. 1).

B. Goals of Intervention

1. To orthopedically correct or minimize the displacement of the alveolar segments.
2. To align the cleft segments to facilitate dental arch development.
3. To facilitate primary lip closure by reducing lip tension over the maxillary segments.
4. To reposition the palatal shelves and reduce the cleft size to facilitate palate repair.

C. Timing of Intervention

1. Referral should be made within the first few days following birth.
2. Treatment should be performed within the first 4 weeks.

D. Types of Intervention

1. Active appliances:
   - Acrylic appliances with internal springs and screws to manipulate the cleft segments
   - Often retained with pins driven into the alveolus
   - Rationale:

     Unilateral cleft—to advance and expand the minor segment while retracting and rotating the major segment

     Bilateral cleft—to expand the lateral segments, allowing for retraction of the premaxillary segment

     Controversial due to the potential damage to developing tooth buds
2. Passive appliances:
   - Acrylic appliances fitting loosely over the segments
   - Retained with the action of the tongue
   - Used in conjunction with extraoral straps
   - Rationale:

     Serve to keep the tongue out of the cleft

     Maintain transverse width while extraoral straps retract the premaxillary segment
   - Treatment often extends into the primary dentition phase
3. Growth guidance appliances:
   - Acrylic appliances that are relieved internally to promote growth guidance
   - No extraoral traction
   - No active expansion of the minor segment in order to allow natural growth to occur and to delay surgery
4. Combination protocol:
   - Loose-fitting passive appliance used in conjunction with extraoral strapping to align major segment

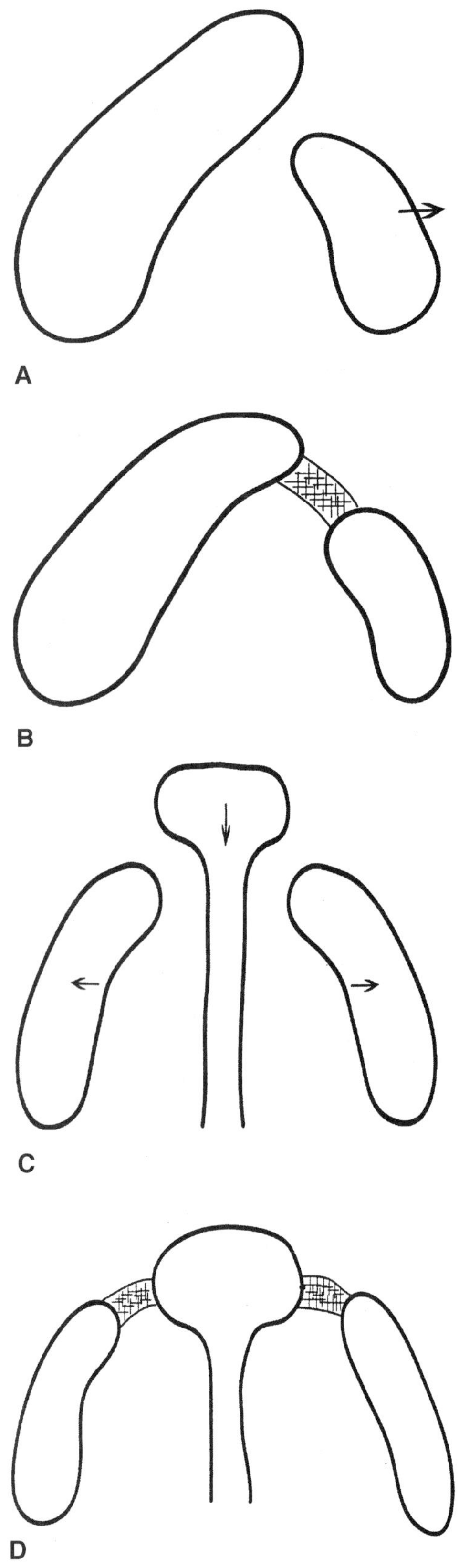

Figure 1 The goal of presurgical orthodontic treatment is to expand the collapsed arch into normal symmetrical arch form. Alveolar bone graft will be followed before the canine eruption. (A) Unilateral cleft with constricted arch. (B) Expanded arch with bone graft (cross-hatched area). (C) Bilateral cleft with constricted arch. (D) Expanded arch with bone graft (cross hatched areas).

- Discontinuance of extraoral strapping when segments are aligned
- A second passive acrylic appliance is used for growth guidance until the time of primary lip closure
- Appliance is maintained as a retainer until the palate is repaired

II. PRIMARY DENTITION

A. Rationale for Treatment

1. Treatment at the time of primary dentition is generally not associated with any major surgical interventions.
2. Orthodontic treatment in the primary dentition has very little effect on the developing permanent dentition. However, correction of posterior or anterior crossbites is important at this time for orthopedic purposes. Many patients with crossbites have associated functional shifts due to the interference of improperly positioned teeth and jaws. These functional shifts in occlusion may eventually result in pathological compensatory growth in the condyles to accommodate the occlusal interferences. Anterior crossbites may result in the inhibition of antero-posterior growth of the maxilla as the mandibular incisors "trap" the maxillary incisors. Treatment therefore focuses on the elimination of both types of occlusal interferences through crossbite correction.

B. Goals of Treatment

1. To correct anterior or posterior crossbites and prevent further collapse of the maxilla.
2. To facilitate maxillary growth.

C. Timing of Treatment

1. When patient is able to cooperate with orthodontic intervention.

D. Types of Treatment

1. For posterior crossbite:
    - Orthodontic expansion appliance (Hyrax-type expansion screw or Quad Helix)
    - Relapse rate is high prior to bone grafting of the cleft
    - Requires long-term retention
2. For anterior crossbite:
    - Minor dental crossbite—active retainer with springs to correct the teeth in crossbite
    - Minor maxillary retrusion—orthopedic face mask with traction applied to the maxillary dentition from an appliance resting for anchorage on the forehead and chin

III. MIXED DENTITION

A. Goals of Treatment

1. To prepare the cleft site for secondary alveolar bone graft surgery.
2. To address collapse of the maxillary arch and posterior crossbite.
3. To address dental malpositions, especially adjacent to the cleft.
4. To regain space for the eruption of remaining permanent teeth or for the restoration of missing permanent teeth.
5. To provide suitable bone for the eruption of the permanent canine teeth.
6. To match maxillary arch form to mandibular arch form.

B. Timing of Treatment

1. Based on dental development rather than chronological age.
2. When the maxillary incisors have nearly completed root development to prevent disruption of the natural development of the root apex.
3. Prior to the eruption of the maxillary canines.

C. Types of Treatment

1. For collapse of the maxillary arch and posterior crossbite:
    - Orthodontic expansion appliance (Hyrax-type expansion screw or Quad Helix)
2. For dental malposition and space regaining.
    - Fixed orthodontic appliances (braces)

        Bands on molars

        Brackets bonded to erupted maxillary incisors, primary canines, and sometimes primary first molars

- Orthodontic treatment should progress through a standard wire sequence, beginning with flexible wires and ending with stiff, larger diameter wires.
- Orthodontic appliances will remain in place for surgery to allow for post-operative stabilization.
- Orthodontic treatment may be continued 8–12 weeks post-operatively.

IV. PERMANENT DENTITION

A. Goals of Treatment

1. To provide functional occlusal relationships.
2. To properly align dentition for aesthetic improvement.
3. To address any remaining skeletal discrepancies.
4. To prepare for orthognathic surgery or soft tissue revisions, if necessary.

B. Timing of Treatment

1. When the full permanent dentition has erupted or is nearly complete in its eruption.

C. Types of Treatment

1. Placement of fixed orthodontic appliances on teeth.
   - To align teeth within the supporting alveolar complex.
   - To coordinate maxillary and mandibular arch form for ideal or functional occlusion.
   - To prepare space if necessary for osteotomies in the event of segmental orthognathic surgery.
   - To provide anchors for intermaxillary fixation following orthognathic surgery.

51

Unilateral Cleft Lip

Steve Lee, M.D., and Court B. Cutting, M.D.
New York University School of Medicine, New York, New York, U.S.A.

I. BACKGROUND

A. Cleft lip is the second most common developmental defect.

B. This defect is characterized by a partition of the upper lip, which may or may not be associated with clefting of the palate and may be either unilateral or bilateral. Significant nasal deformity is usually involved.

C. The incidence of cleft lip varies with ethnicity; it is highest among Asians with approximately 1 in 500 births and lowest in blacks (1 in 2000), with Caucasians in between (1 in 1000).

D. Causes of cleft lip are believed to be multifactorial. Factors that have been linked to cleft lip include genetics, infection, vitamin deficiency, teratogens, and other factors affecting the first trimester of pregnancy.

E. The pathogenesis of cleft lip has generally been thought to result from a failure of fusion of any of the five facial elements—frontonasal process, two lateral maxillary processes, or two mandibular processes of the embryo. More recent evidence, however, has pointed toward the mesodermal penetration theory as the most probable for cleft lip formation. In this theory, the embryonic facial processes are formed by the migration and penetration of the mesoderm into the embryonic epithelial bilayer of the face. If this mesodermal migration fails or is inhibited, clefting results.

F. The primary palate includes the lip, the alveolus, and the hard palate anterior to the incisive foramen. The secondary palate includes the hard palate posterior to the incisive foramen and the soft palate.

II. ANATOMICAL LANDMARKS

Surface anatomy (Fig. 1).

Arteries and musculature (Fig. 2).

III. UNILATERAL CLEFT LIP CLASSIFICATION

For purposes of treatment planning, unilateral cleft lips are classified into one of three groups: microform, incomplete, and complete cleft lip. Cleft lips are considered complete if the defect extends into the nostril floor and incomplete if a bridge of tissue connects the central and lateral lip. This tissue bridge is commonly referred to as a Simonart's band.

A. Microform Clefts

The microform (or forme fruste) cleft lip is the mildest expression of a cleft lip.

1. It is characterized by a groove or crease invading the entire vertical length of the lip.

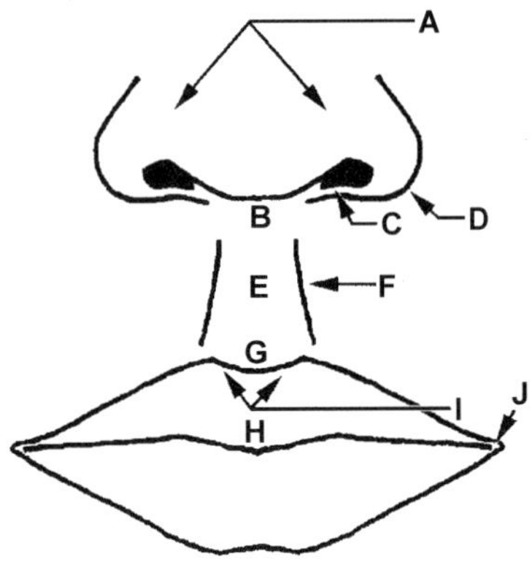

Figure 1 Surface landmarks: (A) alar cartilage prominences; (B) nasal columella; (C) nasal sill; (D) alar base; (E) philtral dimple; (F) philtral column; (G) white roll; (H) philtral tubercle; (I) Cupid's bow; (J) commissure.

2. A vermilion notch, white roll deformity, and vertical lip shortening are also present.
3. Associated nasal deformity may be present and can be more severe than the lip defect.
4. This type of cleft comprises up to 10% of unilateral cleft lip cases.
5. Techniques of repair include straight-line repairs such as the Rose-Thompson method, although others have advocated Millard's rotation-advancement method for better symmetry (Fig. 3).

B. Unilateral Incomplete Clefts

1. Exhibit varying degrees of vertical partition of the lip and alveolus and an intact nasal sill or Simonart's band.
2. The associated nasal deformity should be corrected at the time of lip repair, although the degree of alar mobilization and repositioning varies according to the magnitude of the deformity.
3. Account for 30% of all unilateral cleft lip cases.
4. The technique of choice for this type of defect is Millard's rotation-advancement technique (Fig. 3).

C. Unilateral Complete Clefts

1. Characterized by a division through the lip, alveolus, and nasal sill.
2. Frequently involves the entire palate.

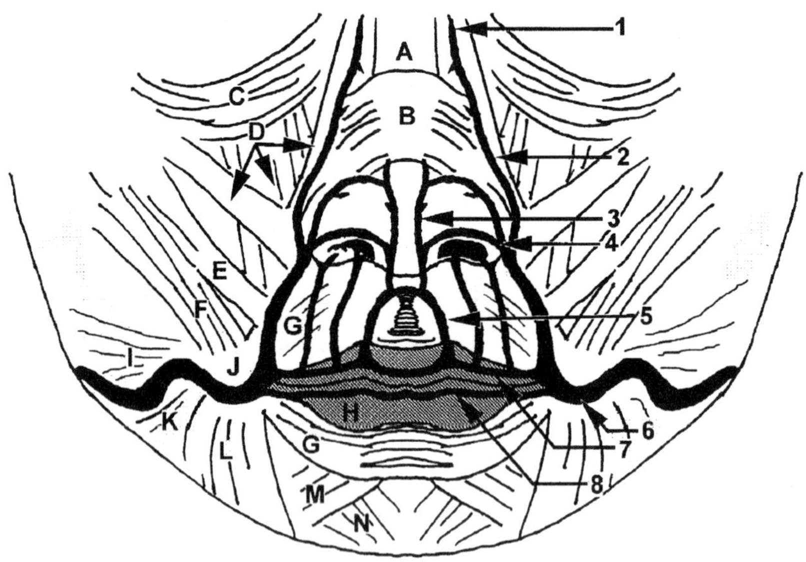

Figure 2 Important arterial supply and musculature of the face. Arteries: (1) Dorsal nasal a.; (2) angular a.; (3) terminal branch of anterior ethmoidal a.; (4) lateral nasal a.; (5) ascending septal branch of superior labial a.; (6) facial a.; (7) superior labial a.; (8) inferior labial a. Muscles: (A) Procerus m.; (B) nasalis m.; (C) orbicularis oculi m.; (D) quadratus labii superiorus m. (angular head, infraorbital head, and zygomatic head); (E) zygomaticus minor m; (F) zygomaticus major m.; (G) orbicularis oris peripheralis m.; (H) orbicularis oris marginalis m.; (I) risorius; (J) modiolus; (K) platysma; (L) depressor anguli oris m.; (M) depressor labii inferiorus m.; (N) mentalis.

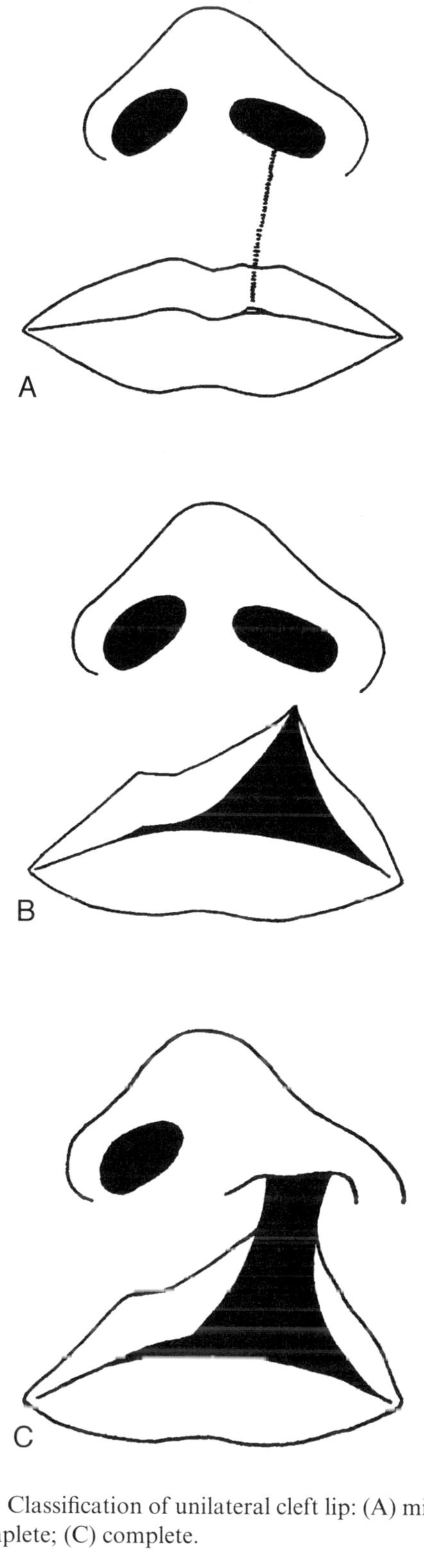

Figure 3 Classification of unilateral cleft lip: (A) microform; (B) incomplete; (C) complete.

3. This type of cleft is the most common, comprising up to 60% of all unilateral clefts.
4. The technique of choice for this type of defect is the rotation-advancement technique (Fig. 3).

IV. PRESURGICAL ORTHODONTIC TREATMENT

A. Presurgical orthodontics (PO) is used to align the maxillary segments and the alveolar arch into a normal position prior to repair. It provides balance and symmetry to the skeletal base, facilitating repair and aiding in feeding.

- Candidates for PO are only those patients with either (1) complete unilateral cleft lip, alveolus, and palate, or (2) cleft lip and alveolus.
- Initiation of PO is usually done during the first or second week following birth, with a maximal response during the first 6 weeks.

B. Three types of PO are currently in use: pin retained (active), molding plate (passive), and nasoalveolar molding (NAM).

- Pin retained:

  Also known as the Latham split appliance, it is a custom-made acrylic-stainless steel appliance that is pinned to the palatal segments in the horizontal processes of the maxilla.

  A transverse stainless steel bar placed just anterior to the prevomerine suture supports mobile arms that lie along both alveolar ridges.

  The posterior end of an activation screw is secured to the appliance, which, in turn, is fastened to the noncleft segment. A nut is threaded to the midpoint of the screw and a wire is looped around the front of the nut and attached to the appliance at the cleft segment. Turning the screw will move the nut forward, pulling the cleft maxillary segment forward and pushing backward the premaxillary area of the alveolar ridge on the noncleft side. Parents are taught to turn the screw (daily) to expand maxillary segments and improve the maxillary alignment.

  Duration of therapy is about 1.5–2 months.

  The results are highly consistent.

- Molding plate:

  A simple custom-made acrylic device similar to a denture without teeth that is retained by undercuts.

  It is designed to maintain posterior transverse dimensions, and it depends on compression to mold the premaxilla.

  Although fairly inexpensive and less invasive, it is also less effective than the pin retained or the nasoalveolar molding methods.

- Nasoalveolar molding:

  A custom-made molding plate with nasal extension.

  It uses acrylic nasal stents attached to the vestibular shield of an oral molding plate to mold the nasal alar cartilages into normal form and position during the neonatal period.

  This method utilizes the malleability of immature cartilage and its ability to maintain a permanent correction of its form.

  The construction is performed by gradual elongation of the nasal stents and the application of tissue-expanding elastic forces that are applied to the prolabium.

  Use of this technique has eliminated surgical columella reconstruction and the resultant scar tissue from the standard of care in the authors' cleft palate center.

V. TIMING OF REPAIR

In general, surgical repair can be carried out at anytime after birth, but most surgeons adhere to the "rule of tens" dictum: is at least 10 weeks old, weighs at least 10 pounds, and has a hemoglobin level of at least 10 g.

VI. OPERATIVE TECHNIQUES

A. Techniques of Choice

1. Many techniques have been devised over the years for the repair of the unilateral cleft lip deformity. Most have fallen out of favor with the exception of the following three techniques that are still in use. They can be divided into two groups: (1) straight-line repairs and (2) Z-plasty repairs.
2. Early simple methods such as the Rose-Thompson straight-line repair are used for mild cases of clefts such as the microform cleft. This repair has the advantage of being easy to master with simple markings and geometry.
3. For more severe cases, however, most surgeons prefer the lower triangular or rotation-advancement methods.

B. Basic Principles

1. Symmetry: regardless of method utilized, the principal goal is to achieve a balanced symmetry of both the repaired and noncleft sides.
2. Primary muscular union: careful dissection of the orbicularis oris bundles from lateral labial elements is required for a tension-free closure. Continuity of the orbicularis is important for soft tissue/skeletal growth and labial movement.

C. Lip Adhesion

1. Lip adhesion, a straight-line muscle approximation, is not a cleft lip repair per se; it is, however, a technique used to enable better alignment of the maxillary arch and alveolar segment.
2. This method effectively closes the nasal sill and upper two-thirds of the lip.
3. It is generally used to transform wide complete clefts into incomplete clefts, which are simpler and easier to correct. In less well-developed regions of the world, this technique is commonly utilized. The authors feel this is an expensive way to provide imprecise presurgical orthopedics (Fig. 4).

D. Straight-Line (Rose-Thompson) Repair

1. This type of repair consists of angled excisions of the cleft edges with primary closure without use of flaps.
2. It is fairly easily mastered. However, its use is currently only acceptable for mild cases of cleft lip.
3. It also has several disadvantages such as a scar contracture, loss of Cupid's bow, asymmetric vermilion tubercle, and no correction of the distorted underlying oral musculature (Fig. 5).

E. Z-Plasty Repairs

For any unilateral cleft lip defect more severe than that of microform clefting, a Z-plasty repair is warranted. The triangular flap (Tennison-Randall) and Millard's rotation-advancement repairs are the two most common repairs today. Whereas the triangular flap repair is

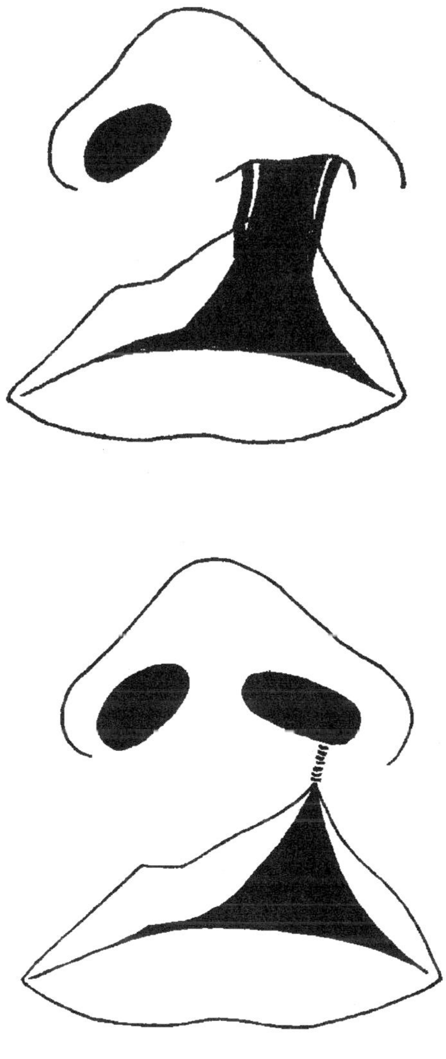

Figure 4 Lip adhesion. Approximation of the pared lips essentially converts a complete cleft into an incomplete cleft lip.

straightforward and relies on precise measurements, the rotation advancement is more technically challenging and requires greater finesse.

1. Anatomical Landmarks

Both the triangular flap and the rotation-advancement repairs share similar anatomical landmarks that are essential for designing the repair (Fig. 6).

A. The peak of Cupid's bow on the noncleft side.

B. The midline; the lowest point of Cupid's bow.

C. The calculated peak of Cupid's bow on the cleft side (distance from A to B).

D. The lateral alar base crease on the noncleft side.

E. The lateral alar base crease on the cleft side.

F. The point on the vermilion border obtained by intersecting a line drawn from E to F, where the distance E–F is equal to D–A.

G. The mid-base of the columella.

H. One should note that in the majority of cases, point B is seldom well defined. In this instance, the total Cupid's bow should be kept narrow; that is, the distance between A and C should be minimized without significant distortion. This is because, postoperatively, the Cupid's bow will be widened somewhat. By keeping Cupid's bow narrow, less vertical discrepancy (G to A minus G to C) will be evident as this will limit the amount of back-cut on any repair.

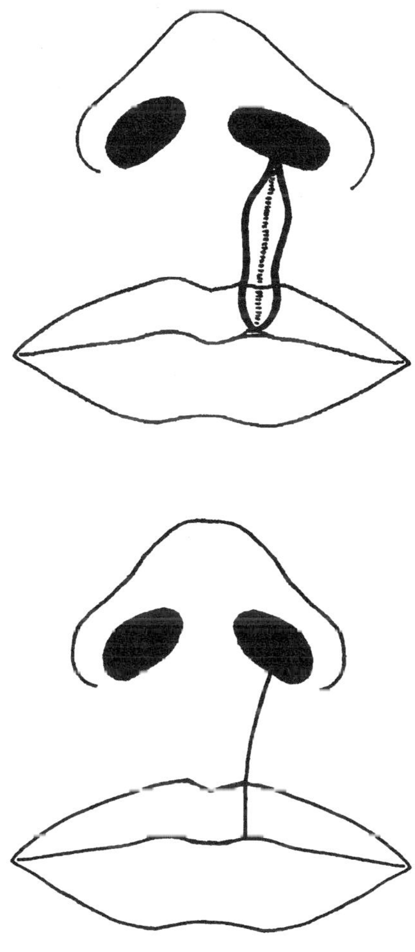

Figure 5 Rose-Thompson straight-line repair. Angled excisions of the cleft edges with primary closure with no use of flaps.

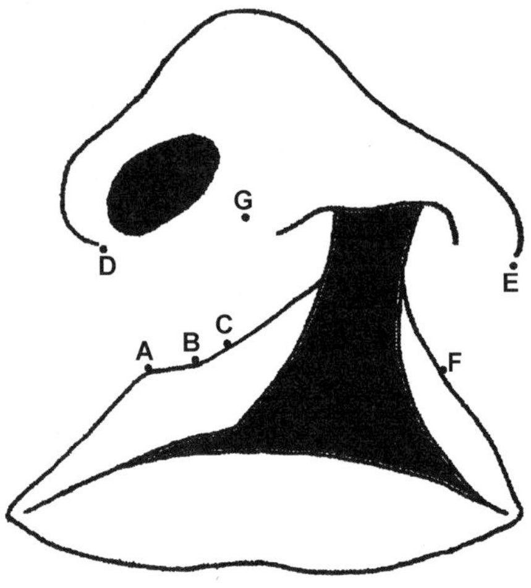

Figure 6 Anatomical landmarks of an unrepaired complete unilateral cleft lip. To find point F, measure distance D to A first, and then measure out the same distance starting from E to the white roll. The point of intersection at the white roll will be point F, making distance D to A = distance E to F.

2. Triangular Flap Technique (Tennison-Randall)

The triangular flap repair, though commonly utilized, is increasingly becoming of historical interest only. The method is a Z-plasty consisting of construction of an equilateral triangular flap on the side of the cleft with its insertion into the constructed gap on the medial element. Precise measurement is essential and straightforward; as such, mastery of this technique is more readily accomplished. It has three main disadvantages: (1) it produces a zigzag scar in the most visible part of the lip; (2) it flattens Cupid's bow; and (3) primary nasal reconstruction is not an integral part of the design (Fig. 7).

3. Rotation-Advancement Technique (Millard)

The classic Millard rotation-advancement method, which has been described as a "cut as you go" technique, is considered to be the gold standard for unilateral cleft lip repair. Its main advantages consists of

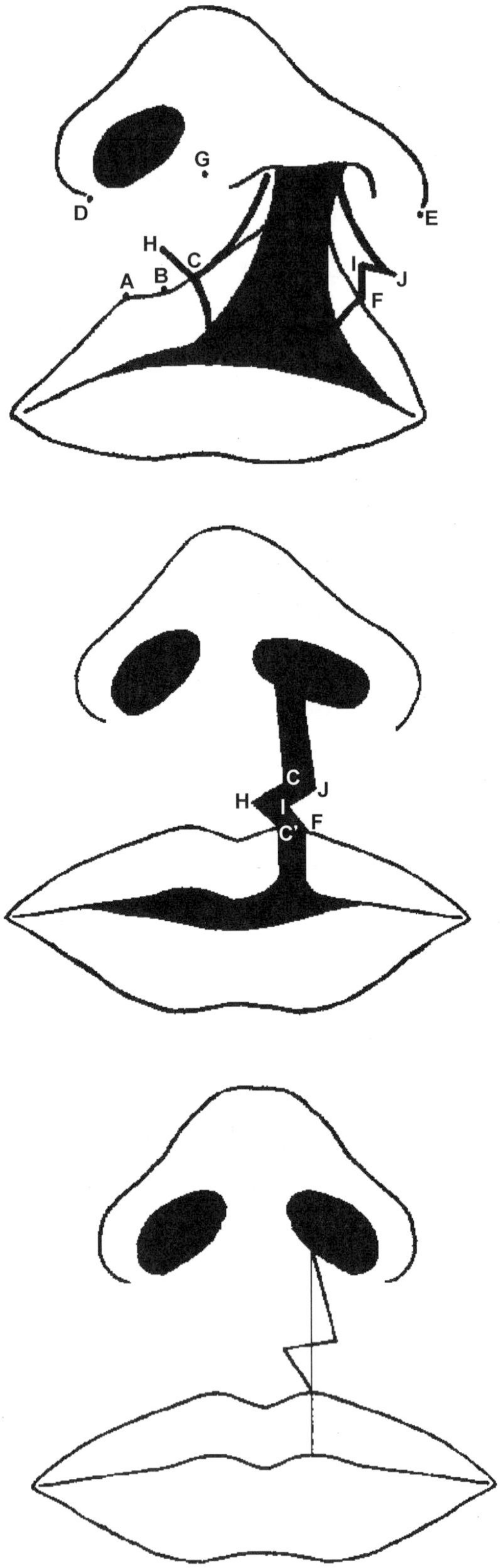

Figure 7 Triangular flap repair. To determine the length of C to H, first find the difference between G to A and G to C (i.e., GA 1−1 GC). The difference is then the length C to H, the back-cut that serves to lengthen the medial lip element. Once CH is obtained, the equilateral triangular flap can then be constructed with FI = IJ = FJ, which are all equal to CH.

placement of tissues in normal positions, creation of a symmetrical Cupid's bow, positioning of scar along the philtral column, preservation of the philtral dimple, and simultaneous primary nasal reconstruction. Its main drawback is its difficulty to master (Fig. 8). The details of the technique are as follows:

A. Construction of the rotation flap—Construction of the rotation flap begins by paring edges of the cleft from point C to the columellar base. This distance is usually shorter by 4–5 mm as compared with the normal (noncleft) side distance of point A to the columellar base. The incision is then further advanced two-thirds of the way along the columellar base and 2–3 mm up on the columella to point W. At this point, the backcut incision, W to X, is carried out medially and parallel to the philtral column on the noncleft side. The rotation flap, now isolated, is then released from the lip. Note that point X may be extended toward point A ("cut as you go") as needed. This maneuver produces a total length required to match to the normal side and situates the Cupid's bow in a symmetrical position.

B. Transposition of the C-flap and insertion of the lateral (advancement) flap—Once the C-flap is obtained, it is measured for transposition into the back-cut so that point Y coincides with point X without tension. This is done by a calculated

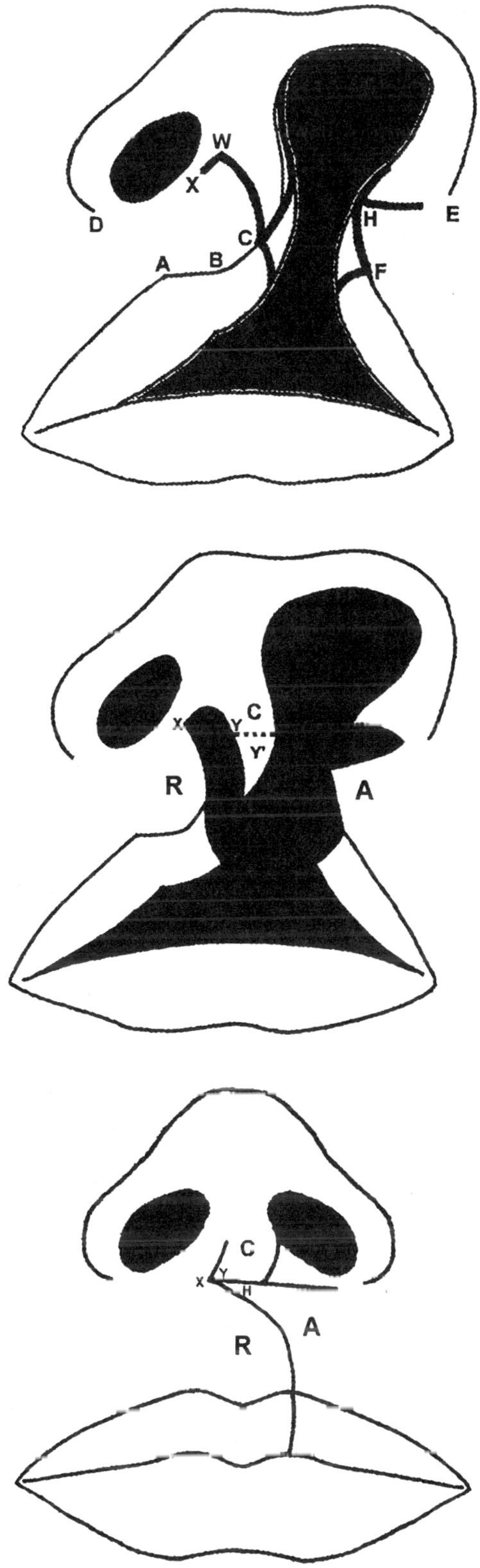

Figure 8 Millard's rotation advancement repair. (Top) Anatomical and incisional landmarks (see also Fig. 6). Point H is the highest point on the lateral lip, where an incision is to be carried out to point E to free the lip from the flared alar base. Point W is 2–3 mm up on the columella and two-thirds the distance across the base of the columella from the cleft side. Point X is where the back-cut is to be extended such that W to A is equal to C to W to X. Also, an important distinction of this technique is that the incision on the upper lateral edge of the medial edge element is extended up to the membranous septum (i.e., from point C up to the septal angle). This maneuver is carried out to aid in reconstruction of the depressed nasal tip. (Middle) The constructed flaps: the rotation flap (R), the lateral advancement flap (A), and the columella flap or C-flap (C). Excision should be made across the measured dotted line on the C-flap so that once the triangular Y-flap is excised, and the resultant C-flap rotated medially, point Y coincides with point X with no tension. (Bottom) The completed repair will reveal a vertical scar along the philtral column crossing the columella base to point X, but should never cross the philtral column on the normal side. Points Y and H are sutured to point X.

transverse excision discarding the Y′ piece. The resultant C-flap is then rotated downward toward X and sutured. A transverse incision freeing the lip from the flared alar base is then carried out to the highest point of the lateral lip, point H. The lateral advancement flap fills in the residual gap with point H coinciding with point X.

C. Oral musculature—Muscles of the lateral lip element must be dissected out completely from the skin and mucosa and transposed down so that, when approximating muscle across the cleft, bulges will not result.

D. Nasal reconstruction—To reconstruct the nasal floor and nasal sill, the incision on the upper lateral edge of the C flap is extended up the nasal membranous septum. From this approach, and from the lateral pyriform aperture, the lower lateral cartilage is dissected away from the overlying nasal tip skin. The cartilage and its nasal mucosal lining is then elevated as a composite flap into normal position and sutured in place with bolsters or absorbable sutures.

VII. POSTOPERATIVE CARE

A. Elbow restraints for 3 weeks.

B. Three weeks of full-strength formula tube feedings via a catheter tip syringe.

C. No nipples for feeding or suckling as they may strain the muscle and skin sutures.

D. Cleansing of wound with half-strength hydrogen peroxide with subsequent application of topical bacitracin ointment.

E. Sutures removed on postop day 7.

52

Primary Repair of Bilateral Cleft Lip and Nasal Deformity

John B. Mulliken, M.D.
Children's Hospital, Boston, Massachusetts, U.S.A.

There are numerous examples in surgical history of how technical advances have allowed complex malformations that once needed multiple procedures to be repaired in a single operation. Primary (often staged) closure of the bilateral cleft lip and secondary correction of the nasal deformity have been largely abandoned. The modern strategy is simultaneous correction of the double labial clefts, alveolar gaps, and nasal deformity, followed by repair of the secondary palate. Evolution to synchronous closure of the primary palate occurred because of: (1) dissatisfaction with results of conventional (multistage) operations, (2) improvements in preoperative maxillary orthopedic manipulation, and (3) recognition that the nasal tip and columella can be constructed by anatomic positioning of the alar cartilages and sculpting the investing skin. Although the principles of single-stage repair of bilateral cleft nasolabial deformity are established, the techniques to achieve this goal continue to evolve.

I. PRINCIPLES

A. *Maintain symmetry*. This is foremost. Even the smallest nasolabial differences on the two sides at the time of closure become more obvious in time.

B. *Secure primary muscular union*. Orbicularis oris bundles are dissected from lateral labial elements to permit tension-free closure. Orbicular continuity is important for soft tissue/skeletal growth and labial movement.

C. *Design philtral flap to be of correct size and shape*. All central labial dimensions are fast growing.

D. *Form the median tubercle and vermilion-cutaneous ridge using lateral labial tissue*. Necessary for normal height/color match and median raphe.

E. *Construct the nasal tip and columella by anatomic placement of alar cartilages*. "The columella is in the nose," hidden because of inferiorly dislocated and splayed alars. There is no need to recruit tissue from the lip and nasal sills.

II. PREOPERATIVE MAXILLARY ORTHOPEDICS

A protrusive, overgrown, labially tilted, and sometimes rotated premaxilla must be positioned to form the platform for simultaneous nasolabial closure.

A. Passive

1. Custom-made semirigid plate retained by undercuts.
2. Designed to maintain posterior transverse dimension.
3. Relies on external elastic compression to mold the premaxilla.
4. Tiny columella can be stretched using a double outrigger and prolabial bar attached to the

molding plate. This is secured to the cheeks with tape.

B. Active

1. Custom-made acrylic–stainless steel appliance (Latham) pinned to maxillary shelves with a staple passed transversely through the premaxilla, just anterior to the prevomerine suture.
2. Elastic chain on each side is connected to the staple, looped around a pulley in the posterior section of the appliance, and attached to a hook on the anterior part of the acrylic plate.
3. Chains are tightened at intervals to retrude the premaxilla.
4. Parents are taught to turn the screw (daily) to expand the maxillary segments.
5. Duration of therapy is about 1.5–2 months.
6. Older removable active appliance for maxillary expansion that relies on passive anterior closure after labial repair.

III. TECHNIQUE

Successful union of bilateral cleft lip and correction of nasal deformity requires an understanding of three-dimensional form and four-dimensional changes that occur during normal growth and that are altered by the malformation. The guiding concept is to construct slow-growing nasal features (protrusion and columellar length) on a slightly large or normal scale and fast-growing labial features and nasal length and width on a small scale. The only exception is the median tubercle, a fast-growing feature made purposively full.

A. Markings (Fig. 1)

1. Nasal: Bilateral rim incisions.
2. Prolabial: Design the philtral flap as a biconcave dart 6–7 mm in length, 3–4 mm in width at peak-to-peak of Cupid's bow, and 2.0 mm at base (columellar-labial junction). Indicate a strip of tissue flanking both sides of the philtral flap. Dimensions are altered slightly for age and familial characteristics.
3. Lateral labial: Peak-points for Cupid's bow are chosen to provide sufficient vermilion height to form the median tubercle and about 3 mm length of white roll on each side. Peak-points are marked at the top of the white roll that become the handle of Cupid's bow. A line is drawn medially from the lateral Cupid's bow peak-point, atop the stripe of white roll, and along the cutaneous vermilion-mucosal junction. Alar base-labial junctions are noted.
4. Tattoo critical anatomic points: base and three distal points of the philtral flap and lateral Cupid's bow peaks and vermilion-mucosal junction line of each lateral labial element.

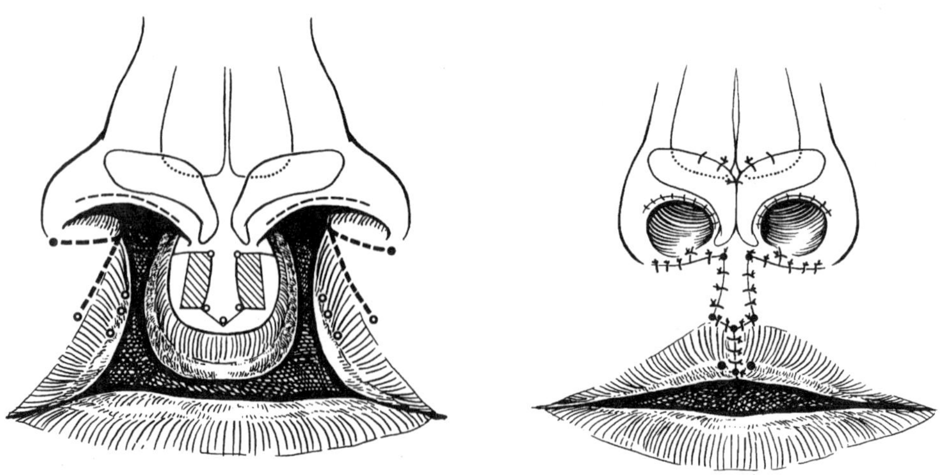

Figure 1 (Left) Markings. (Right) Closure.

B. Dissection

1. Labial: All incisions are initially scored.
2. De-epithelialize tabs alongside the philtral flap and incise/elevate the complex while preserving attachments at the columellar-labial junction.
3. Disjoin each alar base from the lateral labial element and from the piriform aperture.
4. Incise the labial sulci to premolar region and dissect lateral labial elements from the maxilla in the supraperiosteal plane, extending over the malar eminences.
5. Separate white roll–vermilion–mucosal flaps from the cutaneous section.
6. Dissect orbicularis oris muscle layer from the lateral labial elements in both subdermal and submucosal planes.
7. Nasal: Deepen rim incisions and use fine scissors to expose the anterior surface of the dislocated alar domes. Elevate fatty tissue lying between the splayed genua. Vestibular lining is left attached to the underside of the genua and middle crura. Note: "Open rhinoplasty" is an alternative approach to displaced genua. The prolabium and columella are elevated (pedicled on dorsal nasal skin) by dissection either: a) on the anterior surface of the medial/middle crura, or b) through the membranous septum. Former gives better exposure of lower lateral cartilages; both necessitate reconstitution of columellar–labial junctural attachments to the premaxilla.
8. Alveolar clefts: Mucosal flaps are elevated from the lateral and medial sides of the cleft defect to construct nasal floors. Vertically incise opposing gingival margins of the premaxilla and maxillary segments.

C. Closure (Fig. 1)

1. Alveolar Ridge, Muscle, and Median Tubercle

a. Nasal floors are closed first; followed (whenever possible) by gingivoperiosteoplasty.

b. Prolabial vermilion and excess mucosa are trimmed; remaining premaxillary mucosa is sutured to periosteum to form the posterior wall of the gingivolabial sulcus. Close lateral sulci as lateral labial elements are advanced medially.

c. The orbicularis oris muscle is joined, inferiorly to superiorly, with vertical mattress sutures. Uppermost nonabsorbable muscular suture is placed through periosteum of the anterior nasal spine.

d. Lateral white roll–vermilion–mucosal flaps are apposed to construct the superior portion of the median tubercle. Redundant vermilion–mucosal flaps are trimmed bilaterally and joined to form a full median tubercle, align the red-line junction, and construct the anterior wall of the sulcus.

2. Nasal

a. Interdomal mattress suture is placed (untied). This is facilitated by elevating subluxed genua and middle crura with cotton-tipped applicator stick.

b. Genua are suspended to the ipsilateral upper lateral cartilages (near septal junction).

c. Inter-cartilagenous sutures are tied in series.

d. Alae nasi are positioned in both horizontal and vertical axes. Vestibular floors are closed while alar bases are advanced medially. A nonabsorbable horizontal mattress suture is placed from base-to-base to reduce the inter-alar dimension to 23–25 mm.

e. Nostril sills are constructed by trimming flaps at each side of the columellar base and from the tip of each alar flap.

f. Alar bases are secured to underlying orbicularis muscle and premaxillary periosteum to form the normal depression in the lateral nasal sill.

g. Redundant cutaneous crescent is excised from the superior margin of each rim wound (soft triangle) and upper columella. Constructed columella should measure 5–6 mm in length (normal, 3.2 $\pm$ 0.7 mm, age-matched at 0–5 months).

h. The lateral vestibular web is excised (lenticular shape) on the cutaneous side in an axis along the intercartilaginous line. Closing this defect effaces the vestibular web caused by redundant lining and impinging lateral crus.

3. Labial

a. Philtral flap is inset into notch at the top of the constructed median tubercle.

b. Philtral flap is sutured to muscular layer and to simulate the dimple. The ramps on each side of the philtral flap simulate the columns.

c. The superior margins of the lateral labial flaps are trimmed in a cymal (ogee) configuration. This maneuver corrects for tendency to posture alar bases too high and shortens vertically long lateral labial elements. Medial edges of the lateral flaps almost never need adjustment.

d. Labial-sill junction is closed from lateral-to-medial so that the "dog ear" emerges at the philtral column. Note: A 19-gauge polyethylene catheter wrapped in Xeroform® gauze is placed in each nostril. These vented "stents" permit nasal airflow, minimize transnasal swelling, and prevent nasal secretions from macerating the nasolabial wounds.

IV. POSTOPERATIVE CARE

A. An iced-saline gauze sponge is placed on the repaired lip, held in loops of Logan bow, for 24 h.

B. Crusts on the suture line are removed with diluted H_2O_2, as needed, followed by application of a thin layer of aqueous-based antibacterial ointment for 48 h.

C. Nasal plugs are removed 48 h postoperatively.

D. Incisions are kept clean and dry until removal of sutures on postoperative day 4 or 5 (under general anesthetic). Examine infant a few days after suture removal; often nostrils have to be recleaned.

E. Trimmed 1/2 inch Steri-Strip® is applied to healing incisions for 6 weeks.

F. Digital massage is recommended after 6 weeks postoperative.

V. TECHNICAL MODIFICATIONS FOR ANATOMIC VARIANTS OF BILATERAL CLEFT LIP

A. Incomplete Bilateral Cleft Lip and Nasal Deformity

1. Same steps as for complete bilateral cleft labial deformity. Decide whether to ignore fourth principle (see above). If the bilateral labial cleft is minor, with sufficient prolabial muscle, white roll, and vermilion mucosa, the lateral labial elements can be apposed to the prolabial section in a butt joint. If there is an indistinct prolabial white roll and/or deficient vermilion-mucosa, Cupid's bow and the median tubercle should be constructed just as in the complete anomaly.
2. It is tempting to avoid positioning the alar cartilages if not grossly splayed or caudally dislocated. If the columella is short (less than 3 mm), full nasal correction is necessary. Because all philtral dimensions are fast growing, they are made slightly diminutive, and interalar distance should be narrow. Philtral width and alar width, particularly, will broaden.

B. Asymmetric, Complete/Incomplete Bilateral Cleft Lip and Nasal Deformity

Goal is to achieve symmetry—the only advantage that bilateral cleft lip has over its unilateral counterpart. Bilateral asymmetric double cleft presents a spectrum of severity.

1. The tiny cutaneous bridge is severed on the incomplete side and clefts are managed as a bilateral complete deformity.
2. Asymmetric cutaneous bridges permit bilateral synchronous repair.
3. Complete and incomplete (with intact or minor alveolar cleft): Unilateral pin-retained (Latham) prosthesis is used to narrow the complete alveolar gap. Subsequent lip–nasal adhesion on the side of the complete cleft levels the operative field for second-stage, simultaneous, symmetric nasolabial repair. Often, features on the complete cleft side must be overcorrected. Advisable to initially adjust dimensions on the more severe side rather than to match to the repaired incomplete cleft (i.e., do the worst side first).

C. Complete Bilateral Cleft Lip with Intact Secondary Palate

1. Dentofacial orthopedic manipulation is not applicable to this rare anatomic variant of bilateral cleft labial deformity because the premaxilla is rigidly procumbent and often will not fit into the intermaxillary gap.
2. Two alternatives: either repair bilateral labial clefts over protruding maxilla or, better, perform primary premaxillary ostectomy and positioning, and bilateral gingivoperiosteoplasy at time of the synchronous bilateral nasolabial closure.

Warning: Incisions for primary ostectomy and alveolar closure restrict premaxillary blood supply to septal and preserved vomerine mucosa. Primary premaxillary positioning is unlikely to cause midfacial retrusion given the intact secondary palate.

D. Late Presentation of Complete Bilateral Cleft Lip/Palate

1. Child <1 year old: Consider maxillary orthopedics if premaxilla is moldable. If not, proceed to synchronous premaxillary ostectomy/positioning and alveolar and nasolabial closure.
2. Child >1 year old: Maxillary orthopedic adjustment is not possible, and closure over protrusive premaxilla is likely to cause hypertrophic scarring and philtral distortion. Speech is a major concern. At the first stage, combine closure of the secondary palate with primary premaxillary ostectomy/positioning and repair of the alveolar clefts. In an older child, the premaxilla is held with custom-made acrylic plate and secured with bilateral circumzygomatic drop wires. At the second stage, synchronous bilateral nasolabial repair is accomplished without tension. Early surgical positioning of the premaxilla increases likelihood of midfacial underdevelopment. This risk is acceptable considering preferable nasolabial appearance during childhood and adolescence and predictable success of Le Fort I maxillary advancement after completion of skeletal growth or maxillary distraction done earlier.

VI. CONCLUSIONS

Every child born with bilateral cleft lip/palate and nasal deformity should be cared for by a super-specialist. Fewer than 10% of babies born with cleft lip are bilateral, and thus even a busy plastic surgeon will care for only a few such children in a year. Only a few patients can be followed to adulthood. Therefore, every surgeon who accepts this long-term commitment has an obligation to periodically assess results and to continually learn from predecessors, colleagues, and patients in an effort to improve outcome.

53

Secondary Deformities of Cleft Lip Repair

James P. Bradley, M.D., David Staffenberg, M.D., and Henry K. Kawamoto, M.D.
David Geffen School of Medicine at UCLA, Los Angeles, California, U.S.A.

I. INTRODUCTION

The goal of primary cleft lip repair is that the cleft recontruction be undetectable at conversational distance by school age. Failure to reach this goal may be the result of poor planning or technical error and requires correction of secondary deformities of the cleft lip or cleft nose. Secondary deformities vary according to the type of the initial cleft (unilateral, bilateral, incomplete, or complete) and the type of initial repair (rotation advancement, straight-line closure, and triangular or quadrilateral flap). Multiple options are available to correct the various secondary cleft lip and nasal deformities. The procedures selected depend on the risks and reliability of the technique and on the individual surgeon's preference.

A. Guidelines for Initial Cleft Lip Repair

1. Know the normal anatomy.
2. Find the normal landmarks and return them to their normal position.
3. Do not remove any tissue until certain that it will not be useful later.
4. Apply tissue from areas of excess to areas in need.
5. Treat each case individually.
6. Replace lost tissue with similar tissue when prior surgery or growth has been responsible for the loss.

B. Requirements to Avoid Secondary Deformities

1. Accurate skin, muscle, and mucous membrane union.
2. Proper rotation of the deflected lateral orbicularis oris muscle into a horizontal position with its medial components.
3. A symmetric nostril floor and nasal tip.
4. An even vermilion border with reproduction of the Cupid's bow.
5. Slight eversion or pouting of the central upper lip.
6. A minimal scar without contraction.

C. Indication for Surgery

A correctable deformity that, if left unrepaired, is likely to cause psychosocial problems. The surgeon, older patient, or parents of the patient may recognize the anatomic abnormalities.

D. Timing of Secondary Repair

1. In general, initial repair of the cleft lip and nose is done from 3 to 6 months of age, and revisions are done just prior to school age.
2. Secondary revisions should be complete by 6 years of age to facilitate peer interaction.

3. Final nasal revisions are performed in adolescence after near-completion of facial growth and increased patient self-awareness.

II. SECONDARY DEFORMITIES OF THE UNILATERAL CLEFT LIP

A. Unfavorable Scars

Early reoperation is generally not advocated because time must be allowed for optimum healing and lengthening of a contracted lip scar. Scars are unacceptable based on malposition or excessive thickness.

1. Malpositioned scars can be difficult to correct. To avoid this problem in the rotation-advancement repair, the C-flap should fill the rotation defect so the advancement flap can be oriented vertically and the scar can match the contralateral philtral column.
2. Hypertrophic or red, raised, and firm scars appear one month postoperatively and can be treated with taping (pressure) or topical corticosteroids and time.
3. Persistently pink scars can be treated with a pulse dye laser.
4. Wide scars may need to be surgically revised.

B. Discrepancies in Muscle Continuity and Philtral Column

Inadequate approximation of the orbicularis oris muscle fibers can result in a "whistle" deformity, vermilion notch, lateral lip bulge, or alar base groove. Dehiscence or gradual attenuation of the muscle can also occur as the patient ages.

1. Correction is accomplished by repositioning muscle fibers in a horizontal direction.
2. A philtral column and central dimple may be created by incision of the central muscle flaps and transposition or rollover of the flaps to fill in the philtral column area.
3. An Abbe flap in the midline will transpose the lower lip groove to create an upper lip central dimple with scars and ridging along the philtral columns (Fig. 1).

C. Irregularities of Cupid's Bow and the Vermilion Free Border

1. The mucocutaneous line (white roll) should appear continuous and ridged across the cleft repair. Correction includes:
   - Notching may be corrected with Z-plasty to realign the vermilion border and white roll. Another option, the diamond-shaped excision, is often not as desirable because it may result in a straight-line scar and minimal lengthening of the vertically contracted scar.
   - Peaking of the mucosa into the vertical scar may be corrected with a small flap of lateral or medial tissue rotated into the white line to break the vertical scar.
   - Loss of the ridge may be corrected with white roll interdigitation or a free skin graft.

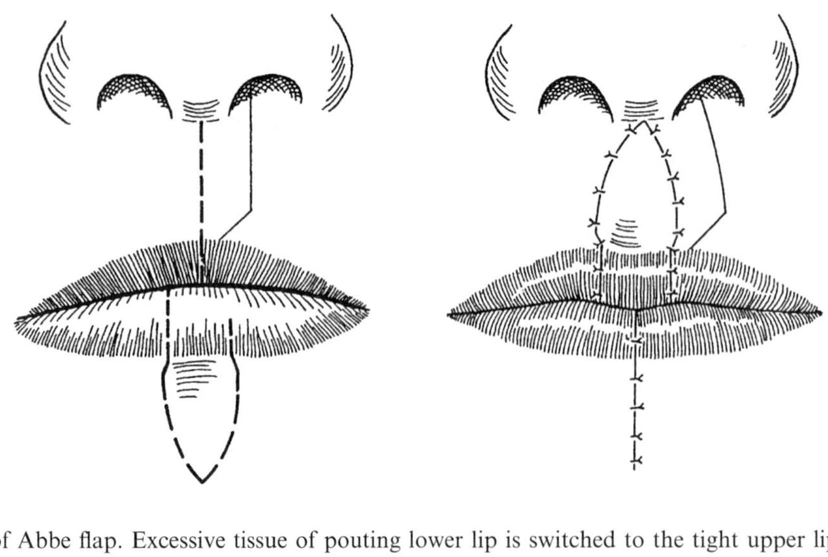

Figure 1 Design of Abbe flap. Excessive tissue of pouting lower lip is switched to the tight upper lip deficient of tissue.

2. Cupid's bow is difficult to correct when absent. One method of correction is with a triangular skin excision just above the mucocutaneous border (Gillies operation).
3. Vermilion free border: Excess bulk on the lateral vermilion can be reduced with an elliptical excision. Lack of fullness of the vermilion can be corrected by:
    - V-Y roll down of the mucosa from the posterior aspect of the lip.
    - Z-plasty to redirect excessive lateral tissue into the deficient notch.
    - Autogenous filler: from locally rotated subcutaneous flaps or from fascial grafts.
    - Wide advancement of the upper lateral sulcus with relaxing incisions along the alveolar margin.
    - Reduction of excess tissue on noncleft side to gain symmetry.
4. Deficient tubercle: Corrected with V-Y advancement of midline mucosa to provide central vermilion bulk.

D. Short Upper Lip

The distance from Cupid's bow to the base of the columella is less on the cleft side. The cause is often failure to adequately lengthen the lip at the time of a straight-line closure or rotation advancement repair. The lip may shorten in the postoperative period, reaching a peak at 6–8 weeks and returning to its original operative length in 6 months. Lip lengthening techniques include:

- Rerotation-advancement with takedown of the muscle.
- Z-plasty close to the nostril sill.
- V-Y advancement flap or use of banked forked flaps.
- Muscle advancements.
- Abbe flap.

E. Long Upper Lip

More commonly found after bilateral cleft repair. In unilateral clefts, this may be seen after triangular repair. Correction involves shortening of the lateral segment by an excision under the alar base and partial derotation of the medial segment.

F. Tight Upper Lip

More common after straight-line repair or triangular repair. The horizontal tightness of the upper lip restrains anterior-posterior facial growth and gives a relative appearance of a pouting lower lip. The Abbe lip-switch flap may be necessary but is a flap of last resort and is used often after bilateral cleft lip repairs (Fig. 1).

G. Secondary Correction after Different Types of Cleft Lip Closures

Secondary deformities may result from a surgeon's mistakes of measurements or misalignment and are not necessarily inherent in the type of closure. However, some deformities are more often seen with certain methods of lip closure.

1. Deformity after straight-line closure: The most common secondary deformity is vertical lip contracture with peaking of the mucocutaneous junction and notching of the vermilion bottom. Corrections include:
    - Transposition flaps: Z-plasty, superior-based flap (Trauner), or inferior-based flap (Ginestet) after excision of the vertical scar.
    - Secondary techniques when sufficient Cupid's bow is present include secondary LeMesurier (quadrilateral), secondary Tennison (triangular), or secondary Millard (rotation-advancement) procedures.
2. Deformity after triangular and quadrilateral flap methods: An inferior triangular flap may result in an asymmetric Cupid's bow and tubercle. The quadrilateral flap may result in a long lip on the cleft side. Secondary corrections of these methods can be difficult, especially if a zigzag scar is present across the philtral column. A rotation-advancement procedure may be necessary.
3. Deformity after rotation and advancement technique: A common problem is shortness of the vertical height. A 6-month waiting period will allow the contracture to relax and the Cupid's bow position to settle. If the lip is still short, then a rerotation with an adequate back-cut may be necessary.

III. SECONDARY DEFORMITIES OF THE BILATERAL CLEFT LIP

A. Central Lip Paucity

This "whistle" deformity may be seen after Manchester repairs because the vermilion of the prolabium, which is histologically different from the true vermilion, is utilized. It is preferable to advance the lateral lip elements and suture the lateral vermilion flaps in the midline. Excess midline vermilion should be left at the initial procedure. If residual deficiency exists, then correction may be achieved by:

1. V-Y advancements
2. Horizontal double V-Y (with subcutaneous muscle flaps if necessary)
3. Bilateral mucosal advancements
4. Lingual flap
5. Vermilion flaps from lower lip
6. Dermal fat grafts

B. Wide Philtrum

At time of surgical revision, excess tissue may be used to lengthen the columella.

C. Deficiency of Labial Sulcus

This leads to a restricted upper lip.

1. To free the lip and correct the deficiency, excise any adhesions and lengthen with a Z-plasty.
2. For an absent upper labial sulcus, a mucosal graft is placed between the premaxilla and upper lip.

IV. UNILATERAL CLEFT NASAL DEFORMITY

A. Pathologic Abnormalities

1. Deflection of nasal tip toward the cleft.
2. Posterior and inferior displacement of the dome of the alar cartilage on the cleft side.
3. Obtuse angle between the medial and lateral crura of the alar cartilage.
4. Obtuse alar-facial attachment.
5. Inward buckling of the ala on the cleft side.

B. Correction

1. Synchronous or at the time of the primary cleft lip repair.
2. Secondary corrective procedure require:
   - Open approach with exposure of the lower lateral cartilages
   - Lengthening of the columella
   - Suturing of the lateral crura at the correct height to create a symmetrical nasal tip
   - Undermining and redraping the skin of the nose
   - Conchal or septal cartilage grafts

C. Complications

1. Nasal stenosis: correct with Z-plasty.

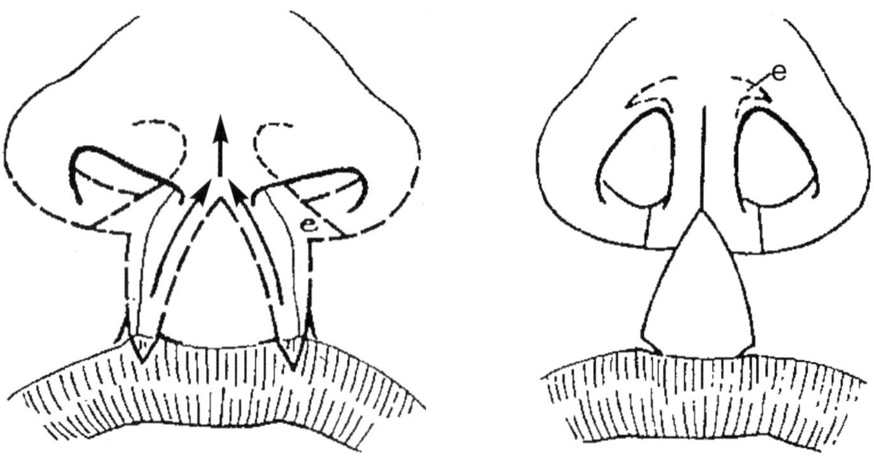

Figure 2 Design of elongation of a short columella after bilateral cleft lip with forked flaps.

V. BILATERAL CLEFT NASAL DEFORMITY

A. Short columella is the prominent deformity. To address this, options include:

- Presurgical columella elongation with nasoalveolar molding device during the neonatal period.
- V-Y advancement of mid-prolabium. If the entire prolabium is used, then an Abbe flap is necessary to fill the upper lip.
- Bilateral forked flaps (Fig. 2).
- The mainstay for correction is recruitment of alar cartilage, columellar strut and nasal tip grafting.

B. Correction of lip deformity is planned with columella lengthening so that enough tissue is allocated for each correction.

VI. SUMMARY

The best chance to obtain the ideal result is at the time of the initial operation. Even with careful planning and meticulous execution of the chosen technique, minor secondary revisions may be necessary. The techniques described have been found to be most useful, but much depends on the individual surgeon's preference.

54

Cleft Palate Repair and Velopharyngeal Insufficiency

James P. Bradley, M.D., and Henry K. Kawamoto, M.D.
David Geffen School of Medicine at UCLA, Los Angeles, California, U.S.A.

I. CLEFT PALATE REPAIR

A. Goal

To close the cleft palate with a technique and timing that results in optimal speech development and minimal midface growth disturbance.

B. Terminology

1. A cleft palate is failure of the lateral palatal shelves to fuse to each other.
2. The incisive foramen is located behind the incisor teeth where the maxillary bones meet the midline premaxilla.
3. The primary palate or prepalatal structures are anterior to the incisive foramen and are abnormal in a cleft lip, either unilateral or bilateral. These structures include the alveolus, lip, and nasal tip cartilages.
4. The secondary palate or palatal structures are posterior to the incisive foramen and include the hard palate, soft palate, and uvula.

C. Classification of Cleft Palate and Association with Cleft Lip

1. Prepalatal clefts should be described as unilateral or bilateral, complete (all the way through structures), or incomplete.
2. Palatal cleft may be described by Kernahan's Y classification as involving one third, two thirds, or all of the hard palate and one third, two thirds, or all of the soft palate.
3. Incidence:
   - Caucasians = 1.4 per 1000 live births.
   - Asians = 2.6 per 1000 live births.
   - African Americans = 0.43 per 1000 live births.
   - Likelihood of a cleft in another child:

     If one first- or second-degree relative (parent or sibling) has a cleft, then 4% likelihood.

     If two first- or second-degree relatives (parent and sibling) have clefts, then 17% likelihood.
4. Unilateral cleft lip and palate: most frequent combination; predominantly on left side; more common in boys than girls.
5. Isolated cleft palate: second most frequent combination; more common in girls.
6. Bilateral cleft lip and palate.
7. Submucous cleft palate—the levator muscle fails to fuse in the midline.
   - Calnan triad of findings in submucous cleft palate—bifid uvula, notched posterior hard palate, and "zona pellucidum" or thin central area at the site of the velar muscular diastasis.
   - Most patients (90%) are asymptomatic.

- Screening is best accomplished by nasopharyngoscopy or video fluoroscopy.

8. Bifid uvula: seen in 2% of Americans. Patients should be followed for speech problems.

D. Timing and Treatment

1. Birth:
   - Feeding—poor suction ability requires special cruciate-cut nipple tip.
   - Presurgical orthopedics or nasal alveolar molding can begin at two weeks of age. A fly-away premaxilla is brought into alignment with the lateral alveolar segments, the flattened cleft-side alar cartilage is elevated, and the columella is elongated.
2. At 3–6 months of age:
   - Cleft lip repair (see Chapter 51).
   - Gingivoperiosteoplasty—controversial whether this decreases the need for subsequent alveolar bone graft or whether subperiosteal undermining leads to mid-face growth disturbance.
   - Myringotomy and grommet tube placement are often performed for hearing acuity problems associated with an increased frequency of otitis media episodes (probably from increased nasopharynx reflux up the eustachian tube secondary to abnormal insertion of the levator veli palatini and tensor veli palatini).
3. At 10–14 months of age: palatoplasty (see techniques below) is performed prior to speech development
4. At 8–12 years of age:
   - Orthodontics for maxillary expansion.
   - Alveolar bone graft from iliac crest is performed when adjacent permanent teeth are erupting.
5. Age of facial skeletal maturity is 15–16 years in females, 17–18 years in males. One may determine skeletal maturity by obtaining wrist x-rays to check for epiphyseal plate closure.
   - Orthodontic therapy is used to correct the malocclusion. If surgical advancement is necessary, presurgical orthodontic preparation is needed to remove dental compensations (see Chapter 41).
   - Maxillary osteotomy and advancement are performed for correction of midface hypoplasia.

E. Palatal Repair Techniques

1. Two-flap palatoplasty with intravelar veloplasty (modified Von Langenbeck) (Fig. 1):
   - Intravelar veloplasty (Braithwaite): Levator muscles are dissected free from the oral and nasal mucosa, released from the palatal aponeurosis and tensor tympani palatini, and then reattached in the midline to each other in anatomic position.
   - The nasal mucosa is closed to itself posteriorly and to the vomer mucosal flap anteriorly.
   - The oral side is closed after mucoperiosteal flaps are raised based on the greater palatine artery. Lateral relaxing incisions are usually left open.
2. Double opposing Z-plasty (Furlow repair) (Fig. 2):
   - Same principles as above except the soft palate is lengthened with two Z-plasties, one on the oral side and a reverse one on the nasal side.
   - The levator muscle on one side is included in a posteriorly based oral mucosa flap, and the levator muscle on other side is included in a posteriorly based nasal mucosa flap.
   - The hard palate is closed similar to the two flap palatoplasty, and with a vomer flap if necessary.
3. V-Y advancement or "push back" of palate (Wardill-Kilner-Veau):
   - The mucoperiosteal flaps of the hard palate are advanced posteriorly and closed to each other centrally to gain anteroposterior palatal length.
   - A major drawback to this technique is that the large exposed areas of membranous bone left to granulate may contribute to maxillary growth disturbances.

F. Complications

1. Perioperative:
   - Respiratory obstruction. This can be a life-threatening risk, especially in patients with Pierre Robin sequence because of retrognathia and macroglossia.

     Make sure patient is fully awake before extubation.

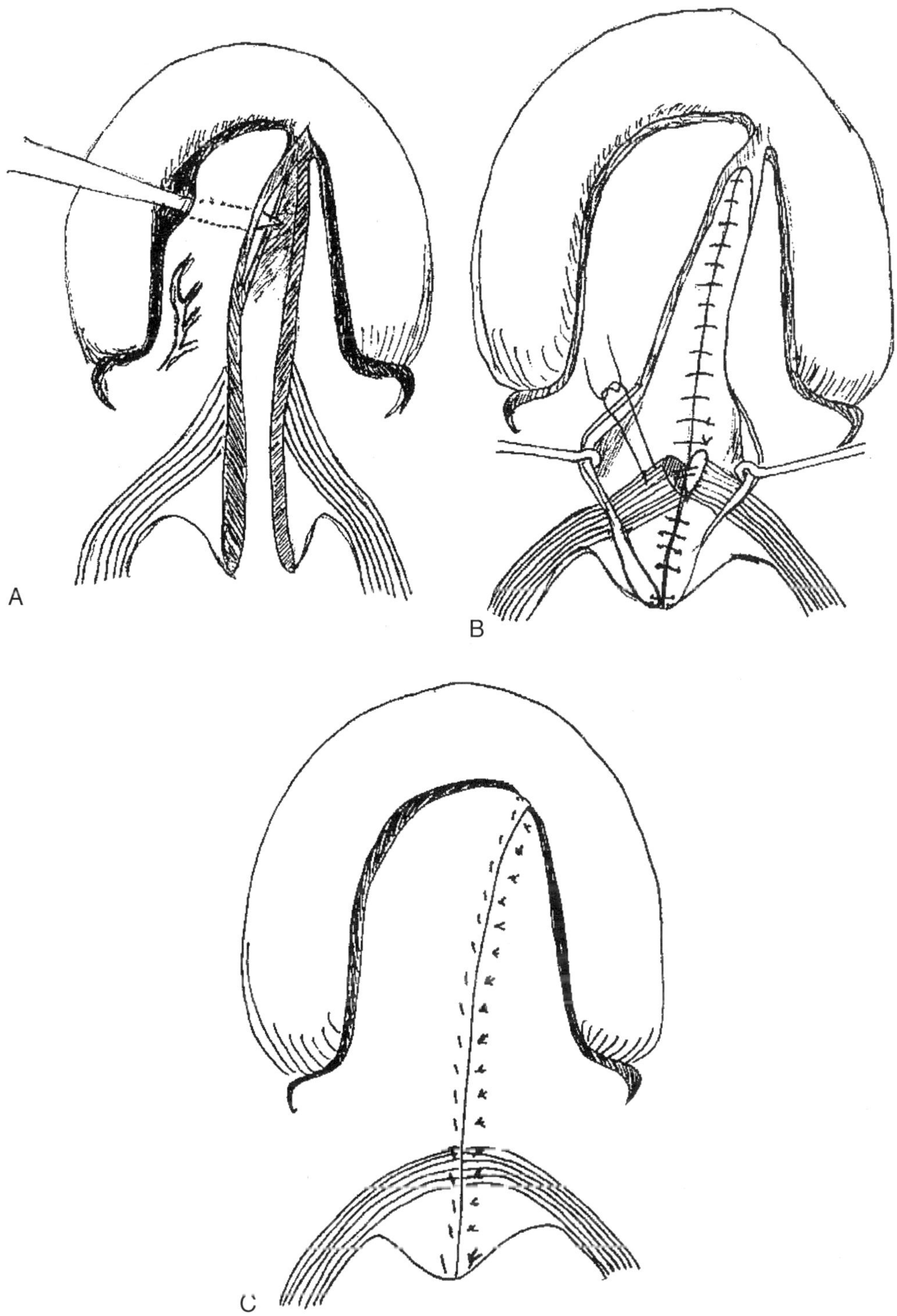

Figure 1 Palatoplasty technique to repair a complete left-side cleft palate. (A) Mucoperiosteal unipedicled flaps, based on the greater palatine artery, are elevated. (B) The nasal floor is repaired with use of a vomer flap anteriorly. Intravelar veloplasty is performed by approximating the levator muscles in the midline after they are freed from the oral and nasal mucosa and released from the palatal aponeurosis and tensor tympani palatini. (C) Vertical mattress sutures are used to close the oral mucosa complete the repair.

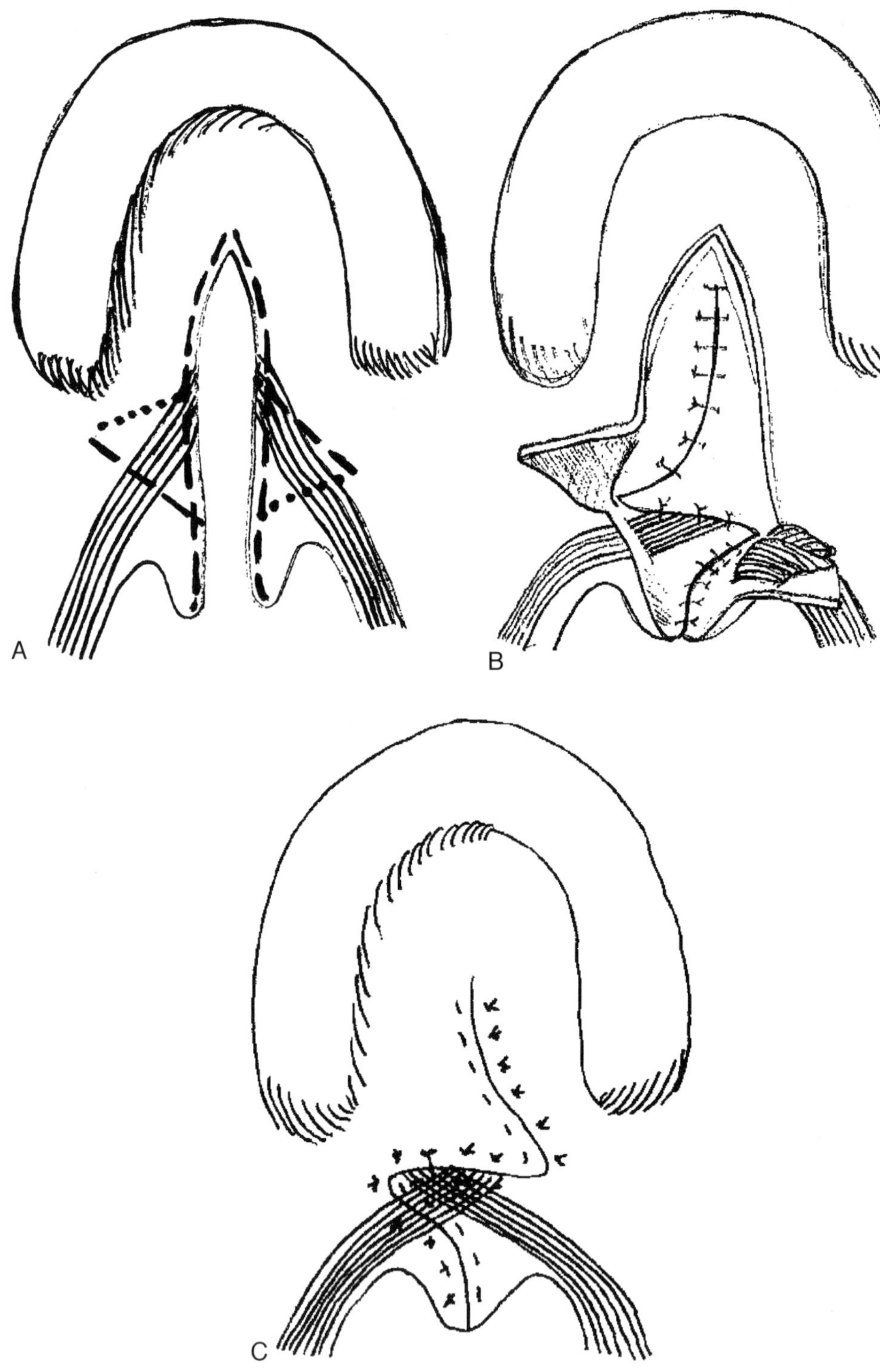

Figure 2 Double opposing Z-plasty technique to close an isolated cleft palate. (A) Incision design includes widely based flaps in the soft palate in the area of the levator muscle and its abnormal insertion. (B) The levator muscle is in the posteriorly based flaps. Nasal mucosa has been closed with a Z-plasty. (C) Repair is completed with the oral side reverse Z-plasty and levator overlap to create a muscle sling.

Tongue suture is placed for 24 hours to allow forced protrusion of the tongue if the patient cannot protect the airway.

Use monitored bed with pulse oximetry; assess patient in recovery room before transfer to floor.

- Bleeding.

2. Late:
   - Palatal fistula: asymptomatic, or associated with speech or feeding problems or dental hygiene.
   - Facial growth disturbance from maxillary scarring.
   - Velopharyngeal incomptence: 1–30% (see below).

5. After pharyngoplasty or pharyngeal flap: Inadequate width of flaps for closure of the sphincter.
6. After adenoidectomy: Without this posterior lymphoid tissue, the velum cannot reach the posterior pharyngeal wall. VPI after these procedures and after maxillary advancement usually resolve in 3–12 months.
7. Enlarged tonsils: Large size may restrict airway in oropharynx and limit palatal elevation.
8. After midface advancement: Patients at risk include those with previous cleft palate repair who demonstrate nasal air escape and some hypernasality before the procedure and those requiring a large maxillary advancement.
9. Neurogenic: Paresis of velopharynx, decreased pharyngeal wall movement.

II. VELOPHARYNGEAL INCOMPETENCE (VPI)

A. Definition

Abnormal coupling of the nasal and oral cavities because the velopharyngeal sphincter cannot close. This leads to hypernasality, nasal emissions, misarticulations (substitution of consonants: e.g., "n" and "m" for "p," "b," "d," "g," and "k"). Occurs in approximately 20% of overall repaired cleft palate patients.

B. Causes of VPI

1. Idiopathic insufficiency of musculature: All elements of the sphincter are working but a tight seal cannot be made because of weakness. Speech therapy is required.
2. Congenital palatal insufficiency: The velum is too short to reach across the posterior pharynx or the pharynx is too large.
3. Submucous cleft palate: Levator muscles fail to unite in the midline. As the palate elevates, the central cleft widens and VPI results in some patients. Nasopharygoscopy is used for screening, and a Furlow double opposing Z-plasty is often used for correction.
4. After repair of cleft palate: The palate may be deficient of tissue or scarred, or the posterior and lateral pharyngeal walls may not move properly.

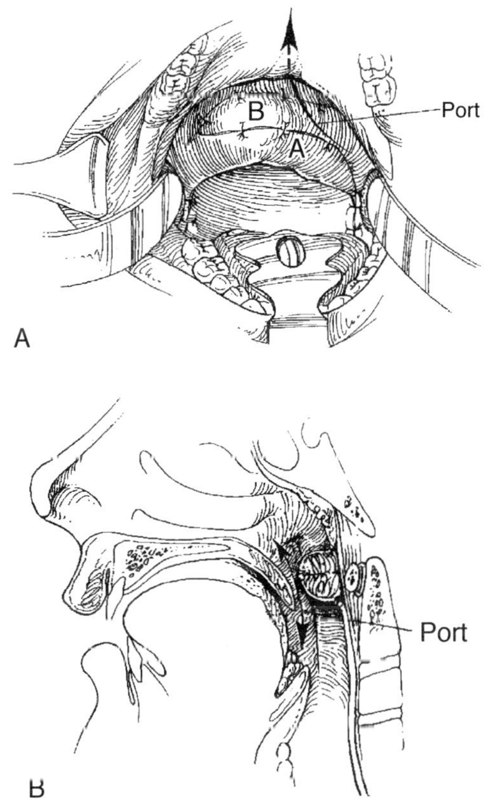

Figure 3 Pharyngoplasty. (A) Operative view through mouth reveals superiorly based pharyngeal flaps that have been sutured together in the posterior midline (note the suture closure of donor sites inferiolaterally). (B) A lateral cross-section schematic demonstrates how the bulk of the pharyngoplasty narrows the port or oronasal air passage.

10. Functional hypernasality: Emotional disturbance inhibits good speech despite competent speech mechanism.

C. Speech Analysis

1. Surgeon and speech pathologist together determine which VPI patients will benefit from surgery.
2. Nasopharyngoscopy or multiview videofluoroscopy can quantitate and localize defects of the sphincter mechanism and assist with surgical procedure planning.

D. Operative Techniques

1. Sphincter pharyngoplasty (Fig. 3):
   - Two superiorly based flaps of the posterior tonsillar pillars and the palatopharyngeus muscle are tranposed from the lateral pharynx to each other across the midline above Passavant's ridge (bulge on the posterior palate above the arch of the atlas).
   - This procedure achieves static and dynamic reduction in the velopharyngeal port.
2. Posterior pharyngeal flap:
   - Central pharyngeal flap with lateral ports.
   - Flap can be superiorly or inferiorly based. Flap should be lined with mucosa from turn-back flaps from the nasal side near the uvula to prevent shrinkage.
   - Port size is usually determined by preoperative study of lateral pharyngeal wall movement:

     If port size is too large, hypernasal speech persists.

     If port size is too small, obstructive sleep apnea results.
3. Palatal lengthening procedures: Double opposing Z-plasty for small central defects.
4. Posterior pharyngeal wall augmentation: prosthetic or autogenous tissue (e.g., costochondral graft). Used if preoperative analysis reveals a small central defect.

E. Speech Therapy

Modification of the secondary superimposed compensatory habit is necessary to improve speech.

55

Microtia

A. Corde Mason, M.D., F.A.A.P.
University of Pittsburgh School of Medicine, Pittsburgh, Pennsylvania, U.S.A.
Michael L. Bentz, M.D., F.A.A.P., F.A.C.S.
University of Wisconsin Medical School, Madison, Wisconsin, U.S.A.

I. TERMINOLOGY (FIG. 1)

A. Auricle or pinna—the external ear.

B. Tragus—anterior projection of cartilage on the pinna that extends back over the opening of the auditory meatus.

C. Antitragus—small cartilaginous projection opposite the tragus that extends forward over the auditory meatus.

D. Helix—the outer curved fleshy ridge of the pinna.

E. Antihelix—cartilaginous depression that parallels the helix along the inferior aspect of the pinna.

F. Microtia—congenitally small or misshapen pinna, often with components absent.

II. ANATOMY

The external ear is composed of an inner elastic cartilage framework covered by perichondrium and a thin skin envelope. There is a scant subcutaneous layer posteriorly.

A. Spatial relationships:

- The ear width is approximately 55% of its height.
- Ear projection measured from the scalp to anterior surface of the superior pole of the helix is 1.5–2.0 cm.
- The superior aspect of the auricle should correspond to the level of the brow superiorly and the base of the columella inferiorly.
- The long axis of the ear is anteriorly rotated 15–20 degrees from the axis of the nose.

B. The vascular supply to the pinna is via branches of the external carotid artery:

- Posterior auricular artery
- Occipital artery
- Superficial temporal artery

C. The lesser occipital and greater auricular nerves supply sensory innervation.

III. EPIDEMIOLOGY

A. The incidence of microtia/anotia ranges from 1 in 500 to 1 in 5000 live births.

B. Males are affected more often than females.

C. Microtia is a unilateral phenomenon in 90% of cases. The right side is affected more so than the left.

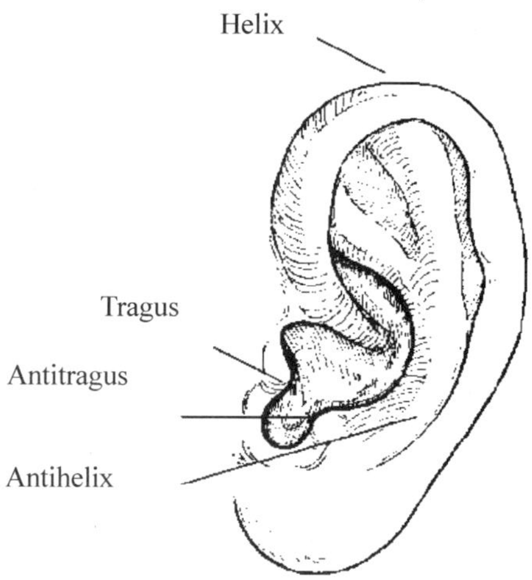

Figure 1 External ear terminology.

D. In 80% of patients, the external auditory canal is atretic or narrow, with associated conductive hearing loss. Approximately 16% of cases have neurosensory hearing loss.

E. 20–40% of patients have associated defects that most frequently involve the face (35%), kidneys (4%), vertebrae, and heart (2.5%).

IV. EMBRYOLOGY

A. The external auditory meatus develops from the dorsal portion of the first pharyngeal cleft at the beginning of the third month of gestation.

B. During the sixth week of gestation, the auricle develops from six mesenchymal proliferations (hillocks) located at the dorsal ends of the first and second branchial arches and surrounding the first pharyngeal cleft. These swellings, three on each side of the external meatus, later fuse and gradually form the resultant auricle. Initially, the external ear is located in the region of the lower neck, but as the mandible develops, the ear ascends the side of the head to the level of the eyes.

C. The auricle assumes an adult configuration by the 20th week and continues its postnatal growth until around 9 years of age. It is 85% of its adult size by age 3.

V. ETIOLOGY

A. The origin of the deformity is not understood. Theories include intrauterine ischemia caused by either an obliterated stapedial artery or a local hemorrhage.

B. No consistent inheritance pattern has been observed.

C. Medications associated with ear deformities include thalidomide, clomiphene citrate, and retinoic acid.

D. Five percent of cases have an immediate family member with a major ear deformity.

E. Parents with two affected children have a risk of recurrence as high as 15% in a subsequent pregnancy.

VI. TREATMENT

A. In general, reconstruction consists of the creation of a framework placed underneath the periauricular skin with several refining soft tissue procedures. Options include:

- Alloplastic materials have not been well received and are plagued with complications, including skin ulceration, infections, extrusion, and rejection.
- Homograft cartilage (maternal, paternal, or banked) resorbs, distorts, or disappears within 18 months.
- The preferred material is autogenous rib cartilage. It affords favorable results, encounters few complications, and withstands trauma.

B. Timing—an important consideration is when to perform the repair. Timing is governed by both psychological and physical considerations:

- The child's concept of body image usually begins to evolve at 4–5 years of age. Psychologically, the child is rarely disturbed with the ear prior to age 7.
- Surgery should be postponed until rib growth affords necessary cartilage volume to permit fashioning of a quality framework.
- By age 6, rib cartilage size is usually sufficient for repair and recognition of the ear as a problem for the child is such that he or she is ready for intervention. At this age, the child is apt to be more cooperative with post-operative care instructions.

C. Preoperative considerations:

- During preoperative planning, one attempts to match the opposite ear with respect to surface topography.

- Consider other facial procedures that may be necessary (i.e., correction of bony deformities, soft tissue deficiency). Specifically, one must take care to preserve the virgin auricular site and keep it free of scar.
- The auricular reconstruction must precede external auditory canal reconstruction when the latter is indicated.

D. Autologous grafting

- There are currently two practiced methods of autologous auricular reconstruction described by Brent in 1980 and Nagata in 1993.
- Classically, the Brent method reconstructs the ear in three or four stages:

  Stage I—A cartilaginous framework is fashioned and placed under a preauricular skin pocket: (1) Rib cartilage from contralateral ribs 6, 7, and 8 is harvested from the chest. Care is taken to maintain the integrity of the chest wall. This is facilitated via preservation of a rim of the upper margin of rib 6. (2) The donor cartilage is carved into the appropriate scaffold shape and size. Perichondrium is preserved. (3) The helix is fashioned from the distal segment of rib 8 and fixed to the framework with nylon sutures. (4) The preauricular skin pocket is created and the scaffold is inset. (5) Drains are placed to suction to prevent hematoma accumulation and to provide negative pressure within the pocket, promoting conformation of the skin flap to the framework.

  Stage II—The lobule is transposed to a more normal position relative to the framework.

  Stage III—The new ear is elevated from the scalp and a retro-auricular skin graft is placed: (1) The neo-pinna is elevated from the head and a skin graft is placed posteriorly to create an auriculocephalic sulcus. (2) Ear projection is maintained by interposition of a wedge of rib cartilage posteriorly. Either a temporoparietal fascial flap or an occipital fascial turnover "book flap" from behind the ear covers the cartilagenous wedge to provide vascular supply to the overlying skin graft.

  Stage IV—The tragus is reconstructed. The tragus can be reconstructed from tissue grafted from the opposite ear. It may also be created as an integral component of the initial scaffold.

- Nagata's technique reconstructs the auricle in two stages:

  In the first stage of reconstruction, a complete framework including the tragus is inserted into the preauricular pocket and the lobule is transposed.

  The ear is then elevated and projected in the second operation.

56

Vascular Malformations and Hemangiomas

Nina J. Lee, M.D., and Nina L. Shapiro, M.D.
David Geffen School of Medicine at UCLA, Los Angeles, California, U.S.A.

I. TERMINOLOGY

A biologic classification has been introduced to define congenital vascular lesions. These lesions were separated into two distinct groups: hemangiomas and vascular malformations.

A. Hemangiomas

Usually not present at birth. Become visible at weeks 4–6 of life. They proliferate rapidly during the first year of life, followed by a slow period of involution. Types of hemangiomas include:

- Superficial hemangiomas
- Deep hemangiomas
- Compound hemangiomas

B. Vascular Malformations

Present at birth. They grow with growth of the child. Types of vascular malformations include:

- Capillary malformations
- Venous malformations
- Lymphatic malformations
- Arteriovenous malformations

II. HEMANGIOMAS

A. Superficial Hemangiomas

Originate in the papillary dermis and appear as a bright red macular or papular skin lesion. Old terminology: strawberry and capillary hemangiomas.

B. Deep Hemangiomas

Originate in the deeper dermal layer (reticular or subcutaneous tissue) and expand the skin without causing a significant color change. Old terminology: cavernous hemangiomas.

C. Compound Hemangiomas

Components of superficial and deep hemangiomas. Old terminology: capillary cavernous hemangiomas.

D. Incidence

Hemangiomas occur in 10–12% of the Caucasian population. They are less commonly seen among Asian and African American infants, and are more common among premature infants <1000 g (22% affected). The male-to-female ratio is 1:6.

E. Etiology

During the proliferative phase, the endothelial cells become plump and undergo frequent division/hyperplasia, resulting in the formation of new vascular channels. During involution, the endothelial cells slowly become less active, flatten in appearance, and undergo apoptosis with the deposition of perivascular fibro-fatty tissue.

F. Embryology

The majority of hemangiomas are solitary lesions in the head and neck that tend to be located along the embryologic fusion plates in the face. The lesions may also follow along the trigeminal nerve dermatome distribution.

G. Clinical Presentation

The lesions are usually not present at birth. A hemangioma is characteristically noticed within the first few weeks of life as a blanched macule. An area of telangiectasia then develops, followed by the characteristic proliferation.

H. Clinical Behavior

In general, 50% of the lesions undergo involution by 5 years of age, and 70% undergo involution by 7 years of age. The involution of a hemangioma can frequently result in a residual scar, area of atrophic or redundant skin telangiectasia, or fibro-fatty tissue requiring corrective surgery.

I. Subglottic Hemangioma

- Incidence—10% of patients with cutaneous hemangiomas will have a subglottic hemangioma, which may or may not be symptomatic. Eighty percent of patients with a subglottic hemangioma will have a cutaneous hemangioma.
- Presentation—usually presents during the first 6–8 weeks of life with the insidious onset of inspiratory or biphasic stridor during crying or feeding. A cutaneous hemangioma should raise the suspicion of a subglottic lesion.
- Clinical behavior—most subglottic hemangiomas tend to be superficial and unilateral, located at the left posterolateral aspect of the subglottis. They can also rarely be located bilaterally or circumferentially. During proliferation they tend to appear as a firm red lesion. They subsequently lighten in color and become softer during involution. These lesions can be diagnosed during endoscopy.

J. Diagnosis

A detailed history is the most important tool in diagnosing a hemangioma versus a vascular malformation. Hemangiomas are usually not present at birth, but then undergo a very rapid period of growth during the first year of life by hyperplasia of the vascular endothelial cells (proliferation). Vascular malformations undergo a slower growth over many years. In addition, only hemangiomas will involute, while vascular malformations will continue to grow.

K. Treatment

1. Cutaneous Hemangiomas

- Observation—lesions that do not result in airway compromise, visual compromise, or systemic compromise may be observed. Reconstructive procedures can be performed following this if involution is incomplete or if significant scarring, epidermal atrophy, redundant skin, telangiectasia, or fibro-fatty tissue deposits remain.
- Steroids—this treatment is only effective during the proliferative phase of the hemangioma. The typical dose is 2–5 mg/kg/day of prednisone or prednisolone for at least 2–3 weeks, followed by an 8- to 10-week tapering period. Side effects, although usually temporary, include growth retardation, appearance of cushingoid features, gastritis, and hyperglycemia.
- Laser therapy—superficial hemangiomas respond better to laser treatment than deeper lesions. Treatments frequently utilize the flashlamp pumped-dye laser with a 585 nm wavelength. Complications are rare and include scarring, hypopigmentation, and postinflammatory hyperpigmentation. Interstitial Nd:YAG laser therapy may be used for both hemangiomas and vascular malformations refractory to other therapies.
- Surgical debulking—hemangiomas develop a surrounding tissue plane during their growth in the proliferative phase, thus allowing easier dissection of the lesion during this time. Instruments to help minimize blood loss such as a thermoscalpel or electrocautery can also assist in surgical resection of the lesions.
- Interferon—this agent can be given for the treatment of hemangiomas at any time in their course. A typical regimen is interferon 3×10^6 units/m^2 body surface area given daily subcutaneously for up to 6–8 months. No tapering of interferon is necessary prior to discontinuation. The reversible side effects included fever, anemia, elevation of liver enzymes, and speech difficulties. A potential irreversible side effect is spastic diplegia.

2. Subglottic Hemangiomas

- Observation—asymptomatic small hemangiomas that obstruct less than 20% of the airway can be observed with frequent examinations. These lesions tend to undergo complete involution.
- Steroids—symptomatic patients or patients with larger lesions should be treated with systemic steroids using a similar regimen as used for cutaneous hemangiomas (see above). During the tapering of the steroid dose prior to discontinuation, careful observations should be performed for rebound growth of the hemangiomas.
- Laser therapy—a CO_2 laser, KTP laser, or Nd:YAG laser can be used to ablate a well-localized lesion. Care must be taken not to injure the cartilaginous larynx during laser treatment.
- Tracheostomy—extensive or deep lesions should be treated with tracheostomy and the establishment of a safe airway until the lesions undergo involution.
- Open resection—surgical resection of a subglottic hemangioma through a cricothyrotomy incision can be performed for localized unilateral lesions.
- Interferon—this agent is rarely used for the treatment of subglottic hemangiomas.

III. VASCULAR MALFORMATIONS

A. Incidence

Male-to-female ratio is 1:1.

B. Etiology

The lesions are composed of congenitally malformed vascular channels, with the site of the malformation determining the type of vascular malformation. The endothelial cells forming the vascular malformations do not increase in number, but the vessels become enlarged and ectatic, causing growth of the lesions.

C. Embryology

Failure of vascular differentiation during the fourth gestational week.

D. Clinical Presentation

Although the vascular malformation itself is always present at birth, the lesions may present at a later time. They tend to slowly enlarge with the patient, although trauma, infection, or hormone changes can cause episodes of rapid growth.

E. Clinical Behavior

These lesions do not undergo an involutional phase. Therefore, vascular malformations will continue to grow in size unless adequate treatment is given.

F. Venular Malformations

These lesions are formed from malformations of the post-capillary venules. Old terminology: port wine stains and capillary hemangiomas.

- Physical examination—venular malformations occur in 0.3% of the population with a 1:1 male:female ratio. They present as a flat erythematous macule and often affect at least one of the dermatomes of the trigeminal nerve (V2 > V3 > V1). The lesions tend to darken and thicken with age, and a cobblestone appearance of the skin may also develop.
- Treatment—these lesions are best treated with lasers. Superficial lesions respond best to treatment. A flashlamp pumped-dye laser can be safely utilized for these lesions.

G. Venous Malformations

The lesions are composed of abnormally developed ectatic and dilated veins.

- Physical examination—although the lesions are present at birth, they frequently present clinically during the first or second decade. The lesions grow as the patient grows. They are soft and compressible and increase in size with increased venous pressure, trauma, and hormonal changes. Venous malformations may also be intraosseous, with the mandible being the most common site affected.
- Radiology—the detection of phleboliths on a radiographic exam is pathognomonic for a venous malformation. In intraosseous lesions, a soap bubble or honeycomb appearance of the bone may be seen. Direct percutaneous puncture of the venous malformation and subsequent injection of contrast can be used to better visualize the entire extent of the lesion. Magnetic resonance imaging (MRI) is the best imaging technique for evaluating venous malformations. MRI reveals signal intensity on T1-weighted images and high signal

intensity on T2-weighted images, with variable gadolinium enhancement.

- Treatment—laser therapy can be used to treat superficial venous malformations. It can also be used as an adjunct to sclerotherapy or surgical resection. Sclerotherapy can be used to treat venous malformations of the lower third of the face and the neck and is used frequently in conjunction with surgical resection. Surgical resection is the only method that can be used to completely remove a venous malformation. This procedure, however, is extremely difficult and involves a high risk of significant intraoperative blood loss due to the very thin walls of the veins forming the lesion.

H. Lymphatic Malformations

Composed of a mass of malformed and dilated lymphatic vessels. Old terminology includes lymphangioma and cystic hygroma (Fig. 1).

- Embryology—failure of vascular differentiation during the fourth gestational week.
- Physical examination—the majority of lesions are diagnosed at birth, and they characteristically grow in size with the patient. A lymphatic malformation presents as a soft, painless, non-discolored soft tissue mass, which can be transilluminated.
- Location—over 90% of lymphatic malformations are found in the neck. The microcystic variety consists of generalized edema with poorly defined borders. These lesions tend to affect the tongue, floor of mouth, and lower face. The macrocystic variety is composed of localized multiloculated cysts and commonly affects the neck.

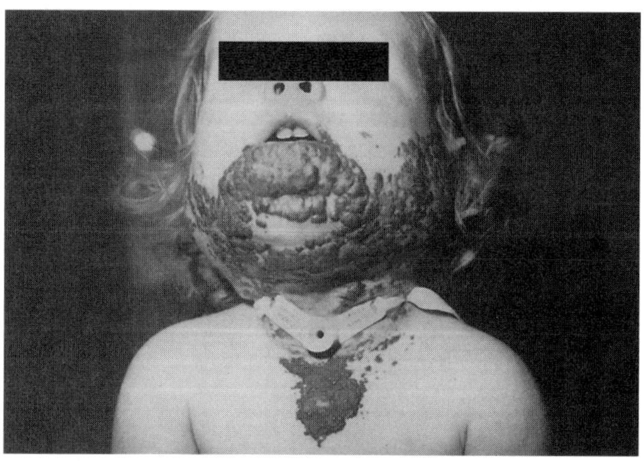

Figure 1 Diffuse cervicofacial hemangiomas with airway obstruction requiring tracheotomy tube.

- Radiology:

  CT scan—after the injection of intravenous contrast material, lymphatic malformations appear as homogeneous, well-defined lesions with attenuation of fluid.

  MRI scan—MRI can better show the extent of the lesion than CT imaging. Lymphatic malformations are heterogeneous in signal on both T1- and T2-weighted images and usually do not show gadolinium enhancement. They appear as low-signal intensity lesions on T1-weighted images and high-signal intensity lesions on T2-weighted images.

  Ultrasound—in the macrocystic variety of a lymphatic malformation, ultrasound can show a multiloculated cystic mass with fibrous septae and poorly defined margins.

- Natural progression—approximately 80–90% of the lesions present within the first 2 years of life. The lesions gradually grow in size with the patient, but rapid periods of growth may occur secondary to hemorrhage or infection. The infection rate of lymphatic malformations is approximately 16%.
- Treatment

  Surgical—lymphatic malformations are difficult to completely resect surgically and thus have a high recurrence rate. The macrocystic variety is easier to remove because it is more localized and loculated than the very diffuse microcystic variety. This type of lesion may recur even following several staged resections.

  Sclerosants—agents effective in the sclerotherapy of lymphatic malformations include bleomycin, doxycycline, and OK-432. These agents cause an inflammatory response and the subsequent contraction of the vessels forming the lesion. As with surgical resection, patients with the macrocystic variety of lymphatic malformations tend to respond better to sclerotherapy than those with the microcystic variety.

  Laser therapy—Nd:YAG laser (interstitial) for lingual lesions.

I. Arteriovenous Malformations

These are congenital lesions composed of multiple fistulas between arteries and veins, resulting in a mass composed of tortuous and dilated arteries and veins (Fig. 2).

- Embryology—arteriovenous malformations are formed from errors in vascular development that occur in the 4th to 6th weeks of gestation.
- Physical examination—the lesions are warm, relatively firm to palpation and not easily compressible, with a violaceous pigment change of the skin or mucosa. A pulsation or thrill may be felt.
- Location—the majority (69%) of the lesions occur in the midface. The most common sites affected are the cheek (31%), ear (16%), and nose (11%).
- Radiology:

  CT scan—this imaging technique can be used to visualize bony changes, asymmetries, or cortical thickening caused by the lesions.

  MRI scan—this is a noninvasive and reliable method of imaging arteriovenous malformations. MRI findings include serpiginous flow voids on both T1- and T2-weighted images resulting from the high-flow lesion. Magnetic resonance angiography (MRA) imaging can also be used to noninvasively create a three-dimensional angiogram, although the information obtained through this method is not as detailed and dynamic as that obtained through conventional (invasive) angiographic methods.
- Natural progression—these lesions are present at birth, but they can become clinically apparent much later in life, not uncommonly during early adulthood. They typically show a slow and relentless growth, which eventually can cause skin ulceration and intermittent hemorrhage to occur.

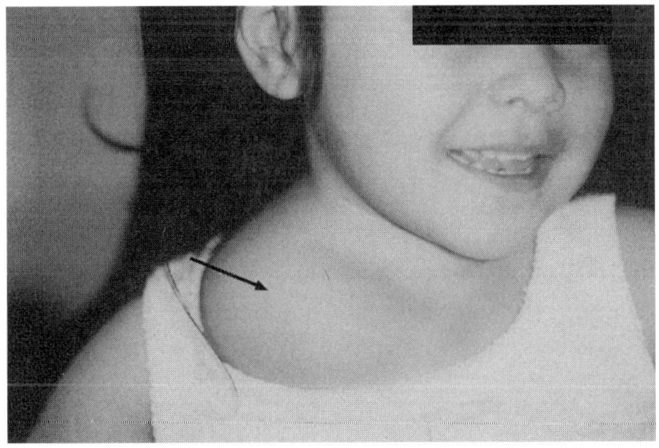

Figure 2 Macrocystic cervical lymphatic malformation (arrow).

- Treatment—combined angiography/embolization/surgery. Surgery alone may result in life-threatening hemorrhage. Angiography/embolization alone may lead to vessel collateralization, and progressive enlargement of the vascular lesion. Embolization can also cause lesion necrosis that can lead to cutaneous necrosis. Ligation of the feeding vessels alone will similarly lead to vessel collateralization and progression of the lesion. Thus, multimodal therapy is indicated. Preoperative angiography and embolization should be performed approximately 24–48 hours prior to surgical resection of an arteriovenous malformation to visualize the extent of the lesion, the blood supply, the nidus of the malformation, collateral circulation, and to reduce intraoperative blood loss. Selective embolization should be performed on distal feeder vessels. This will increase the likelihood of devascularizing the lesion preoperatively.

57

Pediatric Head and Neck Tumors

Robert A. Williamson, M.D., and Nina L. Shapiro, M.D.
David Geffen School of Medicine at UCLA, Los Angeles, California, U.S.A.

I. ANATOMIC CONSIDERATIONS

A. Triangles of the neck (Fig. 1).

B. Nodal groups and lymphatic drainage (Fig. 2).

C. Fascial layers-infectious/inflammatory processes may involve one or more compartments:

- Superficial layer envelops superficial musculature, nodes, and the external jugular (EJ) vein.
- Deep layer subdivides into a superficial investing layer, pretracheal layer, and deep prevertebral layer.

II. TUMOR CLASSIFICATION

A. Congenital Lesions

Branchial anomalies are most common (2nd > 1st > 3rd/4th branchial clefts).

B. 1st Branchial Anomalies (10–15%)

1. External auditory canal (EAC) aplasia/duplication, with or without pinna deformity.
2. Presents as chronic otorrhea or infected cyst.
3. Treatment is excision with dissection of the facial nerve.

C. 2nd Branchial Anomalies (80%)

1. Present from birth to 10 years of age; rarely in adulthood.
2. Typically presents as a neck mass anterior to the sternocleidomastoid (SCM) muscle, with or without inflammation or chronic drainage.
3. Fistula tract originates in the tonsillar fossa.
4. Diagnosis confirmed by computed tomography (CT) or magnetic resonance imaging (MRI).
5. Treatment is antibiotics to reduce inflammation; excision including tract (courses between internal and external carotid arteries, lateral to cranial nerve IX and XII, to the tonsillar fossa).

D. 3rd and 4th Branchial Anomalies

1. Rare.
2. Anterior to the SCM muscle and inferior to 2nd branchial anomalies.
3. Tract is superficial to cranial nerve X and common carotid artery, loops over cranial nerve XII, and opens into the pyriform sinus.

E. Lymphatic/Vascular Malformations (See Also Chapter 56)

1. Etiology is unclear.
2. Embryonic lymphatic spaces coalesce into channels that drain into the venous system.
3. Regional failure of drainage leads to dilatation.
4. Lymphatic malformations:
   - Most common in the head and neck regions.
   - Can be large and can obstruct the airway.

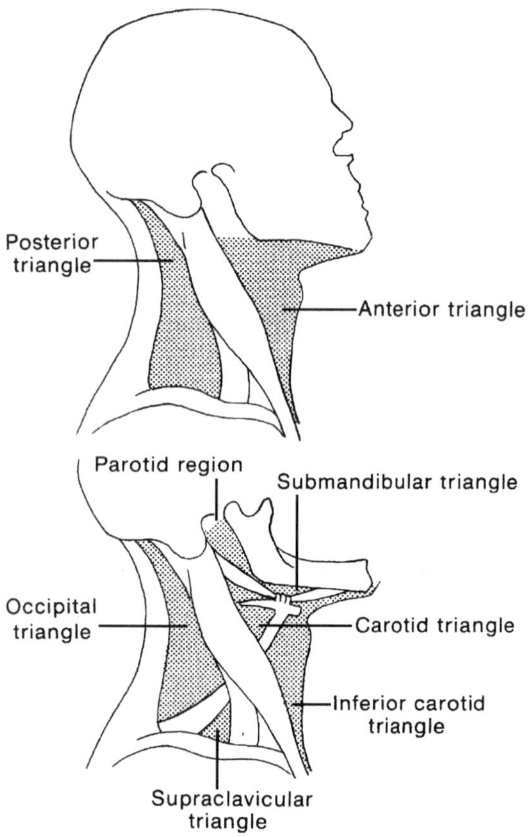

Figure 1 Triangles of the neck. (Adapted from Bluestone CD; Stool SE; Kenna MA. *Pediatric Otolaryngology*. 3rd ed. Philadelphia: WB Saunders, 1996, p. 1472.)

- Present in the perinatal period as large, soft, cystic lesions without inflammation.
- These lesions transilluminate when light is applied to the surface.
- May be asymptomatic or may be large enough to threaten the airway.
- Treatment is to secure the airway if necessary; excision with preservation of vital structures.
- Recurrence following resection is common.
- Sclerosing agents are useful when the lesion approximates vital structures.

F. Congenital Muscular Torticollis

- Unilateral fibrosis of SCM leads to contracture, with palpable fibrous tumor within 10 days after birth.
- Can progress in size
- Head tilts to ipsilateral side, with chin elevating to the contralateral side.
- CT/MRI confirm diagnosis.
- Treatment is passive stretching 4–6 times per day. If conservative therapy fails, the SCM is divided. Untreated, 60–70% will develop craniofacial asymmetry.

III. INFECTIOUS/INFLAMMATORY MASSES

Most common cause of masses/tumors in the head and neck is infection/inflammation. Infection may accompany neoplastic processes due to tumor necrosis or hemorrhage.

A. Cervical Lymphadenopathy (LAD)

LAD is a nonspecific enlargement of a lymph node or nodal group. Most commonly, LAD is due to infection (viral, bacterial, atypical bacterial, fungal, and rarely parasitic in origin).

1. Viral:
   - Adenoviruses, rhinoviruses, and enteroviruses.
   - LAD persists 5–10 days.
   - Epstein-Barr virus (EBV), varicella zoster virus (VZV), and HSV last longer.
   - Treatment is supportive.
   - HIV is also a common cause; 70% develop soft posterior LAD.
2. Bacterial:
   - Staphylococcus and Group A Streptococcus are the most common pathogens, with anaerobes causing 5% of infections.
   - Enteric/Gram-negative bacteria are seen more commonly in the perinatal period.
   - LAD can coalesce, suppurate, and cause local or systemic complications.
   - Ages 1–5 are the most commonly affected.
   - Submandibular and superior deep nodes are the most common locations.
   - Treatment is antibiotics (PO for 10 days, IV if systemic symptoms or large size). Aspiration is performed for small abscesses. Surgical drainage is recommended if large or multilocular nodes, or if patient is toxic.
3. Atypical mycobacterial (e.g., *M. avium intracellulare, M. scrofulaceum*):
   - Nodes are erythematous, nontender, and may drain.

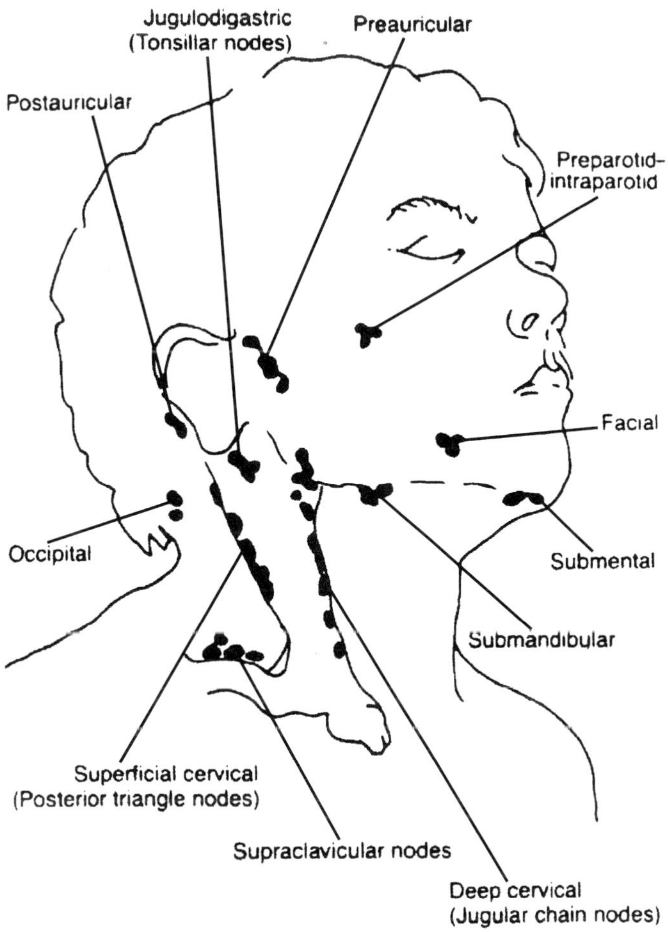

Figure 2 Nodal groups. (From Bluestone CD; Stool SE; Kenna MA. *Pediatric Otolaryngology*. 3rd ed. Philadelphia: WB Saunders, 1996, p. 1513.)

- Unilateral submandibular involvement is common.
- PPD testing is equivocal; diagnosis relies on culture.
- Treatment is antibiotics, with curettage or surgical excision sparing vital structures in some cases.
- Tuberculous LAD (scrofula) is low in the neck and bilateral. PPD is positive; treatment is anti-TB medications.

B. Fascial Space Infections

1. Require aggressive therapy: IV antibiotics and possible surgical drainage.
2. Primary spaces include the peritonsillar, parapharyngeal, retropharyngeal, and prevertebral "danger" space.
3. Can communicate with other sites (e.g., mediastinum) and may compromise the airway.

C. Inflammatory—Kawasaki's Disease

1. Multisystem vasculitis presenting with fever, adenopathy, conjunctivitis, "strawberry" tongue, and rash.
2. Prompt diagnosis and treatment with high-dose aspirin and IV immunoglobulin is required to avoid devastating coronary artery aneurysms and myocardial infarction.

IV. NEOPLASTIC LESIONS

A. 5% originate in the head and neck, and 25% of all malignancies eventually involve the region.

B. Most common sites are: neck > oropharynx > nasopharynx > orbit > salivary glands > face and scalp > auricular region.

C. These present as asymptomatic masses, LAD, otalgia, rhinorrhea or otorrhea, nasal obstruction, hoarseness, or stridor.

D. Mass fixation or firmness, rapid growth, large size, and neonatal onset are more worrisome for malignancy.

E. Posterior masses are malignant more often than anterior masses.

F. Imaging (CT, MRI), biopsy, and examination under anesthesia are important.

A. Benign Tumors

See above causes of nonmalignant masses of the head and neck.

B. Malignant Tumors

1. Hodgkin's Disease (HD)

a. Occurs in adolescence and young adulthood. Rare in children <5 years of age. Male:female ratio is 2:1.

b. >90% of cases originate in lymph nodes; extranodal disease occurs in late stages.

c. Asymmetric, firm, rubbery, and nontender cervical or supraclavicular adenopathy.

d. Mediastinal involvement is common and can obstruct the tracheobronchial tree or superior vena cava.

e. Histology: Reed-Sternberg cells.

f. Categories: nodular sclerosis (2/3 of cases), lymphocyte predominance and mixed (both more common <10 years), and lymphocyte depletion (rare, worst prognosis).

g. Ann Arbor Staging system:

- I—single site
- II—2 sites, same side of diaphragm
- III—sites on both sides of diaphragm, with or without extranodal diseases
- IV—disseminated
- Subtypes—A is no constitutional symptoms, B with constitutional symptoms

h. Staging: CT imaging of the thorax, abdomen, and pelvis. Possible laparotomy for biopsies, and bone marrow biopsy in stages III–IV.

i. Treatment varies with stage:

- Radiation therapy (XRT) for stages I–II
- XRT + chemotherapy for stage III
- Chemotherapy alone for stage IV
- Cure rates are 90% for stages II and I, 35–60% for stages III and IV

2. Non-Hodgkin's Lymphoma (NHL)

a. Most common between 2 and 12 years of age; male > female.

b. Usually presents as asymptomatic LAD in cervical/supraclavicular nodes. Mediastinal nodes are commonly involved, as are extranodal sites.

c. Diagnosis is by biopsy (usually excision).

d. Ann Arbor staging is applied after abdominal CT imaging, bone marrow biopsy, and skeletal survey.

e. Treatment is less effective than for HD and includes XRT for stage I, but relies on chemotherapy for stages II–IV.

f. Prognosis varies with stage, but is less optimistic than for HD.

3. Burkitt's Lymphoma

a. NHL subtype is endemic in Africa and is associated with EBV.

b. Presents as facial or jaw mass.

c. Progresses rapidly.

d. Requires rapid evaluation and treatment with chemotherapy.

4. Rhabdomyosarcoma

a. Most common soft tissue malignancy in children.

b. Represents 50–70% of all sarcomas.

c. Approximately 35% occur in the head and neck and 2/3 of cases present by age 12.

d. Caucasians are affected 4 times more often than non-Caucasians.

e. Histologic subtypes:

- Alveolar—adolescents
- Pleomorphic—adults
- Embryonic—infants and young children
- Botryoid—embryonic variant; affect infants and young children

f. Sites in head and neck: orbit > nasopharynx > middle ear/mastoid > sinonasal areas.

g. Symptoms:

- Progressive unilateral proptosis for orbital tumors.
- Unilateral rhinorrhea.
- Nasal obstruction or otitis media for nasal cavity/nasopharyngeal tumors.
- Skull base and cranial nerve involvement occurs rapidly.

h. CT/MRI and LP are required for evaluation.

i. Metastases occur via lymphatic or hematogenous routes. 8–15% have cervical or distant metastases on presentation (less common in orbital tumors, <5%).

j. Staging system according to Intergroup Rhabdomyosarcoma Study (IRS) protocol:

- Group I: localized disease, complete resection, no regional nodes involved.
- Group II: microscopic residual disease, or regional disease completely resected.
- Group III: incomplete resection; gross residual disease.
- Group IV: metastatic.

k. Treatment (also by IRS) is multimodal:

- Surgical resection is performed to achieve maximal debulking without sacrificing vital structures or function, or to eliminate post-op XRT
- XRT is used for sites not amenable to resection.
- Postop chemotherapy (protocols vary with stage) is given to nearly all patients with head and neck disease.
- Prognosis is best for orbital tumors (2-year survival in Groups I-III is 70–90%, Group IV is 35 40%), followed by non-parameningeal sites (3-year survival is 75% for all groups). Parameningeal sites (e.g., nasopharyngeal, middle ear/mastoid, or infratemporal fossa) have the worst prognosis due to more frequent skull base, meningeal, or CNS involvement.
- Vigilant post-treatment follow-up is needed.

5. Other Sarcomas

Fibrosarcoma, synovial, neurofibrosarcoma, Kaposi's.

6. Thyroid Carcinoma

a. Uncommon.

b. May have history of radiation exposure in the past.

c. Present as asymptomatic, anterior neck mass. Greater than 50% have metastases.

d. Thyroid scan and fine needle aspiration for diagnosis.

e. Treatment is surgical excision. May require nodal dissection and post-operative radioactive I^{131} ablation therapy.

f. Prognosis is good.

7. Salivary Neoplasms

a. Uncommon.

b. Present in adolescence and young adulthood as asymptomatic, firm mass.

c. Pathology and natural history mimic that of adult salivary tumors.

d. Parotid is the most common site.

e. 50% of nonvascular lesions are malignant.

f. Biopsy is required for diagnosis.

g. Treatment is usually surgical excision.

8. Neuroblastoma

a. Most common infant malignancy in children <1 year of age, with 90% <10 years.

b. Head and neck involvement may represent metastasis from abdominal sites.

c. 60–70% of cases have metastases at diagnosis.

d. Primary cervical cases (cervical sympathetic plexus) are rare (<5%).

9. Other Neoplasms

a. Epithelial malignancy is rare.

b. Basal cell carcinoma and melanoma may be familial in xeroderma pigmentosa or dysplastic nevus syndrome.

c. Malignant teratomas are present at birth; 9% occur in the head and neck.

58

Chest Wall and Breast Deformities

Eric W. Fonkalsrud, M.D., Steven R. Beanes, M.D., and William W. Shaw, M.D.
David Geffen School of Medicine at UCLA, Los Angeles, California, U.S.A.

I. EMBRYOLOGY OF STERNAL DEVELOPMENT

A. Sternum appears before the second month of intrauterine development.

B. Develops as bilaterally paired cartilaginous condensations of mesenchyme, independent of the ribs.

C. Condensations migrate toward the midline and fuse.

D. Sternum is divided into three segments:

- Manubrium
- Body (gladiolus)
- Xiphoid

E. Failure of the embryonic sternal bars to meet and fuse in the midline results in a sternal cleft (bifid sternum or congenital sternal fissure).

- May be partial (upper or lower) or complete.
- Ectopia Cordis: Bifid lower sternum associated with the heart being positioned outside the chest wall; one component of pentalogy of Cantrell.

II. PECTUS EXCAVATUM

A. Introduction

1. Pectus excavatum is inherited through either parent, though not clearly as a recessive trait.
2. Occurs in as many as 1 in 500 births.
3. Uncommon in African Americans and Hispanics.
4. Congenital anomaly of the anterior thorax is characterized by a prominent posterior (concave) curvature of the body of the sternum, usually involving its lower half to two thirds, with its deepest point just cephalad to the junction with the xiphoid.
5. Lower costal cartilages bend posteriorly to form a depression.
6. Asymmetry of the defect is common, with concavity slightly deeper on the right.
7. Associated with multiple disorders:
   - Functional heart murmur = 24%
   - Scoliosis = 16%
   - Mitral valve prolapse = 8%
   - Congenital heart disease = 3%

B. Pathogenesis

1. Remains unclear, but not associated with rickets.
2. Several theories have been suggested. The most promising postulate is unbalanced growth in the costochondral regions.
3. Involved cartilages may be fused, bizarrely deformed, or rotated.
4. Resected segments occasionally show disorderly arrangement of chondrocytes, perichondritis, and areas of aseptic necrosis.

C. Symptoms

1. The deformity is apparent soon after birth, progresses during early childhood, and becomes more pronounced during adolescence.
2. Deep inspiration accentuates the deformity.
3. Early childhood—symptoms are uncommon.
4. Early adolescence:
   - Easy fatigability.
   - Decreased stamina and endurance reported by 67% of patients.
5. Moderate to severe deformity:
   - The heart is displaced into the left chest.
   - Pulmonary expansion during inspiration is moderately confined.
   - Wider diaphragmatic excursions are necessary for ventilation during exercise.
6. Related conditions:
   - There is an appreciable incidence of chronic bronchitis, asthma, and bronchiectasis.
   - Respiratory infections are frequent in over one third of patients.
   - At least one fourth of patients experience a compression discomfort in the ower anterior chest.

D. Quantification of Severity

1. Several methods have been proposed, although none are widely accepted. Most include measuring the distance between the sternum and the spine and comparing this to the width of the chest.
   - The distance between the posterior sternum and anterior spine should be measured at the level of the manubrium and also at the level of the maximal lower sternal depression, as noted on a lateral chest x-ray or CT scan.
   - The pectus severity score is determined by measuring the width of the chest divided by the distance between the posterior surface of the sternum and the anterior surface of the spine (normal chest = 2.56).
2. Echocardiographic abnormalities are common:
   - Restricted cardiac stroke volume.
   - Right axis deviation.
   - Mitral valve prolapse is present in approximately 10% of patients.
3. Pulmonary function tests:
   - Almost always in the normal range while at rest; abnormal during exercise (e.g., treadmill, stationary bicycle).
   - Studies have shown an improvement in maximal voluntary ventilation after surgical repair.
   - Previous studies have shown that the restricted cardiac volume and the increased work of breathing that have been reported in pectus excavatum patients can be ameliorated by operative repair. Thus, although the deformity is cosmetically unattractive, the major indication for surgical repair is physiologic.

E. Treatment

1. Operative repair for moderate to severe deformity is preferred between 6 and 19 years of age because of the technical ease, minimal discomfort, short hospitalization, rapid return to full activity, and excellent long-term results.
2. Segments of the deformed costal cartilage are dissected from the perichondrium medially and laterally and removed, carefully preserving the entire perichondrial sheaths and the major portion of the cartilages.
3. The lower deformed portion of the sternum is mobilized, and a transverse wedge osteotomy is made through the anterior table at the level where the sternum begins to depress.
4. The posterior table of the sternum is fractured, but not detached, and then elevated to the desired position, where it is secured with nonabsorbable sutures. Care is taken to maintain good blood supply to avoid necrosis of the distal segment.
5. A thin stainless steel support bar is placed transversely across the anterior chest and wired to a rib on each side to support the inferior-most portion of the sternum.
   - The bar greatly reduces the frequency of recurrent depression.
   - The bar provides immediate stability to the chest, which reduces pain, permits deeper respiratory movements, and allows early discharge.
   - The bar is removed in 6 months as an outpatient procedure.

6. The right pleural space is routinely opened widely for drainage, and a small chest tube is used for 24 hours.
7. Minimal access surgery (Nuss Procedure) is an alternative to the open procedure described above.
   - This procedure involves placing a curved support bar through the chest between the sternum and heart, via two lateral 2.5 cm incisions in the axillary line and forcefully rotating it anteriorly to elevate the sternal defect. The sternal support bar remains in place for at least 2 years.
   - Stated benefits of the procedure include avoidance of an anterior chest wall incision, avoidance of the need to resect costal cartilages, and the avoidance of a sternal osteotomy.
   - Pain with the Nuss procedure is much more severe and hospitalization is longer than with the open surgical repair. Approximately 15–20% require removal of the bar within several weeks because of pain.
   - Approximately 9–33% of all patients in recent series required reoperation for sternal bar complications, including flipping of the bar and iatrogenic carinatum deformity.
   - The morbidity and mortality with this technique is higher, with at least 2 patients having perforation of the heart, with one known death.
   - A relatively small number of the sternal bars have been removed, therefore the long-term results of this technique are not known.

F. Postoperative Care

1. Hospitalization rarely exceeds 3 days and is usually 2 days for younger children.
2. The chest should be protected from direct trauma for 4–6 months.
3. Periosteal regeneration of new cartilage is usually complete within 2 months after the operation.
4. Extensive physical activity using the pectoralis and upper abdominal muscles should be avoided for approximately 8 weeks postoperatively.

G. Results

1. Recurrence rate—fewer than 2% of patients develop recurrence when sternal support bars are used.
2. Complications are infrequent:
   - The main complications include seromas, pleural effusion, atelectasis, and hypertrophic scar.
   - Unintentional pneumothorax occurs in less than 2% of cases.
   - Occasionally, protrusion of one or more upper thoracic costal cartilages occurs, which may warrant later subperiosteal resection.
   - Mortality is less than 0.2% with pectus excavatum repair.

III. PECTUS CARINATUM

A. Introduction

1. Pectus carinatum is characterized by forward projection of the sternum. The resultant appearance is similar to that of the keel of a boat.
2. Protrusion deformities occur approximately 6 times less frequently than depression deformities.
3. The deformity is often mild or imperceptible in early childhood and becomes prominent during early adolescence for 90% of patients. In approximately 10%, the protrusion becomes apparent and symptomatic during the first 2–3 years of life and involves the upper sternum.

B. Pathogenesis

1. Stems from a misdirected growth of costal cartilages. The deformed cartilages push the sternum and xiphoid outward.
2. Two principal types are recognized:
   - Chondromanubrial: less than 10% of cases. The protuberance is maximal in the upper sternum, with the lower portion of the sternum directed posteriorly.
   - Chondrogladiolar: more than 90% of cases. The greatest prominence is in the lower portion of the sternum.

C. Symptoms

1. The majority of symptoms are respiratory.
2. The defect produces a rigid chest with an increased anteroposterior diameter:
   - The thorax is held in a position of partial inspiration with considerable increase in residual air volume.

- Respiratory efforts are inefficient and utilize extensive diaphragmatic excursions.

3. Increased incidence of asthma.

D. Treatment

1. Surgical treatment is variable because of the diversity of carinatum deformities.
2. Main principals for surgical correction of carinatum deformities include:
   - Resection of the segments of the deformed costal cartilage are dissected from the perichondrium both medially and laterally and removed, carefully preserving the entire perichondrial sheaths and the major portion of the cartilages.
   - Making a transverse osteotomy through the anterior table of the sternum and placing a wedge of costal cartilage to secure it in a more downward position.
   - Suprasternal or substernal support bar is used to stabilize the chest in the desired position.

E. Postoperative Care

1. Complications are minor and infrequent, and are similar to those for excavatum patients.
2. Wound catheter is removed in 72 hours.
3. Sternal support bar is removed within 6 months on an outpatient basis.

F. Results

1. Improvement in respiratory symptoms and ability to participate in athletic activities with increased stamina and endurance is almost universal.
2. Improvement is often more dramatic than after pectus excavatum repair.

IV. SKELETAL ANOMALIES

A. Various Deviations from the Normal Pattern of 12 Symmetric Ribs Occasionally Occur

1. Asphyxiating thoracic dystrophy of the newborn (Jeune's disease) is an extreme form of narrow and rigid thorax with multiple cartilaginous anomalies in which the patient experiences progressive respiratory insufficiency. This often results in death.
2. Infants with fusion of ribs or cartilages, or absence of ribs, often have severe limitations in respiratory movement. In association with severe spinal and cardiac defects, Jeune's disease often results in a high mortality rate.
   - Attempts at surgical correction have generally proven unsuccessful.
   - Long-term ventilatory support is often necessary.
   - Chest braces or splints are occasionally helpful.
   - These infants tend to develop recurrent pneumonias, with resultant interstitial fibrosis, pulmonary hypertension, and death.

B. Sprengel's Deformity

1. An anomaly in which the scapula is hypoplastic and fixed in an elevated position.
2. The hypoplastic scapula limits movement of the ipsilateral shoulder.

C. Poland's Syndrome

1. First described by Alfred Poland in 1841.
2. The combination of absence of the pectoralis major and minor muscles, ipsilateral breast hypoplasia, nipple/areola hypoplasia, and absence of segments of two to four ribs. Associated hand anomalies are also common (e.g., brachysyndactyly).
3. Approximate incidence is 1 in 20,000–30,000 live births.
4. Male:female incidence is 3:1.
5. 75% of cases occur on the right side.
6. Etiology is unknown, but is hypothesized to include a primary defect in proximal subclavian artery during fetal development.
7. The majority of the cases are sporadic, although a few familial cases have been identified.
8. Rib grafts from the contralateral thorax are commonly used to stabilize the chest wall during childhood.
9. Muscle flap transfer and breast reconstructions are usually performed during adolescence.

D. Supernumerary Ribs

1. Usually located in the cervical region.
2. May cause vascular compression in adolescence or adulthood.
3. Cervical ribs are associated with thoracic outlet syndrome.

59

Pediatric Genital Reconstruction

Gary J. Alter, M.D.
David Geffen School of Medicine at UCLA, Los Angeles, California, U.S.A.

I. ANATOMY OF THE PENIS

A. Layers

1. Skin—very thin, distensible, and hairless distally.
2. Dartos fascia—the superficial fascia of the penis that is a continuation of Scarpa's and Colles' fascia.
3. Buck's fascia—heavy elastic layer covering the corpora cavernosa and corpus spongiosum. It encloses the deep dorsal vein, dorsal arteries, and dorsal nerves.
4. Tunica albuginea—elastic firm tissue covering the corpora cavernosa.

B. Compartments

1. Corpora cavernosa:
   - The two erectile chambers that contain endothelium-lined spaces or sinusoids that fill with blood, causing an erection
   - Located in the dorsal/lateral portions of the penis
   - A permeable septum divides the two corpora
2. Corpus spongiosum.
   - Compartment that contains spongy tissue and the urethra
   - Located ventral to the corpora cavernosa
   - Connects to the glans or head of the penis
   - Contains the urethra
3. Urethra:
   - Within the corpus spongiosum until the urogenital septum
   - Membranous urethra—located between the bladder neck and the urogenital septum
   - Bulbar urethra—extends from the urogenital septum to the suspensory ligament
   - Penile urethra—distal to suspensory ligament

C. Arterial Supply

1. Internal Pudendal Arterial System—Paired
   a. The deep arterial supply is from the penile artery, which divides into four branches:
      - Bulbourethral artery
      - Urethral artery
      - Cavernous artery—provides increased flow for erection; located within each corpus cavernosum
      - Dorsal artery:

        Found on the dorsolateral surface, outside the tunica albuginea

        Runs within Buck's fascia

        Located between the deep dorsal vein medially and the dorsal nerve laterally

        Enters the glans of the penis distally

2. External Pudendal Arterial System

a. Supplies the skin and dartos fascia.

b. Usually connects to the internal pudendal system only at the coronal sulcus.

D. Venous Supply

1. Superficial—the prepuce, skin, and dartos drain into the superficial dorsal veins, which then subsequently drain into the saphenous veins.
2. Intermediate—the glans, corpus spongiosum, and distal corpora cavernosa drain into the deep dorsal and circumflex veins.
3. Deep—includes the cavernous, crural, and bulbar veins. This complex network of veins drain into the internal pudendal vein.

E. Nerve Supply

1. Dorsal nerves from the pudendal nerves:
   - Paired nerves on the dorsal-lateral penis within Buck's fascia
   - Sensory erogenous nerves to the glans of the penis
2. Cavernous nerves—provide autonomic nerve supply for erections.

II. ANATOMY OF THE SCROTUM

A. Two layers:

- Skin—rugous, well-vascularized skin with sweat and sebaceous glands
- Dartos—nonstriated muscle

III. CHORDEE WITHOUT HYPOSPADIAS

A. Defined as a downward curvature of the penis on erection.

B. Can be painful.

C. Most curves are ventral, but can directed laterally or dorsally.

D. Meatus is found on the glans.

E. Variations:

- Deficient spongiosum—urethra is a thin tube; most severe
- Normal spongiosum with abnormal Buck's fascia and dartos fascia
- Abnormal dartos tethering the penis with normal Buck's fascia, urethra, and spongiosum

F. Surgical correction:

- Artificial erection
- Deglove the penis
- Determine the anatomy
- Skin-dartos defect:

  Mild—usually corrected with degloving and release of the tethering tissue

  More severe—plicate the tunica albuginea on the convex side of the curvature; release the tunica albuginea on the concave side and apply a dermal graft to the corporal defect; reconstruct a short urethra

IV. HYPOSPADIAS

A. Characteristics

1. Defined as an abnormal congenital opening of the urethra upon the undersurface of the penis.
2. Urethral meatus—can be located anywhere from the perineum to the proximal glans.
3. Dorsal hood—secondary to absence of ventral foreskin.
4. Chordee:
   - Ventral curvature
   - Usually less severe the more distal the urethra
5. The glans of the penis is often flat, grooved, or dimpled.

B. Repair

Depends on severity of the hypospadias:

1. Chordee must be corrected prior to performing any definitive urethral repair.
2. Subcoronal meatus:
   - Usually no chordee or chordee is corrected with skin degloving
   - MAGPI—meatal advancement and glansplasty

C. Distal Hypospadias

1. Meatal-based flap (Mathieu procedure):
   - Ventral-based penile shaft skin is flipped distally and sutured to a parallel glans incision

- An intermediate layer of tissue is placed over the suture line
- Glans flaps are then sutured over the urethral closure

2. Tubularized incised urethral plate urethroplasty:
   - Penis skin is degloved
   - Parallel incisions are made on the each side of the urethral plate
   - A midline incision made in the urethral plate from the meatus to the glans tip
   - Urethral plate is tubularized over a catheter
   - Subcutaneous tissue from the dorsal hood covers the urethral closure
   - Glans flaps are closed

D. Mid- and Distal Hypospadias

1. Onlay preputial flaps:
   - Urethral plate is outlined with parallel incisions
   - An island flap is mobilized from the inner prepuce on a dartos pedicle
   - The island flap is transposed ventrally and sutured to the urethral plate
   - Subcutaneous tissue is used as an intermediate layer
   - Glans flaps are closed
2. Tubularized preputial flap:
   - No urethral plate
   - Flap is mobilized from the inner prepuce on a dartos pedicle
   - Flap is tubularized and anastomosed to the proximal urethra and then brought distally
   - Remainder is similar to onlay preputial flap technique

E. Proximal and Complex Hypospadias

1. Severe chordee and proximal urethra.
2. First stage of repair:
   - Circumferential incision at the coronal sulcus
   - Release and correct the chordee (see above), which releases the urethra proximally
   - The glans is divided in the midline to the tip
   - Dorsal foreskin is unfolded and divided in the midline
   - The foreskin is transposed to fill the ventral penis
3. Second stage of repair:
   - Wait 6–12 months
   - Ventral strip is tubularized from the meatus to the tip and then closed
   - Suture line is covered with a tunica vaginalis flap
   - Glans flaps are closed
   - Skin is closed

F. Hypospadias Complications

1. Urethrocutaneous fistula
2. Stricture
3. Diverticula
4. Persistent chordee
5. Urethral positioning too proximal
6. Buried penis
7. Hair within the urethra

G. Repair of Hypospadias Complications

1. Fistula repair
2. Repeat urethroplasty
3. Necessity for graft material to reconstruct urethra:
   - Buccal mucosa
   - Split thickness skin graft urethroplasty, a two-stage operation
4. Cecil operation—temporarily burying the tubularized urethra in the scrotum due to inadequate penile skin

V. CONGENITAL ANOMALIES OF THE SCROTUM

A. Penoscrotal transposition:
   - Usually associated with penoscrotal or perineal hypospadias
   - Correction performed at time of hypospadias repair or in stages

B. Ectopic scrotum

C. Penoscrotal webbing or fusion

VI. EPISPADIAS

A congenital opening of the urethra on the dorsum of the penis or abnormal urethral opening within a fissure of the clitoris.

A. Types:

1. Glanular—defect in covered penis.
2. Severe—penopubic type with incontinence.
3. Complete—associated with bladder exstrophy.

B. Classification:

1. Classified according to the position of the dorsally displaced urethral meatus.
2. Meatus may be located in the glans, penile shaft, or penopubic region.
3. All have various degree of a dorsal chordee.
4. Penopubic type—entire penile urethra is open and bladder neck is gaping.
   - Pubic symphysis is divergent
   - Deficiency of the external urinary sphincter
   - Short penis with severe dorsal chordee
5. Female epispadias:
   - Bifid clitoris
   - Flattening of the mons pubis
   - Separation of the labia
   - Severity ranges from a patulous meatus to a cleft throughout the entire urethral length with an incompetent sphincter

C. Surgical Treatment

1. Goals

a. Reconstruct function and maximize cosmetic appearance:
   - Correct the dorsal chordee
   - Urethral reconstruction
   - Glanular reconstruction
   - Penile skin coverage

b. Repaired at 2 years of age

2. Surgical Procedures

a. Cantwell-Ransley repair

b. Complete penile disassembly

VII. MICROPENIS

A. Normally formed penis that is more than 2 standard deviations below the mean in size.

B. Treatment—possible free flap phalloplasty (see Chapter 96).

VIII. HIDDEN PENIS (BURIED, CONCEALED, INCONSPICUOUS)

A. Multiple Etiologies

1. Abnormally large suprapubic fat pad extending into the scrotum.
2. Dense dysgenetic dartos fascial bands that tether and retract the penis inward.
3. Lack of normal adhesions between Scarpa's and Buck's fascia. The penis retracts into the fat, while the penile skin drapes over the glans and shaft.
4. Removal of too much penile skin on circumcision:
   - Often occurs on congenital buried penis
   - Shaft skin is removed and preputial skin is often kept intact
   - Penis retracts into the suprapubic fat
   - A constricting ring can occur at the circumcision incision line, which buries the penis
   - Secondary circumcision can worsen the condition
5. Chronic inflammation of the penile skin that causes retraction.

B. Operative Techniques

1. Depends on the etiology.
2. Buried penis with adequate normal shaft skin-treatment options include:
   - Suprapubic tacking of the subcutaneous tissue of the penopubic junction to the rectus fascia
   - Possible limited suprapubic lipectomy
   - Tacking of the penoscrotal subdermal dartos fascia to the tunica albuginea, with possible penoscrotal Z-plasty.
3. Buried penis without adequate normal shaft skin-treatment options include:
   - Release circumferential circumcision scar:

     Inner preputial layer may be available for coverage of the penile shaft

Small Z-plasties may be necessary at the circumcision scar

- Thick split thickness skin graft is indicated if insufficient shaft skin is found—performed as a last resort

IX. MAYER-ROKITANSKY-KUSTER-HAUSER SYNDROME

A. Characteristics

1. Developmental deficiency of the Müllerian ductal system.
2. Absence or shortening of the vagina and usually absence of the uterus.
3. May have an increased incidence of renal deformities.

B. Presentation

1. Absence of menses.
2. If uterus present, may present with hematometrocolpos.

C. Surgical Procedures Usually Performed in Mid-Teenage Years

1. Vaginoplasty with full thickness skin graft
2. Pudendal thigh flap
3. Rectosigmoid vaginoplasty
4. Less common:
    - Gracilis myocutaneous flaps
    - Rectus abdominis flap

X. FEMALE AMBIGUOUS EXTERNAL GENITALIA

A. Etiology

1. Female pseudohermaphroditism—most common; due to congenital adrenal hyperplasia:
    - Enzyme defect in normal pathway of steroid biosynthesis
    - Overproduction of androgenic steroids
    - Masculinization of genitalia
2. Other causes:
    - True hermaphroditism
    - Male pseudohermaphroditism
    - Mixed gonadal dysgenesis

B. Timing

Can be as early as 2–3 months old.

C. Surgery

1. Clitoroplasty

a. Goals:

- Feminization
- Preservation of function and sensation
- Cosmetic appearance

2. Procedure

a. Decrease clitoral length and diameter by removing the corporal bodies
b. Decrease size of the glans
c. Recess the glans
d. Preserve the dorsal nerves and vessels of the clitoris
e. Perform vaginal and labial reconstruction at the same time or in a delayed fashion

3. Labioplasty

Labia minora are created from skin of the prepuce and clitoral shaft.

4. Vaginoplasty

a. Flap vaginoplasty to exteriorize a low vagina
b. Pull-through vaginoplasty for high level of vaginal confluence

XI. CONCLUSION

A. Challenging
B. Depends on solid knowledge of anatomy
C. Cosmetic appearance and function should always be considered

60

General Approach to Microsurgery

Reid V. Mueller, M.D.
Oregon Health and Science University, Portland, Oregon, U.S.A.

Balvantray Arora, M.D.
Stony Brook University Hospital, Stony Brook, New York, U.S.A.

Galvin M. Dry, M.D.
Kirkland, Washington, U.S.A.

Nicholas B. Vedder, M.D.
University of Washington, Seattle, Washington, U.S.A.

Since the first microsurgical procedure in 1960, microsurgical techniques have evolved significantly. Microsurgery is surgery performed under magnification provided by an operating microscope. The microscope has led to improved results with conventional operative procedures and to the introduction of new techniques for conditions previously considered irreparable. Microsurgery is clinically applicable in nearly every surgical specialty. In order to achieve success with microsurgery, one must have appropriate instruments and must be facile with the necessary techniques.

I. EVOLUTION

Microsurgery literally means surgery in which a microscope is used. The word microscope is derived from the Greek words *micros* (small) and *skopein* (to view) and includes any instrument that provides an enlarged image of an object. Commercial operating microscopes became available in 1953 and were quickly adopted across numerous surgical specialties.

II. EQUIPMENT

A. Operating Microscope

The operating microscope is necessary for most microsurgical operations. The essential features of an appropriate microscope for the plastic surgeon are:

1. Double-headed system allowing both the surgeon and assistant to view the operative field simultaneously under magnification.
2. A fiberoptic light source.
3. Motorized *x-y* axis control to allow motion of the microscope to different areas of the operative field.
4. Foot-, hand-, or voice-controlled zoom magnification and focusing. Magnification may vary from 4× to 40×, depending on the size of vessels repaired. Magnification at 10× is most common. Surgical loupes are occasionally more practical than an operating microscope, especially for microdissection. Loupe magnification for microsurgery varies from 2.5× to 6×.

5. Interchangeable objective lenses are available to match the working distance and magnification range to the clinical situation. A 200 mm focal length lens is most commonly utilized.

B. Microsurgical Instruments

1. In microsurgery, virtually all surgical movements have been reduced to a pinch mechanism between thumb and index finger, guiding movement by direct vision rather than by "feel."
2. Microsurgical instruments are characterized by small precision tips, lightweight balanced proportions, graded pinch closure, and a dull nonreflective surface.
3. These instruments must be meticulously cleaned, constantly protected, and frequently demagnetized.
4. The essential microsurgical instruments are:
   - Forceps: Jeweler's forceps are available in different lengths and tip diameters.
   - Needle holders: Generally nonlocking with a gently curved tip.
   - Scissors: Both curved and straight should be available. Both dissection scissors and suture scissors are standard on most sets.
   - Vessel dilators: Two general types. The blunt angled probe or "hockey stick" is useful for larger vessels, while a specialized angled forceps tip is more useful for small vessels.
   - Clamps: Reusable and disposable clamps with a range of closing pressures are available. It is generally agreed that closing pressure of greater than 30 g/mm^2 produces marked endothelial trauma, and therefore 30 g clamps or less are used most frequently.
   - Clamp approximators: Two small atraumatic clamps mounted parallel on a rod with an adjustable inter-clamp distance. The primary purpose of approximators is to relieve the tension between retracted vessels, which facilitates a tension-free vascular anastomosis.
   - Irrigators: Angled 27 gauge anterior chamber irrigators used in ophthalmology are excellent irrigators for small digital vessels. For larger vessels, 25 gauge intravenous catheters may be used. The irrigator should be mounted on a 1–3 cc syringe or attached to extension tubing such that the scrub nurse or assistant may operate the syringe while the surgeon cannulates the vessel.
   - Background materials: Blue and green disposable soft plastic mats with millimeter markings help prevent surrounding soft tissue from entangling the suture or obscuring the needle and provide a working surface with good color contrast.
   - Small cellulose sponges: wedges of adsorptive material on small sticks.
   - Instrument cleaning sponge: Soft lint-free cleaning aid. It is important not to use gauze sponges to clean instruments because they will deposit lint on the instruments.
   - Accessory instruments:

     Small vascular hemoclips.

     Suction mat: similar to background material but with attached suction port to evacuate accumulated blood.

     Coagulators: Very fine-tipped bipolar coagulators may be helpful when dividing small vascular side branches during free flap harvest.

C. Microsutures

1. Virtually all microsutures used in plastic surgery are nonabsorbable nylon sutures. Prolene sutures are also used, but these have less strength and are not as easily visualized with the microscope.
2. For most applications, a BV-100 needle or equivalent will work. Tapered needles with a flattened central portion (for easier grasping) are preferred:
   - For vessels 0.5–1.0 mm in diameter, a 75–100 μm needle diameter is preferred.
   - For vessels 1–3 mm in diameter a 100–140 μm needle diameter is preferred.
   - For vessels >3 mm in diameter, a 130–150 μm needle diameter is preferred.
3. Suture should be as fine as possible with sufficient strength for the particular application. The nature and size of the suture depends on the size and consistency of the structure being repaired.

Structure size (mm)	Example	Suture size
Vessels		
0.5 1.0	Digital artery	11-0 or 10-0
1.0–2.0	Gracilis pedicle	10-0 or 9-0
2.0–3.0	Latissimus dorsi pedicle	9-0
	Rectus abdominis pedicle	9-0
3.0–4.0	Radial forearm pedicle	9-0
>4.0		9-0 or 8-0
Nerves		
0.5–2.0	Digital nerve	10-0 or 9-0
3.0–6.0	Median nerve, ulnar nerve	9-0

D. Positioning

1. Microscope should be positioned at a 90° angle to the anastomosis site
2. Surgeon and assistant should be placed 180° opposite to each other
3. Elbows should be flexed to 90°, while the forearms and hands should be on the same plane as the anastomosis site.
4. The ulnar sides of the hands are supported on folded towels.
5. Suturing should be performed with the MP, PIP, and DIP joints of the fingers, while the wrist and forearm remain stable.

III. MICROSURGICAL TECHNIQUES

A. Nerve Repair

1. Nerve repair often requires mobilization of the nerve to achieve tension-free approximation. If mobilization of 1–2 cm of nerve does not provide tension-free approximation, the temptation to pull the nerves together or to flex a joint to relieve tension should be avoided. In these circumstances, an interposition nerve graft is indicated.
2. The ends of the nerve should be sharply debrided back to healthy appearing nerve. The cut ends of the fascicles should be apparent and mushroom or bulge out of the cut end of the nerve. If they are not clearly seen, further debridement is needed. The epineurium should not be retracted away from the cut end or the individual fascicles will splay out.
3. The nerve may be approximated by suturing together any of the anatomic neural layers, but in practical terms only epineurial and epifascicular repairs are used.
4. Epineurial repair:
   - This repair is used for the majority of neural repairs, where motor and sensory fibers are not segregated into separate fascicles.
   - The nerves are aligned by matching epineurial vascular arcades and fascicle patterns, but individual fascicles are not directly approximated.
   - Sutures are placed into epineurium, initially subdividing the circumference of the nerve into thirds. Subsequent sutures may be placed between these initial sutures. Small nerves may only require 3–4 epineurial sutures.
5. Epifascicular repair:
   - This should be used where motor and sensory fibers are segregated into separate fascicles. This is the case, for example, in the median and ulnar nerves within 4 cm of the wrist crease.
   - The epineurium is slit open and the individual fascicles are dissected free for a short distance. One or two sutures are placed into the epifascicular epineurium of the corresponding fascicles. The epineurium is then approximated for strength.
6. Maintenance of approximation:
   - A period of immobilization is often recommended after nerve repair if slight tension is present. This is no substitute for nerve grafting and tension-free repairs, however.

B. Vascular Anastomosis

1. Hand-sewn anastomoses remain the gold standard for approximation of vessels.
2. The sutures can be placed in an interrupted, continuous, or combination fashion with equally good patency.
3. Repair only normal vessel segments. Resect vessel back to atraumatized vessel segments.
4. The basic steps are:
   - Gentle handling of tissues, especially vessels.
   - Dissection and isolation of the vessel from the surrounding tissue. Sufficient vessel

length is mobilized for tension-free repair. Vein graft if insufficient vessel length. Ensure that no kinking or twisting of the vessels exists.

- Ensure adequate inflow from the proximal vessel.
- Application of clamp to interrupt blood flow. Consider irrigation proximally and distally with 10 units heparin/mL prior to clamp application.
- Preparation of vessel—debridement of injured vessel wall (Fig. 1). Remember that avulsion injuries can damage deceptively long segments of vessel.
- Removal of adventitia from cut end of vessel. Any loose strands of adventitia that are entrapped in the anastomosis will be a nidus for thrombus formation.
- Mechanical dilatation with atraumatic vessel dilators to approximately 1.5 times normal.
- Prepared vessel walls and intima must appear normal prior to proceeding with suturing. Repairing injured vessels will result in thrombosis.

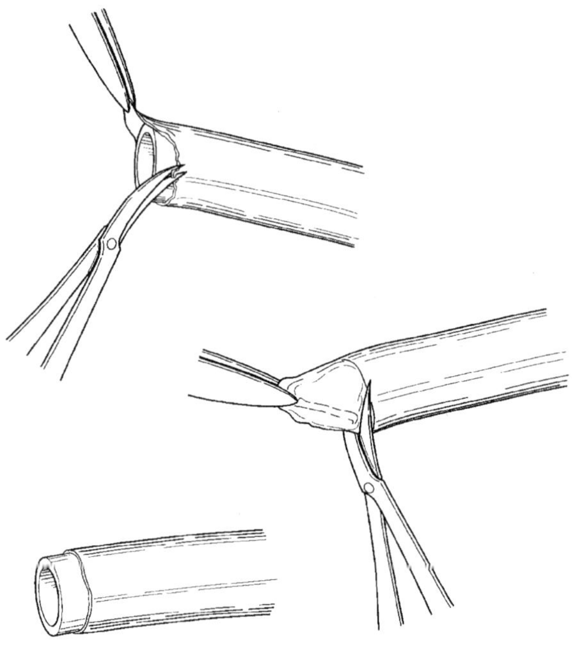

Figure 1 Periadvential tissue is carefully debrided for at least 2 mm from the initimal edge. With care taken not to handle the intima, a sleeve of periadventia is drawn towards the end of the vessel and then transected, leaving a clean initimal lining.

- Placement of sutures—(see below).
- Removal of vascular clamp to reestablish blood flow into the vessel.
- Check for patency. Check for flow across the anastomosis and for perfusion distally. You must be completely satisfied with the flow across the anastomosis and distal perfusion prior to leaving the operating room. It will not magically get better later. If in doubt, reevaluate the vessels and redo the anastomosis or consider a vein graft if necessary.

5. End-to-End Anastomosis (Fig. 2)

   - This repair is the most basic of all vascular anastomoses. Its principles and techniques can be extrapolated to many clinical situations.
   - After preparation of the vessels, sutures are placed 120° apart on the circumference of the anastomosis with subsequent addition of as many sutures as necessary between them. Too few sutures lead to bleeding and thrombosis, while too many cause unnecessary damage to the endothelium.
   - Place the needle through one vessel wall, visualize it in the gap, and then complete through the other vessel wall, using vessel dilators or jeweler's forceps to gently lift the opposite side open. Retrieve the needle in the vessel wall by rotating it out along its curvature, not simply forcing it forward. Avoid placing sutures that capture the back wall of the vessel.
   - After the first two sutures are placed, the clamp is rotated to expose the posterior wall of the vessel. The posterior wall is repaired first. Once the back wall is completed, the clamp is again rotated to expose the anterior wall. The lumen is inspected to ensure that no two-wall sutures have been placed. Placement of the final suture is critical, with care being taken to avoid catching the back wall with the suture. It is common to place the last two sutures as if performing a running suture. The loop between the two sutures is left long and not tightened. The intervening loop is then cut, and both sutures are tied.

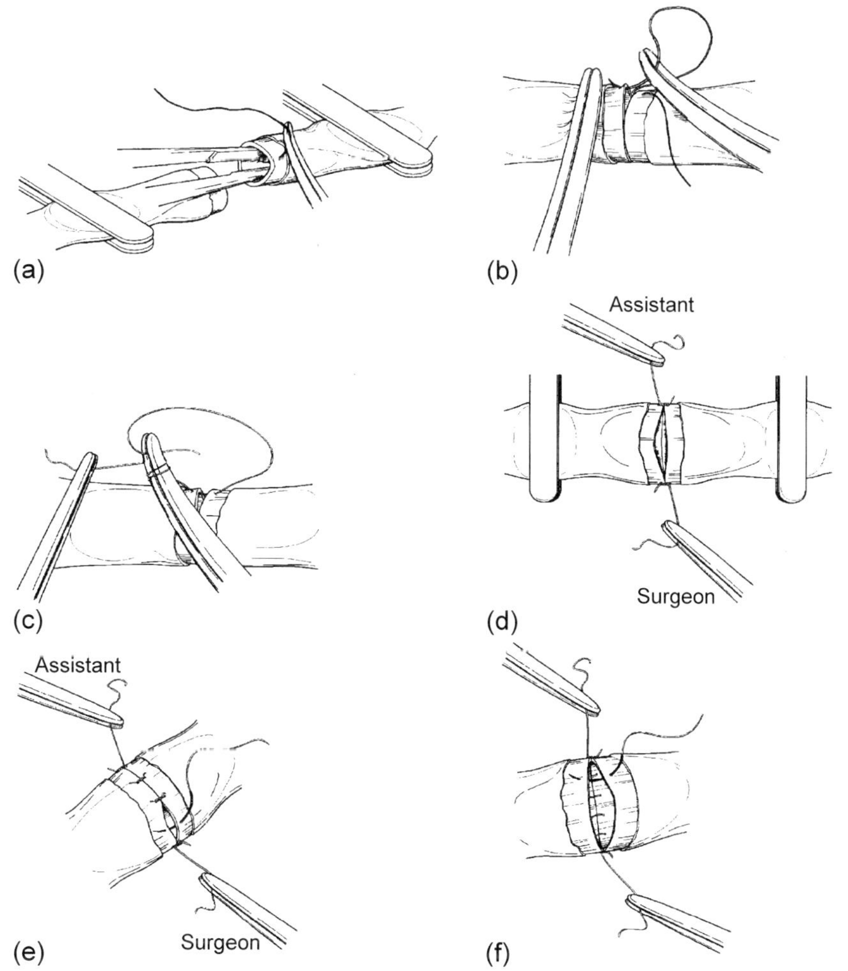

Figure 2 Standard end-to-end microsurgical anastomosis technique. (a) The needle should be aligned parallel to the vessel and the tip should enter perpendicular to the vessel wall. (b) The needle is pushed through the vessel wall, grasped on the other side, and pulled through following the curvature of the needle. (c) A surgeon's knot is placed, using a needle holder and forceps or two forceps. (d) Sutures are placed at 180° to each other and held to expose the lumen. (e) The vessels are rotated and the anastomosis is performed on the first side. (f) The vessel is rotated back to expose the anterior wall. Sutures are again placed to complete the anastomosis.

- Ensure that the needle tip is through all vessel wall layers with eversion of edges.
- Grasp only the adventitial tissues with forceps while suturing. Avoid handling the intima with forceps.
- In arteries, the vessel wall "bite" is 1–2 times the vessel wall thickness back from the edge of the vessel; 2–3 times for veins.
- A surgeon's knot is used for the first throw in arteries, followed by two square knots. A total of three knots is usually sufficient.
- On completion of the anastomosis, the distal clamp is removed first. Observe for back-filling in the vessel across the suture line. Some oozing from the site is normal. The proximal clamp is next removed and the vessel observed for forward flow through the anastomosis. Pulsatile bleeding from the suture line must be repaired with additional sutures. Bleeding from unligated side branches also needs to be controlled.
- Alternative techniques:

  Continuous running suture is acceptable for large vessels with minimal size discrepancy. Two stay sutures are placed at 180° opposite each other. Sutures are then run in continuous fashion down each side. This technique can be performed with either end-to-end or end-to-side anastomoses. Patency rates are equal when compared to interrupted sutures.

Back wall first—used with equal vessel size and when rotation of clamps is not possible or difficult. Begin with suture at point on back wall furthest away from the operating surgeon. Place interrupted sutures until the back wall is completed, then complete the anterior wall in usual fashion.

- Vessel size discrepancies:

  Free tissue transfers and situations requiring vein grafts often mandate end-to-end anastomosis between vessels of differing diameters. If the discrepancy is less than 50%, simple mechanical dilation will usually suffice.

  When faced with large discrepancies, an oblique cut of less than 30° of the smaller vessel is recommended. For two-fold or greater discrepancies, an end-to-side anastomosis or interposition vein graft is preferred.

6. End-to-side anastomosis:
   - This is an extremely flexible means of uniting vessels of markedly different diameters.
   - It is primarily used when the donor vessel cannot be sacrificed for the exclusive perfusion of the transferred tissue. This is a situation commonly seen in the mangled lower extremity with a single vessel supplying foot perfusion.
   - The recipient vessel is cleaned and placed in a double atraumatic vessel clamp.
   - The donor vessel is cut at a beveled angle to increase its diameter.
   - The incision in the primary recipient vessel is usually longitudinal. However, in vessels with thicker walls, excision of incised margins to create an elliptical or circular opening is helpful.
   - A 90° relationship of the two vessels is preferred.
   - The placement of sutures starts at the "toe" and "heel," followed by suturing the back wall or technically more demanding side first. The lumen can then be inspected prior to suturing the front wall.
7. Interposition vein graft:
   - Used when vessel ends cannot be approximated without excessive tension.
   - Greater distensibility allows vein grafts to accommodate size discrepancies better than arterial grafts. This can assist the surgeon in coupling mismatched arteries when a segment is placed end-to-end.
   - Vein grafts are also generally more available as donor vessels than arterial grafts. Common harvest sites include: saphenous, cephalic, basilic, dorsal foot, and hand. Local veins at the operative site are often used as well.
   - Most interposition vein grafts need to be reversed in order to allow flow through the valves.
8. Facilitated approaches to vascular anastomosis:
   - There is an increasing demand for an easier, quicker, less damaging, but reliable procedure to create a vascular anastomosis.
   - Coupling devices:

     Synovis Micro Companies Alliance (Birmingham, Alabama) markets a coupling device with four ring sizes with internal diameters of 1.0, 1.5, 2.0, and 2.5 mm to accommodate vessels of 0.8–3.0 mm diameters. Each vessel end is passed through a ring and the everted vessel wall fixed on protruding pins. The two rings are then united, thereby completing the anastomosis.

     The system is especially suitable for venous end-to-end anastomosis, as thicker arterial walls do not lend themselves as well to this technique. End-to-side anastomoses are possible, but technically more demanding.
   - Stapling and clipping devices:

     Commercial stapling devices crimp small metallic staples onto vessels, taking the place of sutures. These devices have found some application in larger vessels, but are not suitable for small arteries.

The application of these devices requires normal vessels with relatively long, free segments for eversion of the vessel ends for end-to-end anastomosis.

9. Assessment of vessel patency:
   - Direct inspection of vessels under microscope; vessels should appear full and dilated.
   - Check vessels to ensure no kinking or spasm; additionally strip periadventitial tissues or apply topical vasodilators as necessary.
   - Perform "empty and refill" or "distal milk" patency test only if absolutely necessary (technique is traumatic). Grasp and occlude vessel with 2 forceps distal to anastomosis, milk blood from lumen by moving forceps downstream approximately 1 cm, release proximal forceps and observe return of flow through vessel. This test is useful for any vessel of any size.

IV. MONITORING TECHNIQUES

Complications related to thrombosis usually occur within the first 24–48 h. Unrecognized anastomotic failure or failure to act promptly will result in tissue death. In general, the surgeon must identify the problem, return to the operating room, and fix the problem, all within 4–6 h. Therefore, the ideal monitoring technique should provide a continuous recording of tissue perfusion with immediate detection of arterial or venous occlusion. The criteria should be easily interpreted by nursing personnel or junior medical staff. In addition, the ideal system should allow monitoring of both visible and "buried" free flaps.

Tissue	Warm ischemia	Cold ischemia
Skin and subcutaneous	4–6 h	12 h
Muscle	<2 h	6–8 h
Bone	<3 h	24 h

The ability of tissue to survive an initial ischemia-reperfusion cycle decreases with each ischemic episode. Initial ischemia times are listed in the following, but subsequent schemic episodes are progressively less well tolerated. These times underscore the need for prompt identification and correction of anastomotic failure. Most microsurgeons suggest hourly "flap checks" for the first 48 h.

A. Clinical Observation

1. The gold standard for flap monitoring is clinical observation. This includes observation of skin color, capillary refill, tissue warmth, tissue turgor, and dermal bleeding. Blanching, pallor, delayed capillary refill, and loss of turgor are all suggestive of arterial insufficiency. In contrast, a bluish-purple appearance with rapid capillary refill and flap engorgement with oozing of venous blood from the periphery is indicative of venous occlusion.
2. The protocol for clinical observation varies from center to center, and the parameters are open to subjective interpretation, depending on the experience and judgment of the examining physician and staff.
3. Clinical observation cannot be applied to buried flaps unless a segment or island of tissue, termed a buoy flap, is externalized for clinical observation.

B. Doppler Monitoring

1. Doppler monitoring is the most widely used device for monitoring flaps.
2. It is inexpensive and readily available.
3. A triphasic arterial sound can often be differentiated from the smooth whooshing sound of the venous signal. A change in signal quality can quickly detect problems.
4. Doppler monitoring may give a false sense of security for two reasons:
   - The observer will often search for a signal in the vicinity of the pedicle. The signal found may not be the pedicle, but may be a nearby normal vessel of no clinical consequence.
   - Doppler measures only velocity, not flow. Therefore, a recent thrombosis with pulsatile oscillation of a static column of blood will have velocity but no net flow, yielding a Doppler signal that sounds almost normal.

C. Implantable Doppler Probe

1. A small Doppler probe is implanted next to the vein distal to the anastomosis using a Gore-Tex cuff for continuous monitoring. This eliminates several sources of error with the standard Doppler. It also allows continuous assessment of flow both intraoperatively and postoperatively.
2. The wires connecting the transducer to the Doppler machine can be removed by gentle traction after 3 weeks.
3. Helpful in monitoring buried flaps.
4. It is an invasive technique, however, that requires meticulous positioning of the probe. Slight alteration in probe position or dislodgment of the probe may lead to loss of the Doppler signal, mimicking arterial occlusion and leading to false-positive reexploration.

D. Laser Doppler Flowmeter

1. The laser Doppler flowmeter measures the velocity of capillary blood flow in a known volume of tissue and calculates a perfusion index.
2. It provides continuous measurement of perfusion but is very susceptible to movement and positioning of the probe.

E. Fluorescein

1. Fluorescein is used for intraoperative and postoperative monitoring.
2. An intravenous dose of 10–20 mg/kg is given with subsequent visual assessment of fluorescence with a Wood's lamp.
3. Periodic postoperative assessment requires exposed tissue. The procedure involves administration of fluorescein 1.5 mg/kg IV with assessment of baseline, uptake, and washout phases with a quantitative fluorometer.
4. Circulatory embarrassment is indicated by lack of fluorescence or prolonged fluorescence. Poor uptake indicates arterial impairment; slow washout indicates venous impairment.

F. Other Methods

1. Temperature, pH, pulse oximetry, transcutaneous oxygen, and proton washout measurements are primarily of research or historical interest and are not routinely used.
2. Exceptions include use of pulse oximetry in monitoring digital replants and use of temperature probes on large myocutaneous or fasciocutaneous tissue flaps with an exposed skin island. A temperature difference $>3°C$ between the flap skin and the surrounding control skin may indicate vascular compromise.

V. THROMBOSIS

A. Approximately 18–24% of microsurgical anastomoses will require surgical exploration for suspected thrombosis and 66% of these will be salvaged, leading to overall secondary patency rates of 95–98%.

B. There are two risk zones for thrombus formation: the anastomosis itself and the downstream microcirculation. The anastomosis is the highest risk zone for occlusion and is a source of nearly continuous platelet/fibrin emboli that shower the distal microcirculation for the first 30–60 minutes.

C. The platelet metabolite thromboxane A_2 causes vasospasm of the distal circulation, which is also a contributing factor.

D. The majority of failures are related to surgical technique and can be avoided by meticulous attention to detail:

- Avoid suturing the back wall of the vessel, which effectively sutures the anastomosis shut.
- Avoid tension, kinking, or twisting of the pedicle.
- Do not place drains near the pedicle, as they may mechanically compromise flow.
- Obtain good hemostasis to avoid hematoma around the pedicle.
- Debride all potentially damaged vessel segments.
- Avoid tight cutaneous closure.

VI. ANTI-THROMBOTIC THERAPY

The use of anti-thrombotic therapy is variable, and individual physician practices have often been founded on tradition and anecdotal experience rather than strong clinical data. The therapy is divided into prophylactic agents and those used to treat established thrombosis.

A. Prophylaxis

1. Aspirin (Acetylsalicylic Acid; ASA)

a. Inactivates circulating platelets by acetylating the enzyme cyclo–oxygenase.

b. This inhibits production of thromboxane A_2, which is a potent proaggregant and vasoconstrictor.

c. The usual adult dosage is 80–325 mg po/pr daily.

d. Many surgeons start ASA postoperatively and continue it for 4 weeks.

e. Some advocate a preoperative dose for digital replantation.

2. Heparin

a. Potentiates antithrombin III, thus inactivating thrombin and factor XIIa, XIa, and Xa.

b. It is routinely used as an intraoperative irrigant (10–100 U/mL in saline).

c. Some surgeons administer a loading dose of 40 U/kg given before release of clamps following completion of an anastomosis. If there are no complications, heparin is not continued postoperatively.

d. Full heparinization is continued for 5–7 days in patients with replantation of crushed/avulsed parts, in those whose vessels have endothelial damage, or in those with a problem noted at the anastomosis.

e. Continuous low-dose heparin may improve flap survival.

f. For most microsurgical flaps, routine use of heparin is not indicated because of significant complications associated with its use. Complications include bleeding, hematoma formation, and heparin-induced thrombocytopenia.

3. Dextran-40

a. A polysaccharide with antithrombotic, antiplatelet, and rheologic properties.

b. Prior to starting an infusion, a test dose of Dextran-1 (Promit®) is given as a pretreatment to decrease the risk of anaphylactic reactions. The dosage in adults is 20 cc (150 mg/cc) IV over 1–2 minutes, given 1–2 minutes before the IV infusion of Dextran solutions.

c. Dextran 40 is usually administered with a loading dose of 30–40 cc just before microvascular clamps are released. The infusion is then continued at 25–30 mL/h for 5 days, at which time it is discontinued without tapering.

d. Adverse effects include pulmonary edema and renal failure.

B. Topical Vasodilators

1. Lidocaine is most commonly used.
2. Papaverine, a smooth muscle paralytic agent, is a good alternative but has no proven benefit over lidocaine.
3. Magnesium sulfate, nitroprusside, prostaglandins, and chlorpromazine have been reported.
4. Intraarterial injections of priscoline, nitroglycerin, or reserpine are reserved for pathologic vasoconstriction.

VII. COMPLICATIONS

A. General

Those related to the general health of the patient. For example:

1. Pulmonary embolism.
2. Respiratory complications.
3. Neurapraxias secondary to positioning.

B. Local

Those related directly to the microvascular procedure. Local complications are primarily due to vascular problems. Many factors influence failure of microvascular anastomoses:

1. Technical—most common. Examples include both walls sutured together, tension at the suture line, kinking of vessels, traumatic vessel handling, unequal vessel size.
2. Reperfusion—spasm, no reflow, hypercoagulability, cold, acidosis, hypovolemia, blood turbulence.
3. Postoperative—infection, cold, acidosis, extremity position, constrictive dressings.

4. Venous occlusion is more common than arterial occlusion.

VIII. SOLVING PROBLEMS

A. Arterial Problems

1. Findings
   a. Pallor.
   b. Poor or no capillary refill.
   c. Loss of Doppler signal.
   d. No bleeding from needle punctures.
   e. Cold.
2. Vessel Spasm
   a. Causes of spasm of vessel include:
      - Cold.
      - Vessel trauma.
      - Unligated side branch.
      - Physiologic: sympathetic stimulation.
      - Pharmacologic: nicotine.
   b. Intermittent vasospasm may cause sudden episodic impairment of arterial perfusion, especially in small vessels (digital arteries). It may suddenly occur days after the initial procedure, following an otherwise uncomplicated course. It must be differentiated from arterial thrombosis. Failure of nonoperative therapy within an hour must be followed by prompt operative exploration.
   c. Nonoperative treatment:
      - Warm the patient and affected part.
      - Sympathectomy with proximal local anesthetic block
      - Infusion of anastomotic area with small volumes of papaverine or lidocaine 2–4% without epinephrine.
   d. Operative therapy:
      - In general, the anastomosis should be opened to look for thrombus or mechanical explanation for poor perfusion. The vessels should be inspected for kink, twist, external compression, and previously unrecognized damage.
      - If vessel is normal:

        Dilate gently with mechanical distension or hydrodistension.

        Redo the anastomosis.

        Topical application of lidocaine 2–4% or papaverine.

        Keep patient and part warm.

        Coverage with moist gauze and wait.

        Controlled dependency of the part or alteration of the operating table level may be beneficial.
      - If the vessel is abnormal:

        It should be aggressively resected until a normal vessel is reached.

        This may require placement of an interposition vein graft.
3. Treatment of Arterial Occlusion
   a. Correct the underlying cause:
      - Once thrombosis has occurred, the underlying cause must be addressed. This will require operative exploration, inspecting for kink, twist, external compression, mechanical error in the anastomosis, and previously unrecognized damage to the vessels. The anastomosis will often need to be opened and inspected.
      - If damaged endothelium or vessel is suspected, you must resect all suspect vessel segments and possibly place an interposition vein graft.
      - If you can milk thrombus out of distal vessel to reestablish flow, fibrinolytic agents may help. In general, heparin therapy is instituted.
   b. Fibrinolytic agents:
      - These include streptokinase, urokinase, and tissue plasminogen activator. In limited human studies, they have been shown to salvage free tissue transfers when infused locally.
      - Life-threatening allergic reactions and bleeding complications may occur.
      - The addition of heparin or an antiplatelet agent is necessary to prevent rethrombosis.
      - Streptokinase 100,000 IU/h has been infused intraarterially for salvage of failing digital replants.
      - Urokinase (240,000 U/h for 2 h, then 80,000–120,000 U/h until clot lysis occurs

or until a minimum dose of 600,000 U has been given without clinical improvement) has been used as an adjunct to successful limb and digit replantation.

B. Venous Problems

1. Findings:
   - Bluish discoloration of tissue.
   - Tissue swelling and edema.
   - Tissue firmness secondary to increased tissue turgor.
   - Very rapid capillary refill.
   - Dark blood oozing from needle punctures.
2. This is an urgent complication that is no less threatening than arterial occlusion. It demands a quick response (within 1 h).
3. Never had good venous drainage:
   - Occasionally, venous drainage is technically impossible or very poor and no surgical intervention is thought possible. In this situation, you must establish some venous drainage for 7–10 days until new venous outflow pathways become established. Limit interim congestion to prevent tissue death.

     Elevate affected part.

     Create oozing of blood with leeches and/or heparin.
   - Leeches:

     Medicinal leeches (*Hirudo medicinalis*) are commercially available.

     The primary benefit of leeches is not the 5 mL of blood they suck out while attached, but the anticoagulant (hirudin) and vasodilatory effect of leech saliva.

     Leeches usually remain attached for approximately 30 minutes and are regularly applied every 2–6 h to maintain bleeding. The leech bite wound may continue to ooze blood for 4–6 h after the leech has been removed.

     Leeches carry *Aeromonas hydrophila* in their gut. Patients should receive prophylactic antibiotics: fluoroquinolone, trimethoprim/sulfamethoxazole, antipseudomonal penicillin, imipenem, or 2nd, 3rd, or 4th generation cephalosporin.

     Blood transfusions are commonly required after several days of leech therapy.

     Leech therapy should be continued until venous congestion has abated. This may take 7–10 days. If congestion is improved, leech therapy can be stopped and the affected part closely observed for recurrent congestion. This is best done during the day when an experienced staff is more available.
4. If once-good venous drainage is now poor:
   - Primary findings include hematoma, edema, and/or thrombus formation.
   - Sudden onset of new venous congestion suggests that something has compromised outflow. One should consider a wound hematoma compressing the vein (especially if on anticoagulants) or wound edema and tight closure. Thrombus and the same mechanical errors that affect arteries can affect veins.
   - If venous congestion occurs, the part should be elevated aggressively, and the dressing taken down to check for constriction and outflow impairment from a tight dressing.
   - Skin sutures can be removed at the bedside to relieve pressure from edema or hematoma while waiting to go to the operating room.
   - Loss of previously good venous outflow is caused by a mechanical problem or thrombus and should be aggressively explored and treated in a manner similar to arterial problems.

61

Perioperative Care and Monitoring of the Microvascular Surgery Patient

Eric E. Arcilla, M.D.,* Andrew L. Da Lio, M.D., and Prosper Benhaim, M.D.
David Geffen School of Medicine at UCLA, Los Angeles, California, U.S.A.

I. INTRODUCTION

Microvascular surgery has revolutionized the reconstructive surgeon's approach to the management of wounds. Improvements in microsurgical techniques and instruments over the past two decades have resulted in success rates now routinely in excess of 90–95% at most major medical centers. Contributing to this high level of success is the excellent and meticulous perioperative care that is, and must be, accorded to each and every patient undergoing a microvascular surgical procedure. As with any other patient undergoing an operative procedure, the perioperative period is divided into three phases: preoperative, intraoperative, and postoperative.

II. PREOPERATIVE CARE

A. General Considerations

1. Informed consent: The patient should be informed of all aspects of the procedure, including the method of donor flap harvest, recipient-site vessel dissection, flap insetting, possible complications, and functional/morphological changes that may arise in these areas. Most importantly, the patient should be informed of the existence of an alternative reconstructive option, if any, even though this may be less ideal.
2. The patient must be prepared psychologically, since the stress of having a visible and "unnatural-looking" transplanted tissue may be too much for some patients to accept.
3. The cooperation and trust of the patient is important from the outset, as the postoperative course is often long and arduous if the patient proves uncooperative.

B. Medical Considerations

1. Systemic diseases such as diabetes, cardiovascular problems, and renal disease are not contraindications to microvascular procedures. Control of these conditions, however, is essential to minimize anesthetic risks as well as a prolonged postoperative course.
2. Necessary laboratory work-up should be performed, and medical clearance, where appropriate, should be obtained.
3. Current medications must be scrutinized, as they may affect the overall outcome of the operation. In particular, medications that could increase systemic vascular resistance and adversely affect the microvascular anastomoses must be identified. Drugs that affect the patient's bleeding parame-

* *Current affiliation*: University of the Philippines–Philippine General Hospital, Manila, Philippines.

ters, such as aspirin, must be stopped at least 2 weeks prior to the operation, if at all possible.

4. Drug allergies should always be elicited.
5. A history of smoking will affect the patient's capacity for wound healing, at both the recipient and flap-donor sites. Cigarette smoking does not, by itself, increase the risk of anastomotic thromboses or flap failure, but it does increase the risk for other complications (e.g., infection, wound-healing problems, and fat necrosis within the flap). Smoking should be stopped at least 2 weeks before the scheduled operation. Transdermal nicotine patches and nicotine gum should NOT be used.
6. The patient's coagulation status must be examined if there is any suggestion of bleeding tendency or hypercoagulable state, as this may predispose to postoperative hematoma or anastomotic thrombosis, respectively.

C. Flap Donor Site

1. Evaluation of the donor flap preoperatively is important to prevent problems from arising during its harvest. One must be able to determine if the blood supply of the donor flap is intact and whether its harvest would in any way compromise the donor site.
2. Clinical observation and palpation of pulses is still the most reliable and cost-effective means of evaluating the donor flap vascular pedicle (e.g., dorsalis pedis flap, radial forearm flap).
3. Ultrasound Doppler determination may be required in cases where clinical evaluation of pulses is inadequate.
4. An angiogram may sometimes be utilized for the determination of a flap pedicle. In the case of the fibular free flap, the angiogram has proven useful in determining whether harvesting the peroneal artery would be detrimental to the viability of the donor leg, especially in cases of a two-vessel or even one-vessel leg. Some microvascular surgeons routinely obtain an angiogram in all cases of free fibular flaps, while some limit its use to those patients exhibiting signs and symptoms of peripheral vascular disease.

D. Recipient Site

1. Preoperative preparation of the recipient site is just as crucial for the success of a free tissue transfer.
2. In cases of post-traumatic wounds, the wound bed should be adequately debrided of all nonviable tissue. A split-thickness skin graft may also be placed on the open wound while the patient is being prepared for a definitive free tissue transfer reconstruction.
3. Infection at the recipient site must be adequately treated with debridement, regular wound dressing changes, wound cultures, and the appropriate antibiotic regimen.
4. The search for recipient vessels for anastomosis with the use of clinical observation, Doppler ultrasound, and sometimes even angiogram is also desirable but not mandatory. These diagnostic measures are especially helpful in patients who have received irradiation for cancer or who have sustained severe trauma to the lower extremities, either of which may have resulted in vascular compromise.

III. INTRAOPERATIVE CARE AND MONITORING

The primary concerns during this phase are largely based on the patient's general health and vascular status. Microvascular surgery cases may be lengthy and hence expose the patient to the risks of anesthesia, prolonged immobilization, blood loss, and extensive tissue manipulation, often more so than most other types of surgery. In addition, the ultimate success or failure of the free flap depends largely on the anastomosis performed and the condition of the patient during flap harvest and insetting. Numerous postoperative complications can arise from problems encountered intraoperatively.

A. General Considerations

1. Always keep in mind that microvascular surgical procedures may be prolonged.
2. Position the patient appropriately to prevent prolonged traction on nerves (e.g., avoid prolonged arm abduction in breast reconstruction cases to prevent brachial plexus neuropathy).
3. Pressure points should be padded with silicone gel or foam pads to prevent pressure ulcers.
4. Sequential compression stockings should be used to prevent venous stasis, deep venous thrombosis, and pulmonary embolism.
5. Keep the room temperature at 25–28 °C. Warming devices such as the Bair-Hugger or warming blan-

kets should also be used to prevent hypothermia that may induce peripheral vasoconstriction.

6. The patient's hemodynamic status should be optimized, using blood transfusion preferentially for cases with significant blood loss. Serial hematocrit measurements may be required intraoperatively. The urine output should be maintained at a minimum of 0.5 cc/kg/h in order to ensure adequate tissue perfusion.
7. Avoid intraoperative vasoconstrictors. Blood pressure support should be performed by adjusting the level of general anesthetic and through fluid support. Vasopressors that are otherwise commonly used in surgical procedures should be avoided in microsurgical cases to minimize risk of peripheral vasoconstriction, which may jeopardize the microvascular anastomosis.

B. Intraoperative Flap Monitoring

Most postoperative anastomotic complications can be attributed to errors in preoperative planning or intraoperative execution of the free flap transfer. Intraoperative flap assessment immediately following the completion of the flap anastomoses and flap insetting is critical to postoperative success.

1. Assessment of the flap pedicle:
   - The flap pedicle should be of appropriate length relative to the recipient vessel. If too short, tension will decrease blood flow. If too long, kinks or twists may develop.
   - The artery should have a strong palpable pulse distal to the anastomosis. Additionally, a Doppler ultrasound may be used to confirm a strong arterial signal with normal triphasic signal.
   - The vein should be soft and easily compressible. Transient compression of the outflow vein with jeweler's forceps following flap reperfusion should result in slight increased vein turgor or an "engorged" appearance, which immediately resolves with release of the venous compression. In addition, the "milking" test should be performed distal to the anastomosis to confirm brisk refill.
   - Any possible movement of the surgical field, especially near joints, should be tested to confirm adequate range of the flap pedicle during motion without compression or kinking.
   - Closure of the wound over the flap and pedicle should not place any tension or compression on the vessels. Never be hesitant to apply a skin graft to a partially open wound, delay the closure, or increase the length of incisions in order to prevent a thrombosis.
2. Features of an ideal free flap monitoring device include:
   - Continuous recording of flap perfusion.
   - Immediate detection of flap vascular compromise.
   - Easily interpreted by all health care providers, including physicians and nurses.
   - Applicable for monitoring both exposed and buried flaps.
3. One of the best monitoring devices available for intraoperative use is the 20 MHz implantable Doppler probe. This unit uses high-frequency pulsed ultrasound from a Doppler velocimeter. It consists of a single piezoelectric crystal that acts both as a receiver and a sender of ultrasound pulses. It is positioned adjacent to the wall of the artery 1 cm distal to the anastomosis. The Doppler detects triphasic arterial waveform signals, which indicate good arterial inflow. It provides continuous monitoring from the time of the anastomosis until several days into the postoperative period.

IV. POSTOPERATIVE CARE AND MONITORING

The most critical component of this phase of perioperative care is a highly responsible, vigilant, dedicated, and competent staff of nurses and physicians trained in the details of intensive care and microsurgical flaps.

A. Setting

1. The postoperative microvascular patient is initially admitted to the postanesthesia care unit in close proximity to the operating room in the event of an immediate postoperative vascular compromise or hematoma.
2. The Ward/ICU:
   - Hygienic, disinfected room.
   - Supplied with the usual resuscitation equipment and monitoring devices.

- A constant and regulated temperature of 25–28°C. Alternatively, a Bair-Hugger warming machine may be utilized to maintain body temperature. Hypothermia predisposes the patient to peripheral vasoconstriction, with subsequent decreased blood flow to the flap pedicle. If too warm, the patient becomes uncomfortable and restless, which may be detrimental to the flap. Increased insensible fluid losses may also occur, which may result in relative hypovolemia and compensatory peripheral vasoconstriction mediated by an increased sympathetic discharge.
- Quiet surroundings with limitations on visitors.

B. General Considerations

1. Monitoring of vital signs (blood pressure, pulse, respiratory rate, temperature, and mental status) every hour for the first 8 h, then every 2 h for 16 h, then every 4 h.
2. Maintenance of hemodynamic stability. Transfuse blood when necessary to prevent hypovolemia and hypotension, which may secondarily predispose the patient to vasospasm.
3. Maintaining hydration status by increasing IV fluid rates (with or without intermittent boluses), ensuring that urine output remains greater than 0.5 cc/kg/h.
4. Minimizing pain and anxiety with adequate analgesic dosing, which will reduce sympathetic-mediated vasoconstriction. Patient-controlled analgesia (PCA) machines have proved effective, although some surgeons may prefer epidural anesthesia.
5. Careful regulation of ambient temperature to prevent hypothermia or uncomfortably warm temperatures.
6. Maintenance of fluid and electrolyte balance.
7. Encourage the patient to ambulate as soon as possible to prevent atelectasis, deep venous thrombosis, and pulmonary embolism. Early motion and dependency of a lower extremity are prohibited, however, in patients with lower extremity free flaps.
8. Use of incentive spirometry at least 10 times per hour while awake.
9. Sequential compression stockings of the extremities, especially in cases with prolonged bedrest.
10. Drain care and accurate charting of individual drain outputs.
11. The patient is initially kept NPO for the first 12–24 h in the event that an immediate reoperation may be required.
12. Laboratory tests (e.g., hemoglobin, hematocrit, electrolytes, appropriate x-rays) are repeated as necessary.

C. Medications

1. Prophylactic antibiotics are administered up to 24 h postoperatively, unless specific indications are present that require a longer course.
2. Antipyretics, such as acetaminophen, may be given for temperatures reaching 38.5°C.
3. Pain control is usually achieved with use of a PCA machine, but epidural anesthesia is also an option. Caution should be used with epidural anesthesia, however, since a high spinal cord anesthetic level may cause a chemical sympathectomy. This may decrease peripheral vascular resistance with resultant hypotension.
4. The use of anticoagulants and antiplatelet agents remains a highly controversial issue in microvascular surgery, since the only consistent finding in large studies is an increased incidence of hematomas and bleeding complications. There are, however, certain conditions in which their use has been beneficial, including replantation cases, cases of massive trauma to the lower extremities, and cases where anastomotic problems occurred intraoperatively that may have resulted in prolonged flap ischemia, thrombus formation, or embolic episodes. The usual anticoagulants used include Dextran 40, heparin, and aspirin.
   - Dextran 40:

     A derivative of glucose with a molecular weight of 40,000 daltons.

     Decreases blood viscosity by acting as a volume expander.

     Antiplatelet activity by altering the positive charges on the platelet and endothelial cell surfaces.

     Antifibrin effect by binding with fibrinogen.

Usually provided as a 6% dextran solution that comes in 500 mL bottles.

A small percentage of the population may develop a severe hyperallergic or even anaphylactic reaction to dextran. Pretreatment with Promit (Dextran 1), a low molecular weight version of dextran that binds all circulating antibodies to dextran, is usually provided prior to administration of the Dextran 40. Alternatively, a small test dose is given and the patient monitored for hemodynamic stability. Thereafter, a loading dose of 25–40 cc is rapidly infused and a maintenance continuous IV infusion (typically 25 cc/h for a 70 kg male) provided for the next 4–5 days. The effect persists for several hours to days after discontinuation.

Adverse effects include allergic reaction, rash, bleeding, hematoma, renal problems, and volume overload that can result in pulmonary edema, congestive heart failure, and even myocardial infarction. The dextran infusion should be stopped immediately if one or more of these is observed.

- Heparin:

  Mucopolysaccharide.

  Primary mechanism of action is binding with antithrombin III, thereby inhibiting fibrin formation from thrombin.

  Clot-bound thrombin may be resistant to heparin.

  Currently is more commonly used as a local irrigant solution for vessel lumen irrigation during microvascular anastomosis. Not routinely used systemically.

  For IV or IM use, the preparation comes in ampule form of 12,500 units (100 mg/mL). Administration may either be by bolus or slow IV infusion, not to exceed 300 mg per day, but enough to keep the partial thromboplastin time (PTT) at twice the normal level. The effect of heparin is noted 10 minutes after administration and peaks at about 1 hour. It lasts for 4 hours after discontinuation.

  The primary adverse effect is excessive bleeding and/or hematoma formation. In cases of overdosage, protamine sulfate is given in a dose equal to that of the last heparin dose administered.

- Aspirin:

  Acetylsalicylic acid.

  Antiplatelet effect. Mechanism of action is irreversible transacetylation of platelet cyclooxygenase. This prevents production of prostaglandins and thromboxane A_2.

  Action persists for approximately 10 days after discontinuation, requiring new platelets to form to produce fully functional platelets not affected by the previously administered aspirin.

  Usual dose is 80–325 mg daily, either orally or rectally.

  Adverse effects include gastric mucosa irritation, prolonged bleeding, and hematoma formation.

D. Free Flap Care

1. Positioning is critical to ensure that there is neither undue pressure nor tension on the flap and its pedicle. For example, head alignment should suit the location of head and neck free flaps. Arm and shoulder abduction should be tested intraoperatively with free TRAM flaps anastomosed to the subscapular vascular system.
2. Incision lines and drain sites should be kept clean and dry to prevent cellulitis and/or maceration from occurring. This also applies to the donor site wound, which is frequently forgotten or neglected.
3. Dressings should be kept light. Tight circumferential dressings should never be used.
4. Edema in the area of the flap could produce excessive pressure on the pedicle vessels and thus should not be taken lightly. Extremities should be elevated above the level of the heart. If wound edema becomes severe enough to cause tightness of the wound closure, sutures should be released

immediately as necessary to decrease tension on the wound closure.

5. Early detection of hematomas is essential to prevent significant compression of the pedicle. Large hematomas should be evacuated immediately in an operating room setting. The venous anastomosis must be inspected, since venous thrombosis with resulting flap hypertension could be the cause of the hematoma.
6. Early signs of infection should be aggressively managed with frequent dressing changes and empiric antibiotic therapy. These may be replaced with more specific antibiotics once culture results are obtained.

E. Free Flap Monitoring

1. Whether by clinical observation or with the use of monitoring equipment, free flap monitoring should be performed every hour for the first 48 h, then every 2 h for the next 24 h, then every 4 h until discharged.
2. Clinical observation is a very useful method of monitoring flaps with a skin component. Unfortunately, interpretations may be quite subjective and are highly variable. Parameters that are commonly assessed include:
    - Skin color.
    - Capillary refill.
    - Flap turgor.
    - Dermal bleeding/pin prick bleeding.
3. Arterial compromise presents with pallor, capillary refill > 3 seconds, loss of flap turgor, sluggish or absent dermal/pin prick bleeding, or decreased Doppler signal intensity. Venous compromise presents with a bluish-purple discoloration of the flap, a rapid capillary refill < 1 second, engorgement, swelling, increased turgor of the flap, dark blood emanating from pin pricks, or excessive oozing from the flap edges and dermis.
4. Monitoring devices:
    - Temperature monitoring:

      Temperature is a familiar parameter that is easily interpreted.

      Relatively inexpensive adjunct to clinical observation.

      An absolute flap temperature of >30°C is reported to be indicative of a healthy flap.

      More important is the relative temperature difference between the flap and adjacent normal skin. A temperature differential of more than 3°C may signal a failing flap.
    - Surface Doppler ultrasound monitoring:

      An 8 Mhz probe will easily detect the musculocutaneous perforators from the main pedicle to the skin paddle in a typical myocutaneous flap (e.g., TRAM or latissimus dorsi myocutaneous flap). It may also be used to monitor buried flap pedicles in flaps without a skin paddle, although interpretation of signals is sometimes difficult (e.g., difficulty in assessing neck recipient and flap pedicle vessels adjacent to carotid artery in head and neck free flaps).

      May also monitor the patency of the venous outflow by augmentation of venous hum with compression of the flap tissue.

      Relatively inexpensive, easy to use, and easy to interpret.
    - Implantable Doppler ultrasound—discussed above.
    - Pulse oximetry:

      Primarily used in cases of digital replantation.

      Capable of continuously monitoring pulsatile flow and oxygen tension of a replanted digit.

      In replantation surgery, the digital pulse oxymeter has become the standard for postoperative monitoring. A cessation of the pulsatile flow or oxygen saturation of <90–92% is indicative of arterial compromise in a replanted digit.
    - Other less commonly used monitoring techniques:

      Intravenous fluorescein.

      Photoplethysmography.

Electrical impedance plethysmography.

Electromyogram (EMG) and muscle contractility.

F. Flap Ischemia or Vascular Crisis

1. In the event that a free flap vascular crisis is detected, conservative management should first be attempted:

   - Check for possible causes of pedicle compression and reposition the patient if necessary.
   - Remove all dressings.
   - Check for tightness of the skin closure and release sutures as necessary.
   - Determine if there is extensive edema that might necessitate elevation of the involved area, release of sutures, or even a fasciotomy
   - Assess hydration status to rule out hypovolemia; correct accordingly.
   - Check the patient for hypothermia and adequacy of pain control; address any detected problems.
   - Prepare the patient for a possible surgical reexploration.

2. If conservative measures fail after 30–60 minutes or if definite vascular compromise or hematoma is diagnosed, the patient should be immediately brought to the operating room for a reexploration.
3. If a definite vascular pedicle problem is present but the patient cannot be immediately brought to the operating room, there are some temporizing maneuvers that one may perform at the bedside:

   - For an arterial thrombosis, there is no substitute for an immediate reexploration with reestablishment of circulation. Soft tissues will tolerate approximately 4 h of warm ischemia. Inability to reperfuse the flap (no reflow phenomenon) and severe tissue necrosis will occur shortly after this time frame.
   - For a venous compromise, the flap area is elevated above the level of the heart. In extreme cases one may even open the surgical wound to visualize the venous anastomosis, which may then be taken down and the flap allowed to bleed freely intermittently, thus preventing massive venous engorgement. In this scenario, be aware of the patient's hemodynamic and fluid status and have several units of blood available to prevent severe anemia and hypotension.

62

Pedicled Flap and Free Flap Library

Eric E. Arcilla, M.D.,* **and Prosper Benhaim, M.D.**
David Geffen School of Medicine at UCLA, Los Angeles, California, U.S.A.

I. FLAP CLASSIFICATION BY BLOOD SUPPLY

A. Muscle or Musculocutaneous Flaps (Mathes-Nahai Classification)

1. Type I—single dominant vascular pedicle
2. Type II—single dominant vascular pedicle with a single or multiple minor pedicles
3. Type III—two dominant vascular pedicles arising from different main vascular sources
4. Type IV—segmental vascular pedicles
5. Type V—dominant vascular pedicle with secondary segmental pedicles

B. Fasciocutaneous Flaps

1. Type A—direct cutaneous vascular supply
2. Type B—septocutaneous vascular supply
3. Type C—vascular supply coursing through muscle

II. HEAD AND FACE FLAPS

A. Scalp Flap

1. Flap type: fasciocutaneous
2. Pattern of circulation: Type A
3. Vascular anatomy:
    - Dominant pedicles: superficial temporal and occipital arteries and veins
    - Minor pedicles: supratrochlear, supraorbital, and posterior auricular arteries and veins
4. Innervation: supratrochlear, auriculotemporal, postauricular, greater and lesser occipital, great auricular, and third cervical nerves (sensory)

B. Temporoparietal Fascia Flap

1. Flap type: fascial
2. Pattern of circulation: Type A
3. Vascular anatomy:
    - Dominant pedicle: superficial temporal artery and vein
4. Innervation: auriculotemporal nerve (sensory)

C. Temporalis Muscle Flap

1. Flap type: muscle, musculofascial, musculocutaneous
2. Pattern of circulation: Type III
3. Vascular anatomy:
    - Dominant pedicle: deep temporal artery and vein

* *Current affiliation*: University of the Philippines–Philippine General Hospital, Manila, Philippines.

- Minor pedicles: branches of middle temporal artery and vein

4. Innervation: fifth cranial nerve (motor)

D. Median Forehead Flap

1. Flap type: fasciocutaneous
2. Pattern of circulation: Type C
3. Vascular anatomy:
   - Dominant pedicle: supratrochlear artery and venae comitantes
   - Minor pedicles: supraorbital artery and venae comitantes
4. Innervation: supratrochlear and supraorbital nerves (sensory)

E. Standard Forehead Flap

1. Flap type: fasciocutaneous
2. Pattern of circulation: Type A
3. Vascular anatomy:
   - Dominant pedicle: superficial temporal artery and vein
   - Minor pedicles: supratrochlear and supraorbital arteries and venae comitantes
4. Innervation: supratrochlear, supraorbital, and auriculotemporal nerves (sensory)

F. Nasolabial Flap

1. Flap type: fasciocutaneous
2. Pattern of circulation: Type C
3. Vascular anatomy:
   - Dominant pedicle: angular artery and vein
   - Minor pedicle: alar branches of superior labial artery
4. Innervation: trigeminal nerve (sensory)

G. Orbicularis Oris Flap

1. Basis for Abbe flap and Estlander flap
2. Flap type: Muscle, musculocutaneous, musculomucocutaneous
3. Pattern of circulation: Type III
4. Vascular anatomy:
   - Dominant pedicle: superior (upper lip) or inferior (lower lip) labial artery and vein
   - Minor pedicle: medial branch of inferior alveolar artery (lower lip)
5. Innervation: facial nerve (motor); trigeminal nerve (sensory)

H. Facial Artery Musculomucosal (FAMM) Flap

1. Flap type: musculomucosal
2. Pattern of circulation: Type II
3. Vascular anatomy:
   - Dominant pedicles: facial artery, venous plexuses draining to pterygoid plexus, internal maxillary vein posteriorly and facial vein anteriorly
   - Minor pedicles: angular artery and vein, branches of superior labial artery and vein
4. Innervation: supratrochlear, auriculotemporal, postauricular, greater and lesser occipital, great auricular, and third cervical nerves (sensory)

III. CHEST AND BACK FLAPS

A. Deltopectoral Flap

1. Flap type: fasciocutaneous
2. Pattern of circulation: Type C
3. Vascular anatomy:
   - Dominant pedicle: 2nd and 3rd perforating branches of internal mammary artery
   - Minor pedicles: 1st and 4th perforating branches of internal mammary artery
4. Innervation: 2nd to 4th intercostal nerves (sensory)

B. Pectoralis Major Flap

1. Flap type: muscle, musculocutaneous, osteomusculocutaneous
2. Pattern of circulation: Type V
3. Vascular anatomy:
   - Dominant pedicle: pectoral branch of thoracoacromial artery and venae comitantes
   - Minor pedicles: pectoral branch of lateral thoracic artery, perforators from internal mammary and intercostal arteries, and venae comitantes
4. Innervation: lateral pectoral nerve and branches from medial pectoral nerve (motor); 2nd to 7th intercostal nerves (sensory)

C. Pectoralis Minor Flap

1. Flap type: muscle
2. Pattern of circulation: Type III
3. Vascular anatomy:
   - Dominant pedicle: pectoral branch of thoracoacromial artery and branch of lateral thoracicartery
   - Minor pedicle: branch from axillary artery
4. Innervation: medial and lateral pectoral nerves (motor)

D. Trapezius Flap

1. Flap type: muscle or musculocutaneous
2. Pattern of circulation: Type II
3. Vascular anatomy:
   - Dominant pedicle: ascending and descending branches of transverse cervical artery and vein
   - Minor pedicles: branch of occipital artery and vein; dorsal scapular artery and vein; perforators from posterior intercostal artery and vein
4. Innervation: spinal accessory nerve (motor); 3rd and 4th cervical nerves and branches from posterior intercostal nerves (sensory)

E. Scapular Flap

1. Flap type: fasciocutaneous
2. Pattern of circulation: Type B
3. Vascular anatomy:
   - Dominant pedicle: circumflex scapular artery and vein
4. Innervation: lateral and posterior cutaneous nerves from 3rd to 5th intercostal nerves (sensory)

F. Latissimus Dorsi Flap

1. Flap type: muscle or musculocutaneous
2. Pattern of circulation: Type V
3. Vascular anatomy:
   - Dominant pedicle: thoracodorsal artery and vein
   - Minor pedicles: 4–6 perforators from posterior intercostal arteries and lumbar artery and venae comitantes
4. Innervation: thoracodorsal nerve (motor); posterior branches from intercostal nerves (sensory)

G. Serratus Anterior Flap

1. Flap type: muscle, musculocutaneous, or osteomusculocutaneous flap
2. Pattern of circulation: Type III
3. Vascular anatomy:
   - Dominant pedicles: lateral thoracic artery and branches from thoracodorsal artery
4. Innervation: long thoracic nerve (motor); T2–T4 intercostal nerves (sensory)

IV. UPPER EXTREMITY FLAPS

A. Deltoid Flap

1. Flap type: fasciocutaneous
2. Pattern of circulation: Type B
3. Vascular anatomy:
   - Dominant pedicle: posterior deltoid subcutaneous artery from the posterior circumflex humeral artery
4. Innervation: lateral cutaneous branch of circumflex humeral nerve (sensory)

B. Lateral Arm Flap

1. Flap type: fascial and fasciocutaneous
2. Pattern of circulation: Type B
3. Vascular anatomy:
   - Dominant pedicle: posterior radial collateral artery and venae comitantes (branch of the profunda brachii artery)
   - Minor pedicle: radial recurrent artery
4. Innervation: posterior cutaneous nerve of the arm (sensory)

C. Posterior Interosseous Artery Flap

1. Flap type: fasciocutaneous
2. Pattern of circulation: Type B
3. Vascular anatomy:
   - Dominant pedicle: posterior interosseous artery and venae comitantes
   - Minor pedicle: anterior interosseous artery and venae comitantes

4. Innervation: branch of dorsal antebrachial cutaneous nerve and medial antebrachial cutaneous nerve (sensory)

D. Radial Forearm Flap

1. Flap type: fasciocutaneous and osteoseptocutaneous
2. Pattern of circulation: Type B
3. Vascular anatomy:
   - Dominant pedicle: radial artery, venae comitantes, and cephalic vein
4. Innervation: medial and lateral antebrachial cutaneous nerves (sensory)

E. Ulnar Artery Forearm Flap

1. Flap type: fasciocutaneous and osteoseptocutaneous
2. Pattern of circulation: Type B
3. Vascular anatomy:
   - Dominant pedicle: ulnar artery, venae comitantes, and basilic vein
4. Innervation: medial antebrachial cutaneous nerve (sensory)

F. Dorsal Metacarpal Artery Flap

1. A fasciocutaneous flap that may be elevated from any finger based on any of the dorsal metacarpal arteries (usually elevated from the index or middle fingers)
2. Flap type: fasciocutaneous
3. Pattern of circulation: Type A
4. Vascular anatomy:
   - Dominant pedicle: dorsal metacarpal artery
5. Innervation: dorsal sensory branches of radial and ulnar nerves (sensory)

G. First Dorsal Interosseous Flap

1. In contrast to the dorsal metacarpal artery fasciocutaneous flap, a muscle flap (1st dorsal interosseous muscle) based on the first dorsal metacarpal artery
2. Flap type: muscle
3. Pattern of circulation: Type I
4. Vascular anatomy:
   - Dominant pedicle: first dorsal metacarpal artery and venae comitantes
5. Innervation: deep palmar branch of ulnar nerve (sensory)

H. Digital Artery Flap

1. Flap type: fasciocutaneous
2. Pattern of circulation: Type A
3. Vascular anatomy:
   - Dominant pedicle: digital artery
4. Innervation: digital nerve branches of median and ulnar nerves (sensory)

V. ABDOMINAL AND GROIN FLAPS

A. Rectus Abdominis Flap

1. Flap type: muscle and musculocutaneous
2. Pattern of circulation: Type III
3. Vascular anatomy:
   - Dominant pedicles: deep inferior and superior epigastric arteries and veins
   - Minor pedicles: subcostal and intercostal arteries and venae comitantes
4. Innervation: 7th to 12th intercostal nerves (motor); lateral cutaneous nerves from 7th to 12th intercostal nerves (sensory)

B. Superficial Inferior Epigastric Artery Flap

1. Flap type: fasciocutaneous
2. Pattern of circulation: Type A
3. Vascular anatomy:
   - Dominant pedicle: superficial inferior epigastric artery and vein
4. Innervation: 10th to 12th intercostal nerves (sensory)

C. External Oblique Flap

1. Flap type: muscle or musculocutaneous
2. Pattern of circulation: Type IV

3. Vascular anatomy:
   - Segmental pedicles—lateral cutaneous branches of inferior 8 posterior intercostal arteries and venae comitantes
4. Innervation: 7th to 12th intercostal nerves (motor); T3 to T11 lateral cutaneous nerves (sensory)

D. Internal Oblique Flap

1. Flap type: muscle
2. Pattern of circulation: Type V
3. Vascular anatomy:
   - Dominant pedicle: ascending branch of deep circumflex iliac artery and vein
   - Minor pedicles: lateral branches of deep inferior epigastric vessels
4. Innervation: T8 to T12 (sensory)

E. Deep Circumflex Iliac Artery Flap

1. Flap type: musculo-osseous, musculocutaneous, osteomusculocutaneous
2. Pattern of circulation: Type I
3. Vascular anatomy:
   - Dominant pedicle: deep circumflex iliac artery and vein
4. Innervation: T12 (sensory)

F. Groin Flap

1. Flap type: fasciocutaneous
2. Pattern of circulation: Type A
3. Vascular anatomy:
   - Dominant pedicle: superficial circumflex iliac artery and venae comitantes
4. Innervation: lateral cutaneous nerve of T12 (sensory)

G. Pudendal Flap

1. Flap type: fasciocutaneous
2. Pattern of circulation: Type A
3. Vascular anatomy:
   - Dominant pedicle: posterior labial artery and venae comitantes
4. Innervation: pudendal nerve (sensory)

H. Omental Flap

1. Flap type: omentum
2. Pattern of circulation: Type III
3. Vascular anatomy:
   - Dominant pedicle: right and left gastroepiploic artery and vein

I. Jejunal Flap

1. Flap type: small intestine
2. Pattern of circulation: type I
3. Vascular anatomy:
   - Dominant pedicle: jejunal artery and accompanying vein

J. Colon Flap

1. Flap type: large intestine
2. Pattern of circulation: Type I
3. Vascular anatomy:
   - Dominant pedicle: middle colic artery and vein

VI. BUTTOCK AND THIGH FLAPS

A. Gluteus Maximus Flap

1. Flap type: muscle or musculocutaneous
2. Pattern of circulation: Type III
3. Vascular anatomy:
   - Dominant pedicle: superior and inferior gluteal artery and vein
4. Innervation: inferior gluteal nerve (motor); posterior cutaneous nerve and branches from S1–3 and L1–3 (sensory)

B. Anterolateral Thigh Flap

1. Flap type: fasciocutaneous
2. Pattern of circulation: Type B and C
3. Vascular anatomy:
   - Dominant pedicles: septocutaneous branches of descending branch of lateral circumflex femoral artery and venae comitantes

- Minor pedicles: musculocutaneous branches of descending and transverse branches of lateral circumflex femoral artery

4. Innervation: lateral femoral cutaneous nerve (sensory)

C. Lateral Thigh Flap

1. Flap type: fasciocutaneous
2. Pattern of circulation: Type B
3. Vascular anatomy:
   - Dominant pedicles: 1st, 2nd, and 3rd perforators of profunda femoris artery and vein
4. Innervation: lateral cutaneous nerve of thigh (sensory)

D. Medial Thigh Flap

1. Flap type: fasciocutaneous
2. Pattern of circulation: Type B
3. Vascular anatomy:
   - Dominant pedicle: anterior septocutaneous artery and vein from superficial femoral artery
4. Innervation: medial anterior cutaneous nerve of thigh (sensory)

E. Sartorius Flap

1. Flap type: muscle or musculocutaneous
2. Pattern of circulation: Type IV
3. Vascular anatomy:
   - Segmental pedicles: branches of superficial femoral artery and vein
4. Innervation: femoral nerve (motor)

F. Rectus Femoris Flap

1. Flap type: muscle
2. Pattern of circulation: Type II
3. Vascular anatomy:
   - Dominant pedicle: descending branch of lateral circumflex femoral artery and vein
   - Minor pedicles: ascending branch of lateral circumflex femoral vessels and branches of superficial femoral vessels
4. Innervation: femoral nerve (motor)

G. Vastus Lateralis Flap

1. Flap type: muscle and musculocutaneous
2. Pattern of circulation: Type I
3. Vascular anatomy:
   - Dominant pedicle: descending branch of lateral circumflex femoral artery and vein
4. Innervation: femoral nerve (motor); lateral femoral cutaneous nerve (sensory)

H. Vastus Medialis Flap

1. Flap type: muscle and musculocutaneous
2. Pattern of circulation: Type II
3. Vascular anatomy:
   - Dominant pedicle: branch of superficial femoral artery and vein
   - Minor pedicles: branches of descending genicular artery and vein
4. Innervation: femoral nerve (motor); saphenous nerve (sensory)

I. Gracilis Flap

1. Flap type: muscle or musculocutaneous
2. Pattern of circulation: Type II
3. Vascular anatomy:
   - Dominant pedicle: ascending branch of medial circumflex femoral artery and vein
   - Minor pedicles: branches from superficial femoral artery and vein
4. Innervation: anterior branch of obturator nerve (motor); anterior femoral cutaneous nerve (sensory)

J. Tensor Fascia Lata Flap

1. Flap type: muscle, musculocutaneous, musculofascial
2. Pattern of circulation: Type I
3. Vascular anatomy:
   - Dominant pedicle: ascending branch of lateral circumflex femoral artery and vein
4. Innervation: superior gluteal nerve (motor); lateral femoral cutaneous nerve (sensory)

K. Biceps Femoris Flap

1. Flap type: muscle and musculocutaneous
2. Pattern of circulation: Type II
3. Vascular anatomy:
   - Dominant pedicle: 1st to 3rd perforating branches of profunda femoris artery and vein
   - Minor pedicles: branches from inferior gluteal artery and vein and superior lateral genicular artery and vein
4. Innervation: branches of sciatic nerve (motor); posterior cutaneous nerve of the thigh (sensory)

VII. LEG AND FOOT FLAPS

A. Anterior Tibial Artery Flap

1. Flap type: fasciocutaneous
2. Pattern of circulation: Type B
3. Vascular anatomy:
   - Dominant pedicle: septocutaneous branches of anterior tibial artery and vein
4. Innervation: common peroneal nerve (sensory)

B. Tibialis Anterior Muscle Flap

1. Flap type: muscle
2. Pattern of circulation: Type IV
3. Vascular anatomy:
   - Segmental pedicles: branches of anterior tibial artery and vein
4. Innervation: deep peroneal nerve (motor)

C. Fibula Flap

1. Flap type: osseous and osteofasciocutaneous
2. Pattern of circulation: Type IV
3. Vascular anatomy:
   - Dominant pedicle: nutrient artery and vein from peroneal vessels
   - Minor pedicles: periosteal and muscular branches from peroneal vessels
4. Innervation: superficial peroneal nerve (sensory)

D. Extensor Hallucis Longus Flap

1. Flap type: muscle
2. Pattern of circulation: Type IV
3. Vascular anatomy:
   - Segmental pedicles: 6–8 branches from anterior tibial vessels
4. Innervation: deep peroneal nerve (motor)

E. Extensor Digitorum Longus Flap

1. Flap type: muscle
2. Pattern of circulation: Type IV
3. Vascular anatomy:
   - Segmental pedicles: 8–10 branches from anterior tibial vessels
4. Innervation: deep peroneal nerve (motor)

F. Gastrocnemius Flap

1. Flap type: muscle and musculocutaneous
2. Pattern of circulation: Type I
3. Vascular anatomy:
   - Dominant pedicle: medial sural artery and vein (medial head); lateral sural artery and vein (lateral head)
4. Innervation: tibial nerve branches (motor); saphenous nerve for medial head and sural nerve for lateral head (sensory)

G. Soleus Flap

1. Flap type: muscle and musculocutaneous
2. Pattern of circulation: Type II
3. Vascular anatomy:
   - Dominant pedicles: branches from popliteal artery and vein, posterior tibial artery and vein, and peroneal artery and vein
   - Minor pedicles: branches from posterior tibial artery and vein
4. Innervation: tibial and medial popliteal nerves (motor)

H. Sural Artery Flap

1. Flap type: fasciocutaneous
2. Pattern of circulation: Type A

3. Vascular anatomy:
   - Dominant pedicle: direct cutaneous branch from sural artery and lesser saphenous vein
4. Innervation: medial sural cutaneous nerve (sensory)

I. Dorsalis Pedis Flap

1. Flap type: fasciocutaneous
2. Pattern of circulation: Type B
3. Vascular anatomy:
   - Dominant pedicles: septocutaneous perforators from dorsalis pedis artery and first dorsal metatarsal artery, venae comitantes, and long and short saphenous veins
4. Innervation: branches of deep and superficial peroneal nerves (sensory)

J. Extensor Digitorum Brevis Flap

1. Flap type: muscle
2. Pattern of circulation: Type II
3. Vascular anatomy:
   - Dominant pedicle: lateral tarsal branch of dorsal pedis artery and venae comitantes
4. Innervation: lateral tarsal branches of deep peroneal nerve (motor)

K. Abductor Hallucis Flap

1. Flap type: muscle and musculocutaneous
2. Pattern of circulation: Type II
3. Vascular anatomy:
   - Dominant pedicle: proximal branch of medial plantar artery and vein
   - Minor pedicles: branches from medial plantar vessels
4. Innervation: medial plantar nerve (motor); medial plantar nerve (sensory)

L. Abductor Digiti Minimi Flap

1. Flap type: muscle and musculocutaneous
2. Pattern of circulation: Type II
3. Vascular anatomy:
   - Dominant pedicle: proximal branch from lateral plantar artery and vein
   - Minor pedicles: muscular branches from lateral plantar vessels
4. Innervation: lateral plantar nerve (motor); lateral plantar nerve and branches of sural nerve (sensory)

M. Lateral Plantar Artery Flap

1. Flap type: fasciocutaneous
2. Pattern of circulation: Type B
3. Vascular anatomy:
   - Dominant pedicle: calcaneal branches of lateral plantar artery
4. Innervation: medial calcaneal branches of tibial nerve (sensory)

N. Medial Plantar Artery Flap

1. Flap type: fasciocutaneous
2. Pattern of circulation: Type B
3. Vascular anatomy:
   - Dominant pedicle: medial plantar artery and vein
   - Minor pedicles: perforating branches from abductor hallucis and flexor digitorum brevis muscles
4. Innervation: medial plantar nerve (sensory)

O. Great Toe Free Flap

1. Flap type: composite tissue
2. Pattern of circulation: Type A
3. Vascular anatomy:
   - Dominant pedicle: first dorsal metatarsal artery and venae comitantes
   - Minor pedicles: first plantar metatarsal artery and venae comitantes
4. Innervation: medial dorsal cutaneous nerve from superficial peroneal nerve, terminal branch of deep peroneal nerve, proper digital nerve and common digital nerve (sensory)

63

Peripheral Nerve Repair

Janet Baker, M.D.
University of Miami, Miami, Florida, U.S.A.

Ranjan Gupta, M.D.
University of California, Irvine Medical Center, Orange, California, U.S.A.

I. OBJECTIVES OF PERIPHERAL NERVE REPAIRS

A. Maximize the number of axons regenerating across an injury site.

B. Maximize the accuracy of reinnervation by careful realignment of matching fascicles within the nerve (e.g., motor fascicle to motor fascicle, sensory fascicle to sensory fascicle). Detailed nerve maps have been developed for larger nerves to help predict where certain fascicles will rest. For example, in the median nerve, the volar radial segment of the nerve is known to contain the motor branch fibers to the thenar eminence. In the ulnar nerve, the ulnar dorsal segment of the nerve contains the motor fibers to the intrinsic muscles of the hand.

C. Minimize tension and scar tissue formation.

D. Minimize occurrence of postoperative neuroma formation.

II. PRIMARY REPAIR

A. Defined as an immediate repair of the injured or repair within several hours of injury.

B. Primary repair is the treatment of choice for:

- Sharp nerve transection (crushed segments must be excised)
- Clean wound
- Healthy tissue bed
- Appropriate surgical equipment/surgeon/staff
- Patient physically and emotionally stable

III. DELAYED PRIMARY REPAIR

A. Defined as repair of the nerve within 5–7 days of the initial injury.

B. Best with avulsion-type injuries in which the zone of injury is not clear at time of injury. Waiting several days before performing the repair will allow the viable and nonviable segments of nerve to become more clearly identified.

C. If retraction develops at the nerve transection site, direct suture repair may not be possible without excessive tension, thereby necessitating an interpositional nerve graft. Excessive tension on a repair will markedly increase scar tissue formation and decrease overall functional return.

IV. SECONDARY REPAIR

A. Defined as a repair performed more than 7 days from the time of original injury.

V. PRINCIPLES OF NERVE REPAIR

A. Quantitative Pre- and Postoperative Clinical Assessment of Both Motor and Sensory Systems

1. Pinch/grip strength.
2. Static and moving two-point discrimination (test of innervation density). This test is most useful for evaluation of nerve regeneration (e.g., following nerve transection and subsequent repair).
3. Vibration and Semmes-Weinstein pressure stimulus measures (tests of threshold sensation). These tests are most useful for evaluation of decreased function of an intact nerve (e.g., compression neuropathy).

B. Microsurgical Technique

1. Operating microscope provides the best overall view of the surgical field under 6–25× magnification. Some surgeons prefer surgical magnification loupes (2.5–6×) instead of an operating microscope for ease of use.
2. Microsurgical instruments specifically designed for fine sutures and atraumatic handling of tissues.
3. Appropriate microsurgical needles and sutures (e.g., 9-0 or 10-0 nylon sutures).

C. Nerve Repair

1. Tension-free repair is critical to maximize regeneration of nerve fibers across the repair site and to minimize scar tissue formation.
2. Interposition nerve graft or nerve conduit (e.g., vein graft conduit, synthetic absorbable nerve conduit) if tension-free repair is not possible.
3. Extremity must be kept in neutral position following repair. Avoid extreme flexion or extension joint positioning to relieve tension on the nerve repair. If extreme joint positioning is required to relieve tension, it is better to place the joint in a neutral position and to repair the nerve with an interpositional nerve graft or nerve conduit.
4. Primary repair is optimal if clinical and surgical conditions permit.
5. Epineurial repair is performed if fascicles have mixed sensory and motor function without well-defined groups of fascicles or if the nerve is a single small peripheral nerve (e.g., digital nerve).
6. Group fascicular repair is performed when a particular fascicle is recognized as mediating a specific function (e.g., motor fascicle of the ulnar nerve).
7. Motor and sensory reeducation.

VI. TYPES OF NERVE REPAIRS

A. Epineurial Repair

1. Appropriate magnification.
2. Identify proximal and distal nerve ends under tourniquet control to provide a bloodless field.
3. Fascicular or vascular landmarks are identified on the nerve. The surgeon should match the orientation of longitudinal vessels found on the epineurium or match fascicles based on size, location, and shape.
4. Nerve ends are trimmed as necessary to achieve healthy-appearing nerve ends.
5. Epineurial sleeves are joined to oppose contents of the nerve.
6. Minimal pressure or tension or should be present at the completion of the nerve repair.
7. Repair:
   - The first suture is placed at the location on the nerve farthest from surgeon.
   - The second suture is placed 180 degrees opposed from first suture.
   - Uniform tension should be present as each suture is sequentially placed.
   - Additional sutures are placed sparingly to minimize scar formation—only enough sutures should be placed to provide good apposition of the nerve fibers/epineurium and to minimize the number of fibers that protrude outside of the nerve repair boundaries.
   - 8-0, 9-0, or 10-0 sutures are placed using standard microsurgical techniques.

B. Group Fascicular Repair

1. Higher magnification needed.
2. Nerve ends are inspected with respect to size, shape, and location in order to determine alignment of the fascicles.

3. Fascicular groups are aligned, matched, trimmed, and repaired.

C. Individual Fascicular Repair

1. Individual fascicles within a larger group fascicle are dissected and repaired separately.
2. This approach can be difficult (e.g., median nerve has up to 32 individual fascicles) and may engender excessive scar tissue formation within the nerve.

D. Epineurial vs. Fascicular Repair

1. Superiority of one technique has not been proven.
2. Potential benefits of fascicular repair may be lost due to increased surgical manipulation and scar tissue formation.
3. Repair of inappropriate fascicles (mismatched fascicles) results in poor outcome.

VII. FASCICLE MATCHING TECHNIQUES*

A. Intraoperative Nerve Stimulation

1. Positively identifies proximal sensory and distal motor fascicles.
2. Patient cooperation necessary—requires that the procedure be performed under local or regional anesthesia so that the patient may be alert enough to participate in the testing.

B. Histochemical Identification

1. May use up to 9 days from injury.
2. Acetylcholinesterase—present in axoplasm of myelinated motor axons and many unmyelinated axons, not sensory axons.
3. Carbonic anhydrase—present in myelin and axoplasm of sensory axons.
4. Must sacrifice nerve tissue from proximal and distal stumps in order to allow for histochemical testing.
5. 1–2 hours of processing time is required.
6. Patient cooperation is not necessary—general anesthesia is not contraindicated.
7. Is used primarily as a tool in late nerve reconstructions.

*Useful techniques but not routinely performed.

VIII. NERVE GAP VS. NERVE DEFECT

A. Nerve defect—actual amount of tissue lost.

B. Nerve gap—distance between proximal and distal nerve ends. May or may not be associated with a nerve defect (i.e., a simple laceration of a nerve without nerve tissue loss will result in a nerve gap secondary to retraction if not repaired in a timely fashion).

C. Nerve graft—performed when end-to-end repair cannot be performed without excessive tension.

D. Ideal nerve graft features include:

- Large fascicles, little connective tissue
- Separate parallel fascicles
- Large diameter
- Large-caliber axons
- Accessible location
- Little variability
- Little branching
- Minimal donor-site morbidity (expendable donor nerve)

E. Donor nerve graft options include:

- Sural nerve—located in the posterior compartment of the leg, adjacent to the lesser saphenous vein. It can be located easily at the lateral aspect of the ankle, halfway between the posterior border of the lateral malleolus and the anterior border of the Achilles tendon.
- Anterior branch of the medial antebrachial cutaneous nerve.
- Lateral antebrachial cutaneous nerve.
- Terminal branch of posterior interosseous nerve—located at the floor of the fourth dorsal extensor tendon compartment at the distal forearm level.

IX. VASCULARIZED NERVE GRAFTS

A. Role not established.

B. Potential indications:

- Large nerve gaps
- Proximal injuries

- Compromised tissue beds with diminished blood supply
- Large-caliber donor nerve grafts

X. NERVE CONDUITS

A. Usually indicated for nerve defects less than 3 cm in length—best if the defect is less than 2 cm in length.

B. Autogenous vein grafts:

- Vein may be used in its natural orientation or "inside out"
- Advantages:

  Autogenous tissue type—no foreign or synthetic material

  Easily obtained

  Avoids donor site morbidity associated with nerve grafts.

- Disadvantages:

  Requires additional operative time to obtain the vein graft

  Vein graft lacks structural support—is collapsible, which may reduce the amount of nerve regeneration across the conduit

C. Synthetic nerve conduits

- Absorbable—currently available options include collagen type I and polyglycolic acid polymers that ultimately absorb fully over a period of months
- Good structural support—will not collapse
- Primary advantage lack of nerve/vein graft donor site morbidity and "off-the-shelf" availability without requiring additional operative time
- Disadvantages include cost (currently 500–1000 per conduit) and non-autogenous nature of the conduit

64

Anatomy and Embryology of the Hand

Victoria S. Pao, M.D., James Chang, M.D., and Robert A. Chase, M.D.
Stanford University Medical Center, Stanford, California, U.S.A.

I. DEVELOPMENT OF THE HAND

A. Limb development occurs between the third and eighth weeks of gestation.

B. On day 24, upper limb buds (with their mesenchymal core and ectodermal cover) develop from the somatopleuric lateral plate mesoderm at the lower cervical region.

C. The apical ectodermal ridge forms soon after and is essential for differentiation of the limb.

D. By day 33, hand plate, forearm, arm, and shoulder regions are evident. By day 37, the digital plate surrounds the central carpal region.

E. In the fifth week, condensed mesoderm begins to form the skeletal elements.

F. By the sixth week, digital rays are evident. Radial necrotic zones between the digital rays undergo programmed cell death for differentiation of the digits.

G. Between the eighth and twelfth weeks, ossification of the cartilaginous structures occurs. By day 56, all regions of the upper extremity are well defined.

H. After birth, myelination of the nervous system is achieved by 2 years of age. Epiphyses located at the ends of the limb bones gradually ossify until completion of puberty.

II. ARTERIAL ANATOMY

The vascular inflow to the upper extremity and hand is a continuation of the axillary artery to the brachial artery. The brachial artery is palpable just medial to the biceps tendon at the level of the elbow.

A. Radial Artery

1. The brachial artery branches into the radial and ulnar arteries at the bicipital aponeurosis of the elbow.
2. The radial artery continues distally in the forearm between the brachioradialis and flexor carpi radialis muscles. At the wrist, the radial artery is located near the styloid process of the radius, and then travels dorsally across the anatomic snuffbox before penetrating the first dorsal interosseous muscle.
3. In the hand, the radial artery penetrates between the first and second metacarpal bones to create the deep palmar arch.

B. Ulnar Artery

1. The ulnar artery is the other major branch of the brachial artery.
2. Soon after the takeoff of the ulnar artery, the common interosseous artery originates and itself

branches into the anterior and posterior interosseous arteries.

3. The ulnar artery continues in the forearm under the flexor carpi ulnaris muscle.
4. At the wrist, the ulnar artery lies radial to the pisiform, ulnar to the hook of the hamate, and radial to the ulnar nerve. It then travels into the hand through Guyon's canal, deep to the palmaris brevis and the hypothenar fascia. In the hand, it provides the majority of the blood supply to the superficial palmar arch.

C. Superficial Palmar Arch

1. Anastomosis between the ulnar artery and superficial branch of the radial artery.
2. Variations in dominance exist (66% ulnar artery dominance, 30% radial artery, 4% persistent median artery).
3. Digital arteries originate from the superficial palmar arch.

D. Deep Palmar Arch

1. Extension of the radial artery after it penetrates the dorsum of the first web space and gives off the princeps pollicis artery to the thumb.
2. The deep palmar arch forms an anastomosis with the deep branch of the ulnar artery and is the source of the palmar metacarpal arteries.
3. It lies 1.5 cm proximal to the superficial arch in the palm.

E. Dorsal Carpal Arch

1. Anastomosis of radial and ulnar dorsal carpal branches.
2. Provides the arterial supply to the carpal bones.

F. Supplemental Arteries in the Upper Extremity

1. Anterior interosseus artery
2. Posterior interosseus artery
3. Persistent median artery

G. Digital Arteries

1. The digital arteries branch from the superficial palmar arch and lie on the ulnar and radial aspect of each digit.
2. The dominant digital artery to each digit is: (1) thumb and index finger—ulnar digital artery, (2) middle and ring finger—co-dominant digital arteries, and (3) small finger—radial digital artery.
3. An arcade of branches to each digit provides an abundant collateral arterial system.

III. VENOUS AND LYMPHATIC ANATOMY

A. Veins generally follow the arterial pattern in the deep system as venae comitantes.

B. An abundant superficial system of venous drainage also exists. Ultimately, these superficial veins contribute to the cephalic and basilic veins of the upper extremities.

C. Lymphatic drainage terminates in the axillary, supraclavicular, and infraclavicular nodes.

IV. NEURAL ANATOMY

A. Ulnar nerve—branch of the medial cord of the brachial plexus (C8-T1):

- Muscular branches—to flexor carpi ulnaris and flexor digitorum profundus to the ring and small fingers.
- Palmar cutaneous branch—sensation to the hypothenar eminence and medial (ulnar) portion of the palm.
- Dorsal cutaneous branch—sensory; forms the dorsal digital nerves of small finger and ulnar aspect of the ring finger. Also provides sensation to the ulnar half of the dorsum of the hand.
- Superficial branch—sensory; forms the ulnar digital nerve to the small finger and common digital nerve that divides into the small finger radial digital nerve and the ring finger ulnar digital nerve.
- Deep motor branch—supplies the four hypothenar muscles (abductor digiti minimi, opponens digiti minimi, flexor digiti minimi brevis, and palmaris brevis), third and fourth lumbrical muscles, dorsal and volar interossei, adductor pollicis brevis, and flexor pollicis brevis (deep head).

B. Median nerve—from lateral and medial cords of the brachial plexus (C5-T1):

- Muscular branches—supply pronator teres, flexor carpi radialis, palmaris longus, and flexor digitorum superficialis.

- Anterior interosseous branch—innervates the flexor pollicis longus, flexor digitorum profundus to the index and middle fingers, and pronator quadratus. Also provides wrist sensation.
- Palmar cutaneous branch—sensory; supplies the thenar eminence and provides lateral (radial) palmar sensation.
- Recurrent motor branch—innervates thenar muscles [abductor pollicis brevis, opponens pollicis, and flexor pollicis brevis (superficial head)].
- Sensory branches—supply digital nerves to the thumb, index finger, middle finger, and radial aspect of the ring finger.

C. Radial nerve—branch of the posterior cord of the brachial plexus (C6-8):

- Muscular branches—innervate brachioradialis and extensor carpi radialis longus.
- Radial nerve divides into terminal deep and superficial branches at the proximal forearm.
- Deep posterior interosseous nerve—supplies motor branches to the extensor carpi radialis brevis, supinator, extensor digitorum communis, extensor digiti minimi, extensor carpi ulnaris, extensor indicis proprius, extensor pollicis longus, extensor pollicis brevis, and abductor pollicis longus and terminates to supply carpal joint sensation.
- Superficial radial nerve—sensory; provides cutaneous branches and supplies the thumb and radial half of the dorsum of the hand.

V. SKELETAL ANATOMY

A. Wrist

1. The distal radioulnar joint allows pronation and supination of the hand as the radius rotates around the had of the ulna.
2. The proximal carpal row of bones (scaphoid, lunate, triquetrum, pisiform) articulates with the distal radius and ulna, providing the ability to flex and extend the hand and perform radial and ulnar deviation.
3. The distal carpal row (trapezium, trapezoid, capitate, and hamate), along with the second and third metacarpals, for the "fixed unit" of the hand.

B. Phalanges

1. Each digit, except the thumb, is composed of three bones extending from their respective metacarpal (proximal, middle, and distal phalanx).
2. The metacarpophalangeal joint allows flexion, extension, abduction, and adduction of the digit.
3. Radial and ulnar collateral ligaments, along with the volar plates, control joint stability. The collateral ligaments limit lateral motion of the joints. The collateral ligaments are maximally stretched when metacarpophalangeal joints are fully flexed and when interphalangeal joints are fully extended.

VI. MUSCLE ANATOMY

A. Extrinsic Muscles

1. Extensors

a. Extensor muscles lie on the dorsum of the forearm and hand and are innervated by the radial nerve.

b. The brachioradialis (BR) is a flexor of the elbow joint but is included with the extensor muscles because it is supplied by the radial nerve.

c. The BR and the extensor carpi radialis longus (ECRL) originate from the lateral supracondylar ridge of the humerus.

d. The four superficial extensors [extensor carpi radialis brevis (ECRB), extensor digitorum communis (EDC), extensor digiti minimi (EDM), and extensor carpi ulnaris (ECU)] originate from the common extensor tendon that is attached to the supracondylar ridge and lateral epicondyle.

e. The extensors can be divided by function. The extensor carpi ECRL and ECRB and the ECU serve to extend the wrist. The extensor digitorum EDC, extensor indicis proprius (EIP), and the extensor EDM are finger extensors. Three extrinsic extensors assist in thumb motion: abductor pollicis longus (APL), extensor pollicis brevis (EPB), and extensor pollicis longus (EPL).

f. The extensor retinaculum prevents bowstringing of tendons across the wrist. Six extensor compartments exist (listed in anatomic position from radial to ulnar):

1. APL, EPB
2. ECRL, ECRB

3. EPL
4. EDC, EIP
5. EDM
6. ECU

2. Flexors

a. The flexors are located on the volar side of the forearm and wrist.

b. The flexors are innervated by the median nerve, except for the flexor carpi ulnaris (FCU) and the flexor digitorum profundus (FDP) to the ring and small fingers, which are innervated by the ulnar nerve.

c. The flexor carpi radialis (FCR), FCU, and palmaris longus (PL) provide wrist flexion. The digital flexors [flexor digitorum superficialis (FDS), FDP, and flexor pollicis longus (FPL)] pass through the carpal tunnel to provide dual flexion to the fingers and single flexion to the thumb.

d. Flexor digitorum superficialis—bifurcates at the base of the proximal phalanx and inserts into the mid-portion of the middle phalanx.

e. Flexor digitorum profundus—perforates the FDS at Camper's chiasm to run superficial along the length of the proximal and middle phalanges to insert at the base of the distal phalanx. These flexors contribute most of the force for digital flexion. The FDP of the index finger is unique in that it has an independent muscle belly.

f. The flexor pollicis longus inserts at the distal phalanx of the thumb.

g. Pulleys—areas of thickening of the synovial sheaths that enclose the flexor tendons. Pulleys prevent bowstringing of the flexor tendons during flexion. There are five annular (A) and four cruciate (C) pulleys:

- A1—metacarpophalangeal joint; usual site of triggering
- A2—proximal portion of the proximal phalanx
- A3—proximal interphalangeal joint
- A4—middle portion of the middle phalanx
- A5—distal interphalangeal joint
- A2 and A4 are essential to prevent bowstringing
- Cruciate pulleys are flimsy and may be sacrificed

3. Pronators and Supinators

a. The pronator teres originates from the common flexor-pronator origin at the medial epicondyle and inserts at the mid-portion of the radius. It is innervated by the median nerve and is a primary forearm pronator and a weak forearm flexor.

b. The pronator quadratus is a short, wide muscle that spans transversely across the distal radius and ulna. It is also innervated by the median nerve (anterior interosseous nerve) and is a forearm pronator.

c. The supinator originates from the lateral epicondyle of the humerus and inserts on the proximal third of the radius. It is innervated by the deep branch of the radial nerve and is a primary supinator, assisted by the biceps brachii.

B. Intrinsic Muscles

Intrinsic muscles arise and insert within the hand. They can be divided into four groups.

1. Thenar muscles—four muscles:

- Abductor pollicis brevis (APB)
- Flexor pollicis brevis (FPB)
- Opponens pollicis (OP)
- Adductor pollicis (AdP)
- Of note, the APB, OP, and superficial head of FPB are innervated by the median nerve, while the AdP and deep head of FPB are innervated by the ulnar nerve.

2. Hypothenar muscles (all innervated by the ulnar nerve)—four muscles:

- Palmaris brevis (PB)
- Abductor digiti minimi (ADM)
- Flexor digiti minimi brevis (FDMB)
- Opponens digiti minimi (ODM)

3. Lumbricals—four muscles:

- The index and middle finger lumbricals are innervated by the median nerve. The ring and small finger lumbricals are innervated by the ulnar nerve.
- Originate from the flexor digitorum profundus tendons and insert on radial aspect of extensor mechanism, distal to the metacarpophalangeal joint.
- Contribute to flexion of the metacarpophalan-

geal joint and extension of the interphalangeal joints.

4. Interossei:
   - All are innervated by the ulnar nerve.
   - Consist of three palmar interosseous muscles and four dorsal interosseous muscles.
   - Originate from the metacarpals and form the lateral bands (with the lumbricals), acting to flex the metacarpophalangeal joints and extend the interphalangeal joints.
   - They also adduct (volar interossei) and abduct (dorsal interossei) the fingers toward or away from the midline.

65

Examination of the Hand

Tiffany K. Danton, M.D., and Amy L. Ladd, M.D.
Stanford University, Stanford, California, U.S.A.

I. INITIAL HISTORY

A. Examination of the hand begins with the history: identifying the chief complaint and then location, onset, nature, severity, and duration of pain.

B. The presence of numbness or tingling is noted, as is trouble with specific motor tasks such as writing or grasping.

C. The patient's age, gender, hand dominance, occupation, and hobbies are included in the initial assessment.

D. Past history such as the presence of systemic disease, previous trauma, vascular or renal disease, autoimmune disease, and diabetes are also identified.

II. PHYSICAL EXAM

A. General

1. There are several steps in examining the hand. First is observation. Note the presence of scars or lesions, open wounds, swelling, ecchymosis, or bony deformity. Note the posture of the wrist and fingers.
2. Compare the temperature of the skin, and note whether the hands are moist or dry.
3. Check the radial and ulnar pulses and the presence of tenderness over bones, joints, or tendons.
4. Palpate painful areas last so as not to miss other abnormalities (Tables 1 and 2).

B. Range of Motion

Initially, perform a global assessment by asking the patient to make a fist and then straighten or extend all fingers. The metacarpal arch is flat while the fingers are extended. Impaired motion can be caused by dorsal hand edema, scars, adherent extensor tendons, shortened collateral ligaments, or joint abnormalities. Next, assess both active and passive range of motion in each individual digit (Table 3).

1. Metacarpophalangeal (MCP) Joint

a. The thumb MCP joint normally flexes 45–60° and extends to 0°. Hyperextension of the thumb may indicate volar plate disruption at the metacarpal attachment, which can cause the proximal phalanx to sublux dorsally relative to the metacarpal head.

b. A common injury to the thumb is an ulnar collateral ligament tear, often known as a "gamekeeper's thumb" (chronic) or "skier's thumb" (acute). The examiner will be able to demonstrate increased radial deviation at the MP joint compared to the opposite side. Testing is performed by applying stress on both sides of the thumb with the MCP joint in 10–20° of flexion and again in full flexion.

Table 1 Signs of a Closed Fracture

Pain and tenderness over the bone/joint
Swelling, ecchymosis, crepitation
Postural deformity

c. A common injury at the metacarpal joint of the thumb is a Bennett's fracture, an intra-articular fracture at the base of the thumb metacarpal.

d. The finger MCP joint normally flexes to 85° and extends to 0°, compared to the more limited motion of the thumb MCP joint.

e. Finger MCP joint dorsal dislocation may lead to metacarpal head entrapment between the flexor tendon on the ulnar side, the lumbrical muscle on the radial side, and the volar plate.

f. A decreased prominence of the 5th metacarpal head may indicate a fracture of the 5th metacarpal neck ("boxer's fracture"), a common punching injury.

2. Proximal Interphalangeal Joint

a. The finger PIP joint normally flexes to 110° and extends to 0°.

b. Hyperextension of this joint may indicate a ruptured volar plate, long-standing intrinsic muscle còntraction, or loss of the flexor digitorum superficialis tendon.

c. A flexion deformity can result from disruption of the overlying extensor tendon (boutonnière deformity) or from scarring of the flexor tendon or volar plate.

3. Distal Interphalangeal Joint

a. This joint normally flexes to 65° and extends to 0°.

b. The mallet finger deformity occurs with rupture of the terminal extensor tendon, causing flexion of the DIP in the resting position with an inability to actively extend the distal phalanx.

Table 2 Kanavel's Signs of Tenosynovitis

Pain over the affected digit and along the tendon sheath with palpation
Digit held in a flexed posture
Fusiform swelling of the digit
Pain with passive, gentle extension

Table 3 Normal Range of Motion

	Degrees of flexion	Degrees of extension
Finger metacarpal-phalangeal (MCP) joint	85	0
Finger proximal interphalangeal (PIP) joint	110	0
Finger distal interphalangeal (DIP) joint	65	0
Thumb metacarpal-phalangeal (MCP) joint	45–60	0
Thumb interphalangeal (IP) joint	90	0

4. Combination Joint Deformities:

a. The swan-neck deformity (Fig. 1) is identified as PIP hyperextension with DIP flexion. This is seen commonly with rheumatoid arthritis (which causes volar plate laxity and intrinsic tightness), volar plate injuries, and old mallet finger injuries.

b. A boutonnière deformity (Fig. 2) is manifested as PIP flexion with DIP hyperextension. The cause is disruption of the extensor tendon's insertion onto the middle phalanx.

C. Extrinsic Flexors

The extrinsic flexor muscle bellies lie within the forearm, while the tendon insertions are in the hand. This group

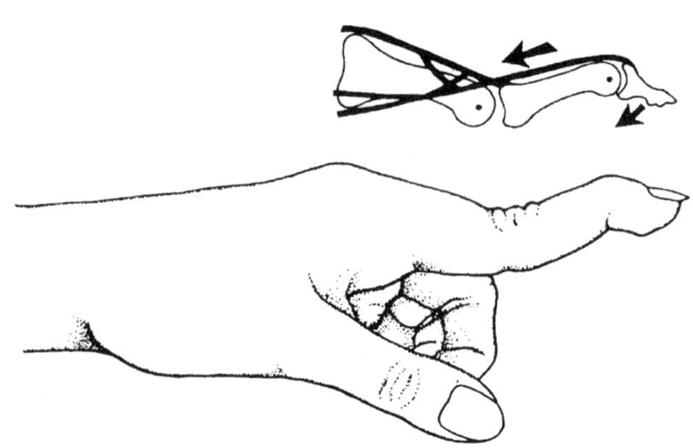

Figure 1 Swan-neck deformity.

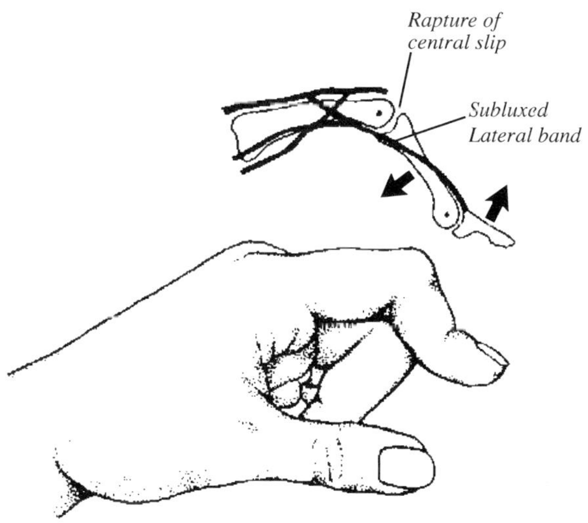

Figure 2 Boutonnière deformity.

includes the flexor digitorum profundus, flexor digitorum superficialis, and flexor pollicis longus for the hand. The extrinsic flexors of the wrist include the flexor carpi ulnaris and flexor carpi radialis muscles.

1. Flexor Digitorum Profundus

a. The FDP flexes both the PIP and DIP joints of the fingers, whereas the flexor digitorum superficialis flexes only the PIP joint.

b. Have the patient make a fist to test the FDP. Isolate the FDP by asking the patient to bend just the tip, or distal phalanx, of each finger while the examiner holds the PIP joint straight to block the FDS (Fig. 3).

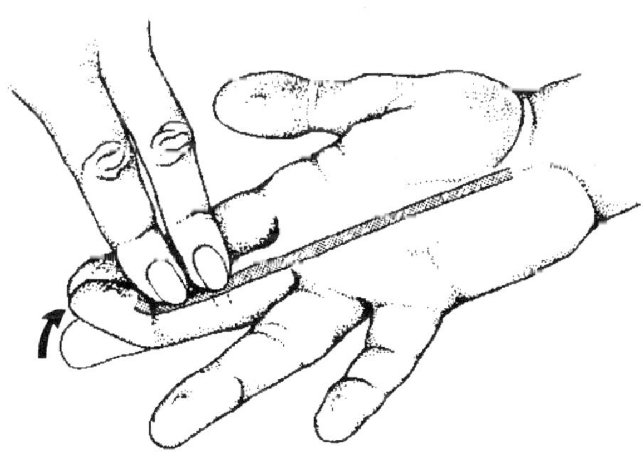

Figure 3 Testing for FDP musculotendinous function.

2. Flexor Digitorum Superficialis

a. The FDS flexes the digits at the PIP joints.

b. To test for the integrity of the FDS tendon, stabilize all but one digit in full extension and ask the patient to bend the free finger to elicit PIP flexion (Fig. 4). With an intact FDS, the PIP joint will flex.

c. The FDS muscle bellies are able to function independently, as opposed to the FDP muscle bellies that act as a unit. This is why DIP flexion is prevented by the extension of the other fingers in this test.

3. Flexor Pollicis Longus

a. The FPL flexes the thumb at the interphalangeal joint.

b. The FPL is tested by asking the patient to flex the interphalangeal joint of the thumb.

D. Extrinsic Extensors

These muscles overlie the dorsum of the wrist and insert onto the dorsal hand. They are arranged into six separate anatomic compartments. Extension of the fingers and thumb at the MCP joints depends upon the extrinsic extensors. At the PIP and DIP joints, extension results from interplay between the extrinsic and intrinsic muscles.

1. Compartment 1

a. The first compartment contains both the abductor pollicis longus (APL) and extensor pollicis brevis (EPB) tendons.

b. The APL inserts onto the thumb metacarpal, where its primary action is abduction. Ask the patient to place his or her hand onto a flat surface

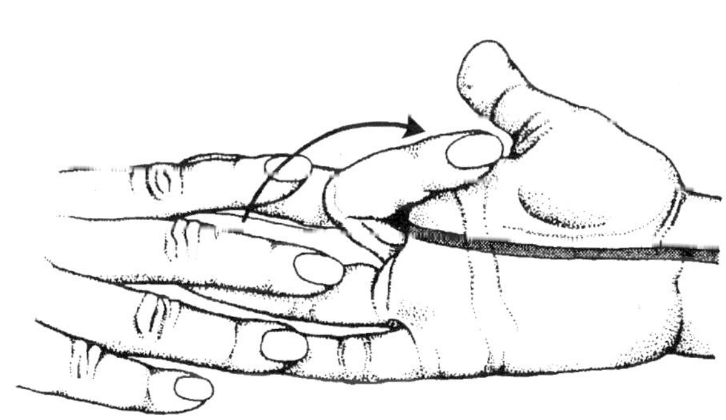

Figure 4 Testing FDS musculotendinous function.

and bring the thumb out to the side (Fig. 5). You should be able to palpate along the taut tendon on the radial side of the wrist going to the thumb.

c. The EPB inserts onto the proximal phalanx of the thumb and primarily extends the MCP joint.

2. Compartment 2

a. This contains the extensor carpi radialis brevis (ECRB) and longus (ECRL).

b. Ask the patient to make a fist while actively extending the wrist, both with and without resistance.

c. One can palpate the tendons over the dorsal wrist, where they insert onto the dorsal base of the index and middle metacarpals.

3. Compartment 3

a. The extensor pollicis longus (EPL) is the only tendon in this compartment.

b. Test the EPL by having the patient place the hand on a flat surface and lifting only the thumb (Fig. 6).

c. The EPL inserts on the dorsal base of the distal phalanx of the thumb, whereas EPB inserts more proximally.

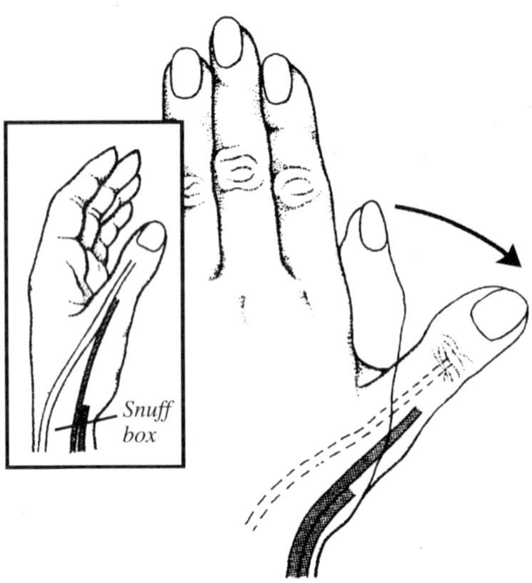

Figure 5 Testing for EPB and APL musculotendinous function.

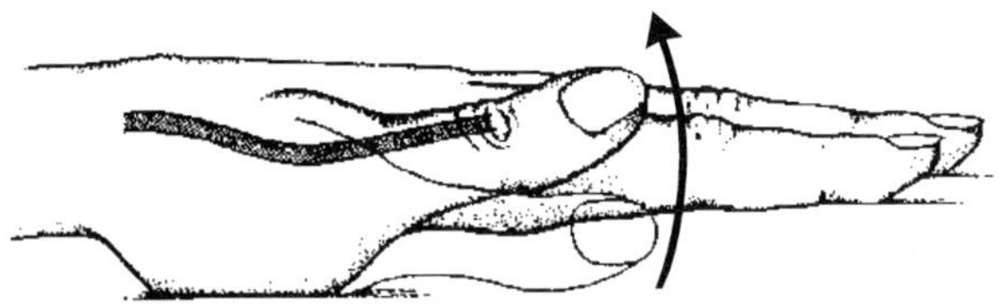

Figure 6 Testing for EPL musculotendinous function.

4. Compartment 4

a. This compartment contains the extensor digitorum communis (EDC) and extensor indicis proprius (EIP).

b. EDC is a series of tendons that share a common muscle belly.

c. Asking the patient to extend all digits tests EDC and EIP. The EIP is tested by the patient's ability to bring the index finger out to extension while the other digits are held in a fist, since the EIP has an independent proximal muscle belly.

5. Compartment 5

a. This compartment contains the extensor digiti minimi (EDM), also known as the extensor digiti quinti (EDQ).

b. Test the EDM by having the patient straighten the small finger while all the others are held in a fist. The EDM has an independent muscle belly from EIP and EDC.

6. Compartment 6

a. This compartment contains the extensor carpi ulnaris (ECU).

b. The ECU inserts onto the dorsal aspect of the 5th metacarpal and acts to extend the wrist.

c. The ECU is tested by having the patient extend the wrist ulnarly as the examiner palpates the tendon just distal to the ulnar head.

E. Instrinsic Muscles

These differ from the extrinsics in that both the muscle origin and tendon insertions lie within the hand. The intrinsic muscles function as flexors of the MCP joints and extensors of the IP joints. They also function as radial and ulnar deviators of the fingers.

Table 4 Flexors and Extensors of the Hand

	Flexion	Extension
Wrist joint	FCR, FCU, PL	ECU, ECRL, ECRB
MCP joints	Lumbricals Interossei	EDC, EIP, EDM, EPB
PIP joints	FDP, FDS FPB, FDM	EDC Lumbricals Interossei
DIP joints	FDP	Lumbricals Interossei
Thumb IP joint	FPL	EPL

1. Thenar Muscles

a. This group includes the abductor pollicis brevis, opponens pollicis, and flexor pollicis brevis.

b. These are palpated over the thumb metacarpal (thenar eminence) and work to pronate or oppose the thumb. This can be tested by asking the patient to touch the thumb and small finger tips together in pulp-to-pulp opposition.

Table 5

Nerves	Motor	Sensory
Median nerve	Pronator teres Pronator quadratus Palmaris longus Flexor carpi radialis Flexor digitorum superficialis × 4 Flexor digitorum profundus × 2 (index, middle) Flexor pollicis longus Index and middle finger lumbrical muscles Thenar muscles: Abductor pollicis brevis Opponens pollicis Superficial belly of flexor pollicis brevis	Volar part of the wrist, thumb, index, middle, and radial side of ring finger—extending to the dorsal DIP joint on all of them
Ulnar nerve	Flexor carpi ulnaris Flexor digitorum profundus × 2 (ring, small) Palmaris brevis Dorsal interosseous muscles Palmar interosseous muscles Ring and small finger lumbrical muscles Adductor pollicis Deep belly of flexor pollicis brevis Hypothenar muscles: Abductor digiti minimi Flexor digiti minimi brevis Opponens digiti minimi	Dorsal and volar aspect of small finger, ulnar side of ring finger Ulnar dorsal half of the hand
Radial nerve	Triceps Anconeus Brachioradialis Supinator Extensor carpi radialis brevis Extensor carpi radialis longus Extensor carpi ulnaris Extensor digitorum communis Extensor indicis proprius Extensor digitorum minimi Abductor pollicis longus Extensor pollicis longus Extensor pollicis brevis	Dorsal thumb, index, middle, and radial side of ring fingers—up to PIP joints Dorsal radial half of the hand Dorsal wrist capsule (posterior interosseous branch)

2. Adductor Pollicis

This muscle originates from the third metacarpal and inserts into the proximal phalanx of the thumb, functioning as an important adductor of the thumb during pinching.

3. Hypothenar Muscles

a. These include the abductor digiti minimi, flexor digiti minimi, and opponens digiti minimi.

b. Ask the patient to abduct the small finger away from the rest of the fingers and palpate contraction of these muscles to test them.

4. Interosseous Muscles

a. The dorsal interossei abduct the fingers while the palmar interossei adduct the fingers. The interossei muscles also flex the MCP joints and extend the IP joints.

b. Having the patient adduct and abduct the fingers tests these muscles. One can isolate the interossei by holding the IP joints in extension while the MCP joints are flexed.

5. Lumbrical Muscles

a. These muscles also flex the MCP joints and extend the IP joints.

b. These can be tested by asking the patient to fully flex the fingers and then move them into extension at the IP joints while the MCP joints are held in active flexion (Table 4).

F. Nerve Exam

1. The median, ulnar, and radial nerves supply both the motor and sensory innervation to the hand. Understanding the anatomic distribution of each nerve aids in identifying which nerve may be injured or dysfunctional (Table 5).
2. Two-point discrimination tests distal sensation for the median and ulnar nerves. This is performed by asking the patient to rest the hand on a flat surface. With the patient's eyes closed, the examiner takes an instrument (such as calipers or a bent paper clip) to determine the smallest distance that the patient is able to distinguish between two points touching the skin. Normal two-point discrimination distance is 2–5 mm in the fingers.

G. Vascular Exam

1. The first step of the vascular exam is the palpation of both the radial and ulnar arteries. The examiner also pinches the fingertips and assesses the nail bed for capillary refill, which is normally less than 3 seconds. Any changes in skin color are noted.
2. The Allen test is an excellent way to assess collateral flow between the radial and ulnar arteries. This is performed by compressing both the radial and ulnar arteries while the patient makes a fist, opening and closing a couple of times to exsanguinate the hand. Next, release the radial artery and check to see that the hand turns pink, which indicates patency of the radial artery with good collateral flow into the ulnar artery vascular territory. Repeat this, except releasing the ulnar artery compression to assess ulnar flow. If the radial or ulnar arteries are difficult to palpate, a Doppler may be useful.
3. The Allen test can also be performed on each of the digital arteries.

66

Diagnostic Imaging of the Hand and Wrist

Peter J. Taub, M.D., and Leanne L. Seeger, M.D.

I. PLAIN RADIOGRAPHS

A. Should be the primary imaging performed in almost every case.

B. Three standard views: posterior-anterior (PA), lateral, and oblique.

C. May require films of the uninvolved extremity for comparison.

D. Evaluate each individual bone in all three views for fractures, dislocations, subluxations, and degenerative changes, and accompanying soft tissue defects.

E. Fractures should be classified on the basis of several descriptive parameters:

- Location: head/condyle, neck, shaft, base
- Intra-articular or extra-articular
- Simple (single fracture line) vs. comminuted (two or more fracture lines)
- Angulation: apex dorsal vs. apex volar
- Fracture configuration: transverse, short oblique, long oblique

II. PHALANGES

A. Each finger is composed of a proximal, middle, and distal phalanx.

B. The thumb only has a proximal and a distal phalanx.

C. Lateral view is useful for identifying angulated fractures of the proximal and distal phalangeal bases (i.e., Mallet-type fracture).

D. Evaluate the subperiosteal surfaces.

E. Erosion (acro-osteolysis) is associated with a number of different entities:

- Connective tissue diseases with vasculitis (scleroderma and Raynaud's disease)
- Hyperparathyroidism
- Trauma
- Frostbite
- Electrical burns

F. Resorption along the radial aspects of the middle phalanges of the index and middle fingers is associated with hyperparathyroidism.

III. METACARPALS

A. Each digit, including the thumb, has a single metacarpal.

B. Each metacarpal is composed of a base proximally, a shaft, a neck, and a head distally.

C. The most common fractures of the hand involve the ulnar-sided metacarpals.

IV. CARPAL BONES

A. There are eight carpal bones arranged in two rows:

- Proximal row (from radial to ulnar)—scaphoid, lunate, triquetrum, and pisiform.
- Distal row (from radial to ulnar)—trapezium, trapezoid, capitate, and hamate.

B. Normal carpal joint spaces are 1–2 mm wide.

C. The two arcs should form two smooth lines on an PA view (Gilula's lines).

- Proximal arc is outlined by the proximal articular surfaces of the scaphoid, lunate, and triquetrum.
- Distal arc is outlined by the proximal articular surfaces of the capitate and hamate.
- Disruption of either of the arcs implies subluxation or dislocation.

D. Carpal instability is identified by abnormal intercarpal angles:

- Scapholunate angle (normal range is 30–60°)—see below.
- Capitolunate angle (normal is 0° with a range of −20 to +10°).
- Radiolunate angle (normal range is 0° to +15°).

E. Carpal height index = Ratio of the distance from the articular surface of the radius to the 3rd metacarpal/Length of 3rd metacarpal (normal range is 0.45–0.60).

F. Lateral view is useful for identifying lunate and perilunate dislocations.

- Lunate dislocation in which there is volar rotation and displacement is referred to as the "spilled tea cup sign."
- The lunate, capitate, and 3rd metacarpal should be in line with one another or at least within 10°.
- Anterior margin of the pisiform should project halfway between the anterior margin of the scaphoid and the lunate.
- Scapholunate angle is formed between the axis of the scaphoid and a line perpendicular to the vertical axis of the lunate.

G. Scapholunate dissociation secondary to a tear of the scapholunate ligament is characterized by palmar flexion of the distal pole of the scaphoid on lateral view, dorsal rotation of the lunate bone, and widening of the scapholunate space on the PA view.

- The "Terry Thomas sign" or "David Letterman sign" is a widened scapholunate space due to disruption of the scapholunate ligament. Widening of the scapholunate space may be increased with a forceful clenched fist, which increases axial loading of the wrist.

H. DISI deformity

- Dorsal intercalated segmental instability pattern of the carpus.
- Due to a tear of the scapholunate ligament.
- Lunate becomes dorsally extended while the scaphoid becomes palmarflexed perpendicular to the long axis of the radius.
- As a result, the scapholunate angle increased above the normal range of 30–60°.

I. VISI deformity

- Volar intercalated segmental instability pattern of the carpus.
- Due to a tear of the lunotriquetral ligament.
- Lunate becomes palmarflexed while the scaphoid becomes dorsiflexed perpendicular to the long axis of the radius.
- As a result, the scapholunate angle decreased below the normal range of 30–60°.

J. Carpal bone fractures

- Most commonly fractured bone is the scaphoid, which may or may not appear on initial radiographs.
- More sensitive studies include CT, MRI, and bone scan.
- Triquetral fractures most commonly occur on the dorsal cortical surface and therefore are best appreciated on a lateral radiograph.

V. DISTAL RADIUS AND ULNA

A. Evaluation requires PA and lateral views. An additional oblique view may demonstrate early erosions of the "bare area" of the metacarpal head due to rheumatoid arthritis.

- Radial height (normal is 11–13 mm).
- Radial inclination (normal is 15–25°).
- Articular fragment incongruity (should be <1 to 2 mm).
- Palmar inclination of the distal radius on the lateral view (normal is 10°).

B. Metaphyseal comminution (expressed as a percent of the sagittal width of the radius).

C. Common fracture patterns of the distal radius include:

- Colles' fracture, in which the distal fragment angulates dorsally.
- Smith's fracture, in which the distal fragment angulates volarly.

D. Ulnar variance:

- Refers to the relative heights of the distal ulna and radius at the radiocarpal joint.
- Measured on a neutral rotation PA view.
- "Ulnar neutral variance" implies an equal height between the articular surfaces of the ulna and radius.
- "Ulnar positive variance" implies that the ulnar articular surface projects more distally than the articular surface of the distal radius. It is associated with tears of the triangular fibrocartilage complex (TFCC) and distal radius fracture malunions resulting in radial shortening.
- "Ulnar negative variance" implies a relatively longer radius. It is associated with Kienböck's disease and lunate impaction.

VI. SPECIAL VIEWS

A. Stress films, including: PA with maximal radial and ulnar deviation, AP and PA of clenched fist, lateral with radial and ulnar tilt, and lateral with maximal flexion and extension.

- May be performed for persistent pain and focal swelling.
- Assess wrist instability, including tears of the proximal row ligaments with or without VISI or DISI deformities.

B. Scaphoid projection view: PA with maximum ulnar deviation of the wrist.

- Indicated in patients with radial-sided pain after trauma.

C. Carpal tunnel view: beam directed 15° toward the palm of the hand with the wrist maximally dorsiflexed and pronated.

- Used to assess injuries to the carpal bones bordering the carpal tunnel (distal pole of the scaphoid, volar margin of the trapezium, pisiform, and hook of the hamate).

VII. PEDIATRIC ISSUES

A. Position of the normal growth plates vary from bone to bone:

- Phalanges—proximal.
- Metacarpals—distal (except the thumb, which is proximal).
- Radius and ulna—distal.

B. Salter-Harris classification of epiphyseal fractures:

- Type I—transverse epiphyseal plate fracture with epiphyseal separation.
- Type II—metaphyseal fragment associated with an epiphyseal plate fracture.
- Type III—fracture through the epiphyseal plate and epiphysis.
- Type IV—fracture through the epiphyseal plate into and including an epiphyseal and metaphyseal fragment.
- Type V—impaction of the epiphyseal plate.

VIII. VIDEOFLUOROSCOPY

A. Performed on both symptomatic and asymptomatic sides.

B. Performed with the wrist in maximal ulnar and radial deviation first with an open hand, then with a clenched fist.

C. Able to detect subtle VISI and DISI deformities.

IX. ARTHROGRAPHY

A. Detects injuries to the TFCC and intercarpal ligaments.

B. Injection of contrast into the radiocarpal joint with resultant opacification of the distal radioulnar joint indicates leakage of dye across the TFCC, consistent with a tear in the TFCC.

C. Contrast extravasation into the intercarpal space indicates a tear of the intercarpal ligaments (scapholunate or lunotriquetral ligaments).

D. Carries a high true-positive rate, but many tears are not symptomatic.

X. BONE SCINTIGRAPHY

A. Utilizes Tc^{99m} bound to methylene diphosphonate, which becomes deposited in areas of increased bone turnover.

B. Half-life is 6 h.

C. Emits gamma radiation that can be detected on a sodium iodine scintillation crystal.

D. Three phases are recognized:

- Blood flow phase is a radionuclide angiogram of the radial and ulnar arteries.
- Blood pool phase at 5–8 minutes.
- Delayed phase at 3–4 h.

E. Possesses a high sensitivity and low specificity.

F. Used for evaluation of reflex sympathetic dystrophy (RSD), which demonstrates increased uptake in all three phases compared to the asymptomatic side.

G. May also use other radiotracers:

- Gallium^{67}—chronic osteomyelitis.
- Indium^{111}—acute osteomyelitis.

XI. ULTRASONOGRAPHY

A. Limited applications in evaluation of the hand.

B. Mainly used to assess fluid collections, such as cysts.

C. Recently, use has been expanded for evaluation of tendons and is especially popular in Europe and Asia.

XII. COMPUTED TOMOGRAPHY (CT)

A. Thin slices are ideal for subtle cortical abnormalities.

B. May better visualize certain lesions:

- Distal radioulnar joint fractures
- Scaphoid and hook of the hamate fractures
- Congenital abnormalities

XIII. MAGNETIC RESONANCE IMAGING (MRI)

A. Based on the spinning properties of the hydrogen atom nucleus.

B. On T1-weighted images, marrow and fat have a high signal intensity (white).

C. On T2-weighted images, cortical bone, ligaments, tendons, and fibrocartilage have low signal intensity (black). Joint fluid, cysts, and edema appear white.

D. Excellent for evaluating the presence of avascular necrosis (Kienböck's and Preiser's disease), which appears as a low signal intensity on both T1- and T2-weighted images.

67

Operating Room Procedures and Anesthesia for Hand Surgery

Yvonne L. Karanas, M.D., and Vincent R. Hentz, M.D.
Stanford University Medical Center, Stanford, California, U.S.A.

I. OPERATING ROOM

A. Set-Up

1. Maximize use of the room.
2. Power sources, electrocautery, and suction devices should be placed on the opposite side of the body from the operative site to allow for easy intraoperative fluoroscopy and use of the operating microscope.

B. Draping

1. Draping should allow the surgeon full access to the entire extremity and allow him/her to move the extremity without contamination.
2. We prefer to use a stockinette to cover the arm up to the tourniquet. Sheets are then placed both under and over the extremity and secured to the stockinette at the level of the tourniquet. This allows the arm to be taken through a complete range of motion without contamination.

II. TOURNIQUET

A. History

The tourniquet was introduced in 1718 by Jean Louis Petit to describe a device to hold pressure on an artery without requiring an assistant. The need for clear visualization of vital structures in the hand during surgery has led to the routine use of tourniquets.

B. Application

1. The arm is covered with cotton padding prior to placement of the tourniquet.
2. Apply the tourniquet snugly to minimize the risk of cuff leakage intraoperatively.
3. A plastic drape is placed at the distal edge of the cuff to prevent the cleansing solution from seeping under the tourniquet, which may result in a chemical burn.
4. The arm is exsanguinated using an Esmarch-Martin rubber bandage, and the tourniquet is then inflated.
5. Alternatively, the arm may be elevated and the brachial artery compressed for 3 minutes prior to tourniquet inflation. The arm should not be exsanguinated in patients with malignancies, compartment syndromes, high-pressure injection injuries, or infections in order to minimize risk of disseminating disease.

C. Pressure

1. The lowest pressure required to occlude arterial flow should be used to avoid posttourniquet paralysis.

2. There is no universally accepted pressure setting. Usually 50–75 mmHg over the systolic blood pressure is sufficient to provide a bloodless field. We use 250 mmHg in adults and 200 mmHg in children.

D. Tourniquet Time

1. The main concerns during tourniquet use are nerve injury due to pressure under the tourniquet and muscle injury due to ischemia.
2. The definitive limits of tourniquet time have not been conclusively defined. The most commonly accepted guidelines advocate 2 h maximum time.
3. If a tourniquet must be reinflated during a prolonged procedure, the tourniquet should be deflated for a period of 5 minutes for every 30 minutes that the tourniquet was inflated (i.e., keep tourniquet deflated for at least 20 minutes after a tourniquet time of 2 h before reinflating).

E. Complications

1. Posttourniquet paralysis: Direct pressure under the cuff is the major source of paralysis. Routine calibration and monitoring of the tourniquet are necessary to avoid the use of excessive pressure.
2. Compartment syndrome.
3. Myopathy.

III. LOCAL AND REGIONAL ANESTHESIA

A. Brachial Plexus Blockade

The brachial plexus may be anesthetized anywhere along its course after exiting the spinal cord. There exists an enclosed perineural and perivascular space that is contained by the investing fascia of the scalene muscles from the transverse processes of the cervical spine to several centimeters distal to the axilla. The plexus can be easily anesthetized anywhere along this fascial sheath. These blocks should be performed by a trained and licensed professional with the appropriate monitoring devices. There are three main approaches to the brachial plexus:

1. Interscalene: The plexus is anesthetized between the anterior and middle scalene muscles at the level of the cricoid cartilage.
2. Subclavian: The plexus is anesthetized in the interscalene groove at the level of the subclavian artery.
3. Axillary: This is the most commonly used technique because it is reliable and has a lower incidence of complications. At the level of the axillary artery, the brachial plexus forms cords that surround the axillary artery. The fascial sheath surrounding the neurovascular structures can be identified by traversing the axillary artery or by eliciting paresthesias. The anesthetic agent can then be delivered into the perineural space. The musculocutaneous and intercostal-brachial nerves must be anesthetized separately.

B. Bier Block Technique

1. A double tourniquet (two cuffs) is placed on the upper arm and a small-bore IV catheter is inserted near the surgical site.
2. The arm is exsanguinated and the distal tourniquet is inflated first to exsanguinate the tissue beneath the distal cuff. The proximal cuff is then inflated, followed by deflation of the distal cuff.
3. Local anesthesia (usually 0.5% preservative-free lidocaine without epinephrine) is injected through the IV catheter to achieve anesthesia of the extremity.
4. After approximately 20–40 minutes, the patient will develop tourniquet pain beneath the proximal cuff, since that region has not been exposed to the anesthetic. At that point, the distal cuff is inflated and the proximal cuff deflated, thereby eliminating the tourniquet pain since the distal cuff is now inflated over an area that has been anesthetized.
5. A Bier block technique can only be used in patients who can safely undergo exsanguination of the arm and when the operation lasts at least 30 minutes. If the tourniquet is deflated earlier than 30 minutes, a large dose of local anesthetic will be delivered systemically, resulting in possible lidocaine toxicity.
6. With supplemental IV sedation, a Bier block can be used in cases that last 90–120 minutes, but is not appropriate for cases of longer duration.

C. Peripheral Nerve Blocks at the Wrist

1. Ulnar nerve: The nerve can be anesthetized at the wrist, where it lies dorsal to the flexor carpi

ulnaris tendon and ulnar to the ulnar artery. The sensory branch can be anesthetized at the level of the ulnar styloid process on the dorsum of the wrist.

2. Radial nerve: The sensory branch of this nerve can be anesthetized by injecting local anesthetic over the dorsum of the forearm 2 cm proximal to the radial styloid process.
3. Median nerve: This nerve lies within the carpal tunnel, just under the transverse carpal ligament at the wrist. Local anesthetic injected at the junction of the vertical mid-palmar and distal wrist creases will achieve anesthesia of this nerve.

D. Digital Nerve Blocks

1. Each digit can be anesthetized by infiltrating local anesthetic around the digital nerves.
2. Epinephrine should be avoided in digital nerve blocks because its vasoconstrictive effects may result in ischemia.
3. The needle can be placed into the web space from a dorsal to volar direction for 1 cm. The anesthetic can then be deposited into the areas adjacent to the bifurcation of the common digital nerves.
4. The dorsal sensory nerves can be anesthetized by injecting local anesthetic on the dorsum of each individual digit.

68

Fingertip Injuries

Rudolf F. Buntic, M.D., and Harry J. Buncke, M.D.
The Buncke Microsurgical Clinic, San Francisco, California, U.S.A.

Fingertip injuries can involve the soft tissue, the distal phalanx, the nail, or the nail bed, all of which may be injured alone or in combination. Although the anatomy and extent of the injury dictate the treatment options, numerous techniques have been described to deal with fingertip injuries. The surgeon needs to formulate a treatment plan together with the patient, taking into consideration the patient's history, occupation, hand dominance, and desired outcome.

I. TERMINOLOGY AND ANATOMICAL CONSIDERATIONS

A. Fingertip—the terminal aspect of the finger, especially the distal half of the distal phalanx, distal tactile surface of the finger, subcutaneous soft tissue, nail, nail bed and distal end of the terminal phalanx.

B. Pulp—the subcutaneous soft tissue of the fingertip composed of fibrous septae separating compartments of vessels, nerves and connective tissue.

C. Open fracture—exposure of fractured bone to the outside environment.

D. Hyponychium—area beneath the distal free margin of the nail, containing numerous lymphatic channels and immune cells. The hyponychium is where the skin and sterile matrix portion of the nail bed join. This site is exposed to frequent trauma, but is very resistant to infection.

E. Paronychium—the skin and soft tissue at the nail edges.

F. Perionychium—the paronychium and nail bed.

G. Eponychium—an epithelium-lined sheath at the nail root.

H. Nail bed—dermal layer beneath the nail.

I. Germinal matrix—proximal third of the nail bed; responsible for nail growth (in conjunction with the proximal nail fold).

J. Sterile matrix—distal two thirds of the nail bed; primarily responsible for nail plate adherence to the underlying nail bed.

K. Lunula—the white line in the nail bed that demarcates the germinal matrix from the sterile matrix. The whitish color is due to cellular nuclei that degenerate at the level of the sterile matrix.

II. DIAGNOSIS

A. History

Factors to consider when evaluating treatment choices include hand dominance, occupation, affected finger(s) (thumb versus other fingers), crush vs. sharp injury, history of smoking, or history of other medical problems that could complicate a reconstructive option.

B. Examination

1. Look for the extent of injury beyond soft tissue. Is bone, joint, or tendon exposed? Is there a fracture or nail bed injury?
2. Entire hand examination: Tendons can be avulsed or ruptured in tip injuries, especially crush-avulsion injuries.
3. Plain x-rays should be taken to demonstrate fractures or foreign bodies, unless there is a clean-cut pulp injury only. Nail bed injuries are often associated with distal phalanx fractures.

III. RECONSTRUCTION PRINCIPLES IN CLOSING FINGERTIP WOUNDS

A. Meticulous technique and minimal debridement of the nail bed.

B. Precise closure of the nail bed with fine absorbable sutures under loupe magnification (e.g., 6-0 plain gut sutures).

C. Maximize sensory return and prevent neuroma formation.

D. Maintain length of the finger and nail bed.

E. Prevent loss of joint function.

F. Treat associated fractures or tendon injuries.

G. Achieve satisfactory aesthetic outcome.

IV. CLASSIFICATION OF FINGERTIP INJURIES

A. Soft Tissue Defects

1. Sharp—require minimal debridement.
2. Crush/avulsion—require more thorough debridement and may delay reconstruction if the zone of injury is not clear.

B. Combination Soft Tissue and Bone and/or Nail Injury

Most fractures, if combined with soft tissue or nail bed injuries, are open fractures.

V. CLASSIFICATION OF ACUTE NAIL BED INJURIES

A. Simple laceration.

B. Stellate laceration.

C. Severe crush injury.

D. Avulsion.

VI. TREATMENT OPTIONS IN SOFT TISSUE DEFECTS

A. Primary Closure

Difficult to do unless the wound is small.

B. Healing by Secondary Intention

1. A good technique for healing of small wounds of the soft tissue with no exposed bone.
2. Generally used with wounds 1 cm^2 or less, but can be used for larger wounds.
3. Watch for bone exposure. Bone exposure requires bone shortening or vascularized coverage. Shortening of bone should be avoided on the thumb—thumb length should be maintained if at all possible. Bone shortening may cause nail deformity.

C. Replantation

1. Very difficult to perform at this distal level because the arteries are extremely small and veins are not available. Occasionally, an artery can be found, but outflow must be established with application of leeches and/or bleeding the nail bed with heparin soaks in combination with systemic heparin therapy.
2. Since bleeding may need to be performed for 5–10 days, blood transfusion may be required.
3. Replantation at this level is usually reserved for pediatric patients.

D. Free Graft of Amputated Part

1. If the amputated part is in reasonably good shape, replantation of the part as a free composite graft can be considered, especially in children.
2. Both the amputated part and stump must be cleaned of nonviable tissue.
3. Some authors advocate cooling the graft with local ice baths placed on the finger until neovascularization occurs.
4. Clean amputations up to 1–1.5 cm in diameter may survive as a composite graft.

E. Split-Thickness Skin Graft

1. Glabrous skin is a good choice.
2. The hypothenar eminence is a common donor site. Such grafts are made up of nonpigmented

skin, like the palmar surfaces of the fingers. If multiple fingers need grafting, other sites can be used.

3. The amputated part, if in good condition, can sometimes be thinned and the skin used as a graft.

F. Local Flaps

1. Atasoy-Kleinert V-Y advancement flap—volar V-Y advancement flap with the proximal extent of the incision just distal to the DIP joint flexion crease. Provides a small amount of soft tissue.
2. Kutler V-Y advancement flap—laterally based ulnar and radial V-Y advancement flaps. Provides a small amount of soft tissue.
3. Moberg flap—large advancement flap of the entire volar soft tissue of the finger with midlateral incisions on radial and ulnar sides of the finger, with or without Z-plasties or a skin graft at the base of the finger. Creation of a Moberg flap is a larger operation that causes soft tissue swelling of the entire finger. It is considered a better option for the thumb than for the fingers. The primary disadvantage is a risk of flexion contracture of the thumb IP joint.

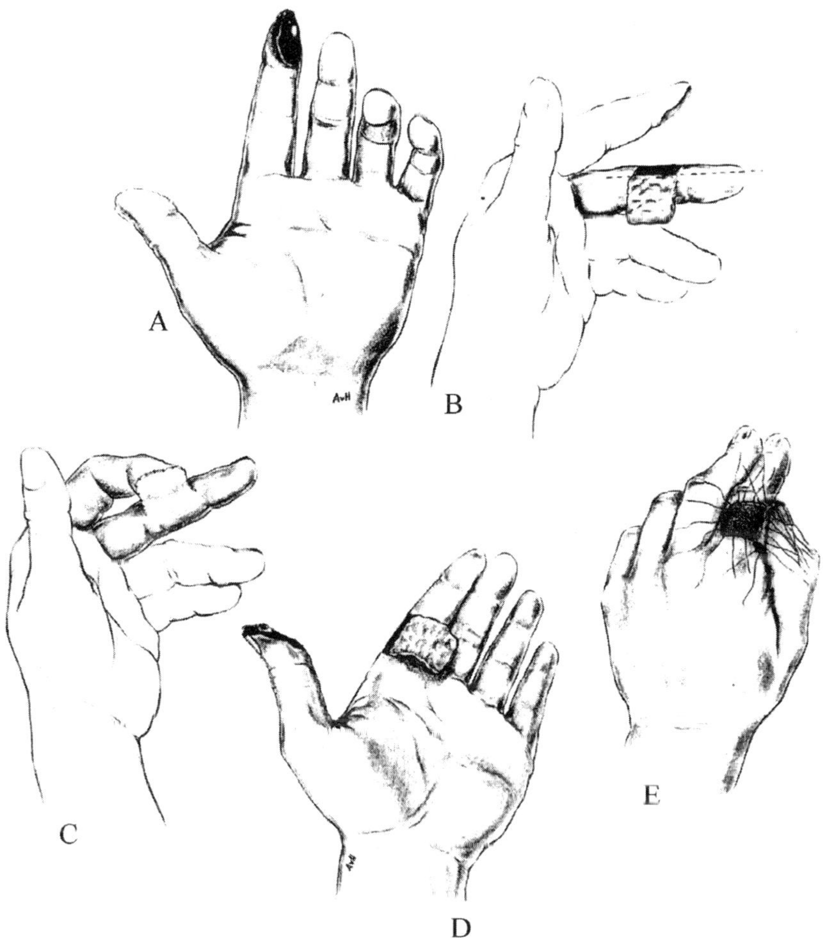

Figure 1 A cross-finger flap is elevated from the dorsal aspect of the middle phalanx and inset over a defect of the index finger. For the thumb, the flap can be elevated from the proximal aspect of the index or long finger. The donor site is skin grafted and the flap is divided at 10–14 days. A = Soft tissue defect of the ulnar side of the index finger distal phalanx; B = Elevation of radial-based cross-finger flap from the dorsal aspect of the middle finger middle phalanx; C = Inset of cross-finger flap on the index finger defect; D = Cross-finger flap elevated from index finger for coverage of thumb defect; E = Inset of index finger cross-finger flap onto thumb. (From Buncke HJ. Fingertip injuries and soft tissue reconstruction. In: Grabb WC, Smith JW, eds. *Plastic Surgery*. Boston: Little, Brown and Company, 1973.)

G. Distant Flaps

1. First dorsal interosseous neurovascular island flap—raised from the dorsal-radial index finger on the radial nerve and first dorsal interosseous artery. Long enough to reach a thumb tip and provide sensation.
2. Cross-finger flap (Fig. 1)—usually elevated from the dorsum of the adjacent finger middle phalanx. The flap is inset on the recipient finger and the donor defect is skin grafted. The flap is divided in 10–14 days.
3. Subcutaneous cross-finger flap—the subcutaneous fascia of the adjacent finger middle phalanx is elevated and inset onto the fingertip defect and used as a recipient bed for a skin graft. The donor site is primarily closed. The flap is divided in 10–14 days.
4. Thenar flap (Fig. 2)—elevated from the thenar aspect of the palm and usually proximally based, although "H"-shaped flaps have been described. Provides glabrous coverage of the index through small fingertips. Design should be wide enough to allow inset without tension. Care needs to be taken to avoid injury to the thumb digital nerves. Donor site may or may not require skin grafting. May be divided in 10–14 days, and the donor skin graft may be excised secondarily.
5. Island pedicle flap (Fig. 3)—neurovascular island flap from the ulnar aspect of the ring or long finger, intended to provide sensate resurfacing of the thumb tip. Technically demanding flap with large dissection and significant donor defect. Donor digit scar contractures are common.
6. Groin flap—raised on the lateral superficial circumflex iliac vessels, usually better suited to

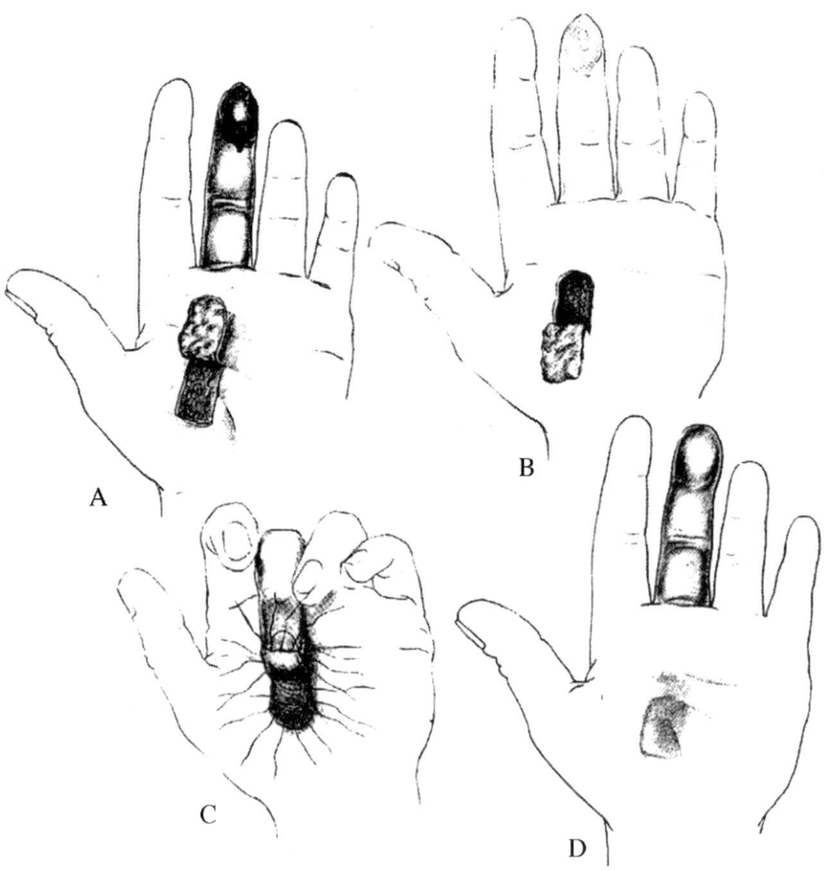

Figure 2 A thenar flap for an avulsion of the middle fingertip. (A) Flap is elevated as a distally based flap. (B) More commonly, the flap is elevated as a proximally based flap. (C) Inset and placement of skin graft with bolster in the defect. (D) After division of flap at 10–14 days. (From Buncke HJ. Fingertip injuries and soft tissue reconstruction. In: Grabb WC, Smith JW, eds. *Plastic Surgery*. Boston: Little, Brown and Company, 1973.)

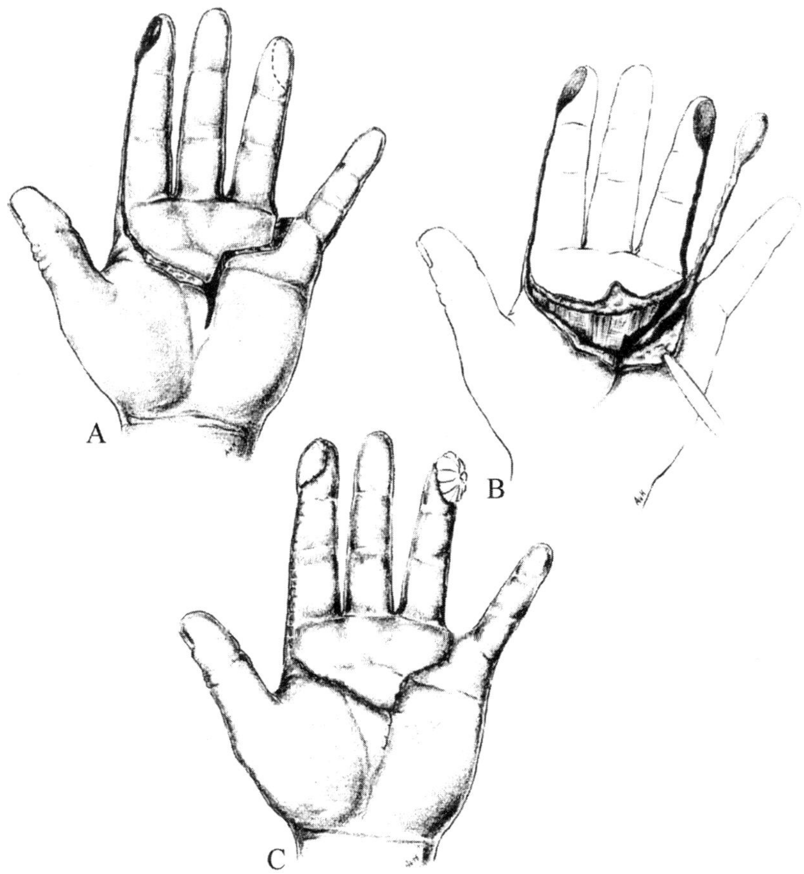

Figure 3 Neurovascular island flap from ring finger can be transferred to radial aspect of index finger or tip of thumb. The donor defect is skin grafted. A = Incisions and design of neurovascular island flap from ring finger for coverage of index finger distal phalanx defect; B = Dissection of the neurovascular pedicle for the neurovascular island flap, based on the ulnar digital neurovascular bundle of the ring finger; C = Inset of the neurovascular island flap onto the index finger defect; the ring finger donor site has been covered with a skin graft and tie-over bolster. (From Buncke HJ. Fingertip injuries and soft tissue reconstruction. In: Grabb WC, Smith JW, eds. *Plastic Surgery*. Boston: Little, Brown and Company, 1973.)

large defects. Easy to elevate. The distal aspect of the flap can be thinned before inset. It is divided in approximately 14 days.

7. Random abdominal or chest tubed flap—random flap raised on the abdomen or chest wall. Should be raised fairly thin so as not to add excessive bulk to the reconstructed finger. It is divided in approximately 14 days.

H. Microvascular Transplants (Free Flaps)

1. Great toe neurovascular island flap—sensory free flap usually reserved for sensate padding and resurfacing of a thumb defect
2. Thenar free flap—sensory free flap nourished by a superficial palmar radial artery and a venae comitans. A 2.5 × 10 cm flap can be harvested.
3. Venous flap—numerous venous flaps can be designed from the volar forearm or foot and used as free flaps to cover fingertip injuries by arterializing the flap. Occasional leeching may be required. A venous flap may be neurotized if taken with a cutaneous nerve.

VII. TREATMENT OPTIONS IN NAIL BED INJURIES AND TUFT FRACTURES

A. Can often be treated in the emergency room with a digital block and use of loupe magnification.

B. Subungual hematoma—evacuated with a micro-cautery or heated paper clip. Micro-cautery is easier to use and more reliable.

C. Simple lacerations—repair with 5-0 or 6-0 plain catgut sutures. Clean the removed nail and replace nail into the nail fold as a splint. The nail can be fixed into position with 4-0 nylon sutures.

D. Stellate lacerations and severe crush injuries—repair meticulously, as for simple lacerations. If the nail was destroyed, use the metal packaging from the catgut suture as a splint, or insert nonadherent gauze in the eponychial fold.

E. Avulsion—in severe avulsions, some of the nail bed is attached to the nail. Free 1–2 mm of nailbed from the nail and suture back into position without freeing completely from the avulsed nail. The nail will act to splint the severely injured bed and repair.

F. Tuft fractures—if not displaced or minimally displaced, can be treated with nail bed repair alone. If displaced and requiring stabilization, use K-wire or 18–20 gauge needle to immobilize the fracture.

VIII. POSTOPERATIVE COMPLICATIONS

A. Treat all hand fingertip and nail bed injuries like any hand injury with appropriate splinting, followed by range of motion exercises as required to reduce stiffness and loss of function.

B. Infection—nail bed injuries and tip injuries can be quite dirty. Antibiotics should be considered.

C. Nail ridges and split nails—may require excision with primary repair or free nail grafting, depending on the size of the injury.

D. Hooked nail deformity—usually caused by loss of distal phalangeal bone support. May need shortening of nail bed or more tip support.

E. Fingertip grafts and flaps can be lost secondary to necrosis, poor flap design and execution, as well as patient noncompliance. Preoperative planning is the best prevention for these complications.

F. Cold intolerance—most patients suffer from some form of cold intolerance after a fingertip injury, varying with the extent of injury. This can be expected to be permanent and patients should be counseled as such, although cold intolerance does tend to improve partially over the first 2 years following the original injury.

G. Neuroma—a painful neuroma can form in more proximal amputations when digital nerves are not padded sufficiently. Nerve resection and retraction at the time of surgery can sometimes prevent this complication. Resection of a neuroma may be required postoperatively if conservative treatment with desensitization fails.

69

Hand Fractures and Dislocations

Holly D. Casey, M.D., and C. Vaughan A. Bowen, M.D., F.R.C.S.(C), M.D.Ch.B.
Foothills Medical Centre, Calgary, Alberta, Canada

I. UNIQUE FEATURE OF HAND INJURIES

Fractures and dislocations in the hand are very common injuries. Biomechanically and biologically, their behavior is similar to fractures in other parts of the body. Specifically, fracture patterns, deforming forces, and fracture healing are no different from fractures elsewhere. A number of factors unique to the hand, however, act to influence, complicate, and/or confuse management decisions.

A. Fingernails complicate management of fractures of the distal phalanx.

B. Other structures are in close proximity to the fractures. The likelihood of neurovascular involvement should always be considered. Management should be designed to minimize the risk of tendon adhesions and joint stiffness.

C. The anatomical feature of multiple parallel skeletal rays may complicate or facilitate management.

D. Good functional results are extremely important. Think about function when treatment is planned. Is it necessary for the fracture to be reduced anatomically to restore function? If not, how much deformity can be accepted before function is affected? Close follow-up is important so that hand therapy, when necessary, can be started as early as possible. Minimize immobilization. When immobilization is needed, the hand should be put into the position of safety: MP joints flexed almost to 90°, IP joints in full extension, and the first web opened widely.

E. Psychological and social factors can be devastating. Hand injuries frequently prevent the patient from returning to work. This often gives rise to a variety of social problems and stresses. These can be compounded if the injury occurred on the job. Be aware of these problems, which need to be managed at the same time as the hand injury.

II. CLASSIFICATION

Classification is essential for describing the injuries and planning treatment. Fractures can be classified as follows:

A. Adult or pediatric: Pediatric fractures can be greenstick or epiphyseal plate fractures. Epiphyseal plate fractures are classified using the Salter-Harris classification.

B. Open (compound) or closed.

C. Traumatic or pathological.

D. Displaced or nondisplaced.

E. Fracture pattern transverse, oblique, spiral, comminuted, or avulsion (Fig. 1).

III. MANAGEMENT

A number of different options are available for the management of any given fracture. Although treatment

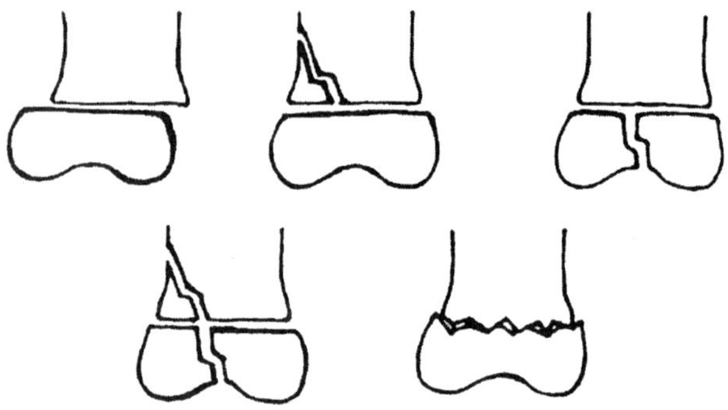

Figure 1 Fracture pattern: transverse, oblique, spiral, comminuted, or avulsion.

must be customized to the needs of each patient, it is important to adhere to the basic principles of reduction, maintenance of reduction, and rehabilitation of function.

Answering the following questions can facilitate decisions concerning the management of specific fractures:

A. Is the fracture in an acceptable position, or is there unacceptable displacement or angulation?
B. If the fracture needs reduction, can it be reduced by closed methods?
C. Once reduced, will the fracture be stable?
D. If the fracture will not be stable once reduced, what has to be done to make it stable?
E. Is recommended treatment acceptable to the patient, and is it available in your location? If fractures have to be immobilized, the hand needs to be put into the "position of safety" with the MP joints flexed to 70–90°, the IP joints in full extension, and the first web space wide open. Immobilization should be for the minimum time necessary. If stiffness occurs, the patient should have early hand therapy.

IV. FRACTURES OF METACARPALS AND PHALANGES

These are most common fractures of the upper extremity. Most fractures are biomechanically stable, but others need reduction and internal fixation.

A. Indications for Operative Intervention

1. Irreducible fracture
2. Malrotation
3. Intra-articular fracture
4. Subcapital phalangeal fracture
5. Open fracture—a relative indication only if the fracture is displaced or angled

B. Indications for Internal Fixation

1. Irreducible fracture
2. Segmental bone loss
3. Polytrauma with hand fracture
4. Multiple hand or wrist fractures
5. Fracture with significant soft tissue injury
6. Intra-articular fractures
7. Replants

C. Considerations of Treatment

1. Location
2. Fracture geometry
3. Deformity
4. Open vs. closed fracture
5. Associated bone and soft tissue injuries
6. Fracture stability
7. Age of patient
8. Occupation
9. Socioeconomic status
10. Systemic illnesses
11. Surgeon's skill
12. Patient compliance

V. METACARPAL FRACTURES (EXCLUDING THUMB)

A. Metacarpal Head Fractures

1. Mechanism—rare injury, due to axial loading or direct trauma, often intra-articular. The index finger is most commonly involved.
2. Diagnosis—three view x-rays (anteroposterior, lateral, and oblique). Brewerton view may clarify fracture pattern around the metacarpal head.
3. Treatment—if nondisplaced, splint for 4 weeks in position of safety. If >25% of the articular surface is involved, or >1 mm step off, may require open reduction and internal fixation. If comminuted, options include immobilization for

2 weeks, skeletal traction, external fixation, or silicone arthroplasty.

B. Metacarpal Neck Fractures/Boxer Fractures

1. Mechanism—a clenched MCP joint strikes a solid object, causing an apex dorsal angulation of the neck due to flexion of the distal fracture segment by the intrinsic tendons.
2. Diagnosis—three view x-rays.
3. Treatment is controversial and is dependent upon the patient, surgeon, and digit involved. Depends on which metacarpal is fractured and its degree of angulation. Ring and small (Boxer) metacarpal neck fractures tolerate angulation of 30 and 40°, respectively. Because of lack of compensatory CMC motion, residual angulation >10–15° in fractures of index and middle finger metacarpal necks are unacceptable. Closed reduction can be done in the ER using the Jahss maneuver after a wrist or hematoma block. Flex the MCP joint 90°, flex the PIP joint 90°, and push the proximal phalanx against metacarpal head upward while applying downward pressure on the metacarpal shaft (Jahss maneuver). If adequate reduction occurs, immobilize for 3–4 weeks in the intrinsic plus or safe position. Follow carefully, as loss of reduction is common. For those fractures with unacceptable angulation or rotational misalignment, reduce the fracture and internally fix using K-wires, plates, or dorsal tension-band wires.

C. Metacarpal Shaft Fractures

1. Mechanism—three types:
   - Transverse—due to an axial load or lateral bending force.
   - Oblique and spiral—oblique fractures are due to lateral bending forces with axial load. Spiral fractures are caused by torsional forces; 5° of malrotation causes 1.5 cm of digit overlap (scissoring or rotational malalignment).
   - Comminuted—direct impact. Often causes shortening of the metacarpal.
2. Diagnosis—three view x-rays.
3. Treatment—closed reduction and immobilization is adequate for most metacarpal shaft fractures with acceptable angulation. Open reduction with fixation is required for open, multiple, unstable, or angulated fractures and scissoring. Options include using K-wires, interosseous wires, plates, lag screws, and external fixation.

D. Metacarpal Base Fractures/Fracture-Dislocations of the CMC Joints

1. Mechanism—due to an axial load or direct blow, often high energy. Less common in index and middle fingers due to lack of motion in the joints. The Baby (reverse) Bennett fracture is a hamate-5th metacarpal intra-articular fracture.
2. Diagnosis—three view x-rays. The ulnar portion of a fifth metacarpal fracture is subluxed proximally and dorsally secondary to the pull of the extensor carpi ulnaris that inserts onto the 5th metacarpal.
3. Treatment—these are inherently unstable fractures that require closed reduction and percutaneous K-wire fixation vs. internal fixation

E. Complications of Metacarpal Fractures

1. Malunion due to angulation, rotation, or shortening.
2. Nonunion from bone loss.
3. Intra-articular damage that causes posttraumatic arthritis (pain and stiffness).

VI. PHALANGEAL FRACTURES (EXCLUDING THUMB)

A. Distal Phalanx Fractures

1. Mechanism—the most common fractures in the hand. The thumb and middle finger are most often involved. Tuft and shaft fractures are usually due to a crushing injury.
2. Diagnosis—three view x-rays.
3. Treatment—depends on location:
   - Tuft fractures—usually involves a laceration of the nail matrix or pulp. Closed fractures may have a subungual hematoma that must be drained with a hot paper clip or needle-point Bovie electrocautery. For open fractures, thoroughly irrigate after removing the nail. Repair nail bed with a fine suture, followed by appropriate immobilization.

- Shaft fractures—if displaced, requires reduction with longitudinal K-wire or screw fixation. Should treat the displaced fracture before repairing the nail bed; failure to do so risks permanent nail deformity.
- Intra-articular fractures:

  Dorsal base (Mallet fracture)—a hyperflexion injury may cause avulsion of a chip fracture that remains attached to the extensor tendon, resulting in an extensor lag at the DIP joint (mallet finger). The first line of treatment is splinting in extension for 6–8 weeks. Compliance is the key! Open reduction with fixation is difficult and usually unnecessary.

  Volar base (flexor digitorum profundus avulsion)—a hyperextension injury may cause a small avulsed fracture fragment, to which the flexor digitorum profundus may still be attached. If present, this may be radiographically visible on a lateral finger x-ray. The profundus may retract all the way into the palm. Treatment requires open reduction with internal fixation.

B. Middle and Proximal Phalanx Fractures

1. Mechanism—crushing injury, direct blow, twisting, or angular forces. The pilon fracture is a comminuted fracture of the middle phalanx proximal articular surface with displaced bone fragments.
2. Diagnosis—three view x-rays.
3. Treatment—if stable or nondisplaced, buddy tape or extension block splinting for 3–4 weeks.
4. Articular fractures:
   - Unicondylar fractures are unstable. Treatment is open reduction and internal fixation.
   - Bicondylar fractures usually need open reduction, internal fixation, and early motion.
   - Comminuted fractures are very difficult to treat. Crushed surfaces may be treated with dynamic splinting or volar plate arthroplasty.
5. Nonarticular fractures:
   - Neck—usually in children. If displaced, requires rigid fixation.
   - Shaft—attempt closed reduction and splinting, if possible. Otherwise, reduction and percutaneous K-wire fixation vs. internal fixation.

C. Complications of Phalangeal Fractures

1. Malunion—four types:
   - Malrotation
   - Volar angulation
   - Lateral angulation
   - Shortening
2. Nonunion.
3. Loss of motion due to tendon adherence and contracture. The PIP joint is most susceptible.
4. Infection—watch pin sites.
5. Flexor tendon rupture or entrapment.
6. Posttraumatic arthritis.

VII. THUMB FRACTURES

A. Extra-articular Thumb Phalangeal Fractures

1. Mechanism—usually direct trauma with angular or rotatory forces.
2. Diagnosis—three view x-rays.
3. Treatment:
   - Distal tuft—usually comminuted and associated with nail injury. Must clean and repair lacerations, drain subungual hematomas, and splint for 3–4 weeks.
   - Transverse shaft—if closed reduction is inadequate, requires open reduction and internal fixation.

B. Intra-articular Thumb Phalangeal Fractures

1. Mechanism—occurs when the partially flexed thumb is axially loaded.
2. Diagnosis—three view x-rays.
3. Treatment—if the fragment is displaced >2 mm or is >25% of the articular surface, the fracture must be reduced with percutaneous K-wire fixation vs. internal fixation.

C. Thumb Metacarpal Fractures

1. Mechanism—head and shaft fractures are due to direct impact or angulatory, rotatory, or torsional forces. These fractures can be intra-articular or extra-articular. Extra-articular fractures with up to 50–60° angulation can be acceptable due to the mobile CMC joint that compensates well for the angulation deformity.
2. The Bennett's fracture is an intra-articular fracture-subluxation at the base of the first metacarpal. A Bennett's fracture occurs when the metacarpal is axially loaded with a partially flexed thumb.
3. Rolando's fracture is traditionally defined as a Y- or T-shaped intra-articular fracture, but now signifies any comminuted intra-articular fractures of the thumb metacarpal base.
4. Diagnosis—three view x-rays. With a Bennett's fracture, the volar ulnar aspect of the base remains fixed due to the anterior oblique ligament. The remaining metacarpal shifts dorsally, proximally, and radially secondary to the pull of the abductor pollicis longus.
5. Treatment:
   - Head—unusual. If displaced, requires reduction and percutaneous K-wire fixation vs. internal fixation.
   - Shaft—extra-articular base fracture can be treated with closed reduction alone in most cases.
   - Intra-articular fractures of the base:

     Bennett's fracture—if the fragment involves < 20% of the CMC joint surface, use closed reduction and pinning. If anatomic reduction is not possible, treat with open reduction with internal fixation.

     Rolando's fracture—treatment depends on degree of comminution. With a few large fragments, open reduction with fixation is possible. Otherwise, skeletal traction may be required.

VIII. PEDIATRIC FRACTURES

Most pediatric fractures are nonepiphyseal (66%). Those fractures that do involve the epiphysis are categorized by the Salter-Harris classification.

A. Salter-Harris I—epiphyseal plate separation due to fracture through the physis. Usually caused by a shearing force in early childhood. Prognosis is good.

B. Salter-Harris II—a metaphyseal fracture fragment associated with an epiphyseal fracture. This is the most common Salter-Harris fracture and is usually found with fractures of the proximal phalanx. Prognosis is also good.

C. Salter-Harris III—fracture through the growth plate and epiphysis. Unless there is early and accurate reduction, prognosis is poor.

D. Salter-Harris IV—fracture through the growth plate and includes a metaphyseal fragment. Fortunately, rarely found in the hand. Prognosis is poor unless good anatomic alignment is established.

E. Salter-Harris V—a crush injury of the epiphyseal plate; highly uncommon in the hand. Beware—initial x-rays may be normal. Poor prognosis.

IX. DISLOCATIONS

A. Proximal Interphalangeal Joint

This is the most common site of ligament injury in the hand. The PIP joint is a hinge joint, with a 100–110° arc of rotation. The joint is stabilized by thick collateral ligaments that pass obliquely and volarly, accessory collateral ligaments, and the volar plate that forms the floor of the joint.

1. Evaluation

   a. Direction—defined by the position of the middle phalanx relative to the proximal phalanx at the moment of joint deformation.
      - Dorsal—caused by hyperextension and longitudinal compression.
      - Lateral.
      - Volar—rare. Due to a rotatory longitudinal compression force on a semiflexed middle phalanx.

   b. Active stability—patient voluntarily moves through the range of motion at the PIP joint. Full range indicates adequate stability. Redisplacement indicates major ligament damage.

   c. Passive stability—test lateral stress of the collateral ligaments in full extension and 30° of flexion. Compare with the normal contralateral joint.

d. X-rays—three views, including a true lateral of the joint. May need stress films (lateral and AP).

2. Grades

a. Mild—microscopic tears, no instability.

b. Moderate—moderate degree of tear and abnormal laxity.

c. Complete—complete tear of the collateral ligaments.

3. Treatment

a. Sprains—splint 2–3 days to control pain and swelling. If stable, early motion.

b. Dislocations:

- Dorsal—decide if dislocation is stable or unstable. Stable dislocations require extension block splinting for 3 weeks. Surgery is necessary for unstable fracture-dislocations in which a closed reduction is not possible. Usually involves fracture of >40% of the volar articular surface. Options include open reduction with fixation or volar plate arthroplasty.
- Lateral—despite complete disruption of the collateral ligaments, ligaments return to their normal position with reduction of the dislocation in almost all cases. Treat with combination of extension block splinting and buddy taping for 3 weeks.
- Volar—check carefully to ensure integrity of the central slip. Splint 2–3 days.

B. Distal Interphalangeal and Thumb Interphalangeal Joints

1. Rare injury due to stability of the joint afforded by insertion of the flexor and extensor tendons.
2. Most frequently a dorsal or lateral dislocation associated with open wounds.
3. These are rarely irreducible. Reduce using longitudinal traction with direct pressure on dorsum of the distal phalanx, and manipulation of the distal phalanx into flexion.
4. Once reduced, immobilize the joint in a dorsal splint for 2–3 days, then begin gentle active motion with buddy taping.

1. Finger Metacarpophalangeal Joint

This is a condyloid joint that most often dislocates in a dorsal or ulnar direction.

a. Dorsal—forced hyperextension, most commonly in the index or small finger:

- Simple subluxation—volar plate remains with the proximal phalanx. Reduce by flexing the wrist to relax the flexor tendons, then simply flex the MCP joint. Apply distally and volarly directed pressure to the dorsal base of the proximal phalanx. Do not convert to a complex dislocation with traction or hyperextension of the joint.
- Complex dislocation—an irreducible dislocation with the volar plate jammed in the joint. Flexion is impossible. Requires open reduction. Immobilize up to 2 weeks.

b. Volar—extremely rare. Attempt closed reduction, but may require open reduction.

c. Lateral—an isolated radial collateral ligament rupture due to forced ulnar deviation with the MCP joint flexed. Immobilize the joint in 30° of flexion for 3 weeks, then buddy tape for 2–3 weeks.

2. Thumb Metacarpophalangeal Joint

a. Most common is gamekeeper's thumb, an avulsion fracture-dislocation from the ulnar base of the proximal phalanx due to the disruption of the ulnar collateral ligament. Occurs when the partially flexed thumb is axially loaded.

b. First line of treatment is immobilization of joint for 6 weeks.

c. If still unstable or if the ulnar collateral ligament is blocked by interposition of the adductor pollicis muscle (Stener lesion), surgical exploration and repair of the ulnar collateral ligament are indicated.

70

Wrist Injuries

David L. Kaufman, M.D., and Heidi Bloom, M.D.
Stanford University Medical Center, Stanford, California, U.S.A.

C. Vaughan A. Bowen, M.D., F.R.C.S.(C.), M.B.Ch.B.
Foothills Medical Centre, Calgary, Alberta, Canada

I. INTRODUCTION

A. The wrist can be regarded as the platform for hand function.

B. The wrist can be the cause of a multitude of clinical problems resulting from developmental anomalies, disease, injury, and overuse. When not working properly, it affects every aspect of a patient's daily activities: work, hobbies, and activities of daily living.

C. The diagnosis of clinical problems involving the wrist can be a formidable task because of its anatomic complexity: multiple carpal bones, complex joints, numerous intrinsic and extrinsic ligaments, flexor and extensor tendons, and the close proximity of important neurovascular structures.

D. The key to successful treatment is making a diagnosis. The key to making a diagnosis is an orderly approach.

II. HISTORY

A. General Features

Sometimes the problem is obvious. Much of the time it is not. Time spent taking a good history will be well rewarded. A good history should suggest the diagnosis. Determine the patient's age, hand dominance, occupation, hobbies, and other interests. The past medical history, family history, social history, and review of systems are also important.

B. Pain

Pain is the usual presenting feature. Ask the following questions about wrist pain:

1. When did it start?
2. How did it start?
3. Where is it located?
4. Does it radiate—if so, where does it go?
5. How severe is it on a 1–10 scale?
6. What kind of pain is it—dull, aching, sharp, burning, throbbing, etc.?
7. Is the pain constant/intermittent or deteriorating/improving with time?
8. What makes it worse?
9. What helps it?
10. Are there any associated features—numbness, tingling, clicking, weakness, etc.?

C. Formulating the Diagnosis

Answering the following questions can help you develop a working diagnosis:

1. Is the problem on the ulnar or radial side of the wrist?
2. What is the anatomical level of the problem: distal forearm, radiocarpal/ulnocarpal joint, proximal carpal row, mid-carpal joint, or distal carpal row?
3. What is the anatomical layer of the problem: skin, subcutaneous, neurovascular, tendon sheath, bone, or joint?
4. Could there be preexisting disease that has been exacerbated by the traumatic episode? Is the preexisting condition congenital or acquired?

III. CLINICAL EXAMINATION

The clinical examination should be used: (a) to verify the working diagnosis, (b) to look for associated features, and (c) to rule out other abnormalities. The exam may also provide useful information about the extent of the problem. Start with a local examination of the wrist. Be systematic, thorough, and detailed. Compare findings with the opposite wrist. After local examination, examine the rest of the region (neck, upper part of the extremity, and hand), looking for referred pain. If necessary, progress to a general examination.

A. Observation

1. Color and texture of the skin
2. Bone and soft tissue deformity
3. Presence of scars, infection, or draining sinuses

B. Range of Motion

1. Active and passive
2. Flexion/extension; pronation/supination; ulnar/radial deviation

C. Palpation

Palpation is the most important tool for making a diagnosis. Palpation should be performed carefully and in a very detailed and systematic manner. Start at the radial styloid and progress to distal radius, Lister's tubercle, DRUJ (distal radio-ulnar joint), distal ulna, ECU (extensor carpi ulnaris) tendon, pisotriquetral joint, hook of hamate, lunate, lunotriquetral joint, triquetrum, body of hamate, triquetrohamate joint, body of capitate, anatomic snuffbox (central, proximal and distal) trapezium, trapezoid, and thumb CMC (carpal-metacarpal) joint.

1. Bone and soft tissue deformity
2. Temperature
3. Tenderness

D. Special Tests

1. Reagan test (lunotriquetral ballottement)
2. Triquetrohamate ballottement test
3. Watson shift test for scapholunate ligament instability
4. Lichtman's test for midcarpal instability
5. Finkelstein's test for de Quervain's tenosynovitis

E. Grip and Pinch Strength

Use a dynamometer and grip gauge. Readings should be compared with the opposite side. Further information can be obtained by doing repeat measures and assessing the REG (rapid exchange grip) curve.

F. Neurovascular Status

This should be assessed on all patients. Test the medial, ulna and radial nerves for both motor and sensory function, as well as looking for features of autonomic dysfunction. Use 2-point discrimination to test sensation.

IV. INVESTIGATION

This should be done in an orderly, focused manner. This type of approach is less expensive, less time consuming, and less likely to lead to false-positive results. In general, investigations are more useful for confirming a diagnosis or mapping out the extent of a problem, rather than for making a diagnosis. Imaging techniques are the most useful investigations for evaluation of wrist injuries, although blood tests and electrodiagnostic studies may also be of value.

A. Plain Radiographs

Radiographic evaluation should begin with neutral rotation PA and lateral views. Images must be standardized if length and angulatory measurements are to be meaningful. Two oblique views may also be obtained if additional information is required.

B. Specialized Radiographs

Specialized radiographs may be helpful to investigate specific regions:

1. Scaphoid views
2. Pisotriquetral view
3. Robert view of the trapezium
4. Dynamic views
5. Carpal tunnel view to rule out hook of hamate fractures

C. Computerized Tomography

CT scanning has largely replaced plain tomography. Useful for:

1. Distal radius fractures (assessing joint surface incongruity; displacement; comminution).
2. Scaphoid fractures (assessing state of union; measuring humpback deformity).
3. Identifying fractures in the distal carpal row.
4. Investigating DRUJ dislocations, subluxations, and instability.
5. Three-dimensional reconstructions can be made from CT images. Although these provide interesting images, they have not appreciably enhanced our diagnostic capability or improved our treatment techniques.

D. Ultrasound

Useful for identifying ganglion cysts. It may have a role in the investigation of tendon lacerations or ruptures.

E. MRI

Use is becoming more common. Can be misleading because of high rate of false positives. Most useful for:

1. Anatomic location and extent of mass lesions (ganglia; tumors)
2. Avascularity of bone (proximal pole of scaphoid; lunate)
3. Tenosynovitis
4. Triangular fibrocartilage complex (TFCC) tears, ligamentous tears, and nondisplaced fractures.

F. Tc99 MDP Bone Scans

These are very useful when a fracture is suspected but cannot be demonstrated on plain radiographs. When used for this purpose, they should be obtained 1–2 weeks after the injury. Early flow images can be useful for confirming diagnosis of reflex sympathetic dystrophy. Late static images are used for identifying presence/absence and sites of bone pathology:

1. Fractures
2. Arthritis
3. Tumors

G. Arthroscopy

Gives direct vision of radiocarpal, ulnocarpal, and midcarpal joint surfaces. Useful for the investigation of:

1. TFCC tears.
2. Ligament injuries.
3. Arthritis.
4. Operative arthroscopy can be used as an adjunct in the treatment of intra-articular fractures of the distal radius.

V. SPECIFIC CONDITIONS

A. Distal Radius Fractures

1. Most common fracture of the wrist.
2. Usually results from a fall onto an outstretched hand.
3. Most fractures are closed.
4. Use radiographs to evaluate:
    - Amount of comminution.
    - Intra-articular extension into radiocarpal and/or distal radioulnar joint.
    - Direction of angular deformity (Colles' fracture or Smith's fracture)

        Colles' fractures are dorsally angulated, often dorsally comminuted fractures of the distal radius that typically result in radial shortening, dorsal angulation, and loss of normal radial inclination.

        Smith's fractures are volarly angulated fractures that typically result in radial shortening, volar angulation, and variable loss of normal radial inclination.

    - Measurement of shortening, palmar tilt, and distal radius inclination.

5. Treatment:

   - Nondisplaced fractures are treated in a cast for 6 weeks.
   - Many different methods are currently used to treat shortened, displaced, or angulated fractures.
   - Smith's fractures, in which there is volar displacement of the distal fragment, are treated by open reduction and volar buttress plating.
   - Extra-articular Colles' fractures require reduction if there is > 4–10 mm shortening, dorsal angulation of over 20 degrees, or significant displacement.
   - Intra-articular fractures require reduction if there is a step-off of >2 mm at the articular surface (CT scan may be needed to evaluate this).
   - In most cases, closed reduction and casting is tried first, although comminution greater than 50% of the diameter of the radius strongly suggests that instability will be a problem. If a satisfactory reduction is obtained, radiographs should be obtained every 1–2 weeks, as loss of reduction is common, especially in the first 2 weeks. Unsuccessful reduction or loss of reduction may require other methods of treatment, such as reduction with internal or external fixation.
   - Acute carpal tunnel syndrome is sometimes seen following distal radius fractures.
   - Other complications include stiffness, posttraumatic arthritis (ulnocarpal, radiocarpal, or distal radioulnar joints), EPL (extensor pollicis longus) rupture, nondissociative carpal instability, and reflex sympathetic dystrophy.

B. Carpal Bone Fractures

It is possible for any carpal bone to be fractured, either as an isolated injury or in association with other fractures and fracture-dislocations of the wrist (greater arc injury).

1. Scaphoid Fracture

a. The most common of the carpal fractures.

b. Typically results from a fall onto an outstretched hand.

c. Most common in young people and frequently presents as a sports injury.

d. Patients usually present with radial wrist pain. There is often no visible deformity, and swelling may be minimal. Tenderness is elicited in the anatomic snuffbox.

e. Radiographs will usually show a fracture. If a scaphoid fracture is suspected but not seen on the plain radiographs, treat the patient for a nondisplaced scaphoid fracture (thumb spica cast) and obtain a Tc99 MDP bone scan in the second week after the injury. A positive scan confirms the diagnosis. Repeat plain x-rays obtained 2–3 weeks following the original injury will sometimes reveal a fracture that was not evident on the initial x-rays (occult scaphoid fracture).

f. Nondisplaced scaphoid fractures are treated in a thumb spica cast until union is achieved (usually 6 weeks). There are many opinions about the type of cast that should be placed (long arm or short arm; wrist in slight flexion or extension; thumb IP joint immobilized or free).

g. Displaced fractures need open reduction and internal fixation. If there is any doubt about displacement or angulation, obtain a CT scan with an oblique cut in the plane of the scaphoid.

h. Long-term complications of scaphoid fractures include nonunion, malunion, avascular necrosis, carpal instability, and posttraumatic SLAC (scapholunate advanced collapse) wrist arthritis.

2. Other Carpal Bone Fractures

a. The mechanism is usually a fall onto an outstretched hand.

b. Patients present with pain localized to the injured area.

c. Radiographs usually show the fracture, although they can be difficult to see, especially in the distal carpal row. If a fracture is present, a Tc99 MDP bone scan will be positive in the second week after injury. A CT scan is the best way to image distal carpal row fractures.

d. Nondisplaced fractures should be casted for 6 weeks. Displaced fractures usually require open reduction and internal fixation.

e. Nonunion of the hook of hamate is a specific complication that frequently causes diagnostic difficulty. Hook fractures are mostly avulsions that occur when a ball is struck forcefully with a bat. Nonunion produces volar and ulnar wrist pain. Palpate the hook for tenderness and the patient will tell you that you have "found the spot." A CT scan will confirm the diagnosis. Treatment is surgical excision of the hook of the hamate.

C. Dislocations and Fracture Dislocations

These variably present from perilunate ligamentous injuries and dislocations (lesser arc injuries) to dislocations associated with fractures of one or more carpal bones (greater arc injuries).

1. Scapholunate Ligament Injuries

a. Injury to the ligamentous support around the lunate progresses with increasing severity of injury in a predictable way. Scapholunate sprains progress to scapholunate dissociation, perilunate dislocation, and dislocation of the lunate. Less severe injuries may present acutely as "wrist sprains" or late as chronic radial wrist pain. Severe injuries present with a strong history of extreme dorsiflexion injury, pain, swelling, loss of function, and visible deformity.

b. Radiographs will demonstrate the ligamentous disruption and/or dislocation. Characteristically, scapholunate disruption will appear as widening between the scaphoid and lunate >3–4 mm (Terry Thomas/David Letterman sign), or as a wedge-shaped appearance to the lunate (piece of pie sign) on PA radiographs. A DISI deformity (dorsal intercalated segment instability—look for a dorsally tilted lunate) or frank dislocation of the lunate volarly (spilled teacup sign) may also be evident on the lateral view.

c. Acute dislocations (within 3–4 weeks) should undergo immediate closed reduction. Percutaneous pinning can be attempted for holding the reduction, but instability is usually severe, and it is usually necessary to do an open reduction and internal fixation to obtain and hold the anatomic position. Immobilization after reduction should be for 8–12 weeks.

d. Scapholunate sprains and mild degrees of disruption can be difficult to diagnose in the emergency situation. Be suspicious when patients present with a wrist injury, pain, and tenderness over the scapholunate area but have normal radiographs. These patients tend to present late with chronic radial wrist pain, exacerbated by activity, but with normal radiographs. The diagnosis of their dynamic scapholunate instability is made if they have a positive Watson shift test, radiographic dissociation on stress radiographs, or disruption seen arthroscopically. Patients with mild symptoms may best be treated conservatively.

e. A number of surgical procedures have been described for treating patients with severe symptoms.

2. Fracture-Dislocations

a. These are severe injuries to the wrist.

b. The trans-scaphoid perilunate fracture-dislocation is the most common form of major arc injury, although almost any combination of fracture and ligamentous injury is possible.

c. Radiographs with the wrist in traction (use finger traps) can be very useful diagnostically. Injuries are treated in the same way as ligamentous injuries (see above), but the fractures are usually internally fixed as well.

3. Ulnar-Sided Ligamentous Injuries

a. Less common and less well understood than the radial-sided injuries.

b. Dorsal ligamentous injuries may be associated with avulsion fractures from the triquetrolunate area, best seen on the lateral radiograph. These are treated with cast immobilization for 6 weeks.

c. Injuries to the lunotriquetral ligament and the midcarpal joint can be difficult to diagnose. There is usually a history of injury with local tenderness, with a positive Reagan test or Lichtman test. A radiographic VISI (volar intercalated segment instability; look for a volar-tilted lunate) is diagnostic. Once diagnosed, treatment of both acute and chronic ulnar wrist instability is similar to that of other wrist ligament injuries.

D. TFCC Tears

1. The TFCC consists of the cartilaginous triangle and supporting ligaments at the distal end of the ulna. It stabilizes the DRUJ and serves as an articulating surface for the ulnar carpus.
2. Injuries are classified as (a) degenerative or traumatic, (b) perforating or avulsion.

3. Patients present with discrete ulnar wrist pain (acute or chronic) that worsens with grip and rotation. Local tenderness on palpation is an important finding.
4. On standardized PA radiographs, there is a strong association with an ulnar-positive variance. Cysts may be seen adjacent to the lunotriquetral joint. Arthrogram and MRI can be helpful in confirming the diagnosis, but arthroscopy is the best method. Be very careful to use clinical features, rather than investigations, to make the diagnosis since degenerative TFCC tears may be present in asymptomatic wrists as early as the 3rd and 4th decades.
5. Acute tears are treated with 4–6 weeks of immobilization. At arthroscopy, central and chronic tears may also be debrided, and some acute peripheral tears may be repairable. In chronic cases, symptoms can be successfully managed with an ulna shortening osteotomy to decompress the ulnocarpal space.
6. Severe injuries to the distal ulna region may result in instability. A CT scan at the level of the DRUJ is the best way to confirm the diagnosis of DRUJ dislocation or subluxation. These injuries need to be aggressively diagnosed and treated in the acute phase, because chronically unstable distal ulnas are very difficult to manage.

E. Tenosynovitis

Tenosynovitis is the correct term for inflammation in tendon sheaths. It can occur in each of the tendons that cross the wrist, usually as they pass through a fibro-osseous tunnel. Tenosynovitis should not be confused with nonspecific musculoskeletal pain related to physical activity, which is confusingly and incorrectly often referred to as "tendonitis."

1. Frictional Tenosynovitis

1. The most common form of tenosynovitis, although the condition may also be associated with systemic disease (e.g., rheumatoid arthritis) or infection (suppurative tenosynovitis).
2. Symptoms include localized discomfort, aggravated by activity and relieved by rest and splinting.
3. On examination, there should be discretely localized swelling, tenderness, and crepitus. Provocative tests (see below) should be positive.
4. Tenosynovitis is usually a clinical diagnosis, although MRI and ultrasound can be useful if there is a need to obtain an image.
5. Treatment should initially be conservative with splinting, change of activity patterns, and nonsteroidal anti-inflammatory medications. If symptoms continue after an adequate period of conservative treatment, local steroid injections can be used (usual maximum number of injections is 2 or 3). Nonresponders may need surgical treatment—usually a compartment release.
6. Tenosynovitis is more common in certain locations than others:

   - de Quervain's tenosynovitis—frictional tenosynovitis in the 1st dorsal extensor compartment (abductor pollicis longus, extensor pollicis brevis) that produces radial wrist pain. Provoked with Finkelstein's test (pain over the first dorsal compartment with the thumb flexed into the palm and ulnar deviation of the wrist—do it gently; it can be very painful). Patients who do not respond to conservative treatment or steroid injections may require surgical release of the first dorsal extensor compartment sheath, including release of a separate deep subcompartment that is often present (usually containing the extensor pollicis brevis tendon).
   - Intersection syndrome—named because it was thought that symptoms came from the anatomical location where the 1st and 2nd extensor compartment tendons crossed. Now thought to be caused by frictional tenosynovitis in the 2nd extensor compartment tendons as they pass though their fibro-osseous tunnel near Lister's tubercle.
   - ECU tenosynovitis—6th extensor compartment frictional tenosynovitis is frequently seen in racquet sport players, especially tennis players. It may present as an acute injury or as a chronic tenosynovitis, chronically subluxing ECU tendon, or an apophysitis at the insertion of the ECU at the base of the 5th metacarpal. Subluxation of the ECU can be provoked by supination with the tendon tensioned by making a tight grip.
   - Frictional tenosynovitis occurs less commonly in other tendons. Look carefully for the appropriate clinical features in locations

where FCR (flexor carpi radialis), finger flexors, FCU (flexor carpi ulnaris), and the other extensors cross the wrist. Be particularly suspicious where there may be a predisposing cause. For example, symptoms may be present in an EPL tendon in a patient who has had a distal radius fracture, or in tendons close to the location of a buried internal fixation device, or in patients engaged in excessive activity (either at work, or related to sports and recreational activities).

2. Suppurative Tenosynovitis

1. A serious condition that has grave consequences because it severely damages tendons.
2. *Staphylococcus* and *Streptococcus* are the most common causative organisms.
3. Treatment in the early cellulitic stage consists of elevation, splinting, and antibiotics.
4. Throbbing pain, especially if it interferes with sleep, is an indicator that pus is present.
5. Suppurative tenosynovitis requires surgical drainage, debridement, and irrigation.

F. Activity-Related Musculoskeletal Pain

1. Many patients complain of musculoskeletal pain related to physical activity. They are often incorrectly and confusingly labeled as having "tendonitis." Cumulative trauma disorder, repetitive strain syndrome, overuse syndrome, occupational arm pain, and many other terms are all used to describe this condition.
2. Characteristically, patients complain of a nonspecific, vaguely localized pain in the arm (patients use their opposite hand to indicate its widespread nature, which cannot be localized and is frequently both dorsal and volar), of insidious onset, variable intensity, aggravated by activity, and not well relieved by rest. It is frequently related to work activities, which are often not strenuous but do tend to be repetitive and dull.
3. The quality of the pain is poorly defined (but seems to be mostly dull and aching in nature), and taking time off work or away from the activity thought to cause the problem is often not associated with relief of symptoms.
4. There is often associated numbness, but this is poorly localized and is not the same as the nocturnal paraesthesia described by patients with carpal tunnel syndrome.
5. On examination, no abnormalities can be found.
6. Investigations also fail to detect any abnormalities (beware of false positives, such as TFCC tears, which do not correlate with the clinical picture).
7. There are many approaches to the management of this condition. When the diagnosis is suspected clinically, we usually do simple screening tests—plain radiographs, sometimes electrodiagnostic tests (if there are symptoms to suggest carpal tunnel syndrome), and a Tc99 MDP bone scan (to rule out musculoskeletal pathology). We do not recommend time off work, as this has not been shown to be beneficial. The mainstay of treatment is education and change of activity patterns. Physiotherapy that includes splinting and various physical modalities is prescribed for acute symptoms, but should not be prolonged. Other modalities of treatment have not been useful. Occasionally, symptoms are severe enough that a change of occupation is necessary.

G. Ganglion Cysts

1. A ganglion cyst can be painful and may be related to an accident. It may result from trauma, although an unrelated injury is often blamed in order to rationalize its presence.
2. The diagnosis is easy if there is an associated swelling, especially if this is in one of the locations normally associated with ganglia, such as the dorsoradial aspect of the wrist or adjacent to the radial artery. Occult ganglia, buried in the wrist capsule, can be difficult to diagnose. They are often in the midline dorsally and may be identified with ultrasound or MRI.
3. Initial treatment is percutaneous aspiration with or without steroid injection, but this approach has at least a 50% recurrence rate. Definitive treatment is by surgical excision.

H. Arthritis

Wrist injuries may aggravate an underlying arthritic condition or may precipitate the diagnosis of a previously unrecognized condition. Posttraumatic arthritis may also result from previous wrist injury. Patients usually present with moderate to severe pain, aggravated by movement, relieved by rest, and associated with stiffness and swelling. On examination there may be swelling, localized tenderness, stiffness and pain on movement, and decreased grip strength. Localizing features may also be present, depending on the specific nature of the condition. Look for underlying disease in patients that present with wrist pain:

1. Kienbock's Disease
    a. Kienbock's disease is defined as avascular necrosis of the lunate.
    b. Etiologically related to an ulnar-negative variance, an end arterial supply to the lunate, and trauma (single incident or repetitive minor trauma).
    c. The diagnosis may be confirmed by plain radiographs, bone scan, and MRI.
    d. Conservative treatment may be tried in the early stages, but surgical intervention is almost always needed eventually. A number of different operations are used depending on the stage of disease and individual surgeon bias. The most commonly used techniques include radial shortening osteotomy and vascularized bone grafting into the lunate.

2. Infective Arthritis
    a. Acute pyogenic arthritis occurs secondary to penetrating trauma or may arise from hematogenous spread. The differential diagnosis includes gout and pseudogout, both of which have physical examination features that also suggest infection.
    b. The joint appears warm and erythematous, with severe pain on passive motion.
    c. *Staphylococcus* and gonococcus are the two most common infecting organisms, but other infections, such as TB, are also seen.
    d. Treatment is immediate arthrotomy, drainage, debridement, irrigation to prevent further destruction of the cartilage, and antibiotics.

3. Degenerative and Posttraumatic Arthritis
    a. Generalized idiopathic osteoarthritis of the wrist is very rare.
    b. STT (scapho-trapezial-trapezoid) joint osteoarthritis is more common and is a differential diagnosis for radial wrist pain.
    c. SLAC (scapholunate advanced collapse) wrist arthritis is a posttraumatic arthritis secondary to scapholunate dissociation and scaphoid nonunion.
    d. Pisotriquetral joint arthritis is a cause of ulnar wrist pain and often results from an old injury.
    e. Clinical features are focused on the affected areas of the wrist but are otherwise no different from those of posttraumatic and osteoarthritis in any other synovial joint.
    f. Conservative treatment may be used for acute exacerbations, but patients also need to be advised about appropriate long-term management for their underlying condition.

4. Other Arthritides
    a. The wrist can be affected by any of the arthritic conditions. It is usually obvious that patients with these conditions have a generalized wrist problem, and that this differs in presentation and appearance from that caused by injury. Trauma, however, may exacerbate symptoms from any affected joint.
    b. Many of these patients have systemic disease and have been previously diagnosed, although on rare occasions wrist pain may develop as the first feature.
    c. Inflammatory arthropathy should be in the differential diagnosis in any patient who presents with generalized wrist pain.
    d. Think of infective (acute and chronic) and noninfective (seropositive and seronegative) conditions in the differential diagnosis.
    e. Conservative treatment may be used for acute exacerbations, but patients also need to be advised about appropriate long-term management of their underlying condition.

71

Flexor and Extensor Tendons

Matthew B. Klein, M.D., and James Chang, M.D.
Stanford University Medical Center, Stanford, California, U.S.A.

I. FLEXOR TENDON ANATOMY

Flexor muscles originate in the volar compartment of the proximal two-thirds of the forearm. There are two flexor tendons for each digit and one for the thumb.

A. Flexor Digitorum Profundus (FDP)

1. Origin = proximal ulna and interosseous membrane.
2. Insertion = palmar base of the distal phalanx.
3. The small, ring, and middle finger FDP muscles have interdigitations and act as a single unit without independent finger motion.
4. FDP innervation:
    - Index and middle fingers = anterior interosseous branch of the median nerve.
    - Ring and small fingers = ulnar nerve.
5. The lumbricals originate from the FDP tendons within the palm.
6. The index and middle finger lumbricals are unipenniform muscles.
7. The ring and small finger lumbricals are bipenniform muscles.

B. Flexor Digitorum Superficialis (FDS)

1. Origin:
    - Humero-ulnar head = medial humeral epicondyle and coronoid process of the ulna.
    - Radial head = proximal shaft of the radius.
2. Insertion = middle phalanx.
3. An independent FDS muscle is present for each digit.
4. Innervation = median nerve.
5. The middle and ring finger FDS tendons are volar to the index and small finger FDS tendons in the carpal tunnel and distal forearm (zones IV and V). This is a useful fact to remember when trying to correctly align multiple tendon lacerations in distal forearm injuries.
6. The FDS tendon divides into two slips at Camper's chiasma, which is located just distal to the MP joint. More distally, the two FDS slips reunite dorsally to separate the FDP from the underlying bone and PIP joint volar plate. The FDS splits again distally to insert onto the middle phalanx as two separate slips. The FDP tendon pierces the FDS tendon from dorsal to volar at Camper's chiasma to proceed more distally.

C. Flexor Pollicis Longus (FPL)

1. Origin:
    - Radial head = proximal radius, interosseous membrane.
    - Accessory head = coronoid process of the ulna or medial epicondyle of the humerus.
2. Insertion = proximal palmar base of the distal phalanx.

3. Located radially within the carpal tunnel:
   - In the palm, FPL located between the adductor pollicis and flexor pollicis brevis
   - Innervation = anterior interosseous branch of the median nerve

D. Flexor Tendon Vincular System

1. Vinculum = mesotenon fold that carries blood supply and nutrition to the tendon. The vincula arise from transverse communicating branches of the digital arteries.
2. Four vincula are present in each of the four fingers:
   - To the FDS tendons:

     Vinculum breve superficialis—located at the neck of the proximal phalanx

     Vinculum longum superficialis—located at the base of the proximal phalanx
   - To the FDP tendons:

     Vinculum breve profundus—located at the neck of the middle phalanx

     Vinculum longum profundus—arises in combination with the vinculum breve superficialis
3. The vincula enter the tendons dorsally. Many advocate that tendon repairs should be performed on the volar portion of the tendon in order to preserve the blood supply provided by these dorsal vincula.

E. Zones

Flexor tendons are divided into zones (Verdan's zones), which reflect the differential outcome following injury.

1. Zone 1—extends proximally from the FDS insertion onto the middle phalanx to the FDP insertion onto the distal phalanx distally.
2. Zone 2 ("no man's land")—extends proximally from the start of the flexor tendon sheath (at the level of the metacarpal neck) to the insertion of the FDS onto the middle phalanx distally.
3. Zone 3—extends proximally from the distal edge of the transverse carpal ligament to the start of the flexor tendon sheath distally.
4. Zone 4—extends from the proximal to the distal edges of the transverse carpal ligament (i.e., within the carpal tunnel).
5. Zone 5—extends proximally from the musculotendinous junctions of the flexor muscles to the proximal border of the transverse carpal ligament distally.
6. Zone T1 (thumb)—extends proximally from the distal end of the A2 pulley to the FPL insertion distally in the thumb.
7. Zone T2 (thumb)—extends proximally from the start of the FPL tendon sheath (A1 pulley) to the distal end of the A2 pulley distally in the thumb.
8. Zone T3 (thumb)—extends proximally from the distal end of the transverse carpal ligament to the proximal edge of the A1 pulley (thenar eminence) distally in the thumb.

II. FLEXOR TENDON INJURY

A. Evaluation

1. A tendon injury should be suspected in any injury of the hand, particularly if there is weakness during motion.
2. A detailed history of the injury is essential, especially in terms of mechanism and timing.
3. Radiographs are important to rule out the presence of a foreign body or fractures.
4. Tetanus immunization status and medical history must be ascertained.

B. Physical Examination

1. Examination of the hand, including inspection of the natural flexion cascade of the digits, is necessary. If a digit is hyperextended compared to other digits, transection of a flexor tendon is likely.
2. Exploration of a tendon injury should be done in a well-lit setting, under loupe magnification, and under tourniquet control of bleeding
3. Neurovascular exam must also be performed.

C. Repair

1. Prerequisites for tendon repair include a clean wound debrided of all devitalized tissue, bony stabilization, and adequate stable soft-tissue coverage. Tendon exposure is achieved either by Bruner incisions or by mid-lateral incisions.
2. Numerous core suture tendon repair methods have been described (e.g., Bunnell, Kessler, modified Kessler, Tajima, Tsuge, Savage, and

Becker). All rely on nonabsorbable suture (usually 4–0).

3. A peripheral epitenon suture (6–0 nylon), in addition to the core suture, has been shown to add additional strength to the repair, to improve external contour of the repaired tendon, and to minimize tendon gapping at the repair site.
4. In zone 1, there is no FDS present. The proximal FDP stump needs to be retrieved. If possible, primary repair is completed. However, if there is insufficient distal tendon, the profundus stump can be reattached to the bone by elevating a periosteal flap from the base of the distal phalanx and placing a pullout suture attached to a button on the dorsal aspect of the nail plate.
5. Zone 2, originally named "no man's land," remains one of the most challenging zones for flexor tendon repair. Assessment and localization of the superficial and profundus stumps is necessary, as is evaluation of digital vessels and nerves. An assessment of tendon sheath injury is also critical. Care must be taken to reorient the superficial and profundus tendons appropriately. Tendon repair is done with an epitenon suture and a core suture. Repair of the sheath may also be necessary.
6. In zones 3–5, primary tendon repair is performed with a core suture; the epitenon suture is optional.
7. Partial lacerations—all suspected lacerations should be explored. If a 50% or greater laceration is present, it should be repaired primarily.

D. Flexor Tendon Avulsion ("Rugger Jersey" Injury)

1. Profundus tendon avulsion occurs most commonly in the ring finger. The injury occurs most often during a football game when, in an effort to make a tackle, the fingers grasp onto the jersey of an opposing player. As the opposing player runs away, the FDP is extended forcibly while in maximal contraction, resulting in an avulsion of the tendon insertion off the distal phalanx.
2. Tendon avulsions have been classified into three types:
   - In type I, the tendon retracts into the palm and there is no active DIP flexion. Treatment consists of tendon reinsertion.
   - In type II (most common), the tendon retracts to the PIP joint. Unlike in type I, one vinculum is intact, which preserves blood supply. Reinsertion is the treatment of choice.
   - In type III injuries, there is avulsion of a large bony fragment. The fragment can be seen radiographically proximal to the DIP joint. Early reinsertion of the fragment with internal fixation is necessary.
3. Postoperative care:
   - Therapy is the cornerstone to a functional outcome.
   - Early mobilization improves tendon healing, reduces scarring, and improves overall functional outcome.

     Kleinert technique uses elastic band traction, which passively holds the finger in flexion but allows active extension within the limits of a dorsal blocking splint.

     Duran technique allows for controlled passive mobilization. A dorsal blocking splint is used to hold the wrist in mild flexion, the MP joints in 45° of flexion and the PIP and DIP joints in full extension. Velcro restraints are removed to allow passive flexion of the MP, PIP, and DIP joints.

E. Staged Tendon Reconstruction

In cases of delayed detection/presentation or a severely damaged flexor tendon system, the use of a silicone tendon implant (Hunter rod) can induce formation of a bed favorable for tendon grafting.

F. Complications of Flexor Tendon Repair

1. Rupture—may require reexploration and repair.
2. Joint contracture.
3. Tendon adhesions—despite adequate repair and early motion, tendon scarring can still occur. Tenolysis may be necessary, but is usually deferred until after a trial of supervised hand therapy and until all post-operative inflammation has subsided (usually at least 6 months following the original repair).

G. Flexor Tendon Wound Healing

1. Flexor tendon nutrition:
   - Through segmental paratenon vessels and longitudinal vessels in the forearm and palm.
   - Through the vincular system in the phalanges.
   - Diffusion plays a greater role than perfusion with regard to tendon nutrition within the tendon sheath.
2. Extrinsic adhesions and fibrosis from sheath and surrounding tissue may *not* be necessary for tendon healing.
3. Intrinsic tendon healing is largely dependent on diffusion. The intrinsic capacity of the tendons to heal is not dependent on extratendinous cells or surrounding adhesions.

III. EXTENSOR TENDON ANATOMY

1. Extensor tendons lie immediately beneath the skin on the dorsal aspect of the hand.
2. Extensor tendons originate from the muscle bellies in the dorsal compartment of the forearm.
3. Extensor tendons are classified into 9 zones, based on location:
   - Zone 1—distal phalanx and DIP joint
   - Zone 2—dorsum of the middle phalanx
   - Zone 3—PIP joint
   - Zone 4—dorsum of the proximal phalanx
   - Zone 5—MCP joint
   - Zone 6—dorsum of the hand
   - Zone 7—wrist
   - Zone 8—distal forearm (distal to musculotendinous junctions)
   - Zone 9—proximal forearm (proximal to musculotendinous junctions)
4. The thumb has its own classification system:
   - T1—IP joint
   - T2—dorsum of the proximal phalanx
   - T3—MCP joint
   - T4—first metacarpal
   - T5—CMC joint and radial styloid process
5. Proximal to the CMC joint—same as for the other fingers.

IV. EXTENSOR TENDON INJURY

A. Evaluation

1. The same steps must be taken as when evaluating flexor tendon injuries with respect to history, mechanism, and tetanus status.
2. Extensor tendon injuries can result from open lacerations, from closed injuries, or from fracture-avulsion injuries.

B. Treatment

1. Exploration of tendon injuries should be done in a well-lit setting, under loupe magnification, and with tourniquet control of bleeding
2. Repair is best done early, within days of the injury. Following injury and prior to repair, the hand is immobilized in a volar or dorsal splint.
3. Treatment is contingent upon zone of injury:
   - Zone 1—zone 1 injuries result in a flexed DIP joint (mallet finger). If the mallet deformity is the result of a closed injury, strict continuous splinting of the DIP joint in extension for 6–8 weeks is the treatment of choice, followed by nighttime splinting for additional 2–4 weeks. Splinting is also effective for most fracture-avulsion injuries. If an open laceration is present, the extensor tendon is repaired by primary repair of the skin and tendon as one combined layer (roll suture technique), since the extensor tendon at this level is quite thin and retains sutures poorly.
   - Zone 2—repair tendon primarily with nonabsorbable sutures, followed by postoperative splinting.
   - Zone 3—disruption of the central slip at the PIP joint with volar migration of the lateral bands can result in a boutonnière deformity. In closed injuries, the boutonnière deformity may not be present initially, but may develop over the ensuing 1–3 weeks. Lacerations in zone 3 may involve the PIP joint space. Tendon lacerations in this area are usually repaired primarily. Closed tendon ruptures are usually treated with extension

splinting of the PIP joint placed in full extension for a total of 6–8 weeks.

- Zones 4–5—primary repair with early postoperative mobilization regimen.
- Zones 6–9—primary repair using nonabsorbable mattress suture. Postoperative splinting (wrist extended 30°; MCP joint flexion; PIP and DIP joint extension) for 4–6 weeks, followed by hand therapy.

4. Partial lacerations—if less than 50% of the tendon is lacerated, treatment consists of splinting.

72

High-Pressure Injection Injuries of the Hand

David Kaufman, M.D., and Kenneth Yim, M.D.
Stanford University Medical Center, Stanford, California, U.S.A.

I. BACKGROUND

A. High-pressure injection injury results from accidental inoculation of foreign material into the hand.

- Most commonly, grease guns, paint sprayers, and diesel jet injectors are the tools involved in the injury. These tools operate at pressures of 100–10,000 psi, which may be increased with nozzle clogging. Pressures of only 100 psi are needed to breach skin integrity.
- Patients tend to be middle-aged male laborers, with an average age of 35 years. The nondominant index finger is the most commonly involved, followed by the palm and middle finger.

B. Amputation rates following injection injury range from 16 to 48%; therefore, prompt treatment to minimize this possibility is essential.

II. PRESENTATION

A. The initial injury is often small and relatively painless, often resulting in a delay in seeking treatment.

B. If untreated, the following clinical picture evolves:

- Within several hours, the digit becomes markedly swollen, discolored, painful, and anesthetic.
- If neglected, ischemia, necrosis, and gangrene with spreading lymphangitis and bacterial superinfection may result.

III. EVALUATION

A. As soon as diagnosis is established, prompt referral to a hand surgeon is essential.

B. Several historical factors must be ascertained, including time from injury, type of material injected, location of injury, and status of tetanus immunization.

C. On physical examination, neurovascular status of the affected part must be determined. The entire upper extremity must be examined, as the zone of injury often exceeds what is clinically expected from the benign appearance of the entrance wound.

D. Plain radiographs should be obtained. Some injected materials are radio-opaque, and films may demonstrate extension not clinically apparent on physical examination. Fractures must also be ruled out.

IV. TREATMENT

A. Emergency department care should include generalized preparations for operative treatment, administration of broad-spectrum antibiotics, tetanus prophylaxis, limb elevation, and radiographic examination of the upper extremity.

B. Corticosteroids are controversial. No controlled studies to date have shown benefit.

C. Operative treatment includes the following measures:

- Treatment is performed with an axillary block or general anesthesia with tourniquet control of the extremity. The arm should not be exsanguinated mechanically. An elevation period of 2 minutes with the brachial artery compressed is followed by tourniquet inflation.
- Bruner or midlateral incisions are used over the affected digits and extended as far proximally as necessary to obtain adequate exposure. Many surgeons prefer midlateral incisions in case the incisions must be left partially open following surgical drainage:

  Neurovascular bundles are identified and carefully preserved.

  All foreign material and nonviable tissue is debrided. Saline irrigation and mechanical debridement are employed. No agent is available to chemically debride/neutralize the injected material without causing damage itself.

  Tendon sheaths, if involved, are opened, irrigated, and allowed to drain.

  If material is in the palm or forearm, the carpal tunnel should be released.

  If the thumb or small finger is involved, the radial and ulnar bursae should be inspected.

  The wounds are then packed open with saline gauze. A loose partial closure is sometimes also used.

  Postoperative radiographic studies are indicated to assess debridement.

  A second-look operation for further debridement may be considered.

V. POSTOPERATIVE MANAGEMENT

A. A regimen of early active motion is essential in order to limit the fibrosis and tendon scarring associated with the intense inflammatory response:

- When not actively involved in hand therapy, elevation, wound care, and splinting in the position of safety (wrist extended at 30°, MP joints at 90° flexion, and IP joints fully extended) are critical to optimal recovery.
- Wounds are allowed to heal by secondary intention.
- Massage may be added to reduce swelling.

B. Hand therapy is probably the single most important factor in the overall outcome of these patients.

VI. BACTERIOLOGY

A. *Staphylococcus epidermidis* is the most common organism cultured from clinically infected injection injuries, followed by polymicrobial culture growth.

B. Broad-spectrum prophylactic antimicrobials are indicated postoperatively.

VII. PROGNOSIS

A. Recent studies have shown that prompt treatment may lower the amputation rate to as low as 16%.

B. With compliance to therapy, the majority of patients are able to return to the same job.

C. In general, prognosis worsens with the following factors:

- Time from injury to surgery—greater than 10 hours places the patient at higher risk for amputation.
- Type and quantity of injectate—paints and solvents are worse than grease and oils.
- Greater pressure of injectate—more injury is sustained with higher pressures.
- The more distal the injury, the higher the risk for complications.
- Presence of secondary infection.

73

Compartment Syndrome

Benjamin Maser, M.D.
Palo Alto Medical Foundation, Palo Alto, California, U.S.A.

I. DEFINITION

Compartment syndrome is a clinical entity that arises from increased tissue pressure within a confined or limited anatomical space, resulting in compromised circulation and decreased function of the tissues contained within the defined space. In the context of the musculoskeletal system, this most commonly occurs within muscular compartments bounded by relatively unyielding muscle fasciae, bones, and/or interosseous membranes.

II. ETIOLOGIES

A. Decreased compartment boundary:

- Excessively tight fascial closure
- Excessive limb traction for reduction of a fracture

B. Increased compartment content volume:

- Hemorrhage or hematoma within the enclosed compartment
- Increased capillary permeability (e.g., schemia-reperfusion injury)
- Trauma
- Intensive muscle use with resultant muscle hypertrophy
- Circumferential burn injury, resulting in circumferential constrictive scar formation
- Intra-arterial injection injury or extravasation injury
- Surgery (e.g., ORIF of fractures)
- Snake bites
- Prolonged exposure to cold temperatures

C. Increased capillary pressure:

- Excessive muscle use
- Venous obstruction

D. Decreased serum osmolarity (e.g., nephrotic syndrome)

E. External pressure:

- Excessively tight dressing or cast
- Prolonged recumbency on a limb

F. Other causes:

- Infiltrated intravenous line
- High-pressure transfusion, as in a trauma resuscitation
- Tumor metastases to muscles within compartments
- Infection
- Acute rhabdomyolysis
- Tendon avulsion
- Excessive tourniquet time during extremity surgery (a form of ischemia-reperfusion injury)
- High-pressure injections (e.g., paint injection injuries)
- Duchenne's muscular dystrophy

III. ANATOMY

A. The forearm contains 3 muscle compartments:

- Anterior compartment: finger flexors (flexor digitorum superficialis and profundus), thumb flexor (flexor pollicis longus), wrist flexors (flexor carpi radialis, flexor carpi ulnaris, palmaris longus), pronator teres, pronator quadratus
- Posterior (dorsal) compartment: finger extensors (extensor digitorum communis, extensor indicis proprius, extensor digiti quinti), thumb extensors (extensor pollicis longus, extensor pollicis brevis), ulnar wrist extensor (extensor carpi ulnaris), long thumb abductor (abductor pollicis longus), and supinator
- Mobile wad: brachioradialis, two radial wrist extensors (extensor carpi radialis longus, extensor carpi radialis brevis)

B. The hand contains 10 muscle compartments:

- Dorsal interosseous muscles (4)
- Palmar interosseous muscles (3)
- Thenar muscle compartment
- Adductor pollicis
- Hypothenar muscle compartment

IV. PATHOPHYSIOLOGY

A. Increased tissue pressure reduces the local arteriovenous gradient and local blood flow, resulting in tissue ischemia of all tissues contained within the compartment.

B. Described by the equation:

$$\mathrm{LBF} = \frac{(P_a - P_v)}{R}$$

where

LBF = local blood flow
P_a = arterial pressure
P_v = venous pressure
R = vascular resistance

V. SIGNS/SYMPTOMS OF COMPARTMENT SYNDROME

A. Persistent pain that increases over time:

- No relief with immobilization of the involved extremity
- Increased pain with passive muscle stretch (e.g., passive extension of the fingers will increase pain in a patient with a volar forearm compartment syndrome)

B. Decreased distal sensation secondary to nerve ischemia

C. Weakness and decreased muscle function

D. Tenseness of the affected compartment on palpation

E. Decreased tissue perfusion or absent pulses (only in severe cases of prolonged duration)

VI. DIAGNOSIS

A. Assess for signs and symptoms as outlined above:

- Pain is the hallmark feature. Increased pain with passive muscle stretch is the most reliable finding on physical examination.
- Neurosensory exam.
- Motor examination with grading of muscle strength.
- Palpate compartments for tenseness.
- Peripheral circulation is *not* a reliable indicator of increased compartment pressure. Tissue color, capillary refill, and temperature can be normal with elevated compartment pressures. Peripheral pulses are rarely absent in compartment syndrome. Normal peripheral pulses do *not* rule out a compartment syndrome!

B. Objective measurement of compartment pressure:

- Used to confirm diagnosis when history/clinical findings are equivocal (e.g., altered mental status, head/spinal cord injury patients, limb ischemia from other causes, peripheral nerve injury patients).
- Techniques include the infusion technique (Whitesides), slit catheter technique (Mubarak), continuous monitoring technique (Matsen), and intracompartmental pressure monitor systems.
- Thresholds for compartment release have been described. However, if a patient is believed to have compartment syndrome based on clinical evaluation, compartment release is indicated regardless of the measured compartment pressure. Commonly used guidelines for compartment release include:

  Compartment pressure >30 mmHg in normotensive patients suspected of having compartment syndrome on physical examination of >8 hours duration or of any uration in uncooperative or unconscious patients.

Compartment pressure <20 mmHg below diastolic blood pressure

Compartment pressure >20 mmHg in hypotensive patients

C. Direct nerve stimulation to discern nerve ischemia from more central lesions.

VII. TREATMENT: SURGICAL FASCIOTOMY OF INVOLVED COMPARTMENTS

A. Technical Tips

1. For release of the anterior forearm compartment, routinely include a carpal tunnel release. This incision is loosely closed at the level of the skin to cover the median nerve.
2. Design incisions to avoid cutaneous nerves and to create well-perfused skin flaps to cover nerves that are exposed by the fasciotomy.
3. Avoid straight-line incisions across joints.
4. Release the epimysium of all individual muscles contained within the compartment. A single fasciotomy of the primary compartment fascia may not adequately release compression of a deeper muscle, which may have an individual tight muscle fascia that also requires release. The epimysium should also be released if muscle bellies appear pale, tense, or avascular.
5. Incision length should span the entire compartment.
6. The dorsal and palmar interosseous compartments may be released through two dorsal incisions, one placed over the 2nd metacarpal and one placed over the 4th metacarpal. The adductor compartment may also be released through the incision over the 2nd metacarpal. The thenar compartment fasciotomy is performed through an incision placed along the radial aspect of the 1st metacarpal, while the hypothenar compartment fasciotomy is approached along the ulnar aspect of the 5th metacarpal.
7. Rubber band or vessel loop laces can be used to keep gentle tension on skin edges to prevent undue retraction and widening of wounds. This will help draw wound edges together and assist in final closure as swelling resolves. In some cases treated in this fashion, a delayed primary closure is possible 4–7 days following the fasciotomy without need for skin grafting.

B. Postoperative Management

1. Splint the extremity (e.g., position of safety in the hand with wrist extended 30 degrees, MP joints flexed at 70 degrees, and IP joints fully extended).
2. Elevation of the extremity.
3. Skin closure or wound coverage with skin grafts 3–5 days after compartment release if a delayed primary closure is not possible.

74

Hand Infections

Matthew Klein, M.D., and James Chang, M.D.
Stanford University Medical Center, Stanford, California, U.S.A.

I. INITIAL EVALUATION—HISTORY

A. The time and mechanism of injury are important to obtain in the history. In addition, the presence or absence of systemic symptoms (fevers, chills, and rigors) is also important.

B. The patient's past medical history, including history of diabetes, peripheral vascular disease, or immunocompromising condition, is similarly important.

C. The patient's tetanus status must be determined. If the wound is a minor clean wound, tetanus toxoid should be administered to patients who have had three or fewer immunization shots, if greater than 10 years has passed since the last tetanus dose, or to patients who are uncertain of their status. For all other wounds, tetanus toxoid must be given to those who have had three or fewer immunization shots if it has been more than 5 years since the last dose or to those who are uncertain of their status. Tetanus immune globulin should also be administered to those who have had three or fewer injections or are uncertain of their status.

II. INITIAL EVALUATION—PHYSICAL EXAMINATION

A. Wound inspection—determine the extent of the wound, cellulitis, drainage, or lymphangitis.

B. Functional status, including both sensory and motor neurologic testing.

C. Radiographic—plain films are important to determine if there is gas gangrene, associated fractures, foreign bodies, or osteomyelitis.

III. PARONYCHIA

A. Acute Paronychia

1. An acute paronychia is an infection of the soft tissue fold around the fingernails.
2. The most common infection in the hand.
3. *Staphylococcus aureus* is the most common infecting bacteria, but mixed flora may be present.
4. Infection can also extend into eponychium.
5. Treatment:
   - Superficial abscesses can be drained with incision. Deeper abscesses may require digital block prior to drainage.
   - The nail adjacent to the paronychia may require excision in severe cases, with an incision made in the nail fold to allow adequate drainage.
   - The abscess cavity is packed initially. The patient is then started on saline soaks and twice-per-day dressing changes.
   - Antibiotics.

B. Chronic Paronychia

1. Chronic paronychia are usually caused by *Candida albicans* infection of the proximal nail fold.

2. Initial treatment is with antifungal agents. If unsuccessful, operative treatment may be necessary.

IV. FELONS

1. Felons are subcutaneous abscesses of the distal volar pulp of a finger or thumb.
2. Felons usually result from a penetrating injury.
3. A patient typically presents with a red, swollen, tender distal phalanx.
4. Surgical drainage is indicated when there is fluctuance in the pulp. Multiple septa within the pulp may cause loculation of the infection. Any drainage procedure must include complete division of all septa to ensure drainage of all loculations.
5. There have been several incisions described for felon drainage, including the fish-mouth incision, the hockey stick (or J) incision, volar transverse, mid-volar longitudinal, and high lateral incision inferior to the lateral border of the nail plate. The high lateral incision and volar incision are usually recommended.
6. Antibiotics that cover *Staphylococcus* are indicated.

V. HERPES SIMPLEX

1. Herpetic whitlow is a viral infection frequently seen in medical or dental personnel.
2. Patient will complain of 2–3 days of burning with no clear etiology until a vesicular eruption occurs.
3. Course is usually self-limited and lasts 2–3 weeks.
4. Treatment consists of pain control and supportive care. Operative treatment is not indicated. Topical antivirals have been recommended in immunocompromised patients.
5. 20% of patients will undergo reactivation.

VI. DEEP SPACE PALM INFECTIONS

A. Web Space

1. Infection usually occurs through a small fissure in the skin between the fingers.
2. Pain and swelling are localized to the web space.
3. Potential for a superficial as well as deep infection needs to be evaluated.
4. An "hourglass" or "collar-button abscess" is a web space infection that extends both dorsally and volarly from the web space. Drainage must include drainage of both components to prevent persistent or recurrent infection.

B. Midpalmar Space

Midpalmar space infections can result from a penetrating wound. These may cause palmar abscesses that spread proximally, flexor tenosynovitis, and may ultimately cause rupture of a flexor tendon.

C. Thenar Space

Thenar space infections arise from penetrating injuries and present with marked swelling of the thenar eminence.

D. Bursa Infections

1. The ulnar bursa is an extension of the flexor digitorum profundus of the little finger. Bursal infection can result from proximal spread of tenosynovitis.
2. The radial bursa is the proximal extension of the tendon sheath of the flexor pollicis longus. Bursal infection can result from proximal spread of tenosynovitis.

E. Parona's Space

Parona's space is located deep to the radial and ulnar bursae and superficial to the pronator quadratus muscle. Infection can occur from extension from the radial or ulnar bursae.

VII. PYOGENIC FLEXOR TENOSYNOVITIS

1. Tenosynovitis is usually caused by penetrating injury, although hematogenous spread to the flexor tendon sheath may also occur.
2. The most common organism is *Staphylococcus aureus*.
3. In the early twentieth century, Kanavel described the classic findings of tenosynovitis (Kanavel's signs):
    - Flexed position of the finger
    - Symmetric enlargement (fusiform swelling) of the entire digit

- Tenderness over the full length of the tendon sheath
- Pain on passive extension

4. If the patient is evaluated within 24–48 h, he or she can be treated with antibiotics, elevation, and immobilization. If this does not succeed, operative drainage is necessary.
5. Operative treatment consists of incision, drainage, debridement, and placement of an irrigation catheter.
    - An incision is made over the proximal extent of the flexor tendon sheath. The tendon sheath is opened proximal to the A-1 pulley.
    - A distal incision is made in the mid-axial line at the level of the DIP joint. A window in the sheath is made distal to the A-4 pulley.
    - The sheath is then irrigated with an 18-gauge angiocatheter or 5 French pediatric feeding tube, which is sutured in place. Irrigation with normal saline should continue for 48 h.

VIII. BITES

Most bites should be left open for drainage.

A. Human Bites

1. *Staphylococcus aureus* and *Eikenella corrodens* are the most common organisms.
2. Treatment is with intravenous antibiotics (penicillin and first-generation cephalosporin), elevation, and immobilization.
3. Human bites that are the result of a clenched fist injury may involve the MCP joint (septic arthritis). Treatment must include surgical exploration of the joint, drainage of the infection, and irrigation. X-rays should also be obtained to detect a foreign body (i.e., tooth fragment).

B. Animal Bites

1. *Pasteurella multocida* is a common microorganism associated with animal bites.
2. Patients require antibiotic coverage (penicillin and first-generation cephalosporin), tetanus immunization, and verification of the animal's rabies immunization status.

IX. CHRONIC INFECTIONS

A. Osteomyelitis

1. Osteomyelitis can be caused by hematogenous spread from a distant source or contiguous progression of a localized infection.
2. Treatment consists of thorough debridement of necrotic bone and long-term antibiotic coverage.

B. Chronic Soft Tissue Infections

1. Biopsy and culture are necessary.
2. Etiology can be aerobic, anaerobic, mycobacterial, or fungal.

X. IMMUNOCOMPROMISED PATIENTS

1. Immunocompromised individuals may present with more widespread infections and with atypical or multiple organisms.
2. These patients need evaluation by a hand surgeon.
3. Treatment requires broad-spectrum antibiotics, culture, and aggressive debridement.

XI. ATYPICAL INFECTIONS

A. Mycobacterial Infections

1. *Mycobacterium marinum*—fresh water lakes, tropical fish tanks, fishermen.
2. *Mycobacterium kansasii.*
3. *Mycobacterium avium intracellulare.*
4. *Mycobacterium tuberculosis.*
5. Diagnosis is established by biopsy, acid-fast bacilli staining, and culture on Lowenstein-Jensen culture media. For *Mycobacterium marinum*, cultures must be performed at 30–32°C.
6. Current drug therapy includes isoniazid, ethambutol, and rifampin.

B. Leech Infections

1. *Aeromonas hydrophila* may be transmitted during leech therapy in microvascular surgery patients.
2. Prophylactic antibiotic treatment with a third-generation cephalosporin is recommended when leeches are required.

75

Tenosynovitis

Aaron Daluiski, M.D., and Prosper Benhaim, M.D.
David Geffen School of Medicine at UCLA, Los Angeles, California, U.S.A.

Tenosynovitis is an inflammatory condition of tendons or tendon sheaths. This condition can grossly be divided into reactive or proliferative tenosynovitis (Table 1). Reactive processes are much more common than are proliferative processes. Reactive tenosynovitis includes trigger digits and extensor tendinitis (e.g., de Quervain's, intersection syndrome, etc). Proliferative disorders are inflammatory and erosive.

I. BASIC ANATOMY

A. Extensors

A total of 12 extensor tendons are present in 6 separate compartments on the dorsum of the hand and wrist. Each compartment has its own synovial sheath (Table 2). Inflammatory conditions associated with each compartment are included in the table. The first and sixth compartments are most commonly affected.

B. Flexors

There are 11 (12 including palmaris longus) flexor tendons that cross the wrist joint. The radial-most (flexor carpi radialis) and ulnar-most (flexor carpi ulnaris) tendons are wrist flexors that are not included within the carpal tunnel. There are nine flexors within the carpal tunnel: flexor digitorum superficialis (FDS) × 4, flexor digitorum profundus (FDP) × 4, and flexor pollicis longus (FPL). These tendons are covered by a double-walled, synovial-lined tube.

1. Eight pulleys are present on each digit: five annular (A1–A5) and three cruciate (C1–C3) pulleys. The thumb (FPL) has two annular pulleys (A1 and A2) and one oblique pulley.
2. The A1 pulley is the causative pulley in trigger digits; it can be sacrificed without loss of function.
3. The A2 pulley is located at the proximal portion of proximal phalanx ("proximal-proximal"), and the A4 pulley is located at the middle portion of the middle phalanx ("middle-middle"). The A2 and A4 pulleys are critical in preventing bowstringing of the tendons and should be preserved if at all possible.
4. Camper's chiasma is the point at which the FDS tendon splits into radial and ulnar slips, allowing the FDP tendon to pass more distally.

II. STENOSING TENDOVAGINITIS

A. Trigger Digits

Trigger digits (stenosing tendovaginitis) produce a snapping sensation of the affected digit with motion. Locking of the digit, usually in flexion, may also occur.

1. Overall incidence = 2.6%.
    - The incidence is higher in patients with diabetes, rheumatoid arthritis, hypothyroidism, gout, and renal disease.
    - More frequent in females (female:male = 4:1).
    - Most commonly affects the thumb, ring finger, or middle finger (least often in the index finger).

Table 1 Types of Tenosynovitis

Proliferative
Rheumatoid arthritis
Crystalline
Deposition
Chronic
Sarcoidosis
Septic
Reactive
1st Compartment (de Quervain's)
2nd Compartment (intersection syndrome)
EPL
ECU
FCR
Linburg's
Other
Epicondylitis

2. Pathology: swelling of the flexor tendons within the sheath secondary to high angular loading of the tendon at the distal edge of the A1 pulley. An increased amount of type III collagen is present in pathologic pulleys.
3. Diagnosis and classification: pain over the A1 pulley with palpable nodule or triggering:
   - Grade I = pretriggering tenderness over the A1 pulley.
   - Grade II = active triggering with full range of motion.
   - Grade III = necessitates passive extension of the digit after the triggering event.
   - Grade IV = fixed flexion contracture.
4. Treatment:
   - Nonoperative: steroid injection is successful in 50–93% of cases, but there is a high recurrence rate:

     Use soluble steroid with local anesthetic.

     The most common combinations are 1 cc of Kenalog 10 (triamcinolone 10 mg/cc) or 1 cc of Celestone (betamethasone 6 mg/cc) combined with 1 cc of 1% lidocaine (total 2 cc).

     25-gauge needle for injection.

     Ethyl chloride as a topical refrigerant is helpful.

     Inject into the flexor tendon sheath, either superficial or deep to the tendons; avoid direct injection into the tendon itself.

     Do not inject locked trigger digits (usually not successful).

     May splint the digit following injection, but this is usually not necessary.

     Maximum of three steroid injections at any one location, spaced at least one month apart from each other. The risk of spontaneous tendon rupture rises with an increasing number of steroid injections.
   - Operative: if the patient has failed several injections, he/she may require surgical release of the A1 pulley.

     Transverse, longitudinal, or oblique incision directly over the A1 pulley.

     Divide the A1 pulley longitudinally.

     Active flexion and extension of the released digit to confirm release; if triggering persists, may require reduction tenoplasty or excision of one slip of the FDS.

     Overall complication rate is 7% (e.g., nerve injury, bowstringing, decreased range of motion, infection).

     For trigger thumbs, the thickened FPL through the A1 pulley occurs at the sesamoid bones, where flexor pollicis brevis attaches. Careful attention must be paid to the radial digital nerve during surgical treatment since it may occupy a superficial position in the subcutaneous tissue in the thumb.

Table 2 Dorsal Compartments of the Wrist (Radial to Ulnar)

Compartment	Tendons	Associated conditions
1	APL/EPB	de Quervain's tenosynovitis
2	ECRL/ECRB	Intersection syndrome
3	EPL	EPL tendinitis
4	EIP/EDC	EIP syndrome
5	EDQ	EDQ tendinitis
6	ECU	ECU tendinitis

Percutaneous A1 pulley release has been described, but is contraindicated for use in the thumb.

B. de Quervain's Tenosynovitis

1. One of the most common causes of radial-sided wrist pain ("washerwoman's sprain"). Also commonly seen in young mothers carrying children 4–12 months of age.
2. Represents a 1st dorsal extensor tendon compartment tenosynovitis: extensor pollicis brevis (EPB) and abductor pollicis longus (APL).
3. Excursion and direction of angle of pull puts these tendons at risk for tenosnovitis.
4. Diagnosis:
   - Tenderness over the radial styloid process.
   - Painful thumb motion (especially extension), occasional crepitation (wet leather sign), or locking are often present.
   - Rule out Wartenberg's syndrome (superficial radial nerve neuritis).
   - Finkelstein's test (Eichhoff maneuver): pain over the radial styloid when the flexed thumb that is held in a clenched fist is ulnarly deviated.
5. Nonoperative treatment: initial treatment includes NSAIDs and splinting for 3–4 weeks continuously in a long opponens splint with the thumb held in abduction. If not successful, injection of the tendon sheath with a soluble corticosteroid is successful in 50–80% of cases.
6. Operative treatment—release of the tendon sheaths of the APL and EPB:
   - The APL usually has several slips (necessary to identify all).
   - The EPB often has a separate sheath that requires separate release (failure of operative treatment is usually due to a missed EPB sheath).
   - Need to identify and protect the radial artery that runs deep to the 1st compartment.
   - Identify and protect the superficial radial nerve.
7. Persistent postoperative pain is often from a neuroma or traction neuritis of the superficial radial nerve.

C. Intersection Syndrome

1. Inflammation of the 2nd dorsal extensor tendon compartment.
2. Misnomer—etiology is not secondary to friction between the 1st (APL/EPB) and 2nd (ECRL/ECRB) extensor compartments.
3. Usually a history of repetitive use; often seen in athletes (weightlifters or rowers).
4. Pain is usually 4 cm proximal to the wrist.
5. Nonoperative treatment: activity modification, splinting wrist in mild extension, NSAIDs; if this fails, corticosteroid injection into the 2nd dorsal compartment.
6. Operative treatment: longitudinal incision with full release of the 2nd compartment without repair of the retinaculum; recommend postoperative splinting for 2 weeks.

D. Extensor Pollicis Longus (EPL) Tendinitis

1. Inflammation of the 3rd extensor compartment ("drummer boy palsy") is quite rare.
2. Diagnosis is based on pain and crepitation over the EPL and pain with resisted extension of the thumb IP joint or passive flexion of the thumb IP joint.
3. Treat with activity modification, splinting, NSAIDs, and possible steroid injection.
4. May require surgical release if refractory to conservative care.

E. Extensor Indicis Proprius (EIP) Syndrome

1. Inflammation of the 4th compartment is rare.
2. Typically attributed to a distal EIP muscle belly passing beneath a tight extensor retinaculum.
3. Diagnosed by pain with full passive wrist flexion and resisted active index finger extension

F. Extensor Digitorum Quinti (EDQ) Tendinitis

1. Rare
2. Etiology thought to be from overuse or presence of an anomalous muscle

G. Extensor Carpi Ulnaris (ECU) Tendinitis

1. Tendinitis of the 6th dorsal compartment
2. The ECU tendon lies in its own fibro-osseous tunnel. It also moves freely over the ulnar head (to allow for unrestricted pronation/supination); this tremendous mobility places the ECU at risk for tendinitis.
3. It is necessary to check for subluxation (increased risk when wrist supinates and ulnarly deviates).
4. Nonperative treatment (splinting and steroids) is effective in half of the patients.
5. Operative treatment is required in the half that fails conservative treatment. The ECU tendon is explored and the retinaculum reconstructed to prevent subluxation. Splint postoperatively.

H. Flexor Carpi Radialis (FCR) Tendinitis

1. Caused by overuse, is more common in females.
2. Tenderness is present over the FCR just proximal to the wrist crease. Must rule out Linburg's syndrome (see below).
3. Nonoperative treatment includes activity modification, splinting, NSAIDs; if this fails, corticosteroid injection is performed around the FCR.
4. Operative treatment is required if nonoperative treatment fails. Release the tendon from proximal to distal; avoid injury to the palmar cutaneous branch of the median nerve. Splint postoperatively for 2 weeks.

I. Flexor Carpi Ulnaris (FCU) Tendinitis

1. Usually secondary to chronic repetitive trauma or calcific tendinitis (which causes a chemical tendinitis).
2. Must rule out the differential diagnosis of pisotriquetral arthritis.
3. Nonoperative treatment includes activity modification, splinting in slight wrist flexion, NSAIDs; if this fails, corticosteroid injection.
4. Operative treatment is sometimes required. Aspiration or open excision of calcium deposits is sometimes indicated. May require pisiform excision with FCU lengthening.

J. Linburg's Syndrome

1. Tenosynovitis secondary to tendinous connection between the FPL and the index finger FDP (found in 25% of cadavers).
2. Linburg's sign is diagnostic (distal forearm pain when the index finger DIP joint is held in extension and patient actively flexes the thumb interphalangeal joint).
3. Nonoperative treatment is rarely successful; usually requires operative resection of the tendinous interconnection.

III. PROLIFERATIVE TENOSYNOVITIS

A. Rheumatoid Arthritis

Rheumatoid arthritis produces a synovitis that affects multiple joints. Tenosynovitis of the hand is common (65–95% of rheumatoid patients are affected). Tendons are commonly involved secondary to the damage caused by the synovial inflammation around the tendon.

1. Extensor surface: swelling and synovitis are easier to detect on the dorsal side of the hand (more extensile with thinner skin):
    - Extensor tenosynovitis is detected earlier and tends to be less painful.
    - Often affects the ulnar border of the wrist.
    - The 4th, 5th, and 6th dorsal compartments are most frequently involved.
    - Higher tendency for rupture than flexor-sided tendinitis.
    - Location of rupture is usually at the distal edge of the extensor retinaculum.
    - Initial management is medical treatment.
    - Tenosynovectomy if indicated if the patient is not responsive to medical management.
2. Flexor surface: can occur at the wrist or at the digits:
    - Early sign of flexor tendosynovitis at the wrist may be median nerve compression secondary to synovitis.
    - Rheumatoid patients have high incidence of trigger digits (4 types of trigger digits in rheumatoid patients, including classic trigger digit as well as trigger-like digit involving synovitis at Camper's chiasma).

- Surgical treatment requires carpal tunnel release and formal flexor tenosynovectomy.
- Digit flexor involvement is variable and may require open surgical treatment.

B. Deposition Diseases

1. Amyloidosis: deposition of low molecular weight protein (β_2-microglobulin) into soft tissues. Tenosynovitis is common in patients with hand involvement:
   - Protein accumulates on the flexor tendons.
   - Most often occurs in patients with renal failure undergoing dialysis (protein is not filtered and accumulates).
   - Clinical findings include swollen digits without erythema or pain.
   - Can cause flexion contractures, triggering, and eventual tendon rupture.
   - Protein deposition mass may cause median nerve compression.
   - Treatment is surgical with decompression of the median nerve (carpal tunnel release) and complete tenosynovectomy.
2. Calcific tendinitis: synovitis occurs secondary to the deposition of calcium into the synovium:
   - Not correlated with serum calcium level.
   - May mimic cellulitis or septic tenosynovitis.
   - Radiographs may reveal calcified masses.
   - Most frequently found in the FCU at its junction with the pisiform bone.
   - Treat with NSAIDs, splint; if an identifiable calcified lesion is detected, may aspirate or drain surgically.
3. Calcium pyrophosphate deposition disease (CPPD)—rare cause of tenosynovitis:
   - Often with associated carpal tunnel syndrome.
   - Radiographs may show calcifications in the triangular fibrocartilage complex.
   - Crystals are positively birefringent and rhomboid-shaped.
   - Treat by excising crystalline deposits and carpal tunnel release.
4. Gout—monosodium urate crystal deposition disease:
   - More common in men.
   - Tenosynovitis may occur without presence of tophi.
   - Can mimic infection or rheumatoid arthritis; may present as an exudative inflammatory reaction.
   - Crystals are negatively birefringent.
   - May occur on the flexor or extensor surfaces.
   - Initial treatment is with medical management of a gouty flair.
   - Excise symptomatic tophi without sacrificing nerve or tendon tissue.
   - May require formal tenosynovectomy.
5. Ochronosis
   - Enzymatic deficiency in homogentisic acid oxidase. This deficiency causes an increase in homogentisic acid with resultant deposition into soft tissues.
   - Characteristic dark-staining deposits can be found in synovium or tendons.
   - May cause triggering.

C. Sarcoidosis

1. Systemic immune-mediated granulomatous disease.
2. More common in women.
3. May cause inflammatory tenosynovitis.
4. Treatment involves resection of offensive granulomata or systemic corticosteriod treatment.

D. Septic Tenosynovitis

IV. OTHER ASSOCIATED INFLAMMATORY CONDITIONS

A. Medial Epicondylitis

1. Inflammation of the flexor-pronator group as it arises off the medial epicondyle.
2. Much less common than lateral epicondylitis.
3. Common in golfers (golfer's elbow) and baseball players.

4. Most commonly affects the dominant arm.
5. Higher incidence in males.
6. Diagnosis: pain at medial elbow increases with resisted pronation and resisted wrist flexion; 20–30% have peri-epicondylar calcifications.
7. Must rule out medial collateral ligament tear, cubital tunnel syndrome (50% coexistence with medial epicondylitis).
8. Flexor-pronator muscle group: inflammation usually involves the FCR and pronator teres (medial epicondyle houses origins for FCR, PT, PL, FDS, and FCU).
9. Nonoperative treatment includes icing, strengthening, NSAIDs, activity modification, and corticosteroid injection into the common flexor-pronator origin at the medial epicondyle.
10. Operative treatment:
    - Medial longitudinal incision over the FCR and pronator teres.
    - Excise granulation tissue (± medial epicondylectomy with preservation of the ulnar collateral ligament).
    - Postoperative splinting in flexion for 2 weeks; no resisted elbow or wrist exercises for 6 weeks; no sports activities for 3–6 months.

B. Lateral Epicondylitis

1. Commonly known as "tennis elbow."
2. Caused by repeated resisted wrist extension.
3. Incidence 1–3%; approximately half of all tennis players develop this, but most cases are in nonathletes.
4. 75% of cases occur in the dominant arm.
5. Onset in the 4th to 5th decades is most common.
6. Diagnosis: tenderness maximally elicited at the lateral epicondyle; pain with resisted wrist extension; must rule out radial tunnel syndrome.
7. Occurs typically in the ECRB tendon (though the lateral epicondyle is the origin of the ECRB, EDC, EDQ, ECU, and supinator).
8. Nonoperative treatment includes wrist stretching (extension), forearm strap (counterforce brace), NSAIDs, physical therapy, iontophoresis, and activity modification.
9. If refractory, corticosteroid injection into the common extensor-supinator origin at the lateral epicondyle is recommended.
10. 95% of patients are successfully treated with excellent results by conservative treatment alone.
11. Operative treatment:
    - 85–95% success rate.
    - Usually recommended for patients refractory to conservative treatment >6 months or recurrences that last >1 year.
    - Lateral incision between ECRL and common extensors; release of ECRB from lateral epicondyle and excision of fibrous tissue with hyaline degeneration (usually no acute inflammation); care to preserve the radial collateral ligament of the elbow joint.
    - Postoperative splinting in flexion for 2 weeks; no resisted elbow or wrist exercises for 6 weeks; no sports activities for 3–6 months.

76

Hand Burns

Kevin M. Ruhge, M.D., and Warren L. Garner, M.D.
Los Angeles County Hospital and University of Southern California Medical Center,
Los Angeles, California, U.S.A.

I. EPIDEMIOLOGY

A. An estimated 2 million people annually suffer burns that require medical attention.

B. Approximately one quarter of these are major burns requiring treatment in a burn center. Of these, a significant number involve the hands, either as the primary area of injury or in combination with other body regions. Since many patients survive large body surface area burns, patients with combined injury are increasingly common.

C. Hand burns are common and hand function is critical for participation in the activities of daily living. Because appropriate and effective treatment is necessary for the optimal result, the American Burn Association has defined an isolated hand burn, in and of itself, as a major burn injury.

D. The distribution of burns has remained relatively unchanged. In children between 1 and 5 years of age, the most common cause is accidental scalding. Among teenagers and young adults, most burns result from accidents with flammable liquids. The most likely adult burn victims are males, and these are often associated with alcohol, drug abuse, or preexisting psychiatric illness.

II. DEPTH OF INJURY

A. Assessment of Injury Depth

1. Assessment of burn depth is based on clinical examination.
2. To support the clinical impression, a detailed history is taken including the type of burning agent, the contact time, temperature (if hot liquid is involved), and the mechanism of injury. These historical facts are helpful in predicting the final depth of injury and the type of care needed.
3. In addition, circumferential areas must be noted and distal perfusion determined.
4. Associated injuries must be ruled out.

B. First Degree Burn

Involves only the epidermis. The skin is characteristically red, dry, and hypersensitive.

C. Second Degree Burn

Epidermis is destroyed. The dermis sustains either superficial or deep injury, but the burn does not extend deep to the dermis. The skin is characteristicaly red, wet, and painful. Blistering often occurs in superficial burns.

D. Third Degree Burn

Both epidermis and dermis are destroyed. The skin is characteristically dry, leathery, and insensate.

III. INITIAL TREATMENT

A. First Degree Burns

No treatment necessary except analgesics and moisturizer over the wound.

B. Second Degree Burns

1. Superficial second degree burns heal within 7–10 days and can be treated with topical antibiotic dressings, most often with silver sulfadiazine (Silvadene).
2. The goal is to prevent desiccation and infection, both of which can convert a partial-thickness injury to ful-thickness skin loss. As an alternative, several types of occlusive dressings are available (e.g., Biobrane, Transcyte). These maintain a moist wound environment, which speeds healing. In addition, they decrease the pain of daily dressing changes.
3. Deep second degree burns have prolonged periods of healing and carry a high risk of hypertrophic scar and contracture formation. In the hand, this can result in significant loss of function. In such cases, these injuries should be treated by excision and grafting.

C. Third Degree Burns

Proper treatment involves excision and grafting. While awaiting operation, local would care with topical antibiotics is essential.

D. Escharotomy

1. Circumferential burns of the upper extremity can result in elevated compartment pressures and decreased distal perfusion. This is evidenced by decreased hand temperature, tightness of the skin, and decreased capilary refill.
2. Compartment pressure can be measured directly using various devices, but clinical examination is sufficient in most patients.
3. Any evidence of circulatory compromise warrants prompt escharotomy.
4. Scalpel incision or electrocautery may be used to perform the escharotomy.
5. On the forearm, a lateral incision from the thenar eminence to the lateral epicondyle and a medial incision from the hypothenar area to the anterior medial epicondyle are made. Care should be taken to avoid injury to the ulnar nerve.
6. Escharotomies of the hands are performed by placing incisions along the ulnar border of the thenar eminence and on the radial border of the hypothenar area.
7. Single incisions are made on the digits—on the radial aspect of the thumb and small finger and on the ulnar aspect of all others. In some cases, paired incisions are necessary for complete release.

E. Outpatient Treatment

Outpatient treatment is appropriate for reliable patients with superficial burns or superficial partial-thickness burns. These patients can be treated with daily application of topical antibiotic agents.

F. Inpatient Treatment

Inpatient treatment is appropriate primarily for individuals with deep partial-thickness and third degree burns, but may also be required for patients with minor injuries who lack adequate capability or social support to care for their wound. These would include children without strong family support, the indigent, someone who is handicapped and lives alone, or one who suffers from a mental disability.

IV. OPERATIVE TREATMENT

A. Surgery

Surgical treatment is appropriate for deep second degree and third degree burns.

1. Devitalized tissue is tangentially excised after first infiltrating the subcutaneous tissue with a 1:1,000,000 solution of epinephrine and normal saline. This accomplishes two goals: it reduces bleeding via vasoconstriction of subcutaneous vessels, and it smoothes and expands the wound, making excision easier and decreasing the risk of tendon injury.
2. Tourniquets can also be used to decrease blood loss.
3. Sheet grafts are used in all but the most extreme cases. It is best to cover the hand and fingers using large sheets of medium thickness (0.012 in.)

skin graft. This decreases the amount of scarring found at skin graft junctions, thereby resulting in better function and cosmetic appearance.

4. After skin grafting, the fingers are wrapped individually with antibiotic-impregnated gauze strips (e.g., Xeroform). This is also placed within the web spaces and on the remaining areas of the grafted hand. Next, a compressive dressing (e.g., Coban) is used again to individually wrap the fingers and hand. This decreases edema and reduces the incidence of seroma formation under the grafts.

B. Splinting

1. Splints are used to maintain position and limit shear. They also help to resist the forces of scar contracture as the wound heals.
2. Splints are placed within 24 hours of injury and in the operating room after surgery. The optimal hand position includes placement of the wrist in neutral position, the MP joints at 90 degrees of flexion, the IP joints at full extension, and the thumb in full abduction and partial opposition.

V. POSTOPERATIVE TREATMENT

A. Elevation

Along with the compressive dressing, elevation will decrease edema and seroma formation. An Osborn sling works well.

B. Graft Inspection

The dressing is removed on postoperative day 2 to allow inspection of the skin grafts. Any hematomas or seromas are evacuated. A new dressing is then placed.

C. Begin Range of Motion Exercises

By postoperative day 4, the grafts are sufficiently adherent to institute light active therapy. By postop day 5, more active range-of-motion exercises (ROM) and passive ROM exercises are begun.

D. Splinting

Maintained continuously until postop day 4, when splinting is changed to nighttime use only. The splits are left in place if there is concern about graft adherence or if the patient is unable to participate in daily therapy. In most patients splinting is stopped or decreased to nighttime only if grafts appear viable and adherent at day 7.

E. Pressure Garments

Pressure has been shown to decrease hypertrophic scar formation. Patients who have undergone excision and grafting as well as those with partial-thickness injury treated nonoperatively are at risk for hypertrophic scarring. Pressure treatment using gloves is also a useful method for protecting fragile grafts during the first months after surgery. If there is good graft adherence, a prefabricated pressure garment is placed on day 7. The patient is measured for custom-fit gloves once edema has resolved and the wound has achieved greater than 90% closure.

VI. RECONSTRUCTION

A. Burn Syndactyly

Contracture and loss of the web spaces can occur to varying degrees as the burn scars contract, shortening the distance along the web space.

1. Prevention—aggressive ROM exercises with frequent abduction exercises and application of pressure at the web spaces when the grafts are well healed.
2. Treatment—pressure garments can be used in an attempt to remodel the scar while it is still immature. Once the scar has matured, surgical treatment is necessary. In most cases, Z-plasties will add length to the scar sufficient to relieve the contracture and restore normal motion. In severe cases or when there is no adjacent normal tissue to rotate, a skin graft may be necessary to add enough length to the scar.

B. Dorsal Hand Contracture

Hypertrophic scar and contracture over the dorsum of the hand can result in contraction and loss of the dorsal hand skin. The result is hyper-extended MP joints and IP joint flexion (ulnar more than radial) that becomes fixed over time.

1. Treatment—pressure garments and hand therapy, including serial casting and dynamic splinting, can be tried initially. If nonoperative treatment fails, surgical intervention is required, consisting primarily of incisional release and grafting or flap resurfacing. It is important to

divide the contracture proximal to the MP joints to insure joint coverage.

C. Boutonnière Deformity

Thermal injury to the PIP joint may result in disruption of the central slip of the extensor tendon, allowing migration of the lateral bands below the center of rotation at the PIP joint. This causes the lateral bands to act as flexors rather than extensors, resulting in PIP joint flexion and DIP joint extension.

1. Treatment—early treatment with splinting and a longitudinal K-wire is often successful. This is kept in place a minimum of 6 weeks, at which time joint stability is evaluated.
2. If initial therapy fails, surgery is required for correction. If skin coverage of the PIP joint is good and the joint is supple, plication of the lateral bands of the extensor tendon or other forms of reconstruction may be attempted. However, it is very difficult to restore normal motion. If skin coverage is marginal, the best solution may be joint arthrodesis.

D. Nail Deformity

Burns affecting the nail bed can cause abnormal nail growth by direct injury to the nail bed or by contracture of the surrounding skin.

1. Treatment:
    - Eponychial fold and surrounding skin contractures—involves surgical release of the nail fold 5–10 mm proximal to the edge of the fold or the contracture on either side of the eponychial fold, followed by mobilization of the fold distally and medially. The proximal defect is covered by rotation of adjacent skin flaps or placement of a skin graft.
    - Bifid nails—injury to the nail bed can induce scar. In some cases, the scar can be excised and the adjacent normal nail bed can be advanced to allow primary closure of the nail bed defect.
    - Severe nail deformity—nail bed obliteration is often the best treatment when surgical options are limited.

VII. CHEMICAL BURNS

A. Pathogenesis

Chemical burns are unique in that injury continues until the substance is diluted or neutralized. Often, damage is greater than it appears upon initial examination. The full extent of tissue loss becomes evident only several days later.

B. Management

Initial treatment involves diluting the chemical by aggressively irrigating the wound with large amounts of water. In rare cases when the specific agent is known, a neutralizing solution may be available. However, most injuries are best treated by prolonged irrigation with tap water. Treatment thereafter is like that of a thermal burn.

C. Hydrofluoric Acid

1. Pathogenesis—fluoride ions diffuse into deeper tissues and cause tissue damage by catalyzing the destruction of cell membranes. The primary symptom is pain in the absence of obvious cutaneous injury.
2. Treatment—after irrigation with copious amounts of water, the fluoride ions are neutralized with application of calcium chloride mixed with KY jelly as a topical gel or injections of subcutaneous 10% calcium gluconate. Relief of pain is evidence of successful neutralization of the fluoride ions.

77

Dupuytren's Disease

Yvonne L. Karanas, M.D., and Vincent R. Hentz, M.D.
Stanford University Medical Center, Stanford, California, U.S.A.

I. DEFINITION

Dupuytren's disease is the abnormal development of progressive fibrosis of the palmar and digital fascia that results in variable flexion contractures of the fingers.

II. HISTORY

Although reported earlier, Baron Guillaume Dupuytren first described the disease in 1831 when he presented three patients with palmar fibromatosis.

III. ETIOLOGY

The cause of Dupuytren's disease remains unknown.

A. Intrinsic theory: pathological changes occur within the normal fascia.

B. Extrinsic theory: the diseased fascia arises in the surrounding tissue by metaplastic transformation.

IV. BIOCHEMISTRY

A. Myofibroblasts derived from local fibroblasts are the source of contraction in Dupuytren's disease. Fibronectin fibrils are present within the diseased tissue and form an attachment site that links the myofibroblast to the connective tissue.

B. As the myofibroblasts contract, the connective tissue is also shortened and joint contracture occurs.

C. Several growth factors, including transforming growth factor-beta one (TGF-β1), may be involved in the pathogenesis of Dupuytren's disease. TGF-β1 promotes myofibroblast differentiation within the palmar aponeurosis from local fibroblasts and increases fibronectin production. Modulation of TGF-β locally may be used in the future to treat Dupuytren's disease.

V. EPIDEMIOLOGY

A. Autosomal dominant transmission with variable penetrance.

B. "Viking" disease with high prevalence in those of northern European descent. However, the disease may be seen in all races.

C. Male predominance.

D. The ring finger is the most common location.

E. Associated factors:

Diabetes mellitus
Alcohol abuse
Epilepsy

VI. DUPUYTREN'S DIATHESIS

Unusual susceptibility or predisposition to Dupuytren's disease. The characteristics of Dupuytren's diathesis include:

A. Onset in relatively young adult patients with a strong family history.

B. Severe or rapidly progressive disease.

C. Ectopic disease:

- Garrod's nodes: knuckle pads on the dorsum of the metacarpal-phalangeal joints
- Lederhose's disease: plantar fibromatosis
- Peyronie's disease: curvature of the penis due to scar tissue in the tunica ablugine a

VII. DIAGNOSIS

A. History

B. Physical exam:

- Thickening, tethering, and pitting of the skin.
- Palpable nodules adjacent to the distal palmar crease and fixed to the skin and deeper structures. Nodules may also be present on the volar aspect of the phalanges.
- Cords within the palm and digits.
- Metacarpal-phalangeal (MCP) joint contractures.
- Proximal interphalangeal (PIP) joint contractures. These may be associated with hyperextension of the distal interphalangeal (DIP) joint (Dupuytren's boutonnière deformity).

C. Differential diagnosis:

- Occupational thickening of the palmar skin (callous)
- Hyperkeratosis
- Inclusion cysts
- Ganglion cysts
- Tumors
- Joint flexion contractures

VIII. INDICATIONS FOR SURGERY

Joint contracture is the main indication for surgery.

A. MCP joint: a 30° flexion contracture becomes an inconvenience to the patient and is readily correctable with surgery.

B. PIP joint: any contracture should be corrected. Full extension may not be attainable in severe cases.

C. Knuckle pads: if painful, they may be treated with excision.

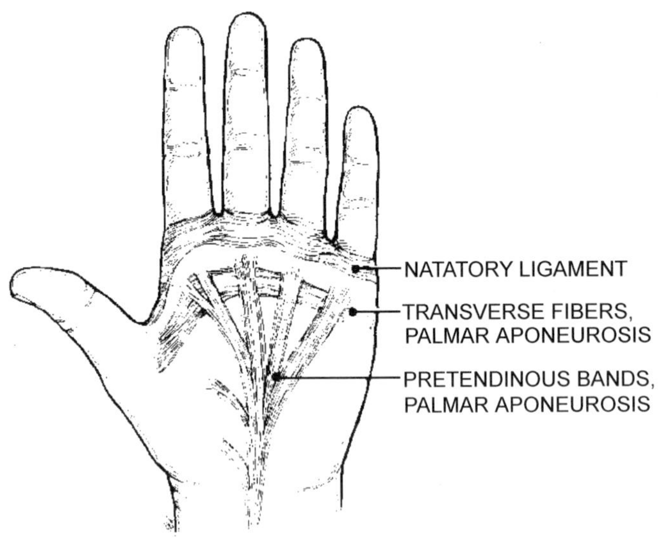

Figure 1 The components of the palmar fascia that become diseased. The pretendinous bands attach to the skin just distal to the distal palmar crease as well as continuing as spiral bands (see Fig. 2). The pretendinous band to the thumb is usually deficient as illustrated, but does on occasion continue into the thumb. Likewise, the pretendinous band to the index finger is often deficient or attaches to the skin on the radial side of the palm. The transverse fibers are at the level of the MP joints of the fingers. Only the portion in the first web space becomes diseased. The natatory ligament sweeps across the distal palm and terminates in the skin at the base of the thumb. (From Hall-Findlay EJ: The radial side of the hand. In: McFarlane RM, McGrouther DA, Flint MH, eds. *Dupuytren's Disease: Biology and Treatment* (The Hand and Upper Limb Series, Vol. 5). Churchill Livingstone, Edinburgh, 1990, pp. 172–175.)

IX. NORMAL FASCIAL ANATOMY (FIG. 1)

A. The Palm

1. Pretendinous bands arise from the palmaris longus and palmar aponeurosis and insert into the dermis between the distal palmar and proximal digital creases. A deeper portion continues into the digit as the spiral band of Gosset.
2. Transverse fibers of the palmar aponeurosis are present proximal to the natatory ligament and deep to the pretendinous bands. These fibers are not traditionally involved in the disease.
3. Natatory ligaments run transversally between the web spaces. In addition, they send fibers that converge with the lateral digital sheet within the digit.

B. The Finger

1. Lateral digital sheet: a condensation of superficial fascia on each side of the digit lateral to the neurovascular bundle. This fascia receives fibers from the natatory ligament superficially and the spiral band deeply.
2. Grayson's ligament: connects the lateral digital sheet with the tendon sheath, passing palmar to the neurovascular bundle (Fig. 2).
3. Spiral band: a continuation of the deep pretendinous band in the palm that surrounds the neurovascular bundle and inserts into the lateral digital sheet dorsal to the neurovascular bundle.
4. Cleland's ligaments: connects the skin to the phalanx, passing dorsal to the neurovascular bundle. They are generally not involved in Dupuytren's disease.

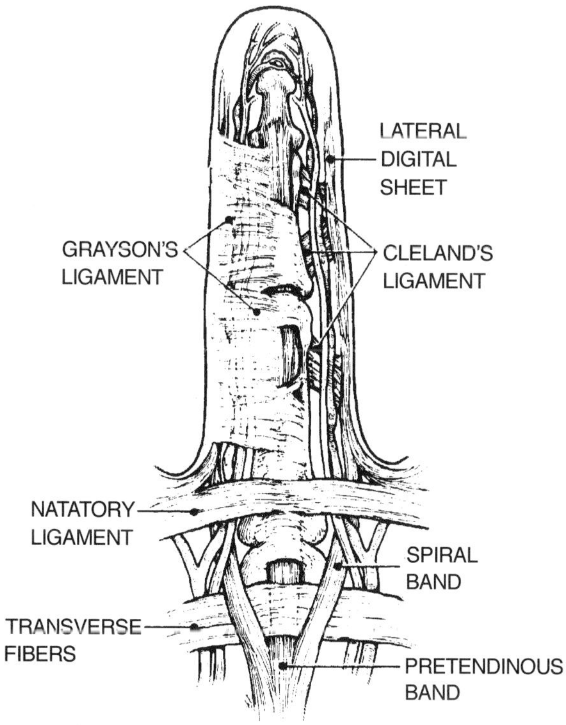

Figure 2 Parts of the normal digital fascia that become diseased. Grayson's ligament is shown on the left. It is an almost continuous sheet of thin fascia and is in the same plane as the natatory ligament. Cleland's ligaments are shown on the right. They do not become diseased. The lateral digital sheet receives fibers from the natatory ligament as well as the spiral band. The spiral bands pass on either side of the MP joint, deep to the neurovascular bundles, to reach the side of the finger. (From McFarlane R. The finger. In: McFarlane R, McGrouther D, Flint M, eds. *Dupuytren's Disease: Biology and Treatment*. Edinburgh: Churchill Livingstone, 1990, p. 159.)

X. PATHOLOGICAL ANATOMY

The bands become cords.

A. MCP Joint Contracture

1. Contracture of the pretendinous cord.
2. No displacement of the neurovascular bundle.

B. PIP Joint Contracture

1. Central cord: arises from the pretendinous cord and passes between the neurovascular bundles to insert onto the tendon sheath or middle phalanx bone. A large nodule may form in this cord proximal to the PIP joint. This cord does not cause displacement of the neurovascular bundle.
2. Spiral cord: arises from the pretendinous cord and continues through the spiral band, lateral digital sheet, and Grayson's ligament, attaching distally to the bone or tendon sheath of the middle phalanx. As the cord contracts, the neurovascular bundle spirals around it and is displaced to the midline. Cleland's ligaments are not involved in Dupuytren's contracture.
3. Lateral cord: arises from the lateral digital sheet and inserts into the skin and onto the tendon sheath distal to the PIP joint via Grayson's

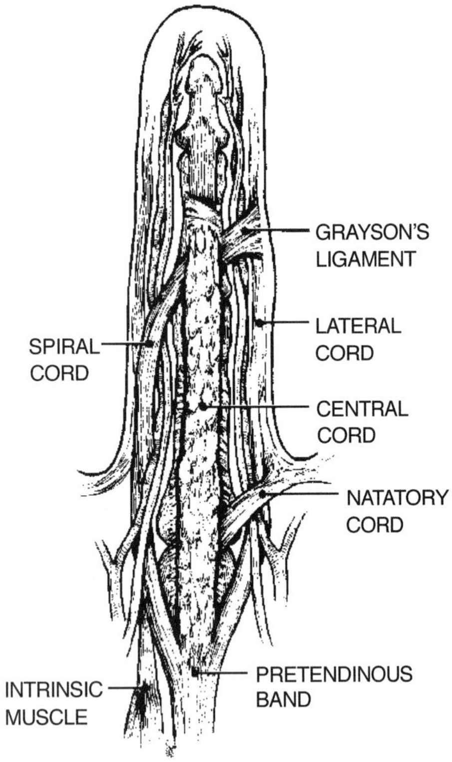

Figure 3 The change in the normal fascia bands to diseased cords. The pretendinous cord causes MP joint contracture and the others PIP joint contracture. When the natatory cord is diseased, it becomes adherent to the pretendinous cord. As it is drawn proximally it appears to bifurcate from the pretendinous cord. Grayson's ligament is diseased in two ways. On the right it is shown simply thickened. On the left it has contributed to the attachment of the spiral cord onto the flexor tendon sheath.

ligament (Fig. 3). This cord may also extend distally to cause DIP joint contracture.

4. Natatory cord: fibrosis of the natatory ligament. Adduction contracture develops; the patient has difficulty spreading the fingers apart.

XI. NONSURGICAL TREATMENT

Nonsurgical treatment has no proven long-term efficacy.

A. Steroid injections.
B. Collagenase injections—may be of benefit in early cases with relatively straightforward pretendinous cords.
C. Splinting.

XII. SURGICAL TREATMENT

A. Fasciotomy

1. The fascia is incised to release the contracture.
2. This procedure is reserved for those patients too ill to undergo surgery. It is associated with a high recurrence rate.

B. Regional Fasciectomy

1. All of the diseased fascia is removed, leaving behind normal fascia. It is unlikely that the disease will recur in the excised areas.
2. New disease, however, may occur in adjacent areas.
3. Bruner or Z-plasty incisions are commonly utilized.
4. Regional fasciectomy is the most commonly performed procedure for the treatment of Dupuytren's disease.

C. Dermatofasciectomy

1. Removal of the skin in conjunction with the diseased fascia.
2. This operation may be considered for patients with aggressive disease due to Dupuytren's diathesis that has recurrent contractures.
3. The skin is replaced with full-thickness skin grafts.

D. Total Fasciectomy

1. Removal of all diseased and normal fascia.
2. This should be considered only for Dupuytren's diathesis patients with extensive disease involving a large portion of the hand.

XIII. POSTOPERATIVE CARE

A. Continuous splinting is used initially until the acute inflammatory response and edema have resolved. Night extension splinting is then used with early active and passive range of motion exercises.
B. Hand therapy is a critical component in the postoperative care of patients with Dupuytren's disease. Patients should begin therapy early after surgery. Patients should understand that therapy is the key to maintaining extension and function of their fingers.

XIV. COMPLICATIONS

A. Wound: hematoma and skin loss frequently complicate surgery for Dupuytren's disease. These complications can be minimized with careful hemostasis and the appropriate use of skin grafts.

B. Nerve injury: excessive traction may cause neurapraxia. Digital nerves may be inadvertently lacerated during fascial dissection or excision.

C. Recurrent contractures of the digits may be caused by:

- Inadequate fascial resection
- Postoperative stiffness
- Recurrent disease

D. Ischemia: injury to the digital arteries may occur during dissection. Patients with PIP con tractures of long duration may have ischemia of the finger with full extension after fasciectomy. Intraoperative examination of perfusion must be performed at the completion of the procedure to ensure that all fingers are perfused.

E. Reflex sympathetic dystrophy complicates 4–8% of procedures. Sympathetic blocks and physical therapy are the mainstays of treatment.

78

Contractures of the Hand

Yvonne L. Karanas, M.D., and Vincent R. Hentz, M.D.
Stanford University Medical Center, Stanford, California, U.S.A.

I. DEFINITION

A. Joint stiffness is defined as decreased range of motion in a joint.

B. The causes of joint stiffness include trauma, infection, edema, prolonged immobilization, and inappropriate splinting.

II. PATHOPHYSIOLOGY

A. Injury to the hand results in edema. The natural tendency of the injured hand is to assume a characteristic position that facilitates the development of edema.

B. The metacarpophalangeal joints (MCP) have the largest potential intracapsular volume in the extended position when the collateral ligaments are lax. This position allows for edema formation within the joint. Full MCP joint extension increases the tone of the flexor tendons, causing the proximal interphalangeal joints (PIP) to be pulled into a flexed position. This posture of MCP extension and PIP flexion is termed the "intrinsic negative" or "intrinsic minus" hand. A hand maintained in this position for a prolonged period of time would develop joint contractures and eventually articular disease.

C. Flexion of the MCP joints and extension of the DIP and PIP joints ("intrinsic plus" position) minimizes joint volume and maximally stretches the collateral ligaments, preventing them from shortening and limiting edema formation within the joint.

III. PREVENTION

A. Appropriate postinjury splinting followed by mobilization at the appropriate time is the most effective means of preventing stiff joints.

B. The hand should be splinted in the intrinsic-plus position with the MCP joints flexed at 80–90° and the PIP and DIP joints fully extended.

IV. ANATOMY

A. MCP Joint

1. Volar plate: this fibrous structure makes up the anterior or palmar capsule of the joint. It is adherent to the volar surface of the proximal phalanx and joined to the metacarpal by a thin membrane. The volar plate is thick and large, but also collapsible enough to permit full flexion of the joint. It is supported laterally by the transverse intermetacarpal ligament. When injured, the volar plate may contract, fibrose, or scar to the surrounding tissue.
2. Collateral ligaments: these structures originate on the dorso-lateral aspect of the metacarpal heads and insert on the volar lateral base of the proximal phalanges. They provide lateral stabil-

ity when the joint is flexed and resist axial rotation of the MCP joints.

B. PIP Joint

The volar plate, collateral ligaments, and the condylar contours of the joint maintain the stability of this joint.

1. Volar plate: a fibrocartilagenous structure that forms the volar floor of the joint. It originates centrally from a thin membrane on the proximal phalanx and from firmer marginal fibers from the lateral aspects of the proximal phalanx. The volar plate inserts onto the volar surface of the middle phalanx. This structure accordions proximally and distally with flexion and extension. Restriction of this sliding will limit flexion and extension of the PIP joint.
2. Chéck rein ligaments: these are abnormal structures that usually develop in association with posttraumatic flexion contractures. Chéck rein ligaments span volarly from the proximal phalanx to the lateral volar plate. They thicken after joint injury and may limit extension of the PIP joint.
3. Accessory collateral ligament and proper collateral ligaments: these structures originate on the lateral aspect of the proximal phalanx and pass volarly to insert on middle phalanx (proper collateral ligament) and volar plate (accessory collateral ligament).

C. DIP Joint

Stiffness at this joint is less common, and its impact on overall hand function is less pronounced.

V. DIFFERENTIAL DIAGNOSIS

A. Limited Flexion

1. Insufficient or adherent dorsal skin
2. Extensor tendon adhesions
3. Intrinsic muscle contracture (lumbrical and interosseous muscles)
4. Contracture of the collateral ligaments
5. Volar plate pathology
6. Bone and joint abnormalities
7. Flexor tendon and/or tendon sheath pathology

B. Limited Extension

1. Volar skin deficiency
2. Fascial contracture
3. Flexor tendon adhesions
4. Volar plate adhesions/contracture
5. Collateral ligament contracture
6. Bone/joint abnormalities

VI. PHYSICAL EXAMINATION

A. Examine skin for signs of skin inadequacy:
   - Scars
   - Burns

B. Extensor adhesions: these can be demonstrated by placing the wrist in dorsiflexion and flexing the MCP and IP joints. The wrist should then be flexed to stretch the extensor tendons. If the MCP and/or IP joints are no longer able to flex, this confirms the presence of extensor tendon adhesions.

C. Intrinsic contracture: when the MCP joints are flexed, the IP joints are passively or actively flexed with ease. If the MCP joints are then extended and the IP joints can no longer flex, an intrinsic contracture is present (intrinsic tightness test).

D. Collateral ligament or volar plate contracture: the joints maintain their stiffness regardless of the position of the adjacent joints.

E. Fascial contracture: palpate the palm and fingers for signs of Dupuytren's disease.

F. Flexor tendon or tendon sheath pathology: adherence of the flexor tendons within the fibro-osseous canal may restrict both flexion and extension.

G. Bony block: exostoses within the joint may inhibit motion. Plain radiographs should be used to confirm the diagnosis.

VII. TREATMENT

A. Splinting

Serial splinting or casting can treat early joint stiffness and prevent progression. Splinting may involve both static and dynamic splints.

B. Therapy

Aggressive physical therapy can be used early at the first signs of joint stiffness once the acute inflammatory response has resolved.

C. Surgery

Surgery is indicated only when aggressive hand therapy has failed to provide any further benefit. Surgical therapy should be designed to address the specific anatomic abnormalities that were identified on physical exam. A dorsal or volar approach will be selected as indicated to address these specific anatomic abnormalities:

1. Dorsal capsulotomy
2. Check rein ligament release
3. Excision of the collateral ligaments
4. Release of tendon adhesions (tenolysis)
5. Release of the contracted intrinsic tendon(s)
6. Release of scar contractures or excision of diseased fascia
7. Removal of bony exostoses that inhibit motion

VIII. POSTOPERATIVE CARE

A. The hand is splinted for the first few days following surgery to allow for resolution of the acute inflammatory process. Once this has resolved, active range of motion must be initiated.

B. Physical therapy is critical to maintain the results obtained in the operating room.

C. Careful patient selection will identify those patients motivated to comply with therapy and likely to have a successful outcome.

79

Hand Arthritis

Alidad Ghiassi, M.D., Prosper Benhaim, M.D., and Roy A. Meals, M.D.
David Geffen School of Medicine at UCLA, Los Angeles, California, U.S.A.

I. OSTEOARTHRITIS (OA)

A. General Considerations

1. OA is a degenerative condition of joints characterized by a primary disorder of hyaline cartilage.
2. Considerable population differences exist in the prevalence of the disease.
3. OA is the most common joint disorder in humans.
4. Age is the most consistent determinant factor in epidemiologic studies.
5. There are also sex, ethnicity, and geographic susceptibilities.
6. Mechanical factors are associated with wear and tear on the joints.

B. Pathophysiology

1. Metalloprotein synthesis by interleukin-1 is implicated in the changes in cartilage matrix.
2. Changes in collagen subtype synthesis are present with increased formation of type II collagen.
3. New subchondral bone formation occurs in the early phases of OA.
4. Enlargement of the joint with osteophyte formation.
5. Advancement of the tidemark with new bone formation in the basal layers of the calcified zone.
6. The abnormal cartilage is abraded in areas of high stress and often the subchondral bone is exposed.
7. Subchondral cysts that are continuous with the cartilage defects are often associated with OA. These cysts can weaken the bone and lead to cartilage collapse.
8. The end result is a stiff, deformed, enlarged, and painful joint.
9. Typically, OA affects the distal interphalangeal joints (Heberden's nodes) and, to a lesser extent, the proximal interphalangeal joints (Bouchard's nodes).

C. Nonsurgical Treatment

1. Initial management in the hand consists of rest, activity modification, and splinting.
2. Anti-inflammatory medications and strengthening programs may aid in pain relief prior to activity resumption.
3. Nonsteroidal anti-inflammatory medications do not change the course of the disease, but do provide pain relief.
4. Occasionally, selective injections of joints with steroids may provide temporary relief.

D. Surgical Treatment

1. Surgical treatment is tailored to the patient's individual needs and symptoms.
2. Surgery is generally indicated for patients with pain refractory to medication, deformity interfering with function, and instability.

3. Distal interphalangeal joint (DIP) involvement can lead to intractable pain, instability, and the formation of problematic mucous cysts along the dorsal aspect of the DIP joint.
4. Heberden's nodes are usually painless nodular enlargements about the distal interphalangeal joint.
5. Surgical intervention for cosmetic improvement of the DIP joints is often fraught with problems.
6. DIP joint fusion in a functional position for painful instability can improve key pinch function.
7. Proximal interphalangeal (PIP) joint painful instability is addressed with either fusion in a functional position or joint arthroplasty.
8. Painful trapeziometacarpal joints are treated surgically with trapezium excision with or without ligament reconstruction, interpositional arthroplasties, or arthrodesis.

II. RHEUMATOID ARTHRITIS (RA)

A. General Considerations

1. RA is a systemic, chronic autoimmune disease with unknown etiology.
2. RA affects more than 1% of the world's population.
3. The annual incidence is 2–4 per 10,000 adult population.
4. Women are affected twice as often as men.
5. Juvenile forms are typically severe and can progress into adulthood.
6. In contrast to osteoarthritis, the proximal joints are more commonly involved (elbow, wrist, and metacarpal-phalangeal joints).

B. Pathophysiology

1. 80% of patients with RA have circulating rheumatoid factor (RF).
2. Several HLA types are associated with the disease (HLA-DR4 and HLA-DR1).
3. Antigen-presenting cells (APC), macrophages, and T cells are major components of RA.
4. T cells (CD4) are the dominant cells in the joint destruction associated with pannus formation.
5. B-cell activation also occurs with production of immunoglobulins (IgG, IgM), which make up the majority of RF.
6. Cartilage-bound immunoglobulins can mediate joint inflammation and destruction.
7. Early in the process, there is injury to synovial tissue with synovial proliferation.
8. With progression, the synovium becomes edematous and hypertrophic.
9. Venous distention, obstruction, and thrombosis lead to perivascular hemorrhage.
10. Direct cartilage destruction is related to the release of collagenase and prostaglandin formation.

C. Etiology

1. The disease occurs in genetically predisposed individuals in response to a pathogenic agent or antigen.
2. Environmental factors, such as infections, may lead to disease formation.
3. Mycobacteria may be the infectious component involved. Mycobacterial heat-shock proteins are elevated in rheumatoid arthritis. However, no mycobacteria have ever been isolated from patients.

D. Natural History

1. Most patients have progressive disease with significant functional loss and morbidity.
2. More than 90% of patients have progression of disease 3–5 years after diagnosis.
3. RF titer levels have poor prognostic significance and do not correlate well with the clinical severity of the disease.
4. The mean life expectancy is reduced by 7 years for men and 3 years for women.
5. Systemic comorbidity (vasculitis, neuritis, pneumonitis, pleuritis, pericarditis) also has significant effects on mortality.

E. Nonsurgical Treatment

1. Goals of nonsurgical treatment include pain relief, reduction of inflammation, and preservation of joint and muscle function.
2. Nonsteroidal anti-inflammatory drugs are used early in therapy: salicylates (aspirin), ibuprofen, ketoprofen, naproxen, diclofenac, and newer cyclooxygenase-2 inhibitors (Vioxx, Celebrex).
3. Hydroxychloroquine (Plaquenil) is an antimalarial drug with anti-inflammatory properties; significant toxicity requires careful monitoring.

4. Gold salts have an anti-inflammatory effect that may produce remissions in some patients; significant toxicity requires careful monitoring.
5. Penicillamine is a chelating agent with an immunosuppressive effect, although its mechanism of action in rheumatoid arthritis remains unknown. It is reserved for severe cases.
6. Methotrexate is one of the most effective immunosuppressants used for rheumatoid arthritis patients. It is reserved for severe cases because of significant toxicity.
7. Corticosteroids (prednisone) have a potent anti-inflammatory agent. Because of significant side effects, they are reserved for severe cases.
8. Infliximab (Remicade) is a potent antibody that blocks the effect of tumor necrosis factor alpha (TNF-α). Dramatic improvements have been noted, but side effects can be serious in certain patients.
9. Etanercept (Enbrel) is a soluble receptor for both TNF α and TNF-β that blocks the effect of TNF. As with infliximab, significant improvement has been observed in patients able to tolerate the medication.

F. Surgical Treatment

1. The goals of surgical treatment for hand involvement are pain control, prevention of progression of disease, restoration or improvement of function, and occasionally cosmetic improvement.
2. The surgical options are preventive, corrective, or salvage in nature.
3. Synovectomies are preventive, while joint arthroplasties and fusions are salvage procedures.

G. Rheumatoid Nodules

1. Occur in 20–25% of RA patients.
2. Are associated with aggressive seropositive disease.
3. Nodules can be symptomatic because of their location (olecranon, posterior surface of the forearm).
4. Steroid injection may cause regression or problematic ulceration.
5. Surgical resection is generally required if symptomatic.
6. Nodules may recur after resection.

H. Rheumatoid Wrist

1. Synovitis of the distal radioulnar joint attenuates the ligaments holding the distal radius and ulna together. This results in supination of the carpus and dorsal subluxation of the ulna.
2. The extensor carpi ulnaris subluxates volarly, increasing the mechanical advantage of radial wrist extensors.
3. This results in radial deviation of the metacarpals and ulnar deviation of the metacarpophalangeal joints.
4. Carpal collapse decreases the efficiency of the extrinsic finger flexors and extensors, resulting in imbalance and finger deformities.
5. Surgical treatment depends on the type and severity of deformity.
6. Surgical options include tendon transfers, synovectomies, soft tissue stabilization, partial wrist fusion, complete wrist fusion, silicone implants, and total wrist arthroplasty.

I. Distal Radioulnar Joint

1. Synovitis of the distal radioulnar joint stretches the capsule and the supporting structures, resulting in joint instability.
2. The instability and joint erosion can lead to extensor tendon rupture.
3. Reconstruction includes resection arthroplasty or fusion and segmental resection of the ulna (Sauvé-Kapandji procedure).

J. Tenosynovitis

1. Tenosynovitis is usually present in rheumatoid hands.
2. The most common site is beneath the extensor retinaculum.
3. Tenosynovectomy is effective when medical control of synovitis cannot be obtained.
4. Tenosynovectomy can also present as rupture of extensor tendons.
5. In the digits, tenosynovitis can cause triggering of the digits and also directly invade the tendons.

K. Flexor Tendon Ruptures

1. Much less common than extensor tendon rupture.
2. Tendon ruptures may be difficult to detect and

should be suspected if patients complain of weakness and volar wrist fullness.

3. Attritional ruptures can also occur from volar wrist osteophytes.
4. Rupture of the flexor pollicis longus tendon over a scaphoid osteophyte is the most common tendon rupture (Mannerfelt syndrome).
5. Treatment includes tenosynovectomy, removal of the attritional source, and tendon reconstruction.

L. Extensor Tendon Ruptures

1. Erosion of the distal radioulnar joint (DRUJ) and sharp bony spikes of the ulna can cause extensor tendon ruptures.
2. It is important to recognize the Vaughn-Jackson caput ulnae (ulnar head) syndrome prior to attritional rupture of tendons.
3. Extensor digitorum quinti rupture may be the first sign of tendon rupture.
4. Treatment includes direct repair, side-to-side transfer, bridge grafting, and tendon transfers.

M. Finger Deformities

1. Treatment of finger deformities depends on the joints involved.
2. DIP joints can usually be fused.
3. PIP joints can be treated with synovectomy, arthroplasty, or fusion.
4. Boutonnière deformities (PIP joint flexion with DIP joint hyperextension) occur as a result of PIP joint synovitis.
5. Swan-neck deformities (PIP joint hyperextension and DIP joint flexion) are caused by terminal extensor digitorum communis tendon ruptures and secondary hyperextension of PIP joints. Rupture of the flexor digitorum superficialis tendon, dorsal subluxation of the lateral bands, and volar plate incompetence at the PIP joint can also result in loss of dynamic stability of the finger and the development of swan-neck deformities.

III. JUVENILE RHEUMATOID ARTHRITIS

A. Inflammatory arthritis affecting the prepubertal age group.

B. Characterized by chronic synovial inflammation and hyperplasia.

C. Three clinical subgroups:

- Systemic (Still's disease)
- Polyarticular
- Pauciarticular

D. Diagnosis is confirmed by clinical and laboratory studies.

E. 20% of patients have positive rheumatoid factor, and 30–40% have positive antinuclear antibodies (ANA).

F. Erythrocyte sedimentation rate (ESR) is usually elevated and can be used to monitor the course of the disease.

G. Hand involvement is most common in the polyarticular variant.

H. Typical patients display wrist flexion with ulnar deviation.

I. Non-operative measures are often recommended for patients with open growth plates.

J. Hand therapy mobilization techniques, splinting, and medical treatment are often recommended.

K. Synovectomy can provide pain relief but does not improve function or motion.

IV. SCLERODERMA

A. Multisystem disease that often affects the hands.

B. Raynaud's phenomenon, flexion deformities of PIP joints, symptomatic calcific deposits in soft tissues, skin ulcers, and septic arthritis are clinical manifestations of the disease.

C. Raynaud's phenomenon is seen in 90% of patients.

D. CREST syndrome (Calcinosis, Raynaud's, Esophageal involvement, Sclerodactyly, Telangiectasia) is associated with anticentromeric antibodies in 80% of patients.

E. Treatment of Raynaud's phenomenon includes supportive measures such as mittens, gloves, hats, and scarves.

F. Digital sympathectomy can be beneficial in selected patients with significant hand ischemia and/or nonhealing digital ulcerations.

G. Calcific deposits should be debrided if they are painful and are eroding through the skin, with or without infection.

V. GOUT

A. Gout is an arthropathy that results from tissue deposition of monosodium urate (MSU) crystals.

B. Gout is a result of sustained hyperuricemia.

C. 20% of patients with hyperuricemia develop gout.

D. Hyperuricemia is the result of either increased synthesis or an elevated kidney threshold for uric acid elimination.

E. Treatment of silent hyperuricemia is not warranted.

F. Tissue deposition of MSU is required for acute attacks.

G. The crystals in the joint cause an acute inflammatory reaction with cell lysis and lysosomal enzyme release.

H. Joint aspiration and fluid examination under polarizing microscope is essential for diagnosis.

I. Intracellular negatively birefringent needle-shaped crystals are diagnostic.

J. Chronic gouty arthritis may closely resemble rheumatoid arthritis.

K. Treatment of acute gout is accomplished with oral colchicine.

L. Prophylaxis is accomplished with allopurinol or probenicid.

M. Surgical management is only indicated when non-operative treatment has failed.

N. Surgery consists of joint debridement, tenosynovectomy, and possible tendon reconstruction/transfer for ruptured tendons.

O. Fusion and arthroplasty may be performed for destructive arthropathy.

VI. PSEUDOGOUT (CALCIUM PYROPHOSPHATE DEPOSITION DISEASE)

A. Calcium pyrophosphate deposition disease (CPPD) is of interest to the hand surgeon because it can resemble septic arthritis.

B. Unlike gout, no biochemical abnormalities are noted.

C. There is generally diffuse dorsal wrist edema.

D. Radiographs reveal chondrocalcinosis. Calcification of the triangular fibrocartilage complex is pathognomonic for CPPD.

E. Diagnosis is confirmed by joint aspiration with weakly positive birefringent crystals.

F. Patients are treated with nonsteroidal anti-inflammatory drugs (NSAIDs) and splinting; they rarely require surgical intervention.

VII. PSORIATIC ARTHRITIS

A. Psoriatic arthritis, considered one of the seronegative spondyloarthropathies, develops in 5–7% of patients with psoriasis.

B. Peripheral joint involvement is noted in 95% of patients with psoriatic arthritis.

C. Arthritis may occur before or after the onset of psoriatic skin manifestations.

D. A significant association between arthritis and development of classic psoriatic nail manifestations (e.g., ridging, pitting) has been observed. Fingers also tend to have fusiform swelling.

E. The primary finding in the hands is DIP joint arthritis with associated nail and skin pathology in the fingers. Multiple joints may be involved in the upper extremities, lower extremities, and spine (oligoarticular disease).

F. X-ray findings include periostitis and a joint arthritis pattern of proximal bone erosion with distal bone osteophyte formation (pencil-in-cup appearance). Severe joint destruction may also be noted (arthritis mutilans).

G. The primary treatment consists of NSAIDs. Severe cases may require treatment with methotrexate, gold, hydroxychloroquine, cyclosporine, sulfasalazine, or TNF blockers.

80

Vascular Disorders

Rudolf F. Buntic, M.D., and Harry J. Buncke, M.D.
The Buncke Microsurgical Clinic, San Francisco, California, U.S.A.

Vascular disorders encompass a broad spectrum of pathology that results in aberrant microvascular perfusion, potentially threatening the viability of the hand or digits.

I. ANATOMICAL CONSIDERATIONS

A. Axillary artery—begins at the first rib and becomes the brachial artery in the upper arm at the lower border of the teres major muscle.

B. Brachial artery—splits into radial and ulnar arteries at the proximal edge of pronator teres, corresponding to the level of the neck of the radius.

C. Radial artery—divides at the wrist into a small superficial palmar artery and a large dorsal radial branch.

D. Dorsal radial artery—dives between the first dorsal interosseous muscles to give rise to a radial digital branch and a major branch to the thumb, often called the princeps pollicis artery. It then continues to form the deep palmar arch. Approximately 12% of the population has radial artery dominance (i.e., ligation of the radial artery will produce ischemia in the radial half of the hand).

E. Ulnar artery—gives off a short common interosseous branch near its origin that divides into anterior and posterior interosseous arteries. In the hand, the ulnar artery divides into superficial and deep branches.

F. Median artery—is usually not present. It is a distal continuation of the anterior interosseous artery into the carpal tunnel. When present, it accompanies the median nerve, often producing a bifid median nerve that is separated by the persistent median artery.

G. Superficial palmar arch—formed by the continuation of the ulnar artery, it runs superficial to the flexor tendons and joins the superficial radial artery. It provides flow to the ulnar digital artery of the small finger and the common digital arteries to the 4th, 3rd, and 2nd web spaces. The superficial palmar arch is incomplete in 20% of patients.

H. Deep palmar arch—is formed by confluence of the dorsal radial artery, 1st web space perforating branch, and the deep branch of the ulnar artery. It lies deep to the flexor tendons.

I. Common digital arteries—three common digital arteries arise from the superficial arch and divide to form digital vessels from the ulnar side of the index finger to the radial side of the small finger. These branches are usually larger than the ulnar digital artery to the small finger and radial digital artery to the index finger, which arise directly from palmar arches. They also have perforating branches that join the deep arch.

J. Patterns of arterial hand anatomy—can be quite variable with radial or ulnar arteries being dominant vessels to the hand. The thumb

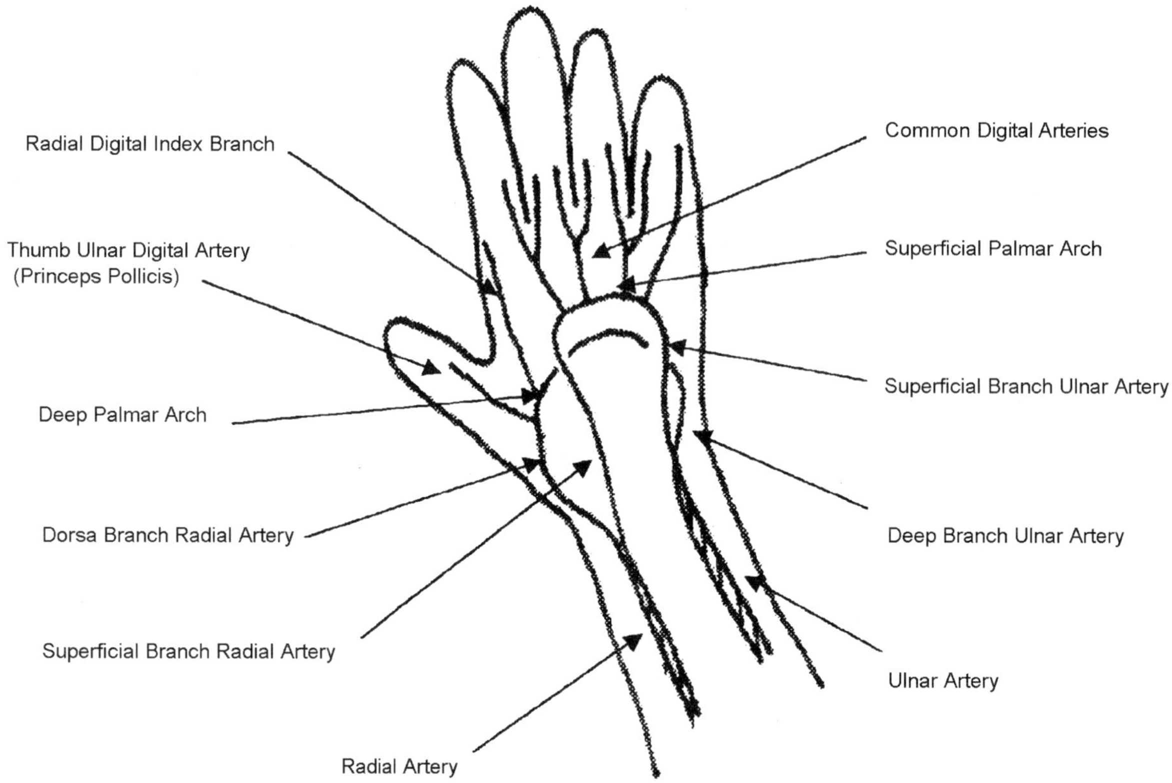

Figure 1 Typical vascular anatomy of the hand displaying the radial and ulnar artery contributions to the deep and superficial arches. The common digital arteries originate from the superficial arch. The main artery to the thumb can be variable but typically arises from the deep branch of the radial artery.

vascular inflow can be quite different from "textbook" descriptions and the concept of a princeps pollicis vessel has been brought into question (Fig. 1).

II. CLASSIFICATION OF VASCULAR DISORDERS

A. Raynaud's Disease

1. Vasoconstriction of digital vessels due to excessive sympathetic nervous system stimulation.
2. Fingers typically become white or cyanotic due to poor distal perfusion.
3. The etiology is unknown and the course is most often benign.
4. Chronicity can, however, result in atrophic changes, painful ulceration, or gangrene.

B. Raynaud's Phenomenon

1. Defined as Raynaud's disease that occurs in association with an underlying medical disorder, such as schleroderma, lupus, or another connective tissue disorder.
2. Arterial narrowing is present due to pathological changes in blood vessels secondary to the underlying medical disorder.

C. Scleroderma (Systemic Sclerosis)

1. A multiorgan (hence systemic) disease process resulting in fibrosis and excessive collagen deposition in tissue.
2. Many organs can be affected, but the skin is most commonly and visibly involved.
3. The disease can be localized or diffuse, but intimal fibrosis generally leads to microvascular disease, Raynaud's syndrome, and symptoms in both the hands and feet.
4. An autoimmune disorder is thought to be responsible.
5. Incidence is greater in women than in men.

D. Buerger's Disease (Thromboangiitis Obliterans)

1. An inflammatory disease of the small- and medium-sized arteries and veins of the extremities.
2. Often seen in men under 40.
3. There appears to be a direct relationship with smoking, and possibly an autoimmune component.
4. Raynaud's phenomenon, claudication, and superficial thrombophlebitis are often present. Limb loss can result.
5. Diagnosis is confirmed by biopsy of an involved vessel.
6. Cessation of smoking is critical.

III. CLASSIFICATION OF VASCULAR DISORDERS

There are numerous causes of vascular disorders of the upper extremity and hand. The following list is based on etiology.

A. Acute Vascular Injury

1. Traumatic:
   - Sharp wounds, penetrating missiles or explosive injuries
   - Crush injuries
   - Severe fractures
   - Joint dislocations
2. Iatrogenic:
   - Radial artery catheterization
   - Drug injection
3. Thrombosis:
   - Atherosclerosis
   - Hypothenar hammer syndrome ulnar artery thrombosis secondary to repetitive trauma against the hypothenar eminence and underlying ulnar tunnel
   - Sepsis/disseminated intravascular coagulation (DIC)
4. Embolism:
   - Atrial fibrillation
   - Myocardial infarction
   - Bacterial endocarditis
5. Compartment syndrome

B. Chronic Vascular Disease

1. Atherosclerosis
2. Thrombosis
3. Embolism
4. Aneurysm
5. Arteriovenous fistula
6. Thoracic outlet syndrome

C. Vasospastic Disease

1. Raynaud's syndrome (Raynaud's phenomenon)
2. Raynaud's disease

D. Congenital Vascular Malformations (Covered Elsewhere)

IV. DIAGNOSIS

A. History

History should include questions that determine the following: acute or repetitive trauma, pain in a finger or hand, bilateral or unilateral symptoms, color changes, ulcerations, cold sensitivity, arteriosclerosis, diabetes, connective tissue disorders, family history, swelling, drug exposure, smoking, numbness, and weakness.

B. Examination

1. Complete exam of the entire upper extremity.
2. Pallor, cyanosis, ulcers, or gangrene indicate poor arterial inflow.
3. Presence and quality of arterial pulses predict site of disease.
4. Evaluate presence of pulsatile masses or bruits.
5. Allen's test helps determine continuity of palmar arches.
6. Adson's test can help exclude thoracic outlet syndrome.
7. Blood pressure differences between the arms can indicate proximal vascular occlusion.
8. A tense forearm with increasing pain during passive extension of fingers and progressive numbness can indicate a compartment syndrome.

C. Diagnostic Testing

1. Pencil Doppler examination is a simple, rapid, and inexpensive way to obtain information

regarding vascular inflow in the entire upper extremity and digits. Most hospital surgical units have pencil Doppler probes available. The Doppler adds to the physical examination by clarifying the presence and level of arterial obstruction and the need for further diagnostic work-up or even emergent exploration. Of particular value is the pencil Doppler's ability to evaluate arterial flow in the ulnar and radial digital arteries of fingers, which can occasionally be difficult to determine with physical examination alone.

2. Doppler ultrasound is another noninvasive method that can aid in diagnosis. Sound waves generated by the diagnostic equipment are reflected from moving intravascular blood cells and are able to differentiate arterial and venous signals. It is primarily capable of evaluating flow and localizing areas of abnormal flow characteristics.
3. Color duplex imaging uses ultrasound and Doppler evaluation to provide color-coded images of vascular flow.
4. Digital plethysmography quantifies flow via the determination of digit volume changes. The most common technique involves the use of air-filled cuffs that are used to measure and generate finger pulse volumes via plethysmorgraphic tracings. The main advantage of this technique is to differentiate between occlusive and vasospastic disease and to assess the significance of any vascular occlusion.
5. Angiography is the most valuable technique for delineating the vascular anatomy and extent or location of disease. It is able to provide the best anatomic detail and to precisely localize structural abnormalities, even in small digital vessels. Access is normally obtained via femoral artery puncture and catheterization of the aortic arch and subclavian vessels via the Seldinger technique. Computer-aided digital imaging and subtraction techniques are able to enhance image quality and remove visual obstruction by bone. In order to obtain the best possible views of the area in question, angiography is best performed with close communication between the radiologist and surgeon. This ensures that critical areas are not cut off from view (e.g., the digital vessels) and that emphasis is placed on the area of suspected pathology. Vasospasm can potentially minimize visualization and can be mistaken for pathology, necessitating the use of a vasodilator such as tolazoline.
6. Compartment pressures—if compartment syndrome is suspected, deep forearm compartment pressures can be measured. Pressure in excess of 30 mmHg generally indicates a need for fasciotomy.

V. SURGICAL TREATMENT OF VASCULAR DISEASE

A. Acute Ischemia or Devascularization

1. Acute ischemia from a traumatic arterial injury with a stab, crush, or avulsion injury requires emergent exploration and repair. Injury to the brachial, radial, and ulnar arteries can cause critical ischemia with impending loss of the extremity (a surgical emergency). Arterial reconstruction is required.
2. Direct arterial repair can be performed in sharp injuries. Hand and finger injuries generally require microsurgical techniques and an operating microscope. All associated nerve, tendon, and bone injuries should be repaired in the same operative session. Bone injuries are usually repaired first, followed sequentially by tendon and vascular repairs. Nerves are usually repaired before soft tissue closure.
3. Vein grafting of arterial defects is performed when primary repair is not feasible or when excessive tension would be placed on primary repairs. Petechial hemorrhages in vessel walls indicate stretch injury that usually requires excision. Vein grafts are reversed to allow forward flow through venous valves.
4. Temporary silastic arterial shunting may be required in extensive injuries where major bone stabilization must be performed and ischemia time is critical (i.e., when forearm muscle is devascularized). The shunts are replaced by primary vessel repairs or vein grafts if primary repair is not possible.
5. Forearm fasciotomy and deep compartment fasciotomies of the hand should be performed if compartment syndrome is suspected or anticipated on reperfusion.

B. Repair of the Nonischemic Injured Vessel

1. Isolated radial or ulnar artery lesions without tendon or nerve injury can be treated with ligatio

if perfusion to the hand is adequate. However, recent evidence indicates single-vessel repairs of the ulnar or radial artery do remain patent in the long term, unlike previous assumptions.

2. If any other injured structure requires intraoperative exploration, single-vessel radial or ulnar artery injuries should be thoughtfully considered for repair.
3. Failure to repair these arterial injuries may also predispose the patient to cold intolerance in the hand.

C. Chronic Ischemia

1. Symptoms, the extent of concurrent cardiovascular disease, and the general health of the patient dictate treatment.
2. Arteriosclerotic lesions of the brachial, radial, or ulnar artery may require saphenous vein interposition grafting.
3. Radial and ulnar artery lesions are best treated by surgery, not by angioplasty. Typically, both radial and ulnar arteries are affected by disease. A complete palmar arch with good distal flow may require only single vessel repair.
4. Arteriosclerotic changes in the hand and finger arteries are difficult to treat and often associated with severe systemic disease and diabetes. Distal vessels must be present on angiography in order for vein grafts to have distal vessels to plug into to achieve the distal arterial reconstruction or bypass. Amputation may be the only option in some cases.
5. Aneurysms and thromboses can be resected and repaired with interpositional vein grafts.
6. The most common upper extremity thrombosis involves the ulnar hammer syndrome (hypothenar hammer syndrome). A thrombosis and/or aneurysm of the ulnar artery at the level of the hook of the hamate is present as a result of repetitive trauma, typically in a manual laborer. Symptoms include hand ischemia, swelling, and pain in the palm and findings of an ulnar nerve compression neuropathy.
7. Embolism in the larger finger, hand, and forearm vessels can be embolectomized with a balloon catheter or sometimes under direct vision via an arteriotomy. Very distal embolism may require infusion of streptokinase or tissue plasminogen activator to dissolve clot and allow reperfusion.
8. Large-vessel acute embolism and reperfusion may result in edema and compartment syndrome requiring fasciotomy. A high index of suspicion must be maintained.

D. Vasospastic Disease

1. Digital sympathectomy can be of value in Raynaud's disease and phenomenon. The common digital and radial/ulnar digital arteries of the affected fingers are stripped of their adventitia and dissected free from their adjacent nerves. This procedure is performed in patients who have a good response to nerve block, as evidenced by increased digital perfusion.
2. Sympathectomy for other connective tissue diseases may not be helpful, depending on the etiology of the digital ischemia.

VI. POSTOPERATIVE MONITORING

A. The fingers should be examined regularly for sensation and capillary refill. Poor capillary refill can indicate thrombosis. Decreased sensation can be a sign of increasing compartment pressures or poor extremity positioning.

B. Pencil Doppler probes can be used to evaluate arterial flow. Doppler examinations can be performed on the digital vessels, radial artery, ulnar artery, or brachial artery.

C. An implantable Doppler probe is used in some centers and can be placed directly on the vessel in question to provide continuous postoperative monitoring of arterial flow.

D. Laser Doppler and temperature probes have also been used to monitor vascular inflow in the hand.

E. Fluorescein dilution test—intravenous fluorescein injection is monitored with a digital readout on a fluorimeter. Failure of fluorescence to rise within the hand indicates arterial occlusion. Failure of fluorescence levels to fall is a sign of venous occlusion.

VII. POSTOPERATIVE COMPLICATIONS

A. The etiology of thrombosis at anastomotic sites is often related to preventable technical errors. Care should be taken in the operating room to use meticulous microsurgical technique. Excessive pressure on repaired vessels and kinking or twisting of repairs or grafts can doom a procedure to failure. Splinting of the hand, forearm, and elbow are critical to avoid pressure and kinking of vessels that would lead to stagnation of blood flow and thrombosis.

B. Recurrent ischemia/thrombosis rates depend on the procedure and nature of the underlying disease process. The first step is always to loosen or remove the dressing to alleviate any areas of possible compression on the extremity vessels. The elbow, wrist, or fingers may require repositioning to eliminate kinks on repaired vessels. If conservative measures fail to reestablish inflow, emergent reexploration is often indicated.

C. When small vessels are repaired, many surgeons recommend postoperative treatment with Dextran-40 and/or aspirin.

D. Infection surrounding a vascular repair in the upper extremity is rare. It can cause potential anastomotic failure and severe hemorrhage and shock. Infection must be managed with appropriate antibiotics and surgical drainage, possibly in conjunction with a muscle flap to protect the anastomosis. Vein grafts and anastomoses can be dressed with moist dressings changed on an intermittent basis and still remain viable for several days.

E. Hemorrhage at the anastomotic site can be minimal in the case of a digit or severe if involving the brachial, ulnar, or radial arteries. In the case of large vessels, hemorrhage must be treated emergently to prevent shock and cardiac arrest.

81

Nerve Injuries

Janet Baker, M.D.
University of Miami, Miami, Florida, U.S.A.

Ranjan Gupta, M.D.
University of California, Irvine Medical Center, Orange, California, U.S.A.

I. NERVE TRUNK DEVELOPMENT

A. Ectodermal origin: nerve trunks arise from neural tube/neural crest with 10,000 cell types in a complex 3D network.

B. Spinal nerves grow into the developing limb bud.

C. Nerves grow into specific muscles and reproducible anatomic locations.

D. Motor neurons:

- Highly target-specific and accurate
- Extracellular matrix in the limb promotes and provides path for growth
- Matrix proteins are important in neural development:

  N-cadherin

  NCAM—expressed on neural ectoderm and axons of differentiated neurons

  Laminin—most effective in promoting neurite growth

  Fibronectin

  Collagen

  Tenacin

E. Axon guidance is a contact-mediated process:

- Inhibitory interactions between the growth cone and surrounding inhibitory molecules restrict growth across a particular surface.
- Selective adhesion between developing neurons and glycoproteins L1, G4, neurofascin, contactin.

F. Growth cones:

- Oriented by diffusable chemotrophic molecules secreted by intermediate or final targets.
- Extracts of denervated muscle have been shown to increase neuron survival and promote neurite extension in vitro.
- Distal stump of transected nerve releases substances that promote and direct regenerating axons.

II. PERIPHERAL NERVE ANATOMY (Fig. 1)

A. Epineurium

1. External epineurium is the outer layer of the peripheral nerve that provides a supportive and protective framework for the nerve.

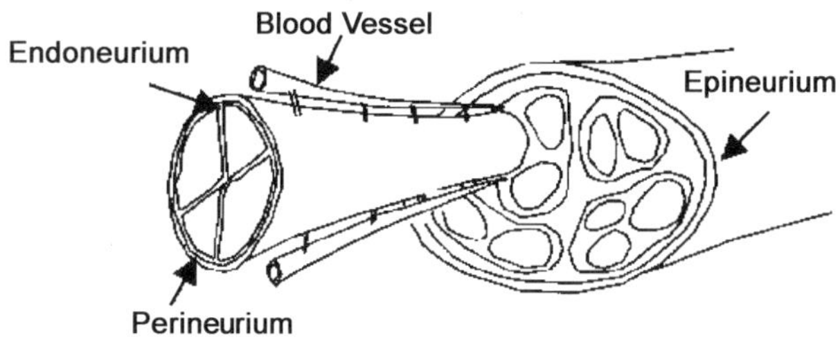

Figure 1 Peripheral nerve anatomy.

2. Internal epineurium surrounds individual fascicles, cushions against external pressure, and allows for longitudinal excursion.
3. Includes a well-developed vascular plexus with channels feeding an endoneurial plexus.
4. Larger amounts of epineurium are found at the level of joints.

B. Perineurium

1. Thin, dense sheath surrounding each fascicle.
2. Is responsible for the blood-nerve barrier (i.e., extension of the blood-brain barrier).
3. High tensile strength that resists up to 750 mmHg pressure.
4. Up to ten layers with flattened mesothelial cells with tight junctions that act as a bi-directional barrier to diffusion.

C. Endoneurium

1. Loose collagenous matrix that surrounds individual nerve fibers.

D. Fascicles

1. Groups of axons packed with endoneurial connective tissue.
2. Smallest unit of a nerve that can be surgically manipulated.
3. Form intertwined plexuses with high variability; not simply a parallel fiber architecture.
4. Structure changes rapidly and often along the length of a major nerve with a maximal unaltered segment length of only 15–20 mm.

E. Blood Supply

1. Well-developed intraneural microvascular plexuses.
2. Intrinsic/extrinsic segmental, longitudinal vessels that run in loose connective tissue surrounding the nerve.

III. CLASSIFICATION OF NERVE INJURIES

Classification of nerve injuries was described initially by Seddon and later modified by Sunderland.

A. Type I—Neurapraxia

1. Focal lesion producing a localized conduction block.
2. May involve a focal area of demyelination.
3. Axon continuity is preserved.
4. No Wallerian degeneration is observed.
5. Reversible (may take 3–4 months).
6. Order of injury: motor, proprioception, touch, temperature, pain.
7. No fibrillation/degenerative changes are seen in affected muscles.

B. Type II—Axonotmesis

1. Axonal damage.
2. Intact endoneurial sheath and basal lamina of Schwann cells.
3. Complete recovery is expected.
4. Fibrillation potentials are noted on EMG with distal atrophy.

C. Type III—Loss of Nerve Fiber Continuity with Intact Perineurium

1. Complete motor and sensory loss.
2. Delayed recovery with inappropriate reinnervation.
3. Endoneurial scarring leads to variable recovery.

D. Type IV—Loss of Nerve Fiber Continuity with Intact Epineurium

1. More severe retrograde degeneration/axonal loss.
2. Extensive intraneural scarring occurs.

3. May require excision and surgical repair or reconstruction with interposition nerve graft.

E. Type V—Complete Nerve Transection (Neurotmesis)

1. At risk for development of a neuroma at the proximal nerve stump.
2. Minimal or no functional recovery is expected.
3. Surgical repair or reconstruction with nerve graft is required.

IV. ETIOLOGY OF NERVE INJURIES

A. Compression

1. Force applied to a nerve changes the cross-sectional dimensions.
2. Acute vs. chronic compression:
   - Time and rate dependency
   - Increased risk of injury with:

     Single or few large fascicles

     Fibers near the surface of the fascicles

     Direct contact with an unyielding surface

     Contained in a compartment with unyielding walls
3. Common nerves at risk:
   - Radial nerve in the musculospiral groove
   - Common peroneal nerve at the fibular head
4. Biologic effects of compression:
   - Increased vascular permeability with edema and hemorrhage
   - Fibrosis
   - Local ischemia
   - Nerve fiber deformation
   - Altered ionic composition of the endoneurial fluid
   - Changes in nerve fiber conduction of action potentials
   - Altered axonal transport
5. Tourniquet recommendations:
   - Maximum tourniquet inflation time of 2 h
   - Maximum upper extremity pressure ≤50–100 mmHg above systolic blood pressure (SBP)
   - Maximum lower extremity pressure ≤2 × SBP

B. Tension/Stretch

1. Deforming force applied along the long axis of a nerve.
2. Acute vs. chronic.
3. Viscoelastic properties:
   - At slow loading rates → 20% elongation
   - At high loading rates → only 2–4% elongation
4. Increased risk of tension or stretch injury with:
   - Single or few large fascicles
   - Scant epineurium
   - Nerve that crosses the extensor surface of a joint
   - Nerves near a joint—increased risk for stretch with joint dislocation
5. Nerve elasticity is determined primarily by the perineurium.
6. Nerves at risk include:
   - Ulnar nerve at the elbow
   - Sciatic nerve at the hip
   - Axillary nerve at the shoulder
   - Common peroneal nerve at the fibular head

C. Double Crush Syndrome

1. Entrapment at one level is commonly associated with symptoms of compression at another level along the same nerve.
2. Endoneurial edema proximally alters axonal transport; decreases delivery of cytoskeletal proteins to distal axon and changes neural circulation distally.

D. Neural Degeneration Within the Zone of Injury

1. Cut ends of the nerve retract.
2. Increased capillary permeability occurs in the first 24 h; maximal at 7–10 days.

3. Histamine/serotonin:
   - Produce swelling of both nerve ends.
   - Axons sprout from the proximal nerve stump and enter the zone of injury. Many of these axons are arrested or deflected.

V. WALLERIAN DEGENERATION

After an axon is transected, the distal stump undergoes the process of Wallerian degeneration to clear axon and myelin debris and to create an environment favorable for nerve regeneration. Breakdown of axoplasm and cytoskeleton is triggered by an increase in axoplasmic calcium.

A. Schwann Cell Response

1. Normal Schwann cells do not divide.
2. Distal segment Schwann cells divide within 24 h of injury with a peak response by 72 h.
3. Bands of Bunger are cytoplasmic processes that interdigitate and line up in rows under the original basal lamina of the nerve fiber.

B. Macrophage Response

1. Macrophages are the primary phagocytes of myelin.
2. Accumulate by 72 h.
3. Early—express MHC class II antigen la and are not phagocytic.
4. Later, penetrate basal lamina, lose antigen la expression, and become phagocytic.
5. Produce interleukin-1 and stimulate Schwann cells to produce nerve growth factor (NGF).

C. Nerve Cell Body Response

1. Alters its metabolic priorities.
2. Decreases neurotransmitter production.
3. Increases protein production (e.g., tubulin, actin, growth-associated proteins).

D. Proximal Segment Response

1. Degenerates if the cell body dies.
2. Regenerates if the cell body survives.
3. Early decrease in ratio of myelin thickness/axon diameter.
4. Late increase in ratio of myelin thickness/axon diameter:
   - This ratio remains smaller than the original preinjury ratio.
   - Conduction velocity does not return to normal.
   - Collateral sprouts from the nodes of Ranvier.
   - Terminal sprouts from tips of the remaining axons.
5. Regenerating unit—growing sprouts from a single axon and from single surrounding Schwann cell and its basal lamina.
6. Axonal regeneration across the zone of injury:
   - Scar tissue between stumps is obstructive to axonal advancement, decreases the number of axons reaching an end organ, delays elongation, and increases misdirection of axons.
   - Within the distal segment, a variable rate of axonal regeneration is observed:

     Based on type/location of the injury

     Regeneration approximately 1–2 mm/day in adults

     Faster and more complete regeneration in young children

     Decreased rate of axonal regeneration in distal regions

E. Axonal Regeneration: Guidance Across Gaps

1. Nerve tubes: arteries/veins/muscle/Millipore/collagen/silicone.
2. Contact guidance: important in early axonal regeneration.
3. Extracellular matrix proteins (collagen, laminin, fibronectin) play a role in cell-cell recognition.
4. Neurotropic factors (e.g., NGF)—promote neurite survival.
5. Axon-promoting factors such as surface-bound laminin, basal lamina of Schwann cells, and endothelial cells.

6. Increased rate of axonal regeneration across a gap has been reported when a nerve guide tube is used to bridge the gap.

VI. NERVE REGENERATION

A. Specificity of Reinnervation

1. Lack of functional recovery with axonal misdirection.
2. Mechanical alignment—surgical.
3. Contact recognition.
4. Neurotropic cues.

B. Neurotropism

1. Diffusion of factors released from distal targets.
2. Factors guide axons to appropriate targets.

C. Neurotrophism

1. Axons grow randomly.
2. Only axons entering the correct pathway/target receive a trophic factor that allows continued regeneration/myelination.

D. Muscle Alteration

1. Contributes to lack of recovery.
2. Loss of motor fibers/units.
3. Loss of ability of muscle fiber to increase in size and reverse atrophy.
4. Long-term denervation results in loss of muscle fibers and increased connective tissue.
5. Consider early tendon transfers.

VII. UPPER EXTREMITY NERVE ANATOMY

A. Median Nerve Anatomy

1. Located medial to the brachial artery at the elbow.
2. Runs between the flexor digitorum superficialis and profundus in the forearm.
3. The palmar cutaneous branch arises approximately 5 cm proximal to the proximal edge of the transverse carpal ligament.
4. The palmar cutaneous branch runs between the palmaris longus and the flexor carpi radialis; it supplies the palmar skin of the thenar eminence.
5. The main median nerve passes under the flexor retinaculum through the carpal tunnel.
6. Distal branches include the median motor branch and the digital nerves to the radial 3-1/2 digits.

B. Radial Nerve Anatomy

1. Located anterior to the lateral epicondyle.
2. Runs between the brachialis and brachioradialis muscles.
3. Branches into the superficial radial nerve and posterior interosseous nerve (PIN).
4. The PIN traverses the supinator prior to sending branches to the extensor muscles (excluding brachioradialis, ECRB, and ECRL).
5. The superficial radial nerve runs under the brachioradialis and emerges between the brachioradialis and the ECRL to supply the dorsal radial aspect of the hand.

C. Ulnar Nerve Anatomy

1. Enters the forearm between the two heads of the FCU.
2. Runs between the flexor carpi ulnaris and flexor digitorum profundus.
3. The dorsal cutaneous branch arises just proximal to the wrist.
4. Enters the hand superficially via Guyon's canal.
5. Superficial branch supplies motor innervation to the palmaris brevis and sensory innervation to the skin.
6. Deep branch passes between the abductor digiti minimi and flexor digiti minimi brevis:
   - Supplies the digital nerves to the ulnar 1-1/2 digits
   - Motor branch supplies the intrinsic muscles of the hand

D. Motor Innervation of the Forearm and Hand

Nerve	Motor	Sensory
Median nerve	Pronator teres Pronator quadratus Palmaris longus Flexor carpi radialis Flexor digitorum superficialis × 4 Flexor digitorum profundus × 2 (index, middle) Flexor pollicis longus Index and middle finger lumbrical muscles Thenar muscles: Abductor pollicis brevis Opponens pollicis Superficial belly of flexor pollicis brevis	Volar part of the wrist, thumb, index, middle, and radial side of ring finger—extending to the dorsal DIP joint on all of them
Ulnar nerve	Flexor carpi ulnaris Flexor digitorum profundus × 2 (ring, small) Palmaris brevis Dorsal interosseous muscles Palmar interosseous muscles Ring and small finger lumbrical muscles Adductor pollicis Deep belly of flexor pollicis brevis Hypothenar muscles: Abductor digiti minimi Flexor digiti minimi brevis Opponens digiti minimi	Dorsal and volar aspect of small finger, ulnar side of ring finger Ulnar dorsal half of the hand
Radial nerve	Triceps Anconeus Brachioradialis Supinator Extensor carpi radialis brevis Extensor carpi radialis longus Extensor carpi ulnaris Extensor digitorum communis Extensor indicis proprius Extensor digitorum minimi Abductor pollicis longus Extensor pollicis longus Extensor pollicis brevis	Dorsal thumb, index, middle, and radial side of ring fingers—up to PIP joints Dorsal radial half of the hand Dorsal wrist capsule (posterior interosseous branch)

82

Compression Neuropathies

Peter J. Taub, M.D., and Prosper Benhaim, M.D.
David Geffen School of Medicine at UCLA, Los Angeles, California, U.S.A.

I. OVERVIEW

A. Etiology may be acute or chronic.

B. Diagnosis depends on:

- Demonstrating that a neuropathy exists
- Localizing the neuropathy with physical examination findings
- Localizing the neuropathy with electrodiagnostic studies

C. Prognosis is often unpredictable until clinical response is observed.

II. CLINICAL EVALUATION

A. History

1. Radiation of pain or paresthesias—location and direction.
2. Progression of symptoms duration and rate.
3. Loss of functional (motor) and/or sensory function.
4. Relation of symptoms to position of the extremity or activities.
5. Past medical history: diabetes mellitus, thyroid disease, rheumatoid arthritis.
6. Social history: occupation, hobbies, hand dominance, tobacco and alcohol use.

B. Physical Examination

1. Detailed sensory testing within the median, ulnar, and radial nerve distributions.
2. Sensibility may be tested in two ways:

- Threshold testing—examines the ability of existing sensory fibers to detect a minimal level of light touch stimulation. This type of testing is most reliable for compression neuropathies.

  Semmes-Weinstein monofilament test—evaluates slowly adapting sensory fibers.

  Vibration—evaluates fast adapting sensory fibers.

- Density testing—through testing of the ability to discriminate two closely positioned stimuli, this test examines the topographic density or concentration of sensory fibers. This type of testing is most reliable for evaluating nerve lacerations and subsequent nerve regeneration; less reliable for compression neuropathies.

  Static 2-point discrimination—evaluates slowly adapting fibers.

  Moving 2-point discrimination—evaluates fast adapting fibers.

3. Detailed motor testing of individual muscle function, including strength testing.
4. Examination for atrophy (late sign).

C. Electrodiagnostic Testing

This type of testing includes a nerve conduction study (NCS) and needle electrode examination (eletromyogram or EMG).

1. Electrophysiologic examination of lower motor neurons.
2. Not a substitute for the physical examination, only an extension of the physical examination. Positive study is helpful to confirm clinical findings; a negative study does not rule out a compression neuropathy (i.e., approximately 6% of patients with carpal tunnel syndrome will have a normal NCS and EMG).
3. Determines location and provides an objective measure of the extent of the compression neuropathy.
4. Often suggests a pathophysiology.
5. Nerve conduction study:
   - Motor NCS: stimulating electrode is placed over nerve and recording electrode is placed over muscle to measure the compound muscle action potential (CMAP).
   - Sensory NCS: stimulating and recording electrodes are placed over sensory nerve to measure the sensory nerve action potential (SNAP).
   - CMAP and SNAP parameters measured include:

     Amplitude: height of the action potential; reflects the number of activated nerve-muscle fiber units.

     Duration: reflects the relative rates of impulse conduction.

     Area: represents a function of amplitude and duration.

     Latency: time (ms) from stimulation to onset of CMAP or SNAP (onset latency) or to negative peak of SNAP (peak latency).

     Conduction velocity: speed of nerve conduction (m/s).

     F wave: late response secondary to stimulation at a distal point; assesses the entire length of the nerve.
6. Needle electrode examination (NEE or EMG):
   - Records the motor unit potential (MUP).
   - Normal muscle will have the following features:

     Demonstrates full interference pattern on maximal effort.

     Many motor units are recruited with a full electrical pattern.

     Individual motor units are not definable.

     No abnormal spontaneous activity at rest; absent positive sharp waves.

     Occasional benign fasciculations.
   - Fibrillation potentials are action potentials of a single muscle fiber:

     Regarded as a sign of denervation (but may occasionally be seen in healthy muscle).

     If reproducible, they indicate lower motor neuron disease: anterior horn cell, nerve root, nerve plexus, and/or peripheral nerve.

     Seen with progressive muscular dystrophy or polymyositis.

     Not seen within the first 14 days after injury.

     Not seen at all with upper motor neuron disease.
   - Denervated muscle after 5 weeks demonstrates: increased irritability, spontaneous activity (numerous sharp positive waves and many fibrillation potentials), and full interference pattern.

D. Radiology

1. Generally of limited value, but sometimes used to rule out cervical rib, deformity, or tumor.
2. MRI is helpful if findings are due to a mass lesion.

III. COMPRESSION NEUROPATHIES OF THE MEDIAN NERVE

A. Possible Sites of Compression

1. Ligament of Struthers, between the supracondylar process of the distal humerus and the fascia of the superficial head of pronator teres (PT). Causes symptoms with the elbow in full flexion (between 120 and 135°).
2. Lacertus fibrosis, which crosses the median nerve at the elbow. Causes symptoms with flexion of the pronated forearm.
3. Within the PT muscle (due to muscle hypertrophy or aponeurotic fascia of the deep surface of the superficial humeral head or the superficial surface of the deep ulnar head of PT). Causes symptoms with resistance to pronation with a flexed wrist, in a position where the flexor digitorum superficialis (FDS) is relaxed.
4. At the arch of the FDS muscle as the nerve passes to the deep surface of the FDS within its fascia. Causes symptoms with resisted flexion of the FDS of the middle finger.
5. Carpal tunnel at the wrist level (carpal tunnel syndrome).

B. Pronator Syndrome

1. Proximal volar forearm pain.
2. Worse with activity and resisted forceful forearm pronation.
3. Predominantly sensory changes: altered sensation in the volar aspect of thenar eminence (palmar cutaneous branch of the median nerve) and the volar aspect of the radial 3-1/2 digits.
4. Signs are not limited to the deep volar compartment of the forearm:
   - Loss of active index finger DIP joint flexion secondary to flexor digitorum profundus (FDP) involvement.
   - Loss of thumb IP joint flexion secondary to flexor pollicis longus (FPL) involvement.
5. Operative treatment includes locating the supracondylar process (5 cm proximal to the medial epicondyle) of the humerus, which may be an accessory origin of the PT through the ligament of Struthers.
   - If the entrapment is here, the ligament is released and the supracondylar process is resected.
   - If the entrapment is more distal to the lacertus fibrosis and entrapment is noted with forearm pronation, divide the lacertus fibrosis.
   - The nerve is then traced distally as it dives into the mass of the PT. The two heads of the muscle at the distal insertion onto the midradius are dissected and the superficial head is reflected medially.

C. Anterior Interosseous Syndrome

1. Sites of potential compression include the fascial bands of the deep head of PT or the tendinous origin of FDS. Some cases may be due to a mononeuritis (Parsonage-Turner syndrome) and are not considered a true "compression neuropathy."
2. Deep proximal volar forearm pain that is worsened by exercise and relieved by rest.
3. Purely motor nerve entrapment (weakness/paralysis):
   - Weakness of thumb IP joint flexion (FPL weakness)
   - Weakness of index finger DIP joint flexion (index finger FDP weakness). The middle finger FDP has crossover innervation from the ulnar nerve with variable weakness of middle finger DIP joint flexion.
   - Pronator quadratus weakness.
4. Unusual pinch with hyperextension of the index finger DIP joint and thumb IP joint (inability of tip-to-tip pinch of the thumb and index finger tips).
5. Diagnosis is made clinically; confirmed by electrodiagnostic studies.
6. Treatment is indicated for failure of conservative management. The nerve is located at the elbow, traced distally and isolated medial to the brachial vessels. The lacertus fibrosis is divided at the pronator teres, preserving small nerve branches to the adjacent muscle bellies.

D. Carpal Tunnel Syndrome

1. Carpal tunnel syndrome is the most frequent upper extremity compression neuropathy.

2. Associated medical risk factors include diabetes, rheumatoid arthritis, hypothyroidism, obesity, pregnancy, and female gender. The most common cause, however, is idiopathic.
3. Repetitive use (e.g., prolonged typing) is simply an aggravating factor.
4. Components of the carpal tunnel include the following:
    - Roof of the carpal tunnel is formed by the transverse carpal ligament.
    - Floor is formed by the carpal bones.
    - Radial side is formed by the scaphoid tuberosity and trapezium.
    - Ulnar side is formed by the pisiform and the hook of the hamate.
    - Contents include the median nerve and 9 tendons (FDS $\times$ 4, FDP $\times$ 4, FPL)
5. Clinical findings include:
    - Female predominance.
    - Peak age incidence is 40–60 years.
    - Pain in the hand, fingers, or forearm that is worse at night and relieved with massage. Frequently, patients awaken at night with painful paresthesias.
    - Hypesthesia or paresthesia in the median nerve distribution (volar aspect of the radial 3-1/2 digits). The volar aspect of the thenar eminence has normal sensation since the site of compression is distal to the take-off of the palmar cutaneous branch from the main median nerve at the distal forearm level.
    - New-onset clumsiness/weakness in the hand.
    - Functional loss includes weakness of the lumbricals to the index and middle fingers, abductor pollicis brevis, opponens pollicis, and flexor pollicis brevis. The primary result is weakness of thumb abduction and opposition.
    - Thenar wasting and decreased sensibility are advanced signs.
6. Diagnostic ("provocative") tests:
    - Tinel's sign: paresthesias in the radial 3-1/2 digits produced by percussion of the median nerve at the carpal tunnel.
    - Phalen's sign: paresthesias in the radial 3-1/2 digits produced by wrist flexion (secondary compression of the median nerve).
    - Median nerve compression test: paresthesias in the radial 3-1/2 digits produced by forceful compression of the median nerve at the carpal tunnel.
    - Semmes-Weinstein monofilament testing of sensory threshold; carpal tunnel syndrome will produce decreased sensation on threshold testing.
    - Strength testing of thumb abduction. Strength testing of FPL and index finger FDP strength to rule out more proximal compression.
    - High false-positive and false-negative rates.
7. Conservative treatment involves activity modification, workstation evaluations, splinting the wrist in neutral or slightly extended position, oral NSAIDs, and injections of steroid and anesthetic mixture into the carpal tunnel:
    - Better for patients with symptoms <1 year and patients with no weakness, intermittent symptoms, normal 2-point discrimination, and <1 to 2 ms latency prolongation on NCS.
    - 80% have transient relief and 20% have relief for 12 months.
8. Indications for surgery include failure of medical therapy, persistence of hypesthesia, thenar atrophy, or the presence of a mass lesion:
    - In dividing the transverse carpal ligament, the surgeon must avoid injury to the palmar cutaneous and median motor branches of the median nerve. Thus, the incision should be just ulnar to the longitudinal axis of the ring finger in the palm and ulnar to the palmaris longus tendon insertion in the distal forearm.
    - Release may also be performed endoscopically ("Agee" and "Chow" techniques).
    - Postoperative NCS improves within 8–12 weeks. However, swelling of the palmar incision is expected for 12–16 weeks and full strength does not return until 6 months postop.

IV. COMPRESSION NEUROPATHIES OF THE ULNAR NERVE

A. Possible Sites of Compression

1. Cubital tunnel:
   - Arcade of Struthers—8 cm proximal to the medial epicondyle.
   - Medial intermuscular septum of the distal arm.
   - Medial head of the triceps muscle.
   - Arcuate ligament of Osborne (cubital tunnel retinaculum).
   - Aponeurosis between the humeral and ulnar heads of the flexor carpi ulnaris (FCU).
   - Anterior subluxation of the nerve at the medial epicondyle.
2. Guyon's canal (ulnar tunnel) at the wrist—ulnar tunnel syndrome.
3. Hook of the hamate (especially with fracture).
4. Compression may also be caused by osteophytes, ganglia, and lipomata.

B. Cubital Tunnel Syndrome

1. Compression of the ulnar nerve at the elbow. Specific sites of compression are listed above.
2. Clinical features:
   - Ulnar-sided forearm and wrist pain.
   - Paresthesias of the hypothenar eminence, ulnar 1/2 of the hand dorsum, and the volar aspect of the ulnar 1-1/2 digits.
   - Abnormal mobility of the ulnar nerve onto or over the medial epicondyle may be palpable.
   - Symptoms are aggravated by full elbow flexion with the forearm in supination (elbow flexion test).
   - Tinel's sign at the medial elbow (seen in 25% of normal people).
   - Weak "key pinch" due to weakness of the adductor pollicis and 1st dorsal interosseous muscles.
   - "Froment's sign"—hyperflexion of the thumb IP joint with hyperextension of the thumb MP joint on attempted tip pinch to compensate for weakness of the 1st dorsal interosseous, 2nd palmar interosseous, and adductor pollicis muscles.
   - "Wartenberg's sign"—abducted position of the small finger secondary to weak adduction of the small finger by the 3rd palmar interosseous.
   - Clawing is not noted with proximal compression of the ulnar nerve.
3. Nonoperative treatment includes NSAIDs and immobilization with an anterior elbow splint at 30° of flexion to avoid elbow flexion.
4. Operative decompression is indicated for patients who fail conservative therapy: persistent sensory disturbances, weakness, muscle atrophy, and objective evidence of moderate-severe nerve compression on NCS. Options for surgery include:
   - Simple decompression (cubital tunnel release).
   - Cubital tunnel release with medial epicondylectomy.
   - Anterior transposition of the ulnar nerve: subcutaneous, submuscular, or intramuscular.

C. Ulnar Tunnel Syndrome

1. Relatively less common compression within Guyon's canal.
2. Anatomic boundaries include the volar carpal ligament radially and the hamate ulnarly.
3. Etiologies:
   - Most common cause is a ganglion cyst arising from the triquetrohamate joint.
   - Thrombosis or aneurysm of the ulnar artery (e.g., hypothenar hammer syndrome secondary to repetitive trauma to the hypothenar eminence).
   - Synovial inflammation.
   - Anomalous muscles.
   - Direct trauma.
4. Clinical features are similar to cubital tunnel syndrome, although clear differences are noted:
   - Clawing of the ring and small fingers is often present in severe ulnar tunnel syndromes.
   - Sensation on the dorsal-ulnar aspect of the hand is normal because the ulnar dorsal

sensory branch to this area originates 5–8 cm proximal to the wrist.

- Negative elbow flexion test.

5. Operative treatment involves release of the volar carpal ligament (roof of Guyon's canal) and is often performed with concomitant carpal tunnel release. A specific release of the pisohamate ligament is also performed to relieve any possible pressure on the ulnar motor branch that passes beneath the pisohamate ligament.

V. COMPRESSION NEUROPATHIES OF THE RADIAL NERVE

A. "Radial Tunnel Syndrome"

1. Compression of the radial nerve from the radial head to the supinator muscle. Compression may involve the radial nerve proper proximally, the superficial radial nerve branch, or the posterior interosseous nerve (PIN) syndrome.
   - The superficial radial nerve supplies sensation to the dorsal-radial aspect of the distal forearm, wrist, hand, and extensor surfaces of the radial fingers.
   - The PIN supplies motor innervation to the digital extensor tendons (extensor digitorum communis, extensor indicis proprius, extensor digiti minimi, extensor pollicis longus, extensor pollicis brevis), wrist extensor tendons (extensor carpi radialis brevis, extensor carpi ulnaris), abductor pollicis longus, and supinator. The extensor carpi radialis longus is innervated proximal to the radial tunnel. The PIN also supplies deep sensation to the dorsal wrist capsule (no skin representation).
2. Potential sites of compression:
   - Fibrous bands anterior to the radiocapitellar joint.
   - Vascular leash of Henry—radial recurrent vessels that supply the extensor carpi radialis longus and brachioradialis muscles.
   - Tendinous proximal margin of the extensor carpi radialis brevis.
   - Arcade of Frohse—proximal edge of the superficial part of the supinator muscle (most common site of compression).
   - Fascial arcade at the distal lateral border of the supinator muscle.
3. Clinical features:
   - Aching in the forearm extensor-supinator muscles that worsens during the day.
   - Weakness of the digital extensor tendons (extensor digitorum communis, extensor indicis proprius, extensor digiti minimi, extensor pollicis longus, extensor pollicis brevis), wrist extensor tendons (extensor carpi radialis brevis, extensor carpi ulnaris), abductor pollicis longus, and supinator. The extensor carpi radialis longus is innervated proximal to the radial tunnel and is usually intact with normal strength.
   - May involve the superficial radial nerve and cause dysesthesias.
   - May be confused with lateral epicondylitis (local anesthetic blocks can differentiate these two).
   - "Middle finger test"—pain with resisted extension of the middle finger with the elbow in full extension.
   - Pain with full flexion of the elbow and supination of the forearm.
4. Nonoperative treatment includes rest and splinting of the extremity.
5. Operative treatment involves release of all possible sites of compression, including the arcade of Frohse and division/ligation of the vascular leash of Henry.

B. Wartenberg's Syndrome

1. Compression of the superficial radial nerve as it emerges from beneath the brachioradialis muscle in the forearm.
2. Clinical features:
   - Persistent pain on the dorsoradial aspect of the distal forearm radiating to the dorsum of the hands and digits.
   - Positive Tinel's sign within centimeters of the radial styloid and over the brachioradialis muscle.
3. Operative release of the superficial radial nerve is indicated for failure of medical therapy.

83

Tendon Transfers

Peter J. Taub, M.D.
New York Medical College and Westchester Medical Center, Valhalla, New York, U.S.A.
Neil F. Jones, M.D.
David Geffen School of Medicine at UCLA, Los Angeles, California, U.S.A.

I. INDICATIONS

A. Restoration of function of paralyzed muscles due to nerve injury (at the peripheral nerve, brachial plexus, or spinal cord level).

B. Restoration of function following tendon rupture or tendon injury.

C. Restoration of balance to a deformed hand.

II. GENERAL PRINCIPLES

A. Soft tissue and bony healing must be complete before considering a tendon transfer. All wounds should be fully healed with resolution of all inflammation (tissue equilibrium).

B. Full *passive* range of motion should be present in all joints to be moved by the transferred tendon.

C. Selection of appropriate donor muscle-tendon unit.

D. Power of the donor muscle is directly proportional to the cross-sectional area of a muscle and can be estimated by the following formula:

$$\text{Power} = 3.65\ \text{kg} \times \text{cross-sectional area}$$

E. Match the amplitude of the donor muscle to the desired function to be restored:

Muscle	Amplitude
Finger flexors	70 mm
Finger extensors	50 mm
Thumb flexor	50 mm
Wrist flexors and extensors	33 mm

F. Direction of the transfer should be in as direct a line of pull as possible.

G. The transferred tendon should perform only one function.

III. LOW MEDIAN NERVE PALSY

A. Defined as an injury to the median nerve distal to the innervation of the extrinsic finger flexors and wrist flexors. The extrinsic flexor tendons innervated by the more proximal portion of the median nerve include the flexor digitorum profundus (FDP) to the index and middle fingers, flexor digitorum superficialis (FDS) to the four fingers, and the flexor carpi radialis (FCR).

B. Motor deficits in a low median nerve palsy include loss of palmar abduction and pronation of the thumb:

- Lumbricals to the index and middle fingers.
- Opponens pollicis (OP).
- Abductor pollicis brevis (APB).
- Flexor pollicis brevis (FPB).

C. Sensory deficits include the palmar aspect of the thumb, index finger, middle finger, and radial half of the ring finger.

D. The four most commonly used tendon transfers to restore thumb opposition (opponensplasties) include:

- Burkhalter transfer: extensor indicis proprius (EIP) to APB transfer.
- Bunnell transfer: FDS of the ring finger to APB transfer.
- Camitz transfer: palmaris longus (PL) to APB transfer. This transfer is performed at the time of carpal tunnel release for low functional-demand patients with chronic compression of the median nerve and denervation of the thenar muscles.
- Huber transfer: abductor digiti minimi (ADM) to APB transfer. Primarily used for children with congenital absence or hypoplasia of the thenar muscles.

IV. HIGH MEDIAN NERVE PALSY

A. Injury to the median nerve proximal to the innervation of the extrinsic finger flexors (FDP to the index and middle fingers, and FDS to all four fingers) and the wrist flexor FCR.

B. Motor deficits include:

- Loss of interphalangeal joint flexion of the thumb—flexor pollicis longus (FPL).
- Loss of PIP and DIP joint flexion of the index and middle fingers (FDP and FDS).
- Loss of thumb opposition, as in a low median nerve palsy.

C. The standard tendon transfers include:

- Brachioradialis (BR) to FPL to restore thumb IP joint flexion.
- FDP of the index and middle fingers sutured to the FDP of the ring and small fingers to restore flexion of the index and middle fingers.
- EIP to APB for thumb opposition.

V. RADIAL NERVE PALSY

A. Motor deficits include:

- Inability to extend the wrist: extensor carpi radialis brevis (ECRB), extensor carpi radialis longus (ECRL), and extensor carpi ulnaris (ECU).
- Inability to extend the fingers: extensor digitorum communis (EDC), EIP, and extensor digitorum quinti (EDQ).
- Inability to extend and radially abduct the thumb: abductor pollicis longus (APL), extensor pollicis brevis (EPB), and extensor pollicis longus (EPL).

B. As a result of the inability to stabilize the wrist in extension, grip strength is decreased. The patient adapts by flexing the wrist to provide some limited extension of the digits through the tenodesis effect.

C. The standard transfer for restoring wrist extension is transfer of the pronator teres (PT) to the ECRB. This transfer is typically combined with one of the three transfers listed below to restore finger and thumb extension.

D. There are three possible transfers to restore finger and thumb extension:

- Jones transfer (FCU transfer):

  FCU to EDC transfer.

  PL to EPL transfer.

- Starr, Brand, and Tsuge transfers (FCR transfer):

  FCR to EDC transfer.

  PL to EPL transfer.

- Boyes transfer (superficialis or FDS transfer):

  FDS of the middle finger to EIP and EPL transfer.

  FDS of the ring finger to EDC of the middle, ring, and small fingers.

VI. LOW ULNAR NERVE PALSY

A. Injury to the ulnar nerve distal to innervation of the extrinsic finger flexors (FDP of the ring and small fingers) and ulnar wrist flexor (flexor carpi ulnaris, FCU).

B. Motor deficits include:

- Clawing of the ring and small fingers (lumbricals to the ring and small fingers).
- Loss of finger abduction and adduction (dorsal and palmar interosseous muscles).
- Loss of synchronous finger flexion: PIP and DIP joints flex before the MCP joints.
- Loss of thumb adduction and index finger abduction (1st dorsal interosseous and adductor pollicis), leading to weak key pinch.
- Abduction deformity of the small finger (3rd palmar interosseous muscle).

C. Claw deformity results from hyperextension of the MCP joint and flexion of the interphalangeal (IP) joints. This is due to an imbalance between unopposed extension of the finger MCP joint by the extrinsic EDC tendon and unopposed flexion of the PIP joint by the extrinsic FDS flexor.

D. Froment's sign is a compensation for weakness of adduction and key pinch strength. Instead of adduction and maintenance of the thumb IP joint in extension during forceful pinch, the thumb IP joint is flexed (FPL via the median nerve) to achieve the substituted equivalent of key pinch.

E. Wartenberg's sign is due to paralysis of the 3rd palmar interosseous muscle. The small finger adapts an abducted posture secondary to the unopposed action of the EDC and EDQ.

F. Sensation is absent on both the radial and ulnar aspects of the small finger and the ulnar half of the ring finger, but present over the ulnar half of the dorsum of the hand. The ulnar dorsal half of the hand is innervated by the ulnar dorsal sensory branch, which arises from the main ulnar nerve at the junction of the proximal two-thirds and distal one-third of the forearm. In most low ulnar nerve injuries, this branch is spared with preservation of sensation to the ulnar dorsal half of the hand.

G. Possible transfers to correct clawing include:

- Stiles-Bunnell transfer: FDS of the middle or ring finger (median nerve innervated) to the radial lateral bands (or A1 pulley or proximal phalanx) of the middle, ring, and small fingers.
- Brand I transfer: ECRB (extended with free tendon grafts) passed dorsally between the intermetacarpal spaces to the radial lateral bands of the middle, ring, and small fingers.
- Brand II transfer: ECRL (extended by free tendon grafts or fascia lata) passed palmarly through the carpal tunnel to the radial lateral bands of the middle, ring, and small fingers and the ulnar lateral band of the index finger.

H. Possible transfers to restore thumb adduction include:

- Bunnell transfer: FDS of the middle or ring finger to adductor pollicis.
- Smith transfer: ECRB (extended with a PL tendon graft) to adductor pollicis.

I. Possible transfers to restore index finger abduction include:

- Neviaser transfer: accessory APL (extended with a PL tendon graft) to the 1st dorsal interosseous tendon.

J. Possible transfer to restore small finger adduction:

- Extensor digitorum quinti (EDQ) to radial collateral ligament of the MCP joint or radial lateral band.

VII. HIGH ULNAR NERVE PALSY

A. Injury to the ulnar nerve proximal to innervation of the extrinsic finger flexors (FDP to the ring and small fingers) and the FCU wrist flexor.

B. Motor deficits include:

- Weakness or loss of DIP joint flexion in the ring and small fingers (FDP).
- Weakness of palmar flexion and ulnar deviation (FCU).
- All deficits of "low" ulnar nerve palsy, except that clawing is not usually seen

because the FDP tendons to the ring and small fingers are weak or paralyzed.

C. Sensory deficits are the same as in a low ulnar nerve palsy, but also include diminished sensation over the ulnar half of the hand dorsum (ulnar dorsal sensory branch).

D. Possible transfers include:

- Side-to-side tenorrhaphy of FDP of the middle finger (median nerve) to the FDP of the ring and small fingers.
- FDS of the middle finger to the FDP of the ring and small fingers.

84

Tumors of the Hand and Upper Extremity

Alidad Ghiassi, M.D., and Prosper Benhaim, M.D.
David Geffen School of Medicine at UCLA, Los Angeles, California, U.S.A.

I. INTRODUCTION

Tumors of the hand can be divided into benign vs malignant tumors and skin, soft tissue, and bony tumors.

A. Benign Lesions

1. Appear as expansive bony lesions on x-rays.
2. Well-encapsulated.
3. Without distant metastasis.
4. Without local recurrence following surgical resection.

B. Malignant Lesions

1. Rapid growth with local infiltration.
2. Atypical cellularity on histologic analysis.
3. Poor cell differentiation on histologic analysis.
4. Distant metastasis.
5. High local recurrence rate following surgical resection.

II. BENIGN SOFT TISSUE TUMORS

A. Ganglion Cyst

1. Ganglions are benign mucin-filled cysts associated with joint capsules, tendons, and tendon sheaths:
   - Most common soft tissue tumor of the hand.
   - Comprise 50–70% of all hand masses.
   - Most common in women between the second and fourth decades of life.
   - Can cause pain and weakness associated with activities.
   - Enlarge with activity and subside with rest—manifested as fluctuation in size of the cyst.
   - X-ray findings are unremarkable.
   - Dorsal wrist, volar wrist, volar flexor tendon sheath, and dorsal wrist occult ganglions account for 90% of these lesions.
   - Other locations include proximal interphalangeal (PIP) joints, extensor tendons, and Guyon's canal.
2. Nonoperative treatment:
   - Digital pressure.
   - Injection of hyaluronidase or steroid (e.g., betamethasone, triamcinolone).
   - Percutaneous needle aspiration and fenestration of the cyst wall.
   - Reassure the patient as to the benign nature of the cyst.
3. Operative treatment:
   - Indicated for persistent symptomatic masses.
   - Ganglion base (stalk) must be completely excised in addition to excision of the cyst itself.

- No need to close the joint capsule following surgical excision of the stalk of the cyst.

4. Complications:
   - Most common complication is cyst recurrence (approximately 8% of cases).
   - Stiffness of joints.
   - Nerve injury.
   - Infection.
   - Tender or hypertrophic scar.

B. Mucous Cyst

1. Mucous cysts are ganglions of the distal interphalangeal (DIP) joint.
2. Occur between middle and old age.
3. Presents as a 3–5 mm mass located adjacent to the extensor tendon.
4. Associated with Heberden's node formation and osteoarthritic changes of the distal or middle phalanges at the level of the DIP joint.
5. Treatment should include removal of the cyst and the underlying osteophyte.

C. Epidermal Inclusion Cyst (EIC)

1. EICs are caused by traumatic injection of epithelial cells into soft tissue or bone, where skin cells begin to produce keratin.
2. Painless swelling that develops over months or years.
3. The most common locations are the pulp of the middle finger and thumb.
4. Usually occurs between ages 20–40, although can develop at nearly any age.
5. Metacarpal involvement is rare (no reported cases).
6. Well circumscribed, firm, slightly mobile.
7. Treatment is marginal excision for soft tissue locations and curettage/bone grafting if located within a bone.
8. Recurrence is uncommon.
9. No malignant transformation has been reported.

D. Lipomas

1. Benign fat tumors located subcutaneously or intramuscularly.
2. Can cause nerve compression if present within the carpal tunnel or Guyon's canal.
3. Long-standing history with slow growth.
4. X-rays show lucent soft tissue shadow.
5. MRI demonstrates tissue signal consistent with fat.

E. Lipofibromatous Hamartomas

1. Benign tumors of the peripheral nerves.
2. Most common in the median nerve.
3. Slow-growing mass with symptoms of nerve compression.
4. Surgical exploration reveals fusiform swelling of the involved nerve without extension into perineural tissue.
5. Mass is intimately associated with the nerve.
6. Partial excision or intrafascicular dissection results in nerve dysfunction.
7. Nerve decompression is generally advocated.
8. Long-term follow-up shows progressive motor loss.

F. Giant Cell Tumor of Tendon Sheath (Pigmented Villonodular Synovitis)

1. Benign soft tissue tumors associated with tendons.
2. Second most common tumor observed in the hand.
3. More common on the volar surface of the fingers and hand.
4. Propensity for radial aspect of the thumb and DIP joints of the fingers.
5. Firm, nodular, and nontender.
6. May be associated with sensory deficit if compressing adjacent digital nerves.
7. May erode underlying bone by direct pressure.
8. Complete excision is recommended.
9. Reported recurrence rate of 5–50%.
10. Malignant transformation in the hand has not been reported.

G. Schwannoma (Neurilemoma)

1. Benign nerve tumor arising from Schwann cells.
2. Most common benign nerve tumor.

3. Well-circumscribed, eccentric, slow-growing, and painless mass.
4. Most commonly on the flexor surface of the forearm.
5. Palpation may produce pain in the involved nerve distribution.
6. Surgically, it can usually be "shelled out" from surrounding intact nerve fascicles.
7. Can be single or multiple.
8. Neurologic recovery can be full.
9. Recurrence is uncommon.

H. Neurofibroma

1. Benign nerve tumor arising from nerve fascicles.
2. Can be solitary or multiple.
3. More commonly associated with neurofibromatosis (von Recklinghausen's disease).
4. Symptoms are similar to schwannoma.
5. Fascicles enter and exit the lesion. Excision of the lesion requires transection of the nerve and subsequent repair vs. reconstruction of the nerve.
6. Motor and sensory loss is common.
7. Risk of malignant degeneration is present in patients with neurofibromatosis.

I. Granular Cell Tumor (Granular Cell Myoblastoma)

1. Extremely rare tumor of neural elements.
2. Painless mass.
3. Excision is curative.
4. Malignant variant has been reported and is very aggressive.

J. Digital Fibroma of Infancy

1. Benign but aggressive fibrous lesion of fingers and toes.
2. 80% arise before 1 year of age.
3. Small dome-shaped mass usually located over the interphalangeal joints.
4. Can lead to progressive joint contracture and angular deformity.
5. Wide excision with skin grafting is recommended.
6. Local recurrence rate can be as high as 60%.
7. No distant metastasis has been reported.

K. Glomus Tumor

1. Vascular and smooth muscle cell tumor arising from the arteriovenous glomus body.
2. Associated with severe pain, cold sensitivity, and tenderness.
3. Typically located in the subungual area.
4. Deep red to blue color with associated nailbed ridging.
5. Treatment requires removal of the nail plate and complete excision.
6. Recurrences are unusual.

L. Nodular Fasciitis

1. Uncommon reactive lesion that can simulate a scar.
2. Usually located along the volar surface of the forearm.
3. Typically characterized as a rapidly growing nodule that has been present for a short time.
4. Can be confused with fibrosarcoma on histology.
5. Marginal excision is required.
6. Recurrence after marginal excision is rare.

III. MALIGNANT SOFT TISSUE TUMORS

A. Epithelioid Sarcoma

1. Most common malignant soft tissue tumor of the forearm and hand.
2. Frequently misdiagnosed.
3. Often presents as a painless nodule that may ulcerate.
4. Metastasis is primarily to regional lymph nodes.
5. Wide excision, radical resection, or amputation is recommended.
6. Chemotherapy and external beam radiation should be considered for large lesions or lymph node involvement.

B. Keratoacanthoma

1. Malignant fibrohistiocytic tumor in sun-exposed areas.
2. Peak incidence in middle-aged patients.
3. Smooth, firm mass growing over 2–4 weeks.

4. Usually small but can reach a diameter of 2 cm or greater.
5. May be associated with ulceration.
6. Can be confused with squamous cell carcinoma.
7. Treatment is excision with modest margins of normal tissue.
8. Recurrence is common.

C. Basal Cell Carcinoma

1. Slow-growing tumors in sun-exposed areas.
2. Lesions have a pink to reddish discoloration with telangiectatic changes.
3. Ulceration and elevation of the border occurs.
4. Fair-skinned people with history of significant sun exposure are at high risk.
5. Treatment is resection with clear margins.
6. Reconstruction requires direct closure or skin grafting.

D. Synovial Sarcoma

1. High-grade soft tissue sarcoma arising in proximity to joints and tendons.
2. Most commonly occurs in the carpus and rarely in fingers.
3. Usually a small mass that is present for years with slow growth history.
4. Soft tissue calcification is present 20–30% of time.
5. 25% have lymph node metastases.
6. Size of lesion is a prognostic factor.

E. Liposarcoma

1. Rare malignant tumor of the hand.
2. Histologic subtypes have been described and have prognostic and clinical significance.
3. May resemble lipoma clinically but is usually painful and rapidly growing.
4. Treatment includes wide excision and possible radiation treatment.

F. Fibrosarcoma

1. Malignant soft tissue tumor of fibrous origin.
2. 30% are in the upper extremity with rare involvement of the hand.
3. Must distinguish from benign aggressive soft tissue tumors.
4. Treatment is wide excision with possible radiation and chemotherapy.

G. Dermatofibrosarcoma Protuberans

1. Low-grade malignant soft tissue tumor arising from the dermis.
2. Painless violet-red nodule that is present for several years.
3. May be associated with ulceration.
4. Treatment includes wide resection with possible external beam radiation.

H. Malignant Fibrous Histiocytoma

1. Rare fibrous tumor of the hand.
2. 20% are found in the upper extremity, with most of those located in the forearm.
3. May arise from both soft tissue and bone.
4. Wide excision is often required.
5. Adjuvant radiation therapy is needed to maximize local control.

I. Malignant Peripheral Nerve Sheath Tumor

1. Malignant soft tissue tumor of neural origin.
2. Includes neurosarcoma and malignant schwannoma.
3. 30% involve the upper extremity.
4. 50% are associated with von Recklinghausen's disease (neurofibromatosis).
5. May arise secondary to external radiation.
6. Wide excision or amputation is required.
7. 5-year survival is 40%, with poor prognosis in patients who also have associated neurofibromatosis.

J. Rhabdomyosarcoma

1. Malignant round cell tumor seen in childhood.
2. Uncommon in the hand.
3. Has poor prognosis.

4. Alveolar type is the most common variant in the hand.
5. Limb salvage with chemotherapy is recommended.

IV. BENIGN BONE TUMORS

A. Enchondroma

1. Benign cartilage lesion found within a bone.
2. Most common primary bone tumor in the hand.
3. Accounts for 90% of bone tumors of the hand.
4. 35% of all enchondromas arise in the hand.
5. Can be monostotic (in one bone) or polyostotic (in multiple bones).
6. Most common incidence is between 10 and 40 years.
7. Proximal phalanx is most common site, followed by metacarpal and middle phalanx.
8. Localized swelling or pathologic fracture are the most common presentations.
9. X-ray findings show lytic lobulated lesion with matrix calcification, cortical thinning, and intact periosteal rim.
10. Small lesions can be observed.
11. Large lesions require curettage and bone grafting.
12. Pathologic fractures may occur; these should be allowed to heal before proceeding with curettage and bone grafting.

B. Multiple Enchondromas (Ollier's Disease)

1. Uncommon nonhereditary lesions of cartilage origin.
2. Usually unilateral, painless masses that produce cosmetic and functional deformity.
3. The risk of malignant transformation into chondrosarcoma or osteosarcoma is 30%.
4. Growth following skeletal maturity and radiographic progression should raise suspicion of malignancy.
5. Patients should be followed closely for malignant transformation.

C. Osteochondroma

1. Osseous growth of a hyaline cartilage cap originating from the physis of the bone.
2. Uncommon in the hand.
3. Distal aspect of the proximal phalanx is the most common hand location.
4. May cause growth deformity.
5. Can be confused with subungual exostosis that has a fibrocartilage cap.
6. Lesions that produce progressive deformity and pain should be removed.
7. No malignant transformation has been reported in the hand.

D. Osteoid Osteoma

1. Benign bone lesion affecting the distal radius and hand.
2. 10% are in the hand and wrist—most commonly found in the carpus and proximal phalanx.
3. Characterized by a deep dull ache that is constant and relieved by NSAIDs.
4. Diagnosis is usually delayed.
5. X-rays demonstrate sclerosis surrounding a central radiolucency less than 1 cm in diameter.
6. Treatment is en bloc excision or curettage of the nidus.

E. Unicameral Bone Cyst

1. Rare simple cyst on the hand.
2. X-rays show lytic metaphyseal lesion with well-defined borders.
3. Treatment includes observation, curettage and bone grafting, or steroid injection.
4. Malignant transformation has not been reported.
5. May present with pathologic fractures.

F. Aneurysmal Bone Cyst

1. Benign aggressive vascular tumor of bone.
2. 3–5% are located in the hand.
3. Most common in ages 10–20 years.

4. Appears as an expansile lesion with cortical thinning on x-rays.
5. Treatment is curettage and bone grafting.
6. Up to 60% local recurrence rate following surgical treatment.

V. MALIGNANT BONE TUMORS

A. Osteogenic Sarcoma

1. Most common malignant primary bone tumor.
2. Rarely seen in the hand.
3. Rapidly growing painful mass.
4. Incisional biopsy followed by wide excision or amputation is advocated.
5. Neo-adjuvant chemotherapy is recommended.

B. Chondrosarcoma

1. Most common malignant primary tumor of the hand.
2. Most common after 60 years of age.
3. X-rays demonstrate stippled calcifications within the lesion.
4. Amputation, limb salvage, and possible chemotherapy are advocated.

85

Replantation

Janet Baker, M.D., Prosper Benhaim, M.D., and Roy A. Meals, M.D.
David Geffen School of Medicine at UCLA, Los Angeles, California, U.S.A.

I. ADVANCES IN MICROSURGERY

A. The first replantation was of an arm in a 12-year-old boy in 1962.

B. The first successful microsurgical digital replantation was in 1965.

C. Operating microscope—Acland 1980.

D. Ultrafine nonreactive sutures.

E. Precision microcaliber needles and instruments with fine tips.

F. Microsurgical technique/training.

II. DEFINITIONS

A. Replantation—reattachment of a completely amputated part.

B. Revascularization—reconstruction of an incomplete amputation that has resulted in devascularization of the involved digit or larger extremity part. Revascularization differs from other extensive nondevascularizing injuries (e.g., circular saw injuries with tendon and bone injury) in that a vascular repair is required to reestablish blood flow to the digit or extremity part in order to maintain tissue viability.

III. GOALS OF REPLANTATION AND REVASCULARIZATION

A. Functional outcome superior to a prosthesis.

B. Cosmetic appearance—appearance of a replanted part is usually better than that of an amputation or prosthesis.

C. Restoration of sensation.

D. Reduction of incidence of cold intolerance.

IV. PREOPERATIVE CONSIDERATIONS

A. Age of the patient.

B. Hand dominance.

C. Occupation.

D. General health, including comorbidities (e.g., coronary artery disease, diabetes, peripheral vascular disease, alcohol use, smoking).

E. Thorough assessment of other associated injuries, especially in patients sustaining multiple trauma.

F. Psychological stability of the patient to assess the ability to comply with postoperative care and rehabilitation protocols.

G. Level of amputation—best results are obtained with replantation of the thumb, hand at the wrist or distal forearm, and finger distal to the FDS insertion (zone I injuries).

H. Type of injury:

- Guillotine amputation—best prognosis overall.
- Crush injuries.

- Avulsion injuries.
- One specific type of avulsion injury is the "ring avulsion" that occurs when a ring on a finger is forcibly pulled off (e.g., entrapment of a ring onto a fence while a person jumps over the fence, causing avulsion of finger soft and/or bony tissues).
- Urbaniak classification of avulsion injury:

  Class I: Circulation adequate

  Class II: Circulation inadequate

  Class II A: Circulation inadequate (arterial injury only)

  Class III: Complete degloving or amputation
- Kay, Werntz, and Wolff classification of avulsion injury:

  Class I: Circulation adequate, with or without skeletal injury

  Class II: Circulation inadequate (arterial and venous), no skeletal injury: (a) only the arterial circulation is inadequate; (v) only the venous circulation is inadequate

  Class III: Circulation inadequate (arterial and venous), with fracture or joint injury: (a) only the arterial circulation is inadequate; (v) only the venous circulation is inadequate

  Class IV: Complete amputation
- Segmental injuries or multilevel injuries.

I. Ischemia time (warm ischemia time, cold ischemia time).

J. Expected chance of part survival.

K. Expected functional outcome.

L. Morbidity to the patient.

M. Total cost to the patient/third party.

V. INDICATIONS/CONTRAINDICATIONS FOR REPLANTATION

A. Indications

1. Thumb amputations.
2. Multiple digit amputations.
3. Partial hand amputations.
4. Any pediatric amputations.
5. Wrist/distal forearm amputations.
6. Single digit amputations distal to the insertion of the flexor digitorum superficialis tendon (Verdan zone I injuries).

B. Relative Contraindications

1. Severely crushed or mangled part.
2. Multiple amputation levels.
3. Comorbid conditions.
4. Atherosclerotic vessels.
5. Mentally unstable patients.
6. Single digit proximal to the insertion of the flexor digitorum superficialis tendon within the flexor tendon sheath (Verdan zone II injuries).
7. Excessively long ischemic time.

VI. ISCHEMIA TIME

A. The maximum ischemia time tolerated depends on the level of amputation and on cold vs. warm ischemia time.

B. Muscle tissue is particularly sensitive to ischemia, making proximal hand or forearm amputation levels much more susceptible to ischemia than distal digit amputations that contain no muscle.

C. In general, ischemia time ideally should be less than 6 h, although successful digital replantation with appropriate cold preservation has been reported >90 h after the original amputation. General guidelines for ischemia time include:

- Proximal amputation level, warm ischemia <6 h
- Proximal amputation level, cold ischemia <12 h
- Distal amputation level, warm ischemia <12 h
- Distal amputation level, cold ischemia <24 h

VII. PRESERVATION OF AMPUTATED PARTS

A. Wrap the amputated part in sterile gauze moistened with Ringer's lactate or normal saline.

B. Place the amputated part that has been wrapped in moistened gauze into a plastic bag, then on ice. It is critical that freezing of the amputated part be avoided. The amputated part should not be in direct contact with ice.

C. Rapid transportation of the amputated part and patient to a medical facility with a trained hand surgeon capable of replantation.

VIII. PREOPERATIVE SURGICAL MANAGEMENT

A. Initial Considerations

1. Decision to proceed with replantation or revascularization.
2. Rapid mobilization of operating room/staff/surgical team.
3. Transportation of patient/amputated part to the operating room.
4. X-rays of the amputated part and proximal amputation stump to assess the extent and pattern of the bone injury.
5. Perform all dissections under loupe or microscope magnification.

B. Handling of the Amputated Part

1. Irrigate and debride the amputated part thoroughly. Remove all foreign material, which is often deeply embedded into the soft tissues and bone.
2. Longitudinal, slightly dorsal midlateral incisions are used to expose the neurovascular structures, tendons, and bone.
3. Isolate and tag the nerves and vessels.
4. Maintain cold ischemia by cooling the amputated part, but avoid freezing any of the tissue.

C. Preparation of the Proximal Amputation Stump

1. Irrigate and debride thoroughly.
2. Longitudinal, slightly dorsal midlateral incisions are used to expose the neurovascular structures, tendons, and bone.
3. Dissect the digital nerves, arteries, and veins. Determine the extent and nature of the damage to the neurovascular structures.
4. In crush and avulsion injuries, long segments of the nerves and vessels may be injured. An injured vessel has a very high risk of postoperative thrombosis, no matter how excellent the anastomosis. It is far better to resect injured vessel segments and to reconstruct such vessels with interposition vein grafts as necessary.
5. If only a short segment of vessel has been injured, a minor degree of bone shortening may be included to facilitate primary repair of the vessels without tension.
6. Resection of injured nerve segments is less commonly required, but should be considered in conjunction with nerve grafts as necessary.
7. If veins are difficult to identify, the arterial anastomosis may be performed first with release of the vascular clamps to allow arterial inflow in order to dilate small veins.
8. Bone shortening (usually <1–2 cm) is routinely used to minimize tension on the nerve and vessel repairs. Excessive shortening is not advised. Vein grafts and nerve grafts should be liberally used to prevent excessive shortening of the bony skeleton.

IX. REPLANTATION

A. Sequence of Techniques

1. Thorough irrigation and debridement.
2. Identification, dissection, and tagging of nerves and vessels.
3. Bone shortening.
4. Rigid internal fixation of fractures.
5. Extensor tendon repair.
6. Flexor tendon repair.
7. Arterial repair.
8. Venous repair.
9. Nerve repair.
10. Wound closure with use of skin grafts as necessary.

B. Bone Shortening

1. Resection of sufficient bone to allow primary approximation of uninjured segments of arteries, veins, and nerves without tension.
2. Digits: 0.5–1 cm.

3. Proximal to hand: 2–4 cm.
4. Avulsion injuries: greater shortening required.

C. Bone Fixation

Rigid internal fixation is preferred to percutaneous K-wire fixation in order to facilitate early motion and to minimize risk of K-wire pin tract infections. Options for fixation include:

1. Single or multiple K-wires.
2. Double parallel K-wires.
3. Crossed K-wires.
4. Interosseous wires (e.g., 90-90 interosseous wiring).
5. Intramedullary rod.
6. Interfragmentary screw.
7. Miniplate/screws.
8. Nonunion rates with different types of bone fixation vary. The highest nonunion rate is seen with crossed K-wires only. An intermediate rate is noted with combined K-wire and interosseous wire techniques. The lowest rate is seen with a perpendicular 90-90 interosseous wiring technique.

D. Extensor Tendon Repair

1. Repair is typically performed with a 3-0 or 4-0 nonabsorbable suture. A core suture technique is commonly used (e.g., horizontal mattress, modified Kessler, or Tajima suture technique).
2. If injured, the lateral bands should also be repaired.

E. Flexor Tendon Repair

1. Repair is usually performed with a multistrand core suture technique (e.g., modified Kessler, Tajima) using a 4-0 nonabsorbable core suture supplemented with a 6-0 epitendinous suture.
2. In zone II injuries, controversy exists with regard to repair of the flexor digitorum superficialis tendon. Repair of both FDS and FDP tendons restores normal anatomy and has the theoretical advantage of better strength. The primary disadvantage of repairing both tendons is increased bulk, which may predispose the digit to postoperative scar formation and tendon adhesions. Many have advocated repair of the FDP tendon only, although there is no consensus on this point
3. Postoperative tendon adhesions are common and may require tenolysis.
4. If tendons are not repairable, a two-stage tendon reconstruction with a Hunter (silicone) rod may be necessary.

F. Arterial Repair

1. Apposition of normal intima to normal intima is critical. Resect injured intima as necessary. Vein graft if necessary.
2. The proximal vessel should have pulsatile blood flow. If not present, an unrecognized intimal injury may have occurred. In such cases, arterial reconstruction with a vein graft may be indicated.
3. In the thumb, the ulnar digital artery is usually larger than the radial digital artery.

G. Venous Repair

1. Finger and hand amputations are best drained through dorsal veins.
2. Venous repairs are often more difficult than arterial repairs, especially in the digits where dorsal veins can be quite small and thin-walled.
3. As with arterial repairs, liberal use of vein grafts is recommended as necessary to minimize tension or to reconstruct segmental defects.

H. Peripheral Nerve Repair

1. Epineurial repairs are performed for digital nerves, while group fascicular repairs are more commonly used for major nerve repairs (e.g., median, ulnar, or radial nerves).
2. Primary repair of nerves is preferred, even if a significant neurapraxia is suspected. Bone shortening may be helpful in reducing tension on the nerve repair.
3. Nerve grafting may be necessary if a segmental defect, severe crush injury, or avulsion is present. Avoid extreme positions (e.g., excessive finger flexion following repair of a digital nerve) simply to avoid the need for nerve grafting. If an extreme position is required, it is better to place a nerve graft.

I. Skin Closure

1. Closure of skin incisions and lacerations should be performed in a loose fashion to allow for postoperative edema. Tight wound closure predisposes the digit to vascular thrombosis.
2. Liberal use of skin grafts is recommended as necessary to minimize excessively tight wound closures.
3. Local flap coverage, if indicated.

X. DIGITAL REPLANTATION

A. Should repair at least one artery/two dorsal veins.

B. Repair two arteries/three veins if possible.

C. If adequate dorsal venous drainage is not possible, options include:

- Repair of volar veins. These veins are more delicate and smaller, making repair difficult.
- Arteriovenous anastomosis—anastomosis of the unrepaired distal digital artery to a dorsal vein proximally.
- Nail plate removal to allow venous oozing from the exposed nail bed. This technique requires anticoagulation with or without use of leeches. Because of anticoagulation, significant hemorrhage may occur and multiple blood transfusions may be necessary.

D. Venous congestion presents clinically with swelling, cyanosis/discoloration, and excessively rapid capillary refill. In such cases, leeches (*Hirudo medicinalis*) may be used to improve venous outflow. Leeches excrete hirudin, a potent local anticoagulant. Use of leeches has been associated with *Aeromonas hydrophila* infections, which can be prevented with third-generation cephalosporin prophylactic antibiotic coverage.

XI. MAJOR LIMB REPLANTATION

A. Extensive muscle debridement is often required, especially in crush or avulsion injuries. Severe crush injuries predispose the patient to myonecrosis and infection.

B. Rapid bony stabilization is indicated to minimize ischemia time.

C. In cases where ischemia time is long, a shunt may be placed rapidly to reperfuse the distal amputation segment. With the shunt in place, other structures may be repaired before formal arterial and venous repairs are performed. The primary disadvantage of a shunt is that it is associated with significant blood loss through oozing from a large raw wound surface.

D. Patients are susceptible to myoglobinuria from myonecrosis and subsequent renal failure. Prophylactic treatment with IV sodium bicarbonate to alkalinize the urine prior to venous anastomosis is indicated.

XII. REPLANTATION IN CHILDREN

A. Skeletal growth continues since growth plates remain open in most cases.

B. On average, 81% of normal length is achieved in a replanted digit or extremity.

C. Functional recovery is generally better than in adults.

D. Static 2-point discrimination of 5–7 mm is the average sensory reinnervation obtained.

E. Cosmetic result following replantation is generally better than that achieved in adults.

F. Survival of replanted digits decreases with:

- Crush/avulsion injuries
- Replantation of severe injuries
- Smaller vessels
- Increased vasospasm (pain/anxiety)

XIII. REVASCULARIZATION

A. Revascularization is technically complex and is commonly as challenging or even more challenging than a replantation procedure. The difficulty often arises from inability to shorten injured structures. Vessels are also frequently injured over a relatively long segment, often necessitating use of interpositional vein grafts for reconstruction of injured vessel segments.

B. Venous drainage may be sufficient if a significant skin bridge is maintained. In these cases, a venous repair may not be necessary.

C. Outcome is similar to that obtained following replantation.

XIV. POSTOPERATIVE CARE

A. The extremity should be elevated above the level of the heart to minimize postoperative edema.

B. Bed rest for the first several days following replantation.

C. Measures to minimize peripheral vasoconstriction include:

- Warm, quiet room
- No nicotine or caffeine (to prevent vasoconstriction)
- Adequate hydration to prevent dehydration and secondary peripheral vasoconstriction
- Adequate pain control to prevent sympathetic discharge

D. Anticoagulation (see Sec. XV details):

- All patients receive daily low-dose aspirin for at least 6 weeks postoperatively.
- Some hand surgeons prescribe a brief 3- to 5-day course of dextran, although consensus is lacking.
- Heparin is not routinely used, since the complications of excessive bleeding, hematoma formation, and thrombocytopenia outweigh the potential benefits in most patients. Heparin is primarily used in cases of vascular thrombosis, recognized problems with the quality of the vessels or anastomosis, and hypercoagulable states.

XV. ANTICOAGULATION

A. Considerations

1. Degree of crush/avulsion.
2. Appearance of vessels prior to and after anastomosis.
3. Use of vein grafts.

B. Goal

Decrease thrombus formation and increase patency rate of microvascular anastomoses.

C. Agents

1. Aspirin—antiplatelet effect.
2. Persantine—inhibits thromboxane A_2 and platelet aggregation.
3. Dextran 40—antiplatelet and heparin-like effects; inhibits normal fibrin formation.
4. Heparin—activates antithrombin III; inhibits platelet aggregation and fibrinogen clotting.
5. Low molecular weight heparins.

D. Dextran

1. Antiplatelet activity.
2. Decreases von Willebrand's factor and platelet adhesion.
3. Causes defective fibrin polymerization and increases lysability of clots.
4. Increases blood volume and blood flow.
5. Colloidal osmotic effect draws interstitial fluid into blood to expand plasma volume.
6. Increases microcirculation by decreasing sludging.
7. Some patients will have a severe allergic reaction to dextran. Prior to administration of dextran, all patients should receive Promit (dextran 1), which acts to bind dextran antibody. Any hemodynamic instability or other allergic reaction observed with Promit should preclude use of dextran.

E. Standard Heparin

1. Inhibition of thrombin and factor Xa are mediated through an antithrombin III effect.
2. Risks include:
   - Bleeding
   - Hematoma
   - Thrombocytopenia

F. Low Molecular Weight Heparin: Enoxaparin (Lovenox)

1. Is one of three low molecular weight heparin (LMWH) medications in current use: others include dalteparin (Fragmin) and tinzaparin (Innohep).
2. Inhibits Factor Xa:
   - Longer half-life
   - Decreased bleeding
3. Antithrombotic potency of low molecular weight heparin in microvascular surgery: influence of

dose and administration on potency rates of crushed arterial anastomoses:

- Topical irrigation of 45 IU is an effective antithrombotic
- Systemic alone—ineffective
- Topical and systemic—no better than topical alone

XVI. OUTCOMES FOLLOWING REPLANTATION

A. Survival rates of approximately 86%. Variables affecting survival include:

- Age
- Number of vessels anastomosed
- Surgeon's experience
- Severity of the initial injury (i.e., guillotine vs. avulsion or crush injury)

B. Cold intolerance:

- Poorly defined
- Cold intolerance is observed in more than 80% of patients following replantation
- Thought to be caused by vascular, neural, metabolic, and hormonal interactions
- Usually resolved or improved by 24 months

C. Factors affecting sensory reinnervation:

- Age—younger patients have a higher potential for sensory reinnervation
- Level of injury—more proximal injuries do worse than more distal injuries
- Mechanism of injury—guillotine vs. crush/avulsion
- Digital blood flow
- Cold intolerance
- Sensory reeducation at the cortical level (best in children younger than 2–4 years of age).

86

Tissue Coverage and Microvascular Reconstruction of the Upper Extremity

Julie A. Melchior, M.D.
Southern California Permanente Medical Group, Baldwin Park, California, U.S.A.

I. INTRODUCTION

A. Soft tissue coverage for appropriate hand injuries can be achieved in a number of ways: primary repair, healing by secondary intention, skin grafting, or flap coverage.

B. Flap coverage of a defect is indicated most often to reconstruct complex wounds with extensive tissue loss, when there are exposed vital structures (bone, tendon, nerve, or blood vessel) to which skin grafts would either fail to adhere or lead to significant scarring and decreased function.

C. Skin grafting has the advantages of relative ease of harvest and technique and wide availability of donor skin.

D. Flap coverage provides greater durability than skin grafts and minimizes contraction and fibrosis:

- A sliding or advancement type flap refers to transfer of skin from an adjacent area without torsion by stretching the skin.
- A transposition or rotation flap transports tissue to an adjacent area while twisting or rotating about a pivot point.

E. Distant pedicle flaps transfer tissue to a remote site by approximating the flap to the defect, on a tubed pedicle, or by microvascular anastomoses.

F. A microvascular free tissue transfer involves moving expendable donor tissue from one part of the body to another, by dividing the vascular pedicle:

- The tissue must be able to survive on a single-pedicled blood supply with an artery and a draining vein.
- The donor vessels of the transplanted part are anastomosed to recipient site vessels to reestablish blood flow.
- Free tissue transfer, compared with local, regional, and distant flaps, has the potential benefit of one-stage reconstruction that does not depend directly on traumatized tissues for blood supply.
- Many free flap donor sites are available throughout the body, allowing for customized selection of appropriate size and tissue characteristics.
- Free tissue transfer also offers the capability to reconstruct a composite defect (including bone, tendon, or nerve).

II. PRINCIPLES OF SOFT TISSUE COVERAGE: THE RECONSTRUCTIVE LADDER

A. Primary Closure

B. Healing by Secondary Intention

1. Wound is not sutured closed, but rather is allowed to develop granulation tissue with dressing changes performed 2–4 times per day.
2. The wound slowly contracts over time, often decreasing the size of a large wound to a relatively small scar.

C. Skin Grafts

1. Split thickness skin graft (STSG):
    - Contains epidermis and a portion of the dermis.
    - Higher survival ("take") rate than full-thickness skin grafts.
    - High degree of ultimate wound contraction, especially if meshed.
    - Most dorsal digital and hand wounds can be covered by a STSG.
2. Full thickness skin graft (FTSG):
    - Contains epidermis and the entire thickness of the dermis.
    - Better sensibility, more durable, and less contractile than STSG. Ideally suited for areas where minimal contracture is desirable (e.g., web spaces of the hands).
    - Palmar hand wounds without exposed underlying structures are usually covered by a FTSG.
3. Keys are secure immobilization and adequate hemostasis.

D. Local Flaps

1. Advancement flap.
2. Rotation (pivot) flap—designed as a semicircular flap.
3. Transposition flap—rectangular flap transposed into an adjacent defect.
4. Interpolation flap—transposition flap used to cover a nearby but not immediately adjacent defect. It is transposed over or under an intervening skin bridge.

E. Distant Flaps

1. Direct.
2. Tubed.
3. Microvascular.

F. Composite Flaps

1. Includes multiple tissue types.
2. May include bone/ tendon/ nerve/ joints.

G. Free Flaps

III. CONSIDERATIONS WHEN CHOOSING A FLAP

A. Size, type, and location of the defect.
B. Size and tissue type(s) of the donor tissue.
C. Vascular pedicle length of the flap.
D. Presence or absence of infection at the defect.
E. Requirements for sensibility.

IV. ADVANCEMENT FLAPS IN HAND SURGERY

A. Atasoy/Kleinert Single V-Y Advancement Flap

1. Single midline palmar flap with initial V-shaped incision that is then closed in a Y-shaped configuration after the flap tissue is advanced distally.
2. Primarily used for coverage of fingertip injuries.
3. Limited size of defect that can be covered (<1.5 cm defect).

B. Kutler Double V-Y Advancement Flaps

1. Two lateral V-Y flaps.
2. Used primarily for coverage of fingertip injuries.

C. Moberg/Snow Palmar Advancement Flap

1. Primarily indicated for coverage of distal thumb injuries.
2. Midlateral incisions are made with elevation of the flap just superficial to the flexor tendon sheath. Flap includes the radial and ulnar digital vessels and nerves.
3. Maximum distal advancement = 1–2 cm.
4. High incidence of interphalangeal joint flexion contracture is observed.

D. Thenar Flap

1. Two-stage random palmar flap used to cover fingertip defects.
2. Risk of PIP joint flexion contracture is significant.
3. Divide flap pedicle at 10–14 days.

V. TRANSPOSITION/ROTATION FLAPS IN HAND SURGERY

A. Z-Plasty

1. Each of two adjacent triangular flaps is transposed to the other's donor site.
2. Consists of three limbs of equal length arranged at 60° angles.
3. Changes the direction of a scar.
4. Length is increased along the central limb of the "Z" at the expense of decreasing width.
5. Four-flap Z-plasty is useful for deepening web spaces; especially useful for correction of adduction contractures of the first web space in the hand.

B. Flag Flap

1. Based on a branch of the 2nd or 3rd dorsal metacarpal artery.
2. Flap is usually located on the dorsum of the index or middle finger proximal phalanx.
3. Main advantage is wide arc of motion (e.g., useful for coverage of adjacent proximal phalanx defect, same finger volar proximal phalanx defect, or distal hand defect at the level of the metacarpal head/neck).

C. Lateral Finger Flap

1. Includes dorsal or lateral skin from the proximal or middle phalanx.
2. Covers traumatic defects of web spaces or the volar/lateral proximal phalanx.

D. Cross-Finger Flap

1. Two-stage transfer that uses dorsal skin from one finger to provide coverage of a defect (usually palmar) on an adjacent finger.
2. Reversed cross-finger flap is used for a dorsal defect on an adjacent finger.
3. Innervated cross-finger flap incorporates the dorsal branch of a digital nerve.
4. Divide the vascular pedicle at 2–3 weeks.

E. Neurovascular Island Flap

1. Transfers tissue from one digit to another on a digital neurovascular pedicle.
2. Wide variety of uses—most often for soft tissue coverage of the thumb or radial side of the index finger (areas that require innervation).
3. Donor sites—ulnar side of the middle or ring fingers.

F. Homodigital Island Flap

1. Originates and terminates on the same digit.
2. Reversed homodigital island flap is used when more advancement is needed.

G. Dorsal Interosseous (Intermetacarpal) Artery Flaps

1. Based on the first or second dorsal interosseous artery.
2. Raised on the dorsum of the middle phalanx of the index finger.
3. First dorsal metacarpal artery flap:
   - "Kite flap," "snuff box flap"
   - Able to restore sensation to the thumb
   - Usually able to reach tip of the thumb
4. Second dorsal metacarpal artery flap:
   - Can be raised as a single or bilobed flap, using the branching vessels of the web space
   - Allows for coverage of proximal defects of adjacent fingers and smaller defects on the dorsum of the hand or wrist
5. Must include the fascia into the pedicle to secure viability of the flap.
6. For dorsal digital defects between the MP and PIP joints, and for coverage of web space defects.
7. Can be reversed in its orientation.

VI. FILLET FLAP

1. Salvage flap of the vascularized soft tissue of an otherwise mutilated digit.
2. Excise phalanges and tendons.

3. Can be used to cover defects on the same digit or adjacent digits.

VII. FOREARM FLAPS

A. Radial Forearm Flap

1. Frequently utilized flap in the upper extremity.
2. Fasciocutaneous flap based on the radial artery, which is located between the brachioradialis and flexor carpi radialis.
3. Allen's test is performed to predict adequate perfusion of the hand after division of the radial artery (in up to 15% of hands, the ulnar artery does not perfuse the radial digits due to an incomplete palmar arch)
4. Versatile:
    - Based proximally to cover defects of the proximal forearm and elbow
    - Reversed (based distally to cover distal forearm, wrist, and dorsal hand defects)
    - Sensate (lateral antebrachial cutaneous nerve)
    - Free flap (thin pliable coverage for dorsum of the hand)
    - Composite flap (may include a segment of radius, lateral antebrachial cutaneous nerve, and/or palmaris longus tendon)
5. Possible disadvantages include donor defect, cold intolerance, transfer of hair, and reduction of forearm strength.

B. Ulnar Forearm Flap

1. Based on the ulnar artery.
2. Theoretical advantages over radial forearm flap include relative lack of hair, and postoperative immobilization not as critical.

C. Posterior Interosseous Artery (PIA) Flap

1. When based proximally, it can reach the elbow.
2. When based distally, it can reach the MP joints on the dorsum of the hand.
3. Technically difficult dissection due to small size and fragility of the PIA.

D. Pronator Quadratus Flap

1. Based on the anterior interosseous nerve/artery.
2. Useful to cover contents of the carpal tunnel.

VIII. ARM FLAPS

A. Lateral Arm Flap

1. Based on posterior radial collateral artery and veins.
2. Standard design can reach the acromion and posterior axilla.
3. Variations include fasciocutaneous free flap (for thicker coverage of a palmar or forearm defect), osteocutaneous free flap, and as a reversed pedicled flap for elbow coverage.
4. Disadvantages include hypesthesia in the distribution of the posterior cutaneous nerve of the arm (if it is divided or harvested when used as a free flap) and highly visible donor site scar.

B. Posterior Arm Flap

Based on a constant branch of the humeral artery.

C. Medial Arm Flap

Based on perforators from the superior, middle, and inferior ulnar collateral arteries.

IX. DISTANT PEDICLE FLAPS

A. Groin Flap

1. Axial flap that can provide a very large skin paddle (up to 10 cm wide; maximal length is from pubis to 5 cm lateral to the anterior superior iliac spine).
2. Supplied by the superficial circumflex iliac artery.
3. Preserve the lateral femoral cutaneous nerve.
4. Pedicle is divided 2–3 weeks after initial flap surgery.
5. Limited by dependent position of the hand during attachment with subsequent edema, prolonged immobilization leading to digit stiffness, hair growth, two-stage procedure, and hyperpigmentation.

B. Anterior Chest Wall Flap

1. On the anterolateral chest wall or infraclavicular region.
2. Based on intercostal vessels or the thoracoepigastric system.
3. Contralateral chest wall flap allows easier immobilization of the extremity with the elbow flexed.

C. Abdominal Wall Flap

1. Termed "epigastric flaps" when above the umbilicus and "abdominal flaps" when below.
2. Most abdominal flaps are inferiorly based random-pattern flaps or axial pattern flaps that are based on the superficial inferior epigastric artery.
3. Length varies from 5 to 18 cm and width from 2 to 7 cm.
4. Useful for coverage of large defects of the distal forearm or hand.

D. Pectoralis Major Flap

1. Based on thoracoacromial artery and perforators from the lateral thoracic artery.
2. Rarely used in the upper extremity.

E. Latissimus Dorsi Flap

1. Based on the thoracodorsal artery and vein.
2. Will reach beyond the olecranon or antecubital fossa.
3. Useful for soft tissue coverage of the shoulder/arm and for functional muscle transfer to restore elbow flexion/extension.

X. FREE MUSCLE FLAPS USED IN THE HAND

A. Rectus Abdominis Flap

1. Good coverage for an extensive circumferential defect.
2. Based on the deep inferior epigastric vessels.

B. Latissimus Dorsi Flap

1. Good coverage for very large defects (up to 25 × 35 cm).
2. Based on subscapular-thoracodorsal vessels.
3. Can be used as a functional motor muscle transfer if the thoracodorsal nerve is included in the transfer and coapted to a recipient motor nerve.

C. Serratus Anterior Flap

1. Based on the subscapular-thoracodorsal vessels.
2. Good coverage for large defects; may be used in conjunction with latissimus dorsi flap for massive defects.

D. Gracilis Flap

1. Can be used as functional muscle transfer, based on the anterior branch of the obturator nerve.
2. Pedicle—ascending branch of the medial femoral circumflex artery.

E. Dorsalis Pedis Flap

1. Based on the dorsalis pedis artery and first dorsal metatarsal artery.
2. Good coverage for dorsal hand defects; provides thin pliable skin.
3. Can be used as a composite transfer by including toe extensor tendons, metatarsal bone, and/or superficial or deep peroneal nerve branches.
4. Primary disadvantage is significant donor site morbidity and scar; poor choice in a patient with peripheral vascular disease.

F. Scapular Flap

1. Based on perforators from the circumflex scapular vessels.
2. Useful when thicker coverage is required.
3. May be used for a palmar or forearm defect.
4. A segment of scapula bone may also be included to make this an osteocutaneous flap when bone is also required for reconstruction.

XI. OSSEOUS FREE FLAPS IN THE HAND

A. Great Toe

1. Based on the first dorsal metatarsal artery.
2. Useful for thumb reconstruction of an amputation distal to the MP joint. Includes two phalanges and a large nail.
3. Greater grip strength than with a second toe transfer.
4. More significant donor site cosmetic defect than with a second toe transfer.

B. Great Toe Wraparound

1. Composite flap of skin, nail, and pulp tissue, with or without the distal phalanx of the great toe.
2. Used to reconstruct partial thumb (or digit) amputations.
3. More aesthetic than a whole great toe transfer; better size match.

C. Second Toe

1. Based on the first dorsal metatarsal artery.
2. Used to reconstruct more proximal thumb amputation levels and to reconstruct nonthumb digits.
3. Can incorporate the metatarsal-phalangeal joint.
4. Makes a triphalangeal, slender thumb.
5. Often utilized for reconstruction of congenital thumb defects.

D. Fibula

1. Based on the peroneal artery and associated venae comitantes.
2. Advantages:

   Length up to 26 cm.

   Excellent structural strength, due to thick cortex.

   Minimal donor site morbidity.
3. Disadvantages:

   Depending on the length of bone used, the vascular pedicle can be short.

   Necessary sacrifice of the peroneal artery (important in patients with lower extremity arterial insufficiency).

E. Iliac Crest

1. Based on the deep or superficial circumflex iliac system.
2. Advantages:

   Long vascular pedicle

   Able to include overlying muscle and skin with limited morbidity
3. Disadvantages:

   Limited amount of transferable bone

   Significant contour deformity at the donor site

   Risk of abdominal wall herniation

XII. OTHER FREE FLAPS

A. Temporoparietal Fascia Flap

1. Thinnest free flap.
2. Good coverage for dorsal hand defects.
3. Provides a suitable gliding surface for underlying tendons.
4. Requires skin graft over the fascial flap.
5. Advantages:
   - Relative predictability of pedicle (superficial temporal artery)
   - Concealed donor scar
6. Disadvantages:
   - Potential for injury to the frontal branch of the facial nerve during flap dissection
   - Scalp alopecia

B. Toe Pulp Neurosensory Flap

1. Used to reconstruct defects of the finger pulp.
2. Consists of glabrous skin and underlying pulp tissue from the great toe or second toe; includes toe digital nerve.
3. The moving two-point discrimination achieved ranges from 3 to 12 mm.

87

Congenital Anomalies

Matthew Klein, M.D., and James Chang, M.D.
Stanford University Medical Center, Stanford, California, U.S.A.

I. EMBRYOLOGY—UPPER LIMB DEVELOPMENT

A. The upper limb develops from the arm bud, which first appears at about 30 days gestation.

B. The limb bud elongates under the influence of the apical ectodermal ridge. Within the limb bud, proximal development occurs before distal structures.

C. Development of individual digits occurs between 5 and 8 weeks gestation.

II. EVALUATION

A. History

1. History of pregnancy.
2. Perinatal events.
3. Family history.
4. Associated anomalies.

B. Examination

1. General appearance.
2. Craniofacial or other syndromic physical deformities (e.g., Apert, Poland, and Holt Oram syndromes).
3. Examination of the feet, as similar deformities may occur in both upper and lower extremities.

C. Radiographic Examination

1. Bilateral radiographs of hands and/or arms.

III. CLASSIFICATION OF HAND ANOMALIES

Seven categories of hand anomalies are recognized (International Federation of Societies for Surgery of the Hand):

1. Failure of formation of parts
2. Failure of differentiation or separation of parts
3. Duplication
4. Overgrowth
5. Undergrowth
6. Congenital constriction
7. Generalized skeletal abnormalities

A. Failure of Formation of Parts

1. Transverse

a. Transverse failures produce congenital amputations:

- Transcarpal and forearm levels are the most common.
- Treatment usually consists of prosthesis or surgical reconstruction (e.g., toe-to-hand transfers) for more distal transverse failures.

2. Longitudinal (Phocomelia)

a. Longitudinal failure of formation results in absence of a portion of the limb with normal components distal to the deleted portion.

b. Phocomelia was common secondary to thalidomide use in the past.

c. Ulnar deficiency or ulnar club hand results from an absence or hypoplasia of the ulna, digital absence, carpal hypoplasia, and absence or hypoplasia of the humerus or shoulder girdle.

d. Radial club hand results from radial deficiency, thumb hypoplasia or absence, radial carpal hypoplasia or absence, and radial hypoplasia or absence. Surgical correction usually includes centralization or radialization of the carpus, followed by index finger pollicization.

e. Cleft hands usually result from absence of central metacarpal shafts.

B. Failure of Separation

1. Syndactyly

a. Failure of normal finger separation leads to syndactyly.

b. Syndactyly is the most common congenital hand deformity. Incidence is 7/10,000 live births.

c. Usually bilateral.

d. Males are affected more frequently than females.

e. Most frequently involves the third web space.

f. Simple syndactyly involves only soft tissue.

g. Complex syndactyly involves some bony fusion.

h. Acrosyndactyly involves fusion of the tips of the fingers.

i. Most commonly treated at 1 year of age—treatment consists of syndactyly release with use of dorsal flap in the web space, zig-zag flaps in the digits, and skin grafting if insufficient soft tissue coverage.

2. Synostoses

a. Failure of differentiation leads to synostoses.

b. Can occur transversely (between digits) or longitudinally between carpus and forearm bones or between radius and humerus.

c. Most often occurs bilaterally.

C. Duplication

1. Polydactyly is common and most frequently affects the 5th digit.

2. Classification:

    - Preaxial refers to the radial aspect of the hand, while postaxial refers to the ulnar aspect of the hand.
    - Type I—involves extra digit attached only by skin bridge.
    - Type II—extra digit contains normal components (e.g. tendons, bones, nerves).
    - Type III—extra digit articulates with an extra metacarpal.

3. Thumb duplication (radial polydactyly):

    - Wassel has classified thumb duplications into seven subtypes. Types 1–6 describe monophalangeal or biphalangeal thumbs, whereas type 7 describes a triphalangeal thumb:

        Type 1: partial duplication of distal phalanx

        Type 2: complete duplication of distal phalanx

        Type 3: complete duplication of distal phalanx + partial duplication of proximal phalanx

        Type 4: complete duplication of distal and proximal phalanges

        Type 5: complete duplication of distal/proximal phalanges + partial duplication of metacarpal

        Type 6: complete duplication of distal phalanx, proximal phalanx, and metacarpal

        Type 7: triphalangeal thumb

    - Wassel type 4 thumb, a single metacarpal articulating with two proximal phalanges, is the most common form of thumb duplication.
    - Correction is by deletion of the more radial digit. In cases where the radial collateral ligament inserts on the digit to be deleted, reconstruction is necessary. The original insertion can be detached from the proximal or distal phalanx with a sleeve of periosteum and joint capsule, which can then be resutured to the retained digit.

D. Overgrowth

1. Macrodactyly:

    - Congenital hamartomas enlarge and give

rise to an abnormally large digit (most frequently the index finger).

- In true macrodactyly, all structures in the digit are enlarged.
- Can be present at birth with subsequent proportional growth or can be normal at birth with subsequent irregular growth.

E. Undergrowth

1. Can affect the entire limb, the entire hand, all digits, or a single digit.
2. Treatment options include prosthesis, web-space deepening, digital reconstruction/transfer, or lengthening.
3. Blauth has classified hypoplasia of the thumb:
   - Grade I—minor hypoplasia with all elements present
   - Grade II—adduction contracture of first web space; laxity of the ulnar collateral ligament; hypoplasia of thenar muscles; normal articulation
   - Grade III—significant hypoplasia; rudimentary extrinsic tendons; skeletal hypoplasia
   - Grade IV—floating thumb ("pouce flottant"), a totally uncontrolled digit attached just proximal to the metacarpophalangeal joint of the index finger
   - Grade V—absent thumb
4. No treatment is required for grade I. Grades III–V are best treated with pollicization of the index finger.
5. Pollicization of the index finger or other radial fingers may be performed. Following division of the metacarpal and flexor/extensor tendons, the digit is rotated 140–160° into the correct position of the thumb. The first dorsal interosseous becomes the abductor pollicis brevis, the first palmar interosseous becomes the adductor pollicis, the extensor digitorum serves as the abductor pollicis longus, and the extensor indicis proprius becomes the extensor pollicis longus.

F. Congenital Constriction Bands

1. Most are presumed to be a result of amniotic bands.
2. Usually present with varying amounts of distal edema, neurologic impairment, and deformity.
3. Treatment is by band excision, usually of half the arm circumference, and Z-plasty to break up the band and to prevent recurrence.
4. Newborn may need emergent release if there is vascular compromise to the hand and limb.
5. Simple, shallow constriction with a viable hand can be released electively.

G. Generalized Skeletal Abnormalities

1. Defects in the hand may occur as a manifestation of a generalized skeletal defect, such as in achondroplasia or dyschondroplasia
2. Madelung's deformity results from disruption of normal growth of the ulnar and palmar portions of the distal radial physis with relative overgrowth and dorsal subluxation of the ulna.

88

Complex Regional Pain Syndrome: Reflex Sympathetic Dystrophy and Causalgia

L. Andrew Koman, M.D.
Wake-Forest University School of Medicine, Winston-Salem, North Carolina, U.S.A.

Reflex sympathetic dystrophy is the generic term given to a group of clinical entities characterized by an unusually prolonged and excessive pain response to an injury. Clinical features vary but typically consist of burning pain, functional impairment, dystrophic changes, and abnormal vasoconstrictive/vasodilatory responses. More recently, the term complex regional pain syndrome and its subclassifications have replaced other terminology to provide a more accurate description of the varied presentations and mechanisms involved in these syndromes.

I. INTRODUCTION

A. Complex Regional Pain Syndrome

1. Type 1—reflex sympathetic dystrophy:
   - Characterized by pain, functional impairment, autonomic dysfunction, and dystrophic changes
   - Without an identifiable nerve lesion
2. Type 2—causalgia:
   - Characterized by pain, functional impairment, autonomic dysfunction, and dystrophic changes
   - With an identifiable nerve lesion
3. Type 3—other pain dysfunction problems.
4. Dystrophic pain may be:
   - Sympathetically maintained
   - Sympathetically independent

B. Pain Dysfunction Syndrome (Dobyns)

This involves excessive pain with functional impairment.

1. Documented associated lesion:
   - Compression neuropathy
   - Neuroma
   - Vascular injury/insufficiency
   - Bony injury
   - Joint injury
   - Functional
2. Undocumented anatomic lesion ("reflex sympathetic dystrophy").

C. Reflex Sympathetic Dystrophy

This is a catchall term.

1. Represents a subgroup of complex regional pain syndrome.
2. Spectrum of dystrophic responses to trauma.

3. The term is used too loosely to be of clinical value.
4. Describes a variety of pain syndromes.
5. Over- and underdiagnosed as an entity.
6. Need objective criteria and improved definition(s).

II. HISTORICAL PERSPECTIVE

A. Silas Weir Mitchell

1. First described reflex sympathetic dystrophy during Civil War (1864).
2. Coined the term "causalgia" (Greek for "burning pain").

B. Sudek

1. "Inflammatory bone atrophy" (1900).
2. Described the fact that osteoporosis is associated with reflex sympathetic dystrophy.

C. Leriche

1. Recognized sympathetic nerve involvement (1916).

D. Spurling

1. Described thoracic sympathectomy as a treatment for reflex sympathetic dystrophy (1928).

E. Roberts

1. Described the difference between sympathetically maintained versus independent pain (1980s).

F. Clinical Subgroups and Syndromes

1. Major causalgia.
2. Minor causalgia.
3. Minor traumatic dystrophy.
4. Major traumatic dystrophy.
5. Shoulder-hand syndrome.
6. Sympathetic-maintained pain syndrome (SMPS).
7. Algodystrophy

III. PHYSIOLOGY OF PAIN

Pain is an unpleasant sensory and perceptual experience associated with actual or potential cellular damage. Painful (nociceptive) information can be:

A. Activated peripherally (transduction):
   - Mechanical
   - Thermal
   - Chemical
   - Ischemic events

B. Transmitted by small myelinated (A-delta) and small unmyelinated C afferent peripheral nerve fibers to the spinal cord, relayed through the dorsal root ganglion to the spinal cord (Fig. 1).

IV. NATURAL HISTORY

A. Observation

1. Departure from the orderly and predictable response of an extremity to surgical or traumatic insult.
2. Transient dystrophic response to injury or trauma is a normal phenomenon. Abnormal prolongation of this response and inability of the patient to modulate or control the pain cycle appears to be the best explanation of reflex sympathetic dystrophy.
3. May result in irreversible end-organ dysfunction, including loss of normal A-V shunt mechanism and permanent alterations in central neurologic responses.
4. Following wrist fracture, stiffness and poor finger function at 3 months correlates with morbidity at 10 years.

B. Clinical Characteristics

1. Pain:
   - Hyperpathia (increased pain at rest)
   - Allodynia (painful response to a nonpainful stimulus)
2. Stiffness.
3. Functional deficit.
4. Trophic changes (autonomic dysfunction).

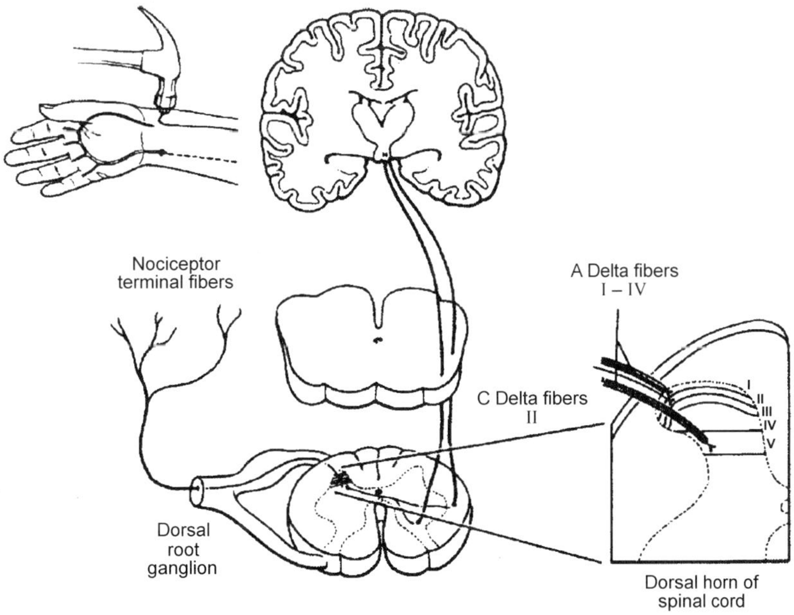

Figure 1 Abnormal central nervous system modulation of afferent sensory stimuli may contribute to the development of a dystrophic response after peripheral "trigger" (hammer striking superficial radial nerve). (From Koman LA and Poehling GG: Reflex sympathetic dystrophy. In: Gelberman RH (ed): *Operative Nerve Repair and Reconstruction*. Philadelphia. J.B. Lippincott Co., 1991, pp. 1497–1523.)

V. PATHOPHYSIOLOGY

Proposed mechanisms fall into two large groups:

A. Peripheral abnormalities.

B. Central neurologic dysfunction:

- Abnormalities of the "internuncial pool"
- Increased activity within the substantia gelatinosa
- Abnormal modulation of wide dynamic range neurons
- Abnormal modulation of afferent signals in higher cortical centers of the brain

C. True pathophysiology may be combination of peripheral and central mechanisms.

VI. CLINICAL PRESENTATIONS

A. Extremely variable in history, physical findings, and diagnostic work-up.

B. History almost always includes surgical or traumatic insult, although the original insult may have been very mild in severity.

C. Clinical diagnosis is made if three or more of the following are noted:

- Pain—intense or unduly prolonged
- Stiffness
- Delayed functional recovery
- Trophic changes often associated with autonomic dysfunction

D. Autonomic dysfunction:

- Vasomotor instability
- Pseudomotor abnormality
- Thermoregulatory changes
- Abnormal nutritional flow with aberrant A-V shunting

E. Presentation:

- After trauma — major or trivial
- Female > male
- Upper extremity and lower extremity
- Identifiable mechanical trigger or etiologic component (e.g., entrapped nerve) found in < 50% of patients

- Possible dependent affect as a personality feature
- Children and adolescents rarely develop reflex sympathetic dystrophy, but often have a severe form if present

F. Signs and symptoms:

- Pain
- Swelling
- Stiffness
- Skin discoloration

VII. DIAGNOSTIC TESTS

A. Plain x-rays:

- Osteoporosis with subchondral resorption (late)
- Up to 30% of patients have no x-ray abnormalities

B. Bone scan:

- Three-phase bone scan recommended
- Controversy:

  a) Kozin—abnormal bone scan in any phase correlates with reflex sympathetic dystrophy

  b) MacKinnon—only third phase (regular bone scan) correlates with reflex sympathetic dystrophy

	Kozin	MacKinnon	Werner
Bone scan specificity	75–85%	96%	92%
Bone scan sensitivity	< 60%	98%	50%

- Bone scan–"positive" dystrophy:

  Recognizable subgroup

  Unknown prognostic significance

  Heterogeneous subgroup without correlation to thermoregulatory (vasomotor) state

- No appropriate major criteria for RSD

C. Thermoregulatory and nutritional blood flow testing.

D. Pseudomotor function.

E. Endurance testing.

F. Diagnostic procedures:

- Stellate ganglion blockade
- Phentolamine test:

  Blocks alpha-adrenergic 1 and 2 receptors

  Relief suggests sympathetic-maintained pain syndrome (SMPS)

- Positive response (relief of symptoms) supports SMPS
- Negative response suggests alternative diagnosis or irreversible peripheral changes with or without central pain

VIII. CLASSIFICATION AND STAGING

A. Staging

1. First stage: 0–3 months, acute edema
2. Second stage: 3–12 months, dystrophic contracture
3. Third stage: > 12 months, atrophic stiffness, osteoporosis

B. Staging and grading are imprecise and can be altered by treatment.

IX. TREATMENT

A. Early Recognition of Possible Complex Regional Pain Syndrome

1. Abnormal postinjury course—"burning," "cutting," or "searing" pain.
2. 80% of those treated within one year of injury show subjective improvement; only 50% of those treated after one year improve.
3. Most effective aspect of treatment of reflex sympathetic dystrophy is early recognition—best results occur if diagnosis and active management are initiated before 6 months.
4. Poor prognosis is correlated with:
   - Initiation of treatment greater than 6 months after onset of symptoms
   - Persistent vasodilatation phase (prolonged A-V shunting)
   - Smoker

Table 1 Antidepressants

Drug	Mechanism of action	Dosage (range)	Common side effects				
			Anticholinergic effects	Seizures	Orthostatic hypotension	Conduction abnormalities	Sedation
Tricyclic antidepressants							
Imipramines (Tofranil®, SK-pramines®)	Blocks reuptake of amines: serotonin + + + + norepinephrine + +	50–75 mg (50–300 mg)	+ + +	+ + +	+ + + +	+ + + +	+ +
Amytriptylene (Elavil®, Endep®)	Blocks reuptake of amines: serotonin + + + + norepinephrine + +	25–75 mg (50–300 mg)	+ + + +	+ + +	+ + +	+ + + +	+ + + +
Doxepin (Sinequin®, Adapin®)	Blocks reuptake of amines: serotonin + + + norepinephrine + +	50–75 mg (50–300 mg)	+ + +	+ + +	+ +	+ +	+ + + +
Despiramines (Norpramine®, Petrofranc®)	Blocks reuptake of amines: serotonin + + + norepinephrine + + + +	50–75 mg (50–300 mg)	+ +	+ +	+ + +	+ + +	+ +
Nortriptyline (Aventyl®, Panelor®)	Blocks reuptake of amines: serotonin + + + norepinephrine + + +	25–50 mg (50–150 mg)	+ + +	+ +	+	+ + +	+ + +
Protriphtoline (Vivactil®)	Blocks reuptake of amines: serotonin + + + norepinephrine + + + +	10–20 mg (15–60 mg)	+ + +	+ +	+ +	+ + + +	+
Tetracyclic antidepressants							
Maprotiline (Ludiomil®)	Blocks reuptake of amines: serotonin + norepinephrine + +	50–75 mg (50–225 mg)	+ + +	+ + + +	+ +	+ + +	+ + +
Atypical antidepressants							
Trazodone (Desyrel®)	Blocks reuptake of amines: serotonin + + + norepinephrine +/−	50–150 mg (50–600 mg)	+	+ +	+ + +	+	+ + +

+ + + +, marked; + + +, moderate; + +, minimal; +, none.

Source: Department of Orthopaedic Surgery, Wake Forest University, Bowman Gray Orthopaedic Manual 1997, L.A. Koman ed. Orthopaedic Press, Winston-Salem, North Carolina

Table 2 Selective Serotonin Reuptake Antidepressants

Drug	Blocks presynaptic serotonin reuptake	Dosage	Common side effects
Fluvoxamine (Luvox®)	Moderate serotonin affinity	Start at 50 mg/day, increase to 100–300 mg/day	Headaches, nausea, sleep disorders
Fluoxetine (Prozac®)	Minimal serotonin affinity	20–80 mg/day	CNS: headache, sleep disorders, agitation GI: nausea Other: chills, weight loss
Paroxetine (Paxil®)	Pronounced serotonin affinity	Initial 20 mg/day Average 20–50 mg/day	CNS: asthenia, sleep disorders GI: nausea Other: male sexual dysfunction
Sertraline (Zoloft®)	Moderate serotonin affinity	Initial 50 mg/day Average 50–100 mg/day (titrate to effect)	CNS: agitation, sleep disorders, headache GI: nausea Other: male sexual dysfunction

Source: Department of Orthopaedic Surgery, Wake Forest University, Bowman Gray Orthopaedic Manual 1997, L.A. Koman ed. Orthopaedic Press, Winston-Salem, North Carolina.

B. Physical Modalities (Usually Combined with Oral Medications)

1. Hand therapy
   - Active and passive range of motion exercises (within limits of pain)
   - Splints
   - Contrast baths (alternating heat and cold)
   - Transcutaneous nerve stimulators
2. Stress loading (Watson)

C. Pharmacologic Intervention

1. Antidepressant medications (Tables 1,2)
2. Anticonvulsant medications (Table 3)
3. Membrane-stabilizing agents (Table 4)
4. Adrenergic agents (Table 5)
5. Others (Table 6)

D. Anesthesia

1. Pharmacologic blockade agents:
   - Guanethidine
   - Clonidine
   - Phentolamine
   - Cortisone sulfate
   - Reserpine
   - Bretylium
2. Pharmacologic blockade methods:
   - Stellate ganglion block—single or continuous (Fig. 2)
   - Axillary or brachial catheter (Fig. 3)
   - Cervical epidural
   - Intravenous

E. Surgical and Ablative Therapies

1. Sympathectomy:
   - Cervicothoracic
   - Periarterial
2. Neurolytic blockade:
   - Phenol
   - Alcohol
3. Implantable stimulators.
4. Neurosurgical:
   - Thalamic stimulators
   - Gray matter stimulators
   - Cingulotomy

F. Psychotropic Therapy

1. Counseling.
2. Biofeedback.
3. Adaptive therapy.

Table 3 Anticonvulsants

Drug	Starting dose, (maximum dose, mg)	Mechanism of action	Side effects: GI	Side effects: Hematologic	Side effects: CNS	Side effects: Other	Contraindications
Phenytoin (Dilantin®)	100 mg tid (up to 400 mg/day)	Membrane stabilization	Nausea Vomiting Constipation Hepatitis Liver damage	Thrombocytopenia Leukopenia Megaloblastic anemia	Nystagmus Ataxia Dizziness Convulsion	Rashes	Liver disease Pregnancy
Carbamazepine (Tegretol®)	100 mg bid (1200 mg/day)	Blocks Na^+ influx across cell membranes	Nausea Vomiting Jaundice Hepatocellular Cholestatic	Aplastic anemia Agranulocytosis Thrombocytopenia	Dizziness Drowsiness Ataxia	Rashes Epidermal neurolysis Congestive heart failure	Bone marrow depression Simultaneous MAO Inhibitors
Valproic acid/valproate (Depakene®)	250 qid (3000 mg/day)	Stimulates GABA production	Nausea Vomiting	Thrombocytopenia Anemias Clotting disorders	Sedation Tremor Hallucinations Headache	Hepatic failure Dysmenorrhea Pancreatitis	Liver disease Pregnancy
Gabapentin (Neurontin®)	600–800 tid (2400 mg/day)	Unknown; assumed to be GABA related	Anorexia Flatulence	Purpura	Somnolence Dizziness Ataxia	Fatigue Hypertension	Care must be taken with renal disease patients

CNS = Central nervous system; GI = gastrointestinal; tid = three times daily; bid = twice daily; NA = sodium; GABA = γ-aminobutyric acid.
Source: Department of Orthopaedic Surgery, Wake Forest University, Bowman Gray Orthopaedic Manual 1997, L.A. Koman ed. Orthopaedic Press, Winston-Salem, North Carolina.

Table 4 Comparative Characteristics of Intravenous and Oral Local Anesthetic Agents Used for Chronic Pain—Membrane Stabilizing Agents

Drug	Dosage	Side effects: Cardiovascular	Side effects: CNS	Side effects: Other	Contraindications
Lidocaine	3 mg/kg (Range 2–6 mg/kg) Note: test dose over 20–30 minutes	Bradycardia, hypotension	Dizziness, nervousness, apprehension, euphoria		
Mexiletine (Mexitil®)	10 mg/kg/day	Palpitations, chest pain, syncope	Dizziness, tremor, headache	Nausea, vomiting	Cardiogenic shock: second or third degree AV block (if no pacemaker)
Tocainide (Tonocard®)	20 mg/kg/day	Hypotension, ventricular arrhythmias	Dizziness; uncommon: encephalopathy and psychosis	Blood dyscrasias, pulmonary fibrosis, nausea, rashes	Second- or third-degree AV block in absence of pacemaker; heart failure

Source: Department of Orthopaedic Surgery, Wake Forest University, Bowman Gray Orthopaedic Manual 1997, L.A. Koman ed. Orthopaedic Press, Winston-Salem, North Carolina.

G. Prevention

1. Most effective treatment for reflex sympathetic dystrophy is prevention.
2. Avoid laceration or entrapment of nerves, known to produce severe pain and disability, which increases dystrophic response acutely.
3. The superficial radial and dorsal sensory branch of the ulnar nerve are most commonly involved.
4. A few moments spent identifying and avoiding at-risk nerves during surgery will significantly reduce the risk of development of postoperative reflex sympathetic dystrophy.
5. Postoperative discomfort "out of proportion" to traumatic insult, especially if manifested by "burning," restlessness, and difficulty sleeping, should be treated to interrupt the "dystrophic cycle."

H. Intervention After Control of Dystrophy

1. Neurolysis of compressed nerves.

Table 5 Adrenergic Agents

	Administration	Action/Mechanism	Side effects
Phentolamine (Regitine®)	IV infusion; 25–30 mg/100 mL saline in 20 minutes	Postsynaptic$_1$ Presynaptic$_2$	Hypotension, cardiac arrhythmias, weakness, nausea, dysrhythmias
Phenoxybenzamine (Dibenzyline®)	Oral: 5–120 mg/day	Postsynaptic$_1$ antagonist Presynaptic$_2$ antagonist$_1 \gg _2$	Orthostatic hypotension
Prazosin (Minipres®)	Oral: 1 mg once at bedtime up to tid	Postsynaptic$_1$ antagonist	Orthostatic hypotension
Terazosin (Hytrin®)	Oral: 1 mg qid	Postsynaptic$_1$ antagonist	Orthostatic hypotension
Clonidine (Catapres®)	Topical, intrathecal, or oral: 1 mg/h patch weekly 1 mg tid initally	Pre-synaptic$_2$ agonist	Dry mouth, drowsiness

IV = Intravenous; tid = three times daily; qid = four times daily.
Source: Department of Orthopaedic Surgery, Wake Forest University, Bowman Gray Orthopaedic Manual 1997, L.A. Koman ed. Orthopaedic Press, Winston-Salem, North Carolina.

Table 6 Injectable Medications

Drug	Methods of administration and usual dosage	Mechanism	Major short-term disadvantages or side effects	Contraindications
Guanethidine sulfate	IV regional up to 30 mg; usually must be repeated	Norepinephrine neuron blocking agent; stabilization of postsynaptic membrane	Orthostatic hypotension	Tricyclic antidepressants
Clonidine	Continuous epidural 10–40 mg/h	Diminishes regional sympathetic outflow by direct action at the spinal cord	Hypotension, transient sedation	Advanced renal insufficiency, AV block
Phentolamine (Regitine)	IV injection 5–15 mg	Alpha adrenergic blocker	Hypotension	
Cortisone sulfate	IV regional 100 mg	Anti-inflammatory		
Reserpine		Norepinephrine inhibitor	Orthostatic hypotension	
Bretylium	IV regional 100–200 mg	Norepinephrine blocking agent; depletion of norepinephrine from terminal vesicles		

Source: Koman LA, Ruch DS, Smith BP, Pollock FE, Poehling GG: Reflex sympathetic dystrophy after wrist surgery. In: Levin LS (ed): Problems in Plastic and Reconstructive Surgery. Philadelphia: J.B. Lippincott Co.

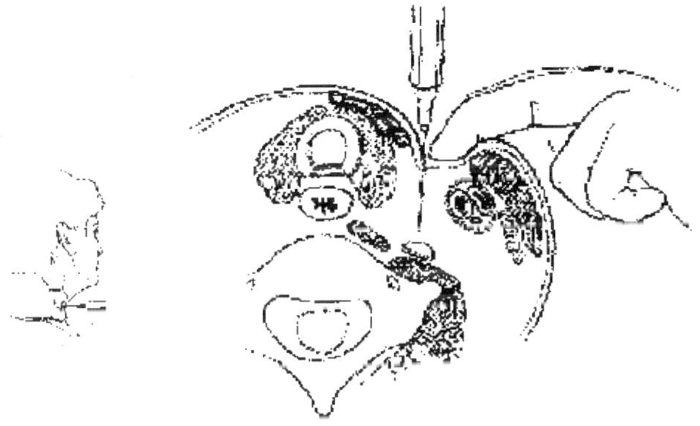

Figure 2 Technique for stellate ganglion block. (From Koman LA and Poehling GG: Reflex sympathetic dystrophy. In: Gelberman RH (ed): Operative Nerve Repair and Reconstruction. Philadelphia: JB Lippincott Co., 1991, pp. 1497–1523.)

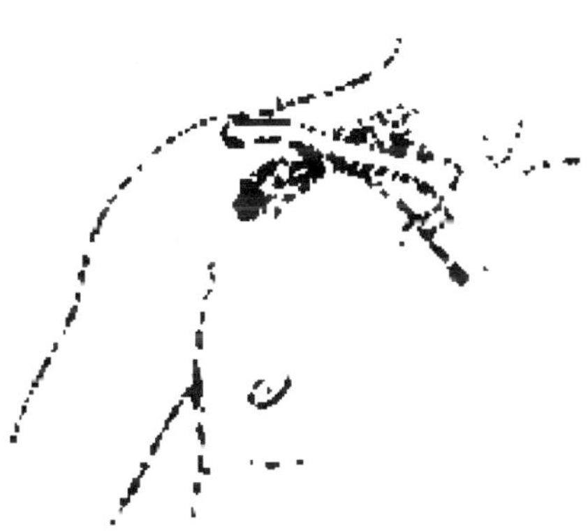

Figure 3 Technique for continuous axillary or subclavian block. (From Koman LA and Poehling GG. Reflex sympathetic dystrophy. In: Gelberman, R.H. (ed): Operative Nerve Repair and Reconstruction. Philadelphia: J.B. Lippincott Co., 1991, pp. 1497–1523.)

2. Release of contracted MP or PIP joints.
3. Prophylactic antidystrophic precautions.
4. Correction of a mechanical lesion.
5. Risk of exacerbating reflex sympathetic dystrophy.

X. SUMMARY

A. Complex pathologic entity characterized by persistent pain, functional deficit, trophic changes, and vasomotor abnormalities.

B. Treatment with a combination of therapeutic approaches aimed at decreasing sympathetic hyperactivity and improving nutritional microvascular blood flow.

C. The most important factor in the clinical approach to reflex sympathetic dystrophy is prompt recognition and aggressive management.

D. Treatment protocols should include:

- Sequential use of existing therapeutic modalities
- Delineation of primary cause, if possible, and its correction or alleviation, if possible
- Local surgical intervention, after control of dystrophic response, to correct primary or secondary mechanical problems (e.g., nerve entrapment)
- Surgical sympathectomy should be employed only if all other techniques have failed

89

Splinting and Immobilization

Renee Portenier, O.T.R., C.H.T.
UCLA Medical Plaza, Los Angeles, California, U.S.A.

Splinting plays a crucial role in the rehabilitation of patients with hand injuries or diseases. Although seemingly straightforward, decisions regarding splint type, splinting material, length of splinting, splint position, and active versus dynamic splinting are actually complex. The art of splinting and splint fabrication has been evolving with the advent of new materials, and, as yet, there is no universally accepted method of classification. Historically, there have been numerous proposed systems of splint classification. This chapter will limit its scope to a brief overview of the purposes of splinting, types of materials, common static splint, and the typical conditions for which they may be utilized. Dynamic splints for tendon injuries will also be reviewed briefly.

I. PURPOSES OF SPLINT APPLICATION

A. Prevent or limit deformity.

B. Support.

C. Protection.

D. Immobilize joints.

E. Mobilize tissue while supporting or immobilizing adjoining tissues.

F. Correct existing deformity.

G. Control for coordination problem.

H. Control or modify scar formation.

II. REASONS FOR STATIC SPLINTING

A. Immobilization:

- Decrease inflammation
- Promote vascularization of skin or bone graft

B. Protection:

- Of healing bone
- Of newly repaired tissues, i.e., tendons, nerves, and ligaments

C. Aid in remolding scar via pressure or stress application to help elongate or shorten tissue.

D. Support or provide mechanical advantage to painful, deformed, and arthritic joints.

III. TYPES OF SPLINTING MATERIAL

A. Prefabricated: can be made from foam and wire, canvas, neoprene or metal.

B. Customized low-temperature thermoplastic materials:

- Thickness ranging from 1/16, 3/32, or 1/8 inch
- Material that softens and becomes moldable at approximately 110–165°F

C. Customized high-temperature materials:

- Typically need to make a cast and a mold
- Material fired at approximately 350°F

D. Cast: made from plaster or fiberglass material.

IV. TYPES OF STATIC SPLINTS

The following is a list of typically used static splints, various names associated with the type of splint (if more than one), diagnoses associated with that type of splint, and the joints and/or motions that are immobilized or limited.

A. Posterior Elbow Splint

1. Limits elbow flexion/extension and forearm pronation/supination.
2. Primary indications for use: biceps brachii tendon repair, cubital tunnel syndrome, and olecranon fracture if casting is not the best option.

B. Anterior Elbow Splint

1. Limits elbow extension and forearm rotation. Blocks elbow flexion.
2. Primary indication for use: cubital tunnel syndrome.
3. Used for static progressive splinting to improve an elbow flexion contracture.

C. Wrist Cock-Up Splint

1. Immobilizes the wrist but allows finger flexion/extension. The thumb is free to move at the MP and IP joints but has limited first CMC joint motion and may not allow full flexion of the small finger MP joint.
2. Primary indications for use: wrist tendonitis, carpal tunnel syndrome, status post–carpal tunnel release, after removal of cast for distal radius fracture for prolonged protection, and unstable wrist due to arthritis.

D. Ulnar Gutter Splint

1. Immobilizes the ring and small fingers.
2. Primary indications for use: fractures of the ring or small finger metacarpals and proximal phalanges; extensor tendon repairs in the ring or small fingers.

E. MP/Wrist Extension Splint

1. Prevents wrist and finger flexion/extension. The splint can be modified to allow partial IP joint flexion.
2. Primary indication for use: extensor tendon repair.

F. Dorsal Blocking Splint

1. Blocks wrist and MP joint extension; IP joints can be strapped into extension.
2. Primary indications for use: flexor tendon repair; nerve or artery repair.

G. C-Bar/Web Space Splint

1. Blocks the first CMC joint motion and maintains first web space width to prevent a thumb adduction contracture. To gain good mechanical advantage, the splint usually extends to the thumb IP joint or to the full length of the thumb; it may also extend to the PIP joint or tip of the index finger.
2. Primary indications for use: median nerve palsy; burn or skin graft in the first web space; status post–index finger pollicization; adduction contractures associated with thumb CMC joint arthritis.

H. MP Flexion Splint

1. Blocks extension of the MP joint and holds the PIP joint in extension. Can allow flexion of fingers. Can be hand based or can extend proximally beyond the wrist.
2. Primary indication for use: Boxer's fracture, metacarpal fractures.

I. Lumbrical Block Splint

1. Dorsally holds the MP joint in flexion and extends to the PIP joint. Allows flexion of fingers.
2. Primary indication for use: ulnar nerve palsy (to prevent clawing of the small and ring fingers).

J. Resting Pan Splint

1. Functional position vs. protective position

K. Position of Safety (Lumbrical Plus) Splint

1. Position of safety: MP joint flexion at 70° with full PIP and DIP joint extension. This position protects against capsular contractures, which occur when MP joints are extended and when PIP/DIP joints are flexed. The lumbrical muscles produce MP flexion and PIP/DIP extension—the "lumbrical plus" position.
2. Primary indications for use: arthritis, burns, metacarpal fractures, coma.

L. Finger Gutter Splint

1. Immobilizes the PIP and DIP joints in a single digit.
2. Primary indication for use: middle and distal phalanx fractures.

M. Finger Dorsal Block Splint

1. Blocks PIP joint extension; can allow PIP flexion or can be strapped to block flexion.
2. Primary indications for use: PIP joint dislocation, volar plate injury.

N. Mallet Finger Splint (Stack Splint)

1. Immobilizes DIP joint in full extension.
2. Primary indications for use: mallet finger deformity, distal phalanx fracture.

O. Hand-Based Volar or Dorsal Splint

1. Holds MP, PIP, and DIP joints in extension.
2. Primary indication for use: status post-Dupuytren's contracture release.

P. Thumb Spica Splint

1. Wrist immobilized and thumb MP joint immobilized in abduction. The IP joint may be left free or added in immobilization if necessary.
2. Primary indications for use: scaphoid fracture, tendon repairs (extensor pollicis brevis, extensor pollicis longus, and/or abductor pollicis longus).

Q. Long Opponens Splint

1. Wrist and thumb MP joint immobilized with inclusion of the thumb IP joint upon request. The thumb is positioned in palmar abduction.
2. Primary indications for use: de Quervain's tenosynovitis, scaphoid fracture.

R. Short Opponens Splint

1. Immobilizes the thumb CMC and MP joints.
2. Primary indication for use: first CMC joint arthritis, gamekeeper's thumb, MP joint sprain.

V. DYNAMIC SPLINTING FOR FLEXOR TENDON INJURIES

A. Postoperative therapy following repair of flexor tendon lacerations must balance the need for immobilization to ensure proper healing of the tendon repair against the need for early motion to minimize scar formation that results in tendon adhesions.

B. In addition, numerous studies have shown that a loaded tendon will heal more rapidly and with greater tensile strength following surgical repair.

C. Within this context, Kleinert (and later modified by Chow) developed a dynamic splinting technique that incorporates a dorsal blocking splint to prevent full extension of the finger MP joints while allowing full extension of the PIP and DIP joints. A rubber band is attached to the fingernail, threaded through a palmar pulley, and attached proximally to a splint at the level of the midportion of the volar forearm. A small degree of tension is applied to the rubber band. The concept is to allow the patient to actively extend the fingers using the intact extensor tendons, while allowing the rubber band to passively flex the finger. In this fashion, the tendon is allowed to glide without active flexion of the repaired flexor tendon, thereby minimizing the risk of tendon rupture. Motion with this type of splinting is initiated within the first 2 days following surgery.

90

Anatomy of the Lower Extremity

Eric E. Arcilla, M.D., Andrew Da Lio, M.D., and William W. Shaw, M.D.
David Geffen School of Medicine at UCLA, Los Angeles, California, U.S.A.

I. EMBRYOLOGY

A. 4th week of gestation: limb buds appear at the ventrolateral aspect of cylindrical body.

B. 5th week of gestation: limbs show regional identity with formation at the beginning of the 6th week of gestation; rudiments of toes can be recognized; development of big toe.

C. 8th week of gestation: digits are separated from one another by cell death at the web spaces.

D. 3rd gestational month: limb is well developed; appearance of nails on the toes.

II. BONES AND BONY LANDMARKS

A. Thigh (Femur)

1. Head:
   - Articulates with the acetabulum of the pelvis
2. Neck:
   - Approximately 5 cm long
   - Connected to the shaft at an angle
3. Greater trochanter:
   - Palpable at the upper lateral aspect of the femur
   - Formed where the upper margin of the neck meets the shaft
   - Serves as attachment for several muscles, notably the gluteus maximus
4. Linea aspera:
   - A longitudinal ridge at the posterior aspect of the shaft
   - In conjunction with the intermuscular septum, serves as an insertion for several muscles
5. Medial and lateral condyles:
   - Distal expansions of the shaft

B. Knee

1. Patella:
   - Triangular-shaped sesamoid bone of the knee encased in the quadriceps tendon
   - Patellar tendon or ligament extends from the apex of the patella to the tibial tuberosity
   - Posterior surface is smooth and articulates with the femoral condyles
   - Functions to protect the knee and prevents chaffing of the quadriceps tendon

C. Leg

1. Tibia:
   - Medial bone of the leg
   - Proximally, has concave medial and lateral condyles that form the tibial plateau for articulation with the femoral condyles

- Tibial tuberosity is found between the condyles anteriorly and serves as insertion of the patellar tendon
- The shaft is mostly subcutaneous medially
- Distally, forms the medial malleolus, the tibial contribution to the talocrural/ankle joint

2. Fibula:
   - Lateral bone of the leg
   - Head of fibula is subcutaneous and palpable superolaterally
   - The common peroneal nerve passes posterior to the fibular head and turns anteriorly across the neck of the fibula
   - Has a thin slender shaft that ends in an elongated prominence (the lateral malleolus), which is the fibular component of the talocrural/ankle joint

D. Foot

1. Tarsal bones (7):
   - Talus—forms the ankle joint with the tibia superiorly and the malleoli laterally and medially
   - Calcaneus—largest tarsal bone; makes up the heel; has a ridge posteriorly for insertion of the Achilles tendon
   - Navicular (scaphoid) bone—located medially, anterior to the talus and posterior to the cuneiforms
   - 3 cuneiforms—medial, intermediate, and lateral; form the distal tarsal row
   - Cuboid—located lateral to the cuneiform bones
2. Metatarsals (5):
   - Metatarsal heads correspond to the ball of the foot
3. Phalanges:
   - 2 phalangeal bones for the great toe
   - 3 phalangeal bones for each of the 2nd to 5th toes

III. JOINTS

A. Knee Joint

1. Composed of two hinge joints:
   - Femoro-patellar joint
   - Femoro-tibial joint—has two articular cartilages: the O-shaped lateral meniscus and the C-shaped medial meniscus
2. Four important external ligaments:
   - Patellar retinaculum—extends medially and laterally to the tibial condyles
   - Lateral (fibular) collateral ligament—from lateral femoral epicondyle to the fibular head; prevents adduction of the leg at the knee
   - Medial (tibial) collateral ligament—from medial femoral epicondyle to the tibial shaft; prevents abduction of the leg at the knee
   - Oblique popliteal ligament—located posteriorly; prevents knee hyperextension
3. Two important internal ligaments:
   - Posterior cruciate ligament—prevents anterior displacement of the femur over the tibia. A torn posterior cruciate ligament elicits a posterior drawer sign (posterior displacement of the tibia)
   - Anterior cruciate ligament—prevents posterior displacement of the femur over the tibia. A torn anterior cruciate elicits an anterior drawer sign (anterior displacement of the tibia)

B. Talo-Crural (Ankle) Joint

1. A hinge joint
2. Formed by the superior articular surface of the talus, which fits into a mortise composed of the tibia, lateral malleolus, and medial malleolus
3. Supporting ligaments:
   - Lateral collateral ligament
   - Medial collateral ligament

IV. FASCIA AND COMPARTMENTS

The lower limb has two primary fascial layers: the superficial and the deep. The deep fascia has invaginations called intermuscular septa that divide the thigh, leg, and foot into compartments. These fascia and septa further serve as muscular attachments, either as origins or insertions.

A. Superficial Fascia

1. In the thigh and leg, the superficial fascia is mainly made up of loose areolar tissue that contains cutaneous nerves and superficial vessels.
2. The superficial fascia of the foot dorsum is loose and thin, while that of the plantar aspect is thickened to provide a tough and durable padding for weight bearing.

B. Deep Fascia

1. Fascia lata:
   - Deep fascia of the thigh
   - Thickened laterally, forming the iliotibial band
   - Divides the thigh into an anterior and posterior compartment through the lateral and medial intermuscular septa
2. Crural fascia
   - Deep fascia of the leg
   - Encircles the leg and blends with the periosteum of the tibia anteromedially
   - Gives rise to the anterior and posterior intermuscular septum, as well as the deep transverse fascia. These divide the leg into anterior, lateral, deep posterior and superficial posterior compartments. The interosseous membrane between the tibia and fibula further separates the anterior compartment from the deep posterior compartment.
3. Plantar aponeurosis:
   - Central portion of the deep fascia of the plantar aspect of the foot
   - Plays a crucial role in the movement of the skin and fat pad of the sole during the gait cycle
   - Gives rise to a medial and lateral intermuscular septum to divide the foot into three compartments: lateral, intermediate, and medial
   - Transverse septae further divide the foot musculature into four layers

V. MUSCULATURE (DISCUSSED AS FLAP USAGE)

A. Thigh

1. Anterior compartment (Table 1):
   - All but one of the anterior compartment muscles are supplied by the femoral nerve (L2–L4)
   - The exception is the tensor fascia lata, which is innervated by the superior gluteal nerve
2. Posterior compartment (Table 2):
   - The hamstring muscles and the ischial portion of the adductor magnus are innervated by the tibial division (L4–S3) of the sciatic nerve

Table 1 Anterior Compartment of Thigh

Muscle	Origin	Insertion	Blood supply/flap type
Rectus femoris	Anterior-inferior iliac spine	Patella	Lateral femoral circumflex artery (Type II)
Vastus lateralis	Posterior proximal femur to lateral lip of linea aspera	Patella	Lateral femoral circumflex artery (Type I)
Vastus medialis	Posterior proximal femur to medial lip of linea aspera	Patella	Lateral femoral circumflex artery (Type II)
Vastus intermedius	Anterior and lateral surface of upper 1/3 of femur and lower lateral intermuscular septum	Patella	Lateral femoral circumflex artery and branches of profunda femoris artery
Sartorius	Anterior superior iliac spine	Medial tibial condyle	Branches from superficial femoral artery (Type IV)
Tensor fascia lata	Anterior lateral iliac crest and anterior superior iliac spine	Iliotibial tract	Lateral femoral circumflex artery (Type I)

Table 2 Posterior Compartment of Thigh

Muscle	Origin	Insertion	Blood supply/flap type
Semitendinosus	Ischial tuberosity	Below medial tibial condyle	1st perforator of profunda femoris artery (Type II)
Semimembranosus	Ischial tuberosity	Posterior medial tibial condyle	1st perforator of profunda femoris artery (Type II)
Long head of biceps femoris	Ischial tuberosity	Lateral side of fibular head	1st perforator of profunda femoris artery (Type II)
Short head of biceps femoris	Femoral shaft	Lateral side of fibular head	2nd/3rd perforator of profunda femoris artery (Type II)
Gracilis	Body and ramus of pubis	Upper medial tibia	Medial circumflex femoral artery (Type II)

- The remainder are innervated by the obturator nerve (L2–L4)

B. Leg

1. Anterior compartment (Table 3):
   - All muscles in the anterior leg compartment are innervated by the deep peroneal nerve (L4–S2)
2. Lateral compartment (Table 4):
   - Both peroneus longus and peroneus brevis are innervated by the superficial peroneal nerve (L4–S2)
3. Posterior compartment (Table 5):
   - All posterior compartment muscle are innervated by the tibial nerve (L4–S3)

C. Foot

1. Dorsal surface muscles: extensor digitorum brevis muscle and extensor hallucis brevis muscle
2. Plantar surface muscles:
   - Superficial layer (Table 6):

     Abductor hallucis and flexor digitorum are innervated by the medial plantar nerve (L4–L5)

     Abductor digiti minimi is innervated by the lateral plantar nerve (S1–S2)
   - Second layer: quadratus plantae and lumbricals
   - Third layer: flexor hallucis brevis, adductor hallucis, flexor digiti minimi
   - Fourth layer: 4 dorsal interossei and 3 plantar interossei

VI. ARTERIES

A. Thigh

1. Obturator artery—from the internal iliac artery, it exits through the obturator foramen and divides into:
   - Anterior branch—supplies muscles of the adductor group

Table 3 Anterior Compartment of Leg

Muscle	Origin	Insertion	Blood supply/flap type
Tibialis anterior	Upper lateral half of anterior tibia	Medial cuneiform bone and 1st metatarsal base	Segmental branches from anterior tibial artery (Type IV)
Extensor hallucis longus	Anterior mid-fibula	Base of distal phalanx of hallux	Anterior tibial artery (Type IV)
Extensor digitorum longus	Lateral condyle of tibia, interosseous membrane and anterior fibula	Middle and distal phalanges of 2nd to 5th toes	Segmental branches from anterior tibial artery (Type IV)
Peroneus tertius	Distal 1/3 of fibula and distal interosseous membrane	Dorsal base of 5th metatarsal	Segmental branches from anterior tibial artery (Type IV)

Table 4 Lateral Compartment of Leg

Muscle	Origin	Insertion	Blood supply/flap type
Peroneus longus	Head and upper 2/3 of fibula	Medial cuneiform bone and base of 1st metatarsal	Peroneal artery (Type II)
Peroneus brevis	Distal 1/3 of fibula	Base of 5th metatarsal	Peroneal artery (Type II)

- Posterior branch—supplies the hamstring group

2. Femoral artery—continuation of the external iliac artery; it enters the femoral triangle of the thigh (femoral triangle: base = inguinal ligament; lateral = sartorius; medial = adductor longus; floor = iliopsoas and pectineus; roof = fascia lata). Branches include:

    - Three superficial branches in the triangle:

        Superficial epigastric artery supplies the hypogastric region of the abdomen

        External pudendal arteries supply the anterior pudendal region

        Superficial circumflex iliac artery supplies the lateral hip region

    - Deep femoral (profunda femoris) artery, the largest branch of the femoral artery, also arises in the femoral triangle. It has two branches:

        Lateral femoral circumflex artery—divides into three branches: ascending, transverse, descending

        Medial femoral circumflex artery—divides into three branches: ascending, transverse, descending

    - Three to four perforating arteries supply the major portion of the hamstring muscles and posterior thigh skin
    - Descending genicular artery—arises medially from the femoral artery in the distal portion of the thigh; divides into two branches:

        Saphenous branch—supplies the superficial tissues of the medial aspect of the leg

Table 5 Posterior Compartment of Leg

Muscle	Origin	Insertion	Blood supply/flap type
Superficial group			
Gastrocnemius	Posterior surfaces of lateral and medial femoral condyles	Calcaneus	Lateral sural artery Medial sural artery (Type I)
Soleus	Head and upper fibula, interosseous membrane, middle 3rd of tibia	Calcaneus	Popliteal artery (Type II)
Plantaris	Distal linea aspera and oblique popliteal ligament	Calcaneus	Main supply = sural artery Minor branches from posterior tibial and peroneal arteries
Deep group			
Flexor hallucis longus	Distal third of posterior fibula	Base of terminal phalanx of great toe	Posterior tibial artery (Type IV)
Tibialis posterior	Posterior shafts of tibia, fibula, and interosseous membrane	Navicular, cuneiform, base of 2nd–4th metatarsals	Posterior tibial artery (Type IV)
Flexor digitorum longus	Posterior surface of tibia shaft	Distal phalanges of 2nd–5th toes	Posterior tibial artery (Type IV)

Table 6 Superficial Layer of Foot

Muscle	Origin	Insertion	Blood supply/flap type
Abductor hallucis	Medial tubercle of calcaneus and plantar aponeurosis	Base of proximal phalanx of great toe	Medial plantar artery (Type II)
Flexor digitorum brevis	Medial tubercle of calcaneus and plantar aponeurosis	Middle phalanx of 2nd–5th toes	Medial and lateral plantar arteries (Type II)
Abductor digiti minimi	Medial and lateral process of calcaneal tuberosity	Lateral side of 5th toe proximal phalanx	Lateral plantar artery (Type II)

Articular branch—anastomoses with the medial superior genicular artery

3. The femoral artery becomes the popliteal artery upon entering the adductor canal. The adductor canal, also known as subsartorial or Hunter's canal, runs between the extensor and adductor muscles and is roofed by the sartorius muscle.

B. Leg and Foot

1. Popliteal artery:
   - Gives off several branches that participate in the geniculate anastomoses around the knee:

     Lateral and medial superior and inferior genicular branches

     Medial genicular branch—supplies the capsule of the knee joint

     Sural arteries descend superficially in the posterior compartment of the leg
   - Gives rise to the anterior tibial artery in the popliteal fossa, which enters the anterior leg compartment with the deep peroneal nerve:

     At the ankle, it gives off anterior medial and lateral malleolar branches

     Dorsalis pedis artery is the continuation of the anterior tibial artery on the dorsum of the foot; it lies between the tendons of the extensor hallucis longus and the extensor digitorum longus muscles. Branches include the (a) lateral and medial tarsal arteries, (b) arcuate artery, (c) metatarsal arteries, which bifurcate into dorsal digital arteries, and (d) deep plantar branch
   - Posterior tibial artery is the direct continuation of the popliteal artery into the posterior compartment:

     Posterior medial malleolar

     Medial calcaneal branch supplies the medial aspect of the heel

     Lateral plantar artery—joins with the deep plantar branch of the dorsalis pedis artery in the first interosseous space to form the plantar arterial arch

     Branches of this arch include the proper digital artery to the lateral side of the fifth toe and four plantar metatarsal arteries. Each of these bifurcates into proper digital arteries to supply the sides of adjacent toes

     Medial plantar artery—supplies the medial side of the plantar portion of the foot
   - Peroneal artery—gives rise to:

     Posterior lateral malleolar branch

     Lateral calcaneal branch, which supplies the lateral aspect of the heel

VII. VEINS

A. Deep Veins

1. These are usually venae comitantes that accompany the arteries of the lower extremity.
2. The venae comitantes of the anterior and posterior tibial arteries form the popliteal vein, which drains into the femoral vein.

B. Superficial Veins

1. These drain into the greater or lesser saphenous veins.

2. The two sets of veins are connected by valved perforating veins, so that blood flow is from superficial to deep veins and moves toward the heart mainly in deep veins:

   - Greater saphenous vein:

     Takes origin in the foot through the medial marginal vein

     Lies in the superficial fascia and ascends along the medial aspect of the leg and thigh

     In the femoral triangle, passes through the fossa ovalis to join the femoral vein

   - Lesser saphenous vein:

     Begins posterior to the lateral malleolus as the lateral marginal vein

     Ascends along the lateral aspect of the leg, freely anastomosing with the greater saphenous vein

     Enters the popliteal fossa and joins the popliteal vein

VIII. LYMPHATICS

A. Lymphatic Vessels

1. Deep lymphatic vessels follow the blood vessels as they course through the limb.
2. Superficial lymphatic vessels run in the superficial fascia.

B. Lymph Nodes

1. Popliteal nodes:

   - Receive superficial lymph vessels from the lateral side of the leg and foot (the area drained by the lesser saphenous vein) and from deep lymph vessels accompanying the anterior and posterior tibial arteries
   - Efferent vessels from the popliteal nodes drain into deep inguinal nodes.

2. Inguinal lymph nodes:

   - Superficial:

     Horizontal group

     Vertical group: receives superficial lymph vessels from the territory drained by the greater saphenous vein. Its efferent vessels drain into deep inguinal nodes

   - Deep:

     Receive lymph from deep vessels in the lower limb that travel alongside arteries, from the superficial inguinal nodes (horizontal and vertical groups), and from the popliteal nodes

     Efferent vessels from the deep inguinal nodes drain into external iliac nodes

IX. NERVES

A. Somatic Sensory Innervation

1. Thigh:

   - Medial aspect—femoral branch of the genitofemoral nerve (L1–L2, anterior)
   - Lateral aspect—lateral femoral cutaneous nerve (L2–L3, posterior)
   - Posterior aspect—posterior femoral cutaneous nerve (S1–S3, anterior and posterior)
   - Anterior aspect—cutaneous branches of the femoral nerve (L2–L4, posterior)

2. Leg and foot:

   - Nearly all by the branches of the sciatic nerve. Exception: cutaneous innervation of the anteromedial portion of the leg by the saphenous nerve, a branch of the femoral nerve
   - Medial aspect—saphenous branch (L4) of the femoral nerve
   - Anterolateral aspect—superficial peroneal branch (L5) of the common peroneal nerve
   - Posterior aspect—sural nerve (S2), formed by the tibial and common peroneal nerves
   - Middle and lateral aspects of the plantar foot, including the small toe—lateral and medial plantar branches (S1) of the tibial nerve

B. Motor Innervation

See Musculature section.

91

Acute Lower Extremity Trauma

Nolan S. Karp, M.D., and Sheel Sharma, M.D.
New York University Medical Center, New York, New York, U.S.A.

Advancements in microsurgical reconstruction, fracture management, and tissue transfer have greatly increased the options for limb salvage in severe lower extremity trauma. The primary goal of the reconstructive surgeon must be to salvage an extremity that is more functional than an amputated leg with a prosthesis.

I. ANATOMY

A. Several anatomic features unique to the lower extremity should be taken into consideration prior to reconstruction. These include:

- Bipedal ambulation is possible even with significant muscle loss.
- The lower extremity is prone to edema, deep vein thrombosis, and venous stasis.
- Atherosclerosis affects the lower extremity more than the upper extremity.
- The tibia is largely subcutaneous, which renders it susceptible to exposure following injury. This often necessitates specialized soft-tissue coverage.
- Normal plantar sensation is essential for weight bearing and tactile position sense. Intact plantar sensation, therefore, is one of the key determining factors in lower extremity salvage.
- The fibular shaft is an excellent source of vascularized bone graft and can be sacrificed without significant morbidity.

B. Anatomic compartments of the leg—the deep fascia of the leg invests the muscles of the leg into four discrete compartments (Fig. 1, Table 1).

II. COMPARTMENT SYNDROME

A. When the interstitial pressure within an osseofascial compartment increases enough to compromise the microcirculation, myoneural necrosis may result. This is called *compartment syndrome* and can occur in any compartment following trauma. The compartment needs to be decompressed immediately to prevent ischemic tissue necrosis.

B. The typical signs of compartment syndrome are:

- Pain out of proportion to the injury.
- Pain on passive flexion and extension of the foot.
- Palpably swollen or tense compartments.
- Loss of pulses is usually a late sign. The presence of a pulse does not rule out a compartment syndrome.

C. Diagnosis is confirmed by measuring compartment pressures. This can be done with commercially available units or simply by connecting a saline-flushed 18-gauge needle introduced into the compartment to a transducer. Pressures greater than 30 mmHg are a strong indication for fasciotomy.

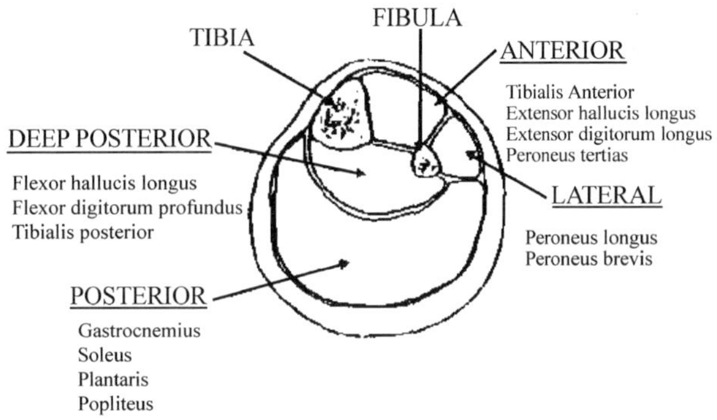

Figure 1 Cross-sectional anatomy of the leg. (From *Grabb & Smith's Plastic Surgery*, 5th Edition. Philadelphia: Lippincott Williams & Wilkins, 1997, p. 1034.)

D. Four-compartment fasciotomy should be performed whenever there is suspicion of compartment syndrome. The morbidity of a fasciotomy is far less than the morbidity of ischemic tissue necrosis.

III. FRACTURE CLASSIFICATION

The Gustilo classification is the most widely accepted classification for open tibial fractures (Table 2).

IV. MANAGEMENT OF THE MANGLED EXTREMITY

A. The management of complex lower extremity injuries requires a team approach involving the trauma, orthopedic, and plastic surgeons.

Table 1 Compartments of the Leg

Compartment	Muscle
Anterior	Tibialis anterior
	Extensor hallucis longus
	Extensor digitorum longus
	Peroneus tertius
Lateral	Peroneus longus
	Peroneus brevis
Superficial posterior	Gastrocnemius
	Soleus
	Popliteus
	Plantaris
Deep posterior	Flexor hallucis longus
	Flexor digitorum longus
	Tibialis posterior

Table 2 Gustilo Classification for Open Fractures

Type	Wound
I	<1 cm long
II	>1 cm long, but without extensive soft tissue disruption
III	Extensive soft tissue disruption
	Open segmental fracture
	Traumatic amputation
IIIA	Adequate soft tissue coverage of bony fragments
IIIB	Soft tissue loss, with bone exposure and periosteal stripping
IIIC	Arterial injury requiring repair

B. An algorithm should be utilized to best manage the complicated aspects of these injuries (Fig. 2).

V. INITIAL EVALUATION

A. Severe mutilating injuries to the lower extremity are usually associated with life-threatening injuries. The airway, breathing, and circulation are first managed as per established ATLS protocols.

B. Once the patient has been stabilized, a careful, multiteam assessment of the vascular, nerve, bone, and soft-tissue injuries is carried out to determine if the extremity is salvageable.

C. The initial evaluation should address the following questions:

- Are there injuries to the major vessels of the leg? Does the extremity require revascularization, and is it technically feasible? The use of a Doppler aids in the assessment of the vessels of the limb.
- Is there nerve injury in the extremity? Is sensation intact to the foot? It is extremely important to evaluate the peroneal and tibial nerves, since complete disruption of these nerves may be a relative contraindication to extremity salvage.
- Is the bone reconstructable? The orthopedic surgeon, based on x-rays and clinical evaluation, best determines this issue.
- Is the soft-tissue defect treatable? A good assessment of the soft-tissue defect is best made only after debridement of the nonviable tissue in the operating room.

D. If the initial evaluation determines that the extremity is unsalvageable, an amputation is

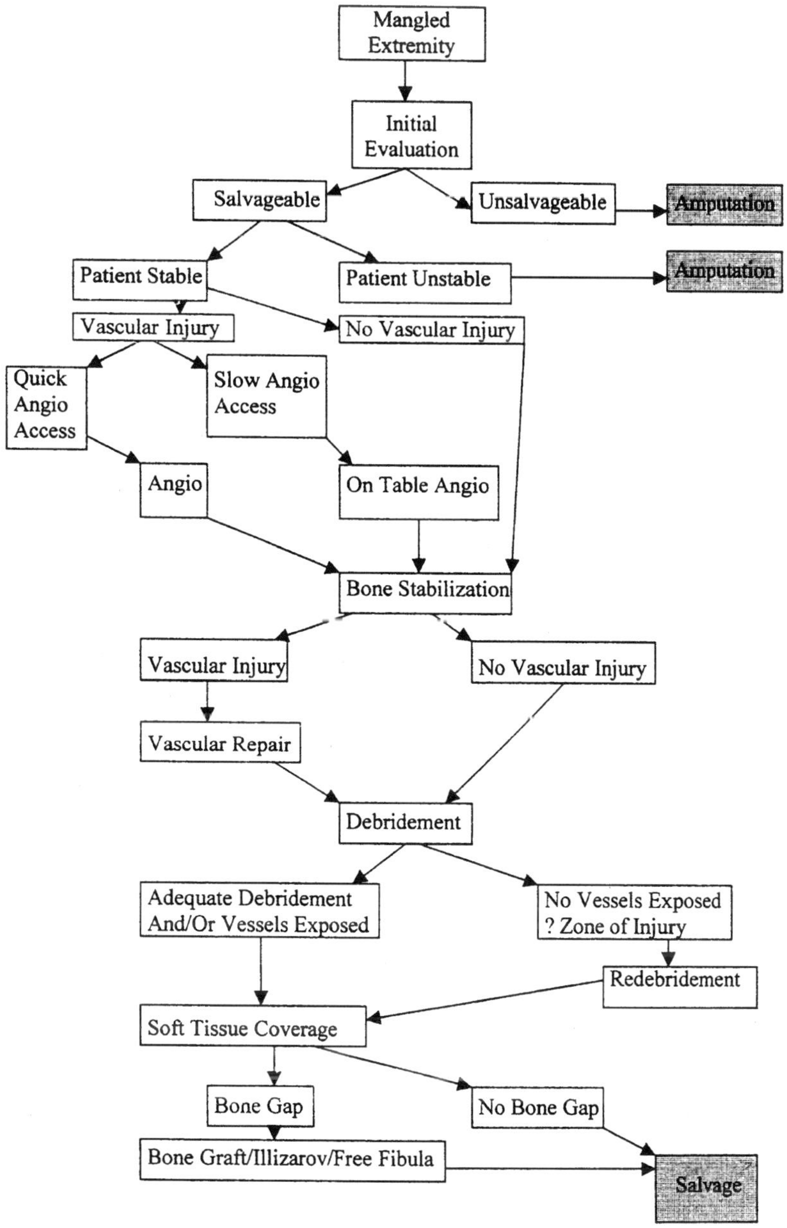

Figure 2 Algorithm for the treatment of lower extremity trauma. (From *Grabb & Smith's Plastic Surgery*, 5th Edition. Philadelphia: Lippincott Williams & Wilkins, 1997, p. 1036.)

indicated. If the extremity is salvageable, a reconstructive plan is formulated.

VI. THE RECONSTRUCTIVE PLAN

A. The first issue to be addressed is the extent of vascular injury. A decision needs to be made whether the patient should have an angiogram prior to surgery. Active arterial bleeding and compartment syndrome are relative contraindications to a preoperative angiogram.

B. Once in the operating room, the first step is usually stabilization of the bone injury. If revascularization is required, the stabilization must be done quickly. If stabilization is not possible in a timely manner, a vascular shunt is placed to minimize the ischemia time. If the vascular repair is performed prior to the orthopedic work, disruption of the anastomosis with bone manipulation is likely.

C. The vascular injury is repaired after bone stabilization. Full four-compartment fasciotomy must be performed in all lower extremities at risk for compartment syndrome following revascularization.

D. All nonviable tissue must then be debrided. If the vascular repair is exposed after debridement, immediate soft tissue coverage must be performed. If no vital structures are exposed, a second debridement should be performed prior to definitive flap coverage of the bone or orthopedic hardware. Ideally, soft tissue coverage is completed quickly (within 72 h from the time of injury). This is associated with a much lower microsurgery complication rate and decreased risk of osteomyelitis.

VII. FRACTURE MANAGEMENT

A. Traction is only used when the patient is too hemodynamically unstable to undergo formal stabilization and fixation.

B. Cast immobilization is only an option in closed injuries or after soft-tissue coverage is obtained and healed. Occasionally, a cast can be made with a window to allow for wound care.

C. Intramedullary nails:

- Reamed nails provide rigid fixation by tight fitting of the prosthesis within the medullary canal. The reaming of the canal results in complete loss of the endosteal blood supply. These nails are only useful in minimally comminuted bones without significant periosteal stripping. This technique is rarely used in the massively traumatized extremity.
- Nonreamed nails do not take up the entire medullary canal, and therefore do not require stripping of the endosteal blood supply. They offer many of the advantages of reamed nails (i.e., stable fixation with early ambulation) without the decreased blood supply to the bone. Nonreamed nails are very effective in Gustilo I, II, and IIIA tibial fractures. In cases of Gustilo IIIB fractures, early soft tissue coverage is required.

D. Internal fixation with plates and screws allows good alignment and relatively rigid fixation of fractures:

- This technique often requires extensive soft tissue and periosteal stripping. This results in decreased blood supply to the wound.
- Early coverage with local or free flaps is required.
- This technique is not indicated in cases where serial debridements are required to assess the soft tissue.

E. External fixation is usually the technique of choice in the severely injured lower extremity:

- External fixation provides fairly rigid fixation with minimal soft tissue stripping and interference with bone blood supply.
- The external fixation devices usually allow good exposure for local wound care.
- Careful planning of the pin placement is required so that future flap surgery is not obstructed.
- Pin tract care needs to be meticulous to avoid pin tract infections.
- Hybrid fixators can be designed to allow conversion to bone lengtheners to deal with bone gaps.

VIII. NERVE INJURY

A. Peroneal nerve injury results in foot drop and loss of sensation on the dorsum of the foot. Static foot splinting or tendon transfers are usually performed to correct the foot drop. The loss of sensation on the dorsum of the foot is usually not a major problem.

B. Tibial nerve injury is much more devastating. The loss of sensation on the plantar surface of the foot results in loss of position sense and can lead to chronic ulceration in the foot.

C. If possible, nerve injuries to the lower extremity should be repaired at the time of the injury. If a nerve graft is required, this should only be performed when a healthy soft tissue bed is assured. Therefore, nerve grafting is often best performed in a delayed manner.

D. Nerve injuries to the lower extremity are associated with poor prognosis. This is due to the long distance from the spinal cord and the long distance from the nerve repair to the motor endplate.

IX. SOFT TISSUE MANAGEMENT

A. Split-thickness skin grafts are used to cover exposed muscle, periosteum, paratenon, and occasionally short segments of vessels or nerve:

- Generally, skin grafts are adequate to cover Gustilo IIIA fracture wounds.
- Skin grafts alone are never adequate to cover Gustillo IIIB or IIIC fracture wounds.

B. Local flaps can be muscle or fasciocutaneous flaps:

- Local flaps are used to cover exposed bone, nerves, or vessels.
- Small defects in the proximal two-thirds of the leg can often be covered with local flaps. Gastrocnemius and soleus muscles are the local muscle flaps most frequently used in the lower extremity:

  The medial or lateral gastrocnemius muscle can be used to cover defects of the proximal third of the leg. The gastrocnemius blood supply arises from the sural vessels above the knee. Therefore, the gastrocnemius muscles can be used to cover the knee or proximal tibia.

  The soleus or hemi-soleus muscle may be used to cover defects of the middle third of the leg. A segment of muscle much larger than the defect must be raised.

  The functional defect resulting from sacrifice of one gastrocnemius muscle or the soleus muscle is usually minimal.

  The tibialis anterior muscle may also be used to cover small wounds of the anterior tibia. This muscle has a segmental blood supply and should be used as a bipedicle flap with the tendon left intact. The tibialis anterior is an important muscle in foot dorsiflexion and should not be transected.

- There are no local flaps available to cover wounds of the distal one-third of the leg. Microvascular free flap is usually necessary.
- Fasciocutaneous flaps are usually proximally based. The length of the flap should not exceed 1.5 times the base of the flap. Even small defects require a large flap to achieve closure. Fasciocutaneous flaps are not suitable to cover large defects that require well-vascularized tissue. A skin graft is almost always needed to cover the flap donor site.

C. Free tissue transfer is utilized for large wounds of the lower extremity with exposed bone, hardware, nerves, or tendons. Free flaps are also indicated for wounds in the distal third of the leg:

- Adequate debridement of the wound is essential prior to coverage.
- The rectus abdominis and the latissimus dorsi muscles are the most commonly used free flap donor sites for the lower extremity.
- Recipient vessels should be out of the zone of injury to minimize the risk of postoperative thrombosis in the recipient vessels.

D. Cross-leg flaps are are rarely used today. The cross-leg flap is used when a recipient artery is not available for free tissue transfer. The cross-leg flap requires prolonged immobilization of both extremities and never has as good a blood supply as free tissue transfer.

X. BONE GAPS

A. Nonvascularized cancellous bone grafts are utilized when the bone gap is less than 6 cm and the bed is well vascularized.

B. Vascularized bone grafts (i.e., usually fibula, but occasionally iliac crest) are utilized for bone gaps greater than 6 cm.

C. Bone transport or lengthening may be used for bone gaps 6 cm or longer. This may be accomplished in one of two ways. In the first method, the bone gap is maintained and then a segment of bone is transported to obliterate the gap. The other option is to reduce the gap by shortening. After bone healing, the extremity is lengthened to match the length of the other leg.

92

Chronic Wounds of the Lower Extremity

Christopher E. Attinger, M.D.
Georgetown University Medical Center, Washington, D.C., U.S.A.

I. INTRODUCTION

A chronic wound in the lower extremity occurs because the body is unable to heal the wound due to overwhelming injury, infection, inadequate blood flow, an ineffective immune system, or poor nutrition. The key to healing the wound is to determine its etiology, optimize the patient's wound-healing ability, and then apply the appropriate medical, topical, and/or surgical procedures.

II. CHRONIC WOUNDS NEED A TEAM APPROACH

Chronic wounds usually originate secondary to trauma of some type. Preexisting conditions such as diabetes, vascular insufficiency, venous stasis disease, lymphedema, vasculitis, steroid use, radiation, or hematological abnormality all inhibit subsequent healing. Chronic wounds can also originate from osteomyelitis, cancer, or abnormal dermatological condition or they can be factitious in nature. Because of the myriad of possible causes for chronic ulcers, it is critical to assemble a team to address each component of the treatment necessary for the wound to heal.

A. Wound Expert

The team leader is a wound care specialist. He or she diagnoses the ulcer etiology, coordinates appropriate referrals, and directs the overall wound care. This person can be any of the physician specialists listed below.

B. Infectious Disease Specialist

This specialist coordinates the treatment of the infectious component of the ulcer. He or she assesses culture results and prescribes the appropriate antimicrobial, antifungal, or antitubercular medications.

C. Vascular Surgeon

This surgeon helps assess the vascular flow of the leg and determines the most effective way to restore diminished or obstructed arterial flow. He or she must be experienced in distal revascularizations using autogenous veins, in situ techniques, short below-the-knee bypasses, and distal bypasses to pedal vessels. Expertise in endovascular techniques is essential. This individual also addresses venous disorders, including valvular incompetence or venous thrombosis.

D. Orthopedic Surgeon

This surgeon determines the best way to treat the bony skeleton when it is fractured, has osteomyelitis, or has developed structural abnormalities. He or she should be experienced in the use of external fixators, internal fixation, and bone transport (Ilizarov technique). Orthopedists with additional foot and ankle training are very useful in treating the skeletal abnormalities that develop in diabetics, such as Charçot joint collapse.

E. Podiatrist

The podiatrist guides the preventive foot care of diabetics so that skin breakdowns do not develop. If surgically trained, podiatrists can also manage the surgical aspects of foot and ankle wounds.

F. Plastic Surgeon

The plastic surgeon helps address the soft tissue defects that the wound and its subsequent debridement create. Many combinations of wound closure techniques are available, including primary closure, skin graft, local flap, pedicled flap, and/or microsurgical free flap.

G. Hyperbarist

Sometimes the wound requires hyperbaric oxygen treatments to help convert the chronic wound into a healing wound.

H. Medical Specialists

1. A rheumatologist skilled in treating vasculitis is critical for treatment of vasculitic ulcers.
2. A dermatologist is very helpful in treating pyoderma gangrenosum or other complex dermatologic problems.
3. A diabetologist is essential in helping control serum glucose levels in diabetics with poor control of serum glucose levels.
4. A hematologist is necessary to help optimize whatever blood dyscrasia underlies the existence of certain ulcers.

I. Physical Therapist

This professional guides the physical rehabilitation of the patient. The therapist is also skilled in placing contact casts for neuropathic plantar ulcers that help redistribute the weight over the whole foot while the patient heals.

J. Pedorthetist

Treatment of foot ulceration often requires special shoewear while the ulcer is healing and accommodative orthotics and shoes when it has healed. The pedorthetist uses the foot pressure measurement of an F-Scan or other similar devices during gait to design the optimal shoe-wear that equalizes weight distribution over the whole foot during gait.

K. Prosthetist

The prosthetist helps make the prosthesis for the amputated limb when salvage has not been possible. This includes short foot amputations (e.g., Chopart and Syme amputations) as well as below- and above-knee amputations.

III. DIAGNOSIS

The diagnosis can often be established with a thorough medical history and physical examination. Adjunctive tests are often necessary to confirm the diagnosis.

A. History of Present Illness

1. A good history about the current wound should be obtained. Establish when the ulcer began, why it began, and how it was previously treated.
2. If surgery was performed, obtain the previous surgeon's name and old operative notes. In trauma cases, a good history can help establish the extent of the initial trauma.
3. If a previous flap was used for coverage, it can help determine what reconstructive options remain.
4. Results of any tests previously performed are useful: recent vascular testing, angiograms, x-rays, nuclear medicine studies, culture results, pathology, etc.
5. Determine the patient's current tetanus status.

B. Past Medical History

1. Conditions that may affect the patient's ability to heal must be elicited:
    - Decreased local blood flow: arteriosclerosis, venous obstruction, radiation, vasculitis
    - Poor nutrition: cancer, diabetes, GI abnormality, vegetative state, psychiatric condition
    - Abnormal immune system: autoimmune disease, blood dyscrasia, infectious disease, malnutrition, diabetes, renal failure
    - Poor oxygenation: lung disease, heart failure or shunting, smoking, etc.
    - Medications that might impede healing: steroids, beta-blockers, or chemotherapy

2. The patient's primary care physician should be available to update the medical history and clear the patient for surgery.
3. A history of the patient's medication allergies and current medications should also be obtained.

C. Physical Exam

1. The Wound

a. The size of the wound should be measured along its longest length and widest width in centimeters. Initial and all subsequent measurements should be recorded. The depth of the wound as well as the type of tissue exposed (bone, tendon, muscle, fascia, fat, dermis, and/or epidermis) should also be recorded.

b. The quality of the wound (type of exposed tissue, percent and quality of granulation tissue, amount of fibrinous cover, necrotic or desiccated tissue, dry or wet gangrene) is recorded.

c. The wound is probed with a metal probe. If bone can be palpated at the base of the wound, there is an 85% chance that osteomyelitis is present.

d. The surrounding tissue is then examined to determine the extent of erythema, induration, bogginess, and edema. The border of erythema is delineated with indelible ink and dated so that the success of subsequent therapeutic intervention can be assessed.

e. If the wound is infected or purulent, the proximal and distal areas of possible spread should likewise be examined.

f. Evaluate for proximal lymphadenopathy.

2. The Vascular Exam

a. Determine the quality of local blood supply. The femoral, popliteal, dorsalis pedis, and posterior tibial pulses should be palpated. Each individual pulse should be quantified as strong, medium, or weak. Avoid confusing one's own pulse with that of the patient's by comparing the patient's extremity pulse with the patient's wrist pulse.

b. If the pulses are not palpable, a Doppler exam should be performed. If the sound is triphasic, the flow is excellent. If signals are biphasic, flow may be adequate. If monophasic, further study is required.

c. The presence of tortuous serpentine veins or obvious incompetent perforators should be noted. Venous stasis disease often coexists with arterial disease. The arterial exam is, therefore, very important in a patient with obvious venous disease.

3. Lower Extremity Biomechanical Exam

a. The range of motion of the major joints of the lower extremity should be documented. Attention should be directed toward flexion contractures of the knee and ankle. If the knee lacks the final 15° of extension, it loses its ability to lock in during the stance phase of gait. This means that the leg can never relax because the quadriceps has to be continually active to prevent the leg from buckling.

b. The Achilles tendon tends to shorten in diabetics because elevated glucose levels bind to collagen of the Achilles tendon, which makes it less flexible. In turn, this places additional stress on the midfoot and forefoot. Normally, a patient should be able to dorsiflex his or her foot 10° beyond neutral. If the patient can only do this when the knee is flexed, this implies that the gastrocnemius portion of the Achilles tendon are tight. If the patient cannot dorsiflex the foot 10° or more with the knee straight or flexed, then both the soleus and gastrocnemius portions of the Achilles tendon are tight.

c. Other abnormalities [e.g., flat or rocker bottom foot, varus or valgus foot, hammertoes or hallux valgus (bunion)] should likewise be documented.

4. Lower Extremity Neurological Exam

a. Sensation within the major nerve territories of the lower extremity should be evaluated and documented. This is especially important in the neurosome (area sensed by a given nerve) that contains the ulcer.

b. When there has been trauma to the area, sensation above and below the area of damage has to be documented. Look for frank nerve damage by checking for a Tinel's sign at and distal to the area of trauma.

c. Evaluate for a compressive neuropathy by percussing over the peroneal tendon at the fibular head and over the posterior tibial nerve at the tarsal tunnel.

d. To assess the patient's protective sensation in a given area, a 5.07 Semmes-Weinstein filament, which applies 10 g of pressure, is used. If the patient cannot sense the pressure from this filament over a given neurosome, then he or she has lost protective sensation there and can develop a neuropathic ulcer.

5. Physical Exam

A routine physical exam should be performed and should include vital signs, weight, cardiac, pulmonary, abdominal, vascular, neurological, and musculoskeletal exams.

D. Tests

Tests should be ordered carefully to rule in or rule out specific diagnoses. Most wounds can be adequately evaluated by x-rays and noninvasive vascular studies only.

1. X-ray: The underlying bone skeleton should be examined for abnormal pathology: fracture, dislocation, osteomyelitis, and foreign body. Osteomyelitis can only show up radiographically as late as 3 weeks after it is clinically present.
2. Culture: If the patient is insensate, the wound should be debrided and a deep-tissue culture sent for aerobic and anaerobic testing. Fungal and special cultures should be obtained if there is any suspicion that these may be present.
3. Biopsy: If there is suspicion of cancer, vasculitic ulcer, pyoderma gangrenosum, or other recognized pathology, a biopsy of the ulcer should be obtained. This can be done with a simple punch biopsy. Discuss with the pathologist how much tissue is needed, whether it should include normal tissue at the ulcer's edge, and the storage medium it should be sent in (saline, 10% formalin, etc.).
4. Chemistry and hematology:
   - A basic chemistry screen should be ordered to assess glucose levels and kidney function.
   - If there is congestive heart failure or liver disease, liver enzymes should be ordered.
   - If malnourishment is suspected, albumin and prealbumin should be ordered.
   - For ulcers due to vasculitis, a rheumatological panel should be ordered. Half of the patients with vasculitic ulcers also have an underlying coagulopathy. A coagulation profile should therefore be ordered to determine whether anticoagulation will eventually play a role in the healing of the ulcer.
   - An appropriate hematological screen should be ordered for suspected blood dyscrasias: thrombocytosis, granulocytosis, sickle cell disease, hemophilia, etc.
5. Noninvasive vascular testing:
   - Arterial Doppler examinations are important to document the quality of blood flow because an ankle-brachial index (ABI) is notoriously unreliable in patients with calcified vessels. The quality of the arterial tracing at the level of the superficial femoral artery in the thigh, the popliteal artery, anterior and posterior tibial vessels in the lower leg, the posterior tibial vessel at the ankle, the dorsalis pedis on the dorsum of the foot, and the digital vessels at the toes can help pinpoint the area of narrowing or occlusion. An absolute pressure of 30 mmHg at the level of the toes usually indicates sufficient blood flow to heal a wound.
   - Tissue oxygen measurements can also to document the quality of vascular supply to the skin. These are usually compared to a reference point, commonly over the chest. It is important to document the transcutaneous oxygen tension (TcP_{O_2}) around the ulcer. Pressures of 40 mmHg or higher reflect sufficient blood flow to heal the wound. Pressures of 30–40 mmHg may be sufficient to heal the wound. Pressures less than 30 mmHg require further vascular work-up, as the wound is unlikely to heal.
   - Venous testing can evaluate obstruction of the superficial or deep venous system. It can document valvular incompetence in the superficial and deep system as well as the presence of incompetent perforators linking the two.
6. Nuclear scans: Routine bone scans are notoriously unreliable because they are positive in any area where there is a chronic wound or active arthritis. However, they can be very useful to rule out osteomyelitis in areas away from the wound. Technetium scans are more selective for osteomyelitis; HMPAO scans are the most selective.
7. MRI: MRI can be very sensitive in determining the presence and extent of osteomyelitis if the radiologist reading the studies is experienced in assessing

bone pathology. They are also useful in evaluating tumor size, metastasis, and lymphadenopathy.

8. Angiogram:
   - Angiograms are usually ordered by the vascular surgeon prior to planning repair of the diseased vascular tree. They can also be ordered by the plastic surgeon if planning to repair the wound defect includes using a microsurgical free flap.
   - The risk of renal damage necessitates that this test should only be ordered if it will affect the outcome of the wound.
   - Patients with allergy to iodine should be prescreened by the angiographer so that proper precautions can be taken (prehydration and steroids).
   - The angiographer/vascular surgeon should be experienced in endovascular techniques. Good communication between the vascular surgeon and angiographer is key to making sure that the optimal sequence of events is carried out: angiogram, endovascular dilation $\pm$ vascular bypass.
   - With the ever-improving quality of imaging with magnetic resonance angiography (MRA), angiography-related problems may become obsolete within a few years.

IV. PREPARING THE WOUND FOR CLOSURE

The key to healing a chronic wound is to convert it into an acute wound. Chronic wounds are arrested in the inflammatory phase of wound healing. Their surfaces have chronically high protease levels that overwhelm local growth factors. By debriding the wound back to normal tissue, wound healing can start anew. The wound-healing team's job is to then provide and main tain the optimal environment for the wound. The wound can subsequently go through the normal wound-healing phases until it heals by secondary intention or successfully accepts coverage (i.e., delayed primary closure, skin graft, pedicled flap or free flap).

A. Debridement

1. Immediate debridement should only occur in the setting of wet gangrene or necrotizing fasciitis. Debridement can otherwise be delayed until the diagnosis has been established and until the steps to improve the local environment are underway. For example, debriding an ischemic wound before revascularization will only serve to increase the wound size, as the new surface is likely to desiccate and die. Debriding a vasculitic wound before anti-inflammatory medications are optimized will only increase the size of the wound as well.
2. Pyoderma gangrenosum wounds are better treated with medication and topical therapy rather than surgical debridement.
3. Debridement should be performed as often as necessary until the wound is clean and ready for reconstruction.
4. Topical debriding agents can be used when a minimal amount of tissue has to be removed and the patient tolerates surgical debridement poorly. However, these debriding agents can themselves also be painful.
5. Between debridements, topical antibiotics can reduce the bacterial load: silver sheeting (Acticoat©) or silver-sulfadiazine works well for all wounds, Bactroban© for MRSA, gentamicin ointment or diluted acetic acid for *Pseudomonas* infections, and bacitracin for minimally infected wounds. Patients can develop an allergy to these ointments, which should be discontinued if allergies develop. Topical steroids can help treat the allergic skin reaction that may occur around the ulcer.

B. What to Debride

Aggressive debridement back to normal tissue is key. One should only be limited by vital structures, such as neurovascular bundles.

1. Soft tissue: Resect back to bleeding tissue. The presence of clotted veins in the subcutaneous tissue signifies that further debridement is necessary. The skin edges should have pinpoint bleeding and the subcutaneous fat should be bright yellow.
2. Fascia, tendon: All stringy and soft tendon or fascia should be debrided back to solid tissue with normal tissue integrity. When dealing with large tendons (e.g., Achilles tendon), the tendon should be shaved back until glistening tendon fibers appear and the normal firm texture is felt. The tissue that covers the tendon above and below the ulcer should be explored to make sure that all the necrotic tissue has been removed.

3. Cartilage: Exposed cartilage at the base of the wound should be removed. However, if fresh healthy cartilage is exposed in the process of debriding and the wound is to be immediately covered, it need not be removed.
4. Bone: The bone should be burred or cut back to healthy bleeding bone. When dealing with a large bone, it is best to burr it with a cutting burr until punctate bleeding is seen (Papineau sign). If cutting smaller bone, serial slices should be made until there is hard, bleeding bone. Bone sequestra should likewise be removed because they act much like a foreign body.
5. Foreign body: All foreign bodies should be removed from the wound bed if possible. This includes fixation devices, joint implants, sutures, mesh, and synthetic vascular grafts. This may not always be possible when dealing with vascular grafts or orthopedic fixation hardware. In those cases, the debridement is coordinated with the appropriate surgeon.

C. When Is the Wound Ready to Close?

When all the abnormal parameters surrounding the wound have been corrected and when all signs of acute inflammation have disappeared, the wound is ready to close. Alternatively, it can then also be treated topically so that it can heal by secondary intention.

1. Erythema: The wound itself should have no surrounding erythema. Cellulitis should not be confused with dependent rubor due to ischemia or recent local surgery. If surrounding erythema goes away immediately with elevation of the extremity, the wound has dependent rubor. If erythema persists, inflammation still exists.
2. Induration: The wound edges should have minimal, if any, induration. Wrinkled skin lines at the wound's edge are one of the most reliable signs that inflammation has largely resolved. Induration, however, may be absent in patients who lack good immunologic responses (i.e., renal failure, steroid dependence).
3. Pain: Pain should have subsided in a wound with resolving inflammation. Decreasing pain, however, is a less reliable indicator than resolving erythema or induration.
4. Fresh granulation tissue within the wound: Indicates sufficient blood supply and a hospitable environment for the wound to go through the remaining stages of wound healing.
5. Neo-epithelialization at wound's edge: The presence of new epithelium at the wound's edge reflects a healthy wound that is on its way to healing by secondary intention.
6. If quantitative bacterial cultures are available, a bacterial concentration of $<10^5$ bacteria per gram of tissue signifies that the wound is ready to be successfully skin grafted.

D. Promoting Healing by Secondary Intention

A healthy healing wound should decrease in surface area by at least 10–15% per week. The optimal dressing to allow the most rapid epithelialization is a moist dressing, usually a gel of some type. If the wound is on the plantar aspect of the foot, that portion of the foot should be unweighted. If the wound is at a mobile portion of the leg, the involved joint should be immobilized.

E. Adjuncts to Help the Wound Heal

Several adjuncts can help a wound that fails conservative therapy to heal:

1. Platelet-derived growth factor: This gel is effective in diabetic wounds when they are well vascularized, clean, and regularly debrided. Curetting the coagulum off the wound before applying the growth factor is important because the coagulum contains proteases that can digest the applied growth factor before the latter can have an effect. Covering the growth factor with a dressing that inactivates proteases (Promogram by Johnson & Johnson, Skipton, U.K.) maximizes the growth factor effect on the wound.
2. Temporary coverage: Xenograft (pigskin) or allograft (cadaver skin) provides an excellent temporary dressing. Their advantage is that they provide an excellent temporary moist dressing that is inexpensive. If the temporary graft initially "takes" before it is rejected immunologically, the underlying recipient bed is adequately vascularized for a split-thickness skin autograft to successfully take.
3. Cultured skin substitutes: While these are not skin graft substitutes per se, they provide a moist covering that produces the whole array of local growth

factors at the wound site. They have been effective in healing diabetic and venous stasis ulcers.

4. Hyperbaric oxygen:
   - Hyperbaric oxygen improves the oxygen concentration at the wound's edge and thus increases the oxygen gradient between the edge and center of the wound. The higher the gradient, the more successfully it can promote angiogenesis, collagen synthesis, and neo-epithelialization.
   - Hyperbaric oxygen is only effective if there is adequate vascular inflow. Before undergoing hyperbaric oxygen treatment, candidates should undergo an oxygen challenge test that shows a rise in the local tissue oxygen pressure after exposing the lungs to increased oxygen content. Breathing 100% oxygen should lead to >10 mmHg rise in tissue oxygen levels. Diving in a chamber at 2 atmospheres pressure should increase the tissue oxygen level to above 300 mmHg. Otherwise, the treatment is unlikely to be effective.
   - Hyperbaric oxygen and platelet growth factor work synergistically, proving to be more effective together than when compared to use of either agent alone.
5. Subatmospheric pressure dressings (VAC by KCI, San Antonio, Texas): Negative pressure applied directly to a wound via a closed suction mechanism decreases peri-wound edema, stimulates angiogenesis and sterilizes the wound. The combined effect of all three actions accelerate the formation of healthy granulation tissue over the wound bed provided there is adequate blood flow and the wound has previously been appropriately debrided. The VAC can be used to primarily heal a wound by secondary intention or to prepare a wound for subsequent soft tissue reconstruction.

V. CLOSURE TECHNIQUES

Although the individual techniques have been covered in other chapters, it is important to point how they can be adapted for optimal results in the lower extremity.

A. Delayed Primary Closure

Because the leg consists of circumferential tissue around a bone pillar, it is easy to apply excessive circumferential pressure when a wound is closed too tightly. Check distal blood flow with a Doppler if there is any suspicion that a tight closure may have compromised blood flow.

B. Skin Graft

1. This is the simplest of all coverage techniques, provided that the underlying bed has healthy granulation tissue and all signs of inflammation are gone.
2. Split-thickness skin grafts 0.015 inch thick are usually sufficient.
3. If the wound is on the lower leg, an Unna boot dressing allows the patient to ambulate immediately postoperatively.
4. If the area is around the ankle or foot, then immobilization with a posterior splint or external fixator and non-weight bearing for 2 or more weeks is critical for the graft to take successfully.
5. If the graft is on the plantar aspect of the foot, there should be no weight bearing until the skin graft has matured (usually 6 weeks).
6. To ensure the highest possible skin graft take (>95%), the skin graft should be covered with a subatmospheric dressing during the first 3 to 5 days.

C. Pedicled Flaps

These flaps work well if their vascular pedicle is intact and if they were not involved in the initial trauma, infection, or radiation field. Otherwise, the flaps are stiff and difficult to dissect. In addition, the vascular pedicle is usually very intolerant of any twisting or turning that occurs when the flap is transposed into its new position. The complication rate can be as high as 40%.

D. Microsurgical Free Flap

1. The microsurgical free flap is the most complex reconstruction that paradoxically carries the highest success rate (>95%).
2. A good recipient artery and vein(s) must be present to which the flap vessels can be anastomosed.
3. Muscle flaps with or without skin work best to cover osteomyelitis and the sole of the foot. Good donor muscles include the gracilis, rectus abdominis, serratus anterior, and latissimus dorsi muscles.

4. Fasciocutaneous and cutaneous free flaps work equally well or better elsewhere. Flaps that are frequently used include the radial forearm, lateral arm, lateral thigh, and parascapular flaps.

VI. TYPES OF CHRONIC WOUNDS

The list below, without being exhaustive, includes the most common causes of chronic wounds. Note that infection usually plays a role in all these ulcers. Trauma, however slight, is usually the initiating factor superimposed on one of the conditions listed below.

A. Diabetic Wounds

These are the majority of lower extremity wounds seen in wound clinics today. Neuropathy is frequently present. The lack of sensation and biomechanical gait abnormality are the most frequent contributing factors. In addition, vascular insufficiency is present in approximately 30–60% of cases. Because of poor medical care, diabetics face a 50% chance of major amputation when they present with an ulcer. After major amputation, they face 50% mortality and 50% chance of contralateral amputation within the ensuing 5 years.

1. Neuropathy

a. Diabetics are prone to develop neuropathy because of abnormal glucose pathways leading to accumulation of sorbitol within the nerves. The nerves not only function more inefficiently but also tend to swell. This increase in diameter leads to compression of the nerves as they pass through narrow anatomic channels (i.e., tarsal tunnel). The combination of nerve swelling and a tight tunnel (double crush syndrome) leads to severe neuropathy affecting the sensory, autonomic, and motor pathways.

b. Patients can lose sensation in the lower extremity (>40% after 20 years of diabetes). This then robs them of early warning signs that damage is occurring from excessive shear, tight shoes, or foreign body (thumbtack, pebble, or even a large callous). If the patient cannot feel a 5.07 Semmes-Weinstein filament, then he or she cannot sense 10 g of pressure and has essentially lost protective sensation. The patient will need orthotics and careful follow up by podiatry to prevent future breakdown.

c. Neuropathy also involves the autonomic system. The patient loses the ability to sweat and the skin is poorly lubricated. Cracks can easily develop in the skin, providing an entry point for bacteria. Frequent lubrication should be part of the regular care of all diabetic feet.

d. Finally, neuropathy involves the motor nerve supply to the lower leg and intrinsic muscle of the foot. When the anterior or lateral leg muscles are involved, abnormal gait and excessive local plantar pressures result. When the intrinsic muscles weaken, hammertoes develop. This places excessive pressure on the head of the metatarsals during gait. The dorsi-flexed PIP joints are at risk from shear forces when in a tight toe box. Surgical correction of hammertoes, as well as shoe modification with a rocker bottom sole and large toe box are important prophylactic measures.

2. Biomechanical Abnormality

In addition to the biomechanical abnormalities that can occur from motor neuropathy (see above), excess glucose binds to collagen of the Achilles tendon. As a result, the tendon loses its flexibility and tightens. The patient is subsequently unable to dorsiflex the foot beyond neutral, which places excessive weight on the forefoot during gait. This leads to breakdown of the plantar forefoot and can lead to Charçot collapse of the midfoot. Achilles tendon lengthening can correct this problem if performed before secondary deformities develop.

3. Vascular Insufficiency

a. The vascular disease in diabetics tends to be infrapopliteal at and distal to the trifurcation of the popliteal artery. As such, a distal bypass is frequently necessary if there is insufficient distal perfusion.

b. Absence of palpable pulses suggests insufficient blood flow. The ankle-brachial index is not useful in diabetics because the calcifications present in the vessel wall make the readings difficult to interpret. Toe pressures greater than 30 mmHg or tissue oxygen levels higher than 40 mmHg suggest sufficient blood flow.

c. More reliable is a triphasic Doppler signal over the dorsalis pedis or posterior tibial artery.

d. If there is any question as to the adequacy of the blood flow, the patient should be referred to a vascular surgeon specializing in distal revascularization.

4. Infection

Diabetic infections tend to be polymicrobial: Gram positive, Gram negative, and anaerobic. After obtaining a deep culture, broad coverage should be started. The coverage can be narrowed as soon as definite culture results are obtained.

5. Amputations

a. Most ulcers that involve bone usually require limited amputations. The focus should be on removing the least possible amount of tissue to maintain a biomechanically stable foot. Heel ulcers can often be taken care of with a limited Calcaneus resection and delayed primary closure.

b. Toe amputations should generally be at the metatarsal-phalangeal joint level if the proximal phalanx is involved. If more than two toes are removed, a transmetatarsal amputation should be considered. An Achilles tendon lengthening should accompany the procedure to prevent lateral plantar forefoot breakdown.

c. Shorter foot amputations (i.e., Lisfranc amputation at the cuneiform-metatarsal joint or Chopart amputations at the tarsal-cuneiform joint) should be accompanied by an actual Achilles tenectomy because these amputations otherwise tend to go into an equina-varus deformity that will break down anterolaterally. Close consultations with the pedorthetist and prosthetist are necessary to prevent future breakdown.

d. If a major amputation cannot be avoided due to an uncorrectable and unstable skeletal abnormality, a below-the-knee amputation should be performed.

B. Vascular Insufficiency

1. Advanced atherosclerosis leads to obstruction of the vascular tree to the lower extremity. The decreased blood flow and consequent oxygen delivery are insufficient for the leg muscles to function normally. This initially leads to claudication (pain on ambulation). Further decrease in blood flow leads to ischemic ulcers and gangrene.
2. The occlusion can be at the aortic, iliac, femoral, popliteal, or distal arteries.
3. Ischemic lower legs appear atrophic with cool feet, shiny hairless skin, and dependent rubor. Proximal pulses may be present or absent, while distal pulses are absent. Doppler signals over the main distal arteries are usually monophasic.
4. Noninvasive arterial Doppler studies show inadequate blood flow. They can pinpoint the location of the obstruction by determining the level at which the signal deteriorates.
5. Referral to a vascular surgeon experienced in distal revascularizations is the first step in getting the ulcer healed. Once the leg is revascularized, the wound can be treated in the ways described above.

C. Venous Stasis Disease

1. Chronic venous insufficiency is present in over 20% of working men and women. Varicose veins (protuberant greater or lesser saphenous veins with incompetent valves), incompetent perforator veins (veins connecting the superficial and deep venous system), and/or occlusion of the deep venous system all are potential contributors to the disease.
2. Deep venous disease is far more frequent than superficial varicose veins or incompetent perforators.
3. Increased venous pressure results both from exercising muscle (as high as 200 mmHg) and from the static column of uninterrupted blood from the heart to the lower leg. The high pressure leads to local accumulation of white blood cells and chronic inflammation in the lower leg. The skin itself becomes discolored and pigmented while the tissue becomes chronically indurated (liposclerosis). Combined with chronic swelling, this leads to skin breakdown and chronic ulceration. Remember that atherosclerosis can coexist with venous stasis disease and that both should be evaluated.
4. The resultant symptoms vary from a pulsating sense of pressure, burning, and/or a feeling of heaviness. These symptoms are relieved with leg elevation or elastic support.
5. Surgical treatment is effective in cases where the superficial system (greater and lesser saphenous vein) or incompetent perforators are involved. This can now be done endoscopically, minimizing surgical incisions in areas that are difficult to heal. The superficial veins can be stripped and the incompetent perforators can be ligated. Unfortunately, there is no highly successful surgery for

deep vein incompetence as venous valve transplants are fraught with complications.

6. In the postoperative period, the leg should be dressed with either an Unna boot or a 4-ply dressing. The 4-ply dressings are more effective than the Unna boot in applying increased long-term pressure to the entire lower leg. When the wound has healed, it is most important that the patient wear pressure stockings in the 30–40 mmHg range thereafter. If the pressure stockings are worn continuously, the recurrence rate can be as low as 17% over the next 3 years. If not worn regularly, the recurrence is 100% at 1 year.

D. Lymphedema

1. Whether the lymphedema is congenital or acquired, the result is a massively swollen leg that has decreased skin blood flow, stagnant lymph fluid, and increased susceptibility to secondary infection.
2. Surgical therapy has been disappointing, including the Charles procedure where the entire soft tissue overlying the fascia is removed and replaced with skin grafts.
3. The most successful treatment is referral to a lymphedema clinic, where the patients are started on lymph-press pumps and elaborate leg-wrapping techniques. If recurrent bouts of cellulitis occur, the patient should be referred to an infectious disease specialist for possible chronic bacterial suppression.

E. Osteomyelitis

1. Chronic bone infection manifests itself by chronic sinus tracts that fail to close despite appropriate local wound care.
2. A history of previous trauma is usually present.
3. Residual hardware or bone sequestrum often contributes to the draining sinus.
4. When dealing with the long bones or the hind- or mid-foot, the care should be coordinated by both the orthopedic and plastic surgeons. The infected bone is removed and cultured, the bone on either end is stabilized by external fixation, and the defect is closed either primarily or with a muscle-based flap.
5. The defect itself can be filled with methyl methacrylate beads containing antibiotics. When the wound has achieved stable coverage and is sterile off of systemic antibiotics, the beads can be removed and the bone defect repaired with bone graft or a bone transport mechanism (Ilizarov technique).

F. Cancer

1. Skin cancer or metastatic cancer can cause a nonhealing ulcer. Always think of cancer as a possible diagnosis when evaluating a chronic ulcer. If there is any suspicion that it may be cancer, a biopsy of the ulcer should be obtained.
2. A Marjolin's ulcer (malignant squamous cell carcinoma) can arise from a chronic wound or scar that has been present for years.
3. When extensive resections are mandated, limb salvage can be achieved when the care is coordinated between an orthopedic oncology surgeon and a plastic surgeon. If the major vessels are involved, a vascular surgeon may also be necessary.

G. Radiation

1. Treatment for cancer of the lower extremity often includes radiation therapy. The radiation permanently damages the local blood supply, rendering the affected tissue ischemic and prone to breakdown. When skin does break down, it is difficult to heal because of insufficient local blood flow.
2. Local flaps are usually ineffective because they or their vascular pedicles lie within the zone of radiation.
3. Pretreating the wound with hyperbaric oxygen stimulates angiogenesis at the edges of the radiated field.
4. The radiated tissue should then be excised and replaced with a microsurgical free flap. As much of the radiated tissue should be removed as can be replaced by the free flap.

H. Vasculitis

Auto-destruction of the dermal vessels secondary to immunological abnormalities occurs with patients who suffer from rheumatoid arthritis, lupus, scleroderma, and other collagen-vascular diseases. In addition, there is often an arterial spastic component to the disease (Raynaud's syndrome). These ulcers are treated medically with calcium channel blockers, steroids, and antineoplastic drugs. The medical management of these patients should be directed by a rheumatologist.

I. Hematologic-Based Ulcers

1. Ulcers can be due to abnormal hematologic conditions that affect blood flow in capillaries: thrombocytosis, blood dyscrasias, sickle cell disease, etc.
2. They can also affect the function of white blood cells in fighting infection (e.g., granulocytosis, leukemia).
3. Abnormal clotting may also be present (e.g., hemophilia, antithrombin III deficiency, protein C deficiency).
4. The care of these wounds should be coordinated with a hematologist.

J. Pyoderma Gangrenosum

This dermatological condition causes skin breakdown and is associated with ulcerative colitis or Crohn's disease. It is also seen with internal cancers. Care is best provided by a dermatologist, as surgery is singularly unrewarding.

K. Factitious

When all possible causes of a given wound have been ruled out, consider self-mutilation as the cause for the wound chronicity. It is often difficult to confront a patient with this diagnosis. A psychiatrist can be very helpful in this respect.

93

Lymphedema

James P. Watson, M.D.
David Geffen School of Medicine at UCLA, Los Angeles, California, U.S.A.

Lymphedema is the physical manifestation of inadequate clearance of protein-rich fluid from the interstitial space. This results in a pathologic build-up of both fluid and protein in the extracellular space. The underlying cause may be either a congenitally malformed lymphatic system (primary lymphedema) or injury to the lymphatic vessels from infection, radiation, surgery, or other trauma (secondary lymphedema).

I. CLASSIFICATION OF LYMPHEDEMA

A. Primary Lymphedema

All cases of lymphedema that are either congenital or of unknown etiology are called primary lymphedema. These are subclassified by age of onset into one of the following types:

1. Lymphedema congenita—onset at birth or before puberty. This includes cases with a genetic history of lymphedema, which is called Milroy's disease (sex-linked dominant inheritance pattern). Only 5% of primary lymphedema patients have a positive family history, however.
2. Lymphedema praecox—onset between puberty and 35 years of age. This is the most common type of primary lymphedema, accounting for 80% of cases.
3. Lymphedema tarda—onset after 35 years of age. This accounts for 10–15% of primary lymphedema cases. The lymphedema may present late in life with no apparent cause or precipitating event.
4. Syndromes with primary lymphedema:
   - Yellow nail syndrome is a triad of yellow, dystrophic nails, primary lymphedema, and bilateral pulmonary effusions.
   - Klippel-Trenaunay syndrome is a slow-flow, complex, combined capillary–lymphatic vascular malformation that is associated with extremity lymphedema in 25% of cases.

B. Secondary Lymphedema

This accounts for the majority of lymphedema cases in the United States and worldwide. The cause appears to be scarring and fibrosis of preexisting (normal) lymphatics or direct injury by surgery or trauma. These are subclassified not by age of onset, but by etiology. Although there are hundreds of causes, the most common worldwide include the following:

1. Infection—the parasite *Wucheria bancrofti* (filariasis) damages the lymphatic system by direct infestation of lymph nodes. Other agents include tuberculosis, lymphogranuloma, actinomycosis, cat scratch fever, snakebites, and insect bites.
2. Surgery—lymphadenectomy surgery for breast, prostate, melanoma, and other cancers is the most common cause of lymphedema in developed countries. It may occur in 10–40% of breast cancer cases treated with mastectomy and 5–10% of cases treated with lumpectomy, axillary node dissection, and postoperative radiotherapy. The onset of lymphedema is often delayed, and

the risk increases significantly with the addition of postoperative radiation. Lower extremity arterial reconstructive surgery may also cause secondary lymphedema.

3. Radiation—high-dose radiation for cancer therapy can cause lymphedema alone or may precipitate lymphedema in patients who previously had lymphadenectomy surgery.
4. Cancer—although lymphedema is usually a late manifestation of cancer, it may be the first presenting sign of primary cancer or recurrent cancer involving the lymph system (lymphoma), invading the lymph system (lymphatic spread), or impeding lymph flow by a mass effect (extrinsic compression).

II. INCIDENCE AND NATURAL HISTORY

1. Worldwide incidence is approximately 140 million.
2. Primary lymphedema:
   - Most common type—lymphedema praecox
   - Female:male = 3:1
   - Most common limb—left leg
   - Most common age of onset—menarche
3. Secondary lymphedema:
   - Most common cause worldwide—filariasis
   - Most common cause in United States—breast cancer therapy
4. Most common event precipitating the onset of lymphedema—cellulitis.
5. Natural history of lymphedema:
   - Onset—usually gradual in onset (exception: edema due to cancer).
   - Latency period—the time between birth (primary) or injury (secondary) and manifestation of edema is extremely variable.
   - Precipitating events—precipitating events that cause the onset of lymphedema can often be identified. Common precipitating events include cellulitis, air travel, intravenous catheters, tourniquets, extremity surgery, and minor trauma (abrasions, lacerations, ingrown toenails, etc.).
   - Prognosis—lymphedema may remain stable for decades, but usually gradually worsens over a period of years. Avoidance of precipitating events, lifestyle modification, and appropriately aggressive therapy can slow or prevent the natural course.

III. DIAGNOSIS AND WORK-UP

A. History

Most cases of lymphedema can be diagnosed by history and physical examination alone. A thorough history will usually reveal the cause of secondary lymphedema, although a long interval of time may occur between the initiating event and the actual occurrence of lymphedema. A family history will be helpful in cases of Milroy's disease. The following specific issues should also be discussed:

1. History of cellulitis/lymphangitis—bacterial soft tissue infections often precipitate the manifestation or worsening of preexisting primary or secondary lymphedema. Minor skin trauma (splinters, cuts, periungual infections, insect bites) as potential etiologies should be identified for purposes of lifestyle modification.
2. History of prior diagnostic studies—most patients present with a variety of negative test results, such as venous ultrasounds or CT scans. Prior lymphographic x-ray studies performed with radiopaque dye can actually cause further damage to the lymphatics and may precipitate worsening of the lymphedema.
3. History of prior treatment—most patients present with a prior history of failed attempts to control their edema. This history is vital to developing a treatment protocol that is aggressive enough to control their edema successfully.

B. Physical Examination

Pitting edema is the classic finding in early lymphedema, regardless of etiology. The distal extremity (hands, ankles) are usually affected first. Proximal migration of the edema coincides with a measurable increase in limb diameter and volume, which can be compared to the opposite extremity as a reference. Specific items that should be documented or evaluated include the following:

1. Presence of cellulitis or lymphangitis.
2. Skin quality—chronic erythema and thick, hyperkeratotic changes occur in longstanding lymphedema.
3. Body weight—weight gain occurs with lymphedema.

4. Photographic documentation.
5. Limb circumference measurements at multiple levels.
6. Limb volume (by water displacement in a cylinder).
7. Presence of open wounds or lymphocutaneous fistulae.
8. Examination for local cancer recurrence or new cancer (e.g., lymphangiosarcoma occurs after longstanding postmastectomy lymphedema—Stewart-Treves syndrome).

C. Differential Diagnosis

Many other chronic diseases can cause peripheral edema and can confuse the physician caring for the patient with lymphedema. As a consequence, many patients with lymphedema are misdiagnosed, and patients with other underlying disease are often labeled as lymphedema. In general, bilateral lower extremity edema is usually due to systemic disease (cardiac, renal, hepatic, malnutrition). Unilateral edema is more likely due to venous disease, lymphedema, or more unusual conditions. Lymphedema can coexist with venous insufficiency as well. Other causes of extremity swelling that are often misdiagnosed as lymphedema include the following:

1. Obesity—extremity obesity is often diagnosed as lymphedema. Patients with underlying lymphedema often become obese due to difficulty with ambulation or performing exercise. For this reason, lymphoscintigraphy is often needed to exclude or diagnose lymphedema in obese patients.
2. Lipedema—lipedema is a term used to describe patients with symmetric, idiopathic ankle swelling with no accompanying foot edema. The swelling is due to fat deposits without other signs of lymphedema (skin changes, cellulitis, etc.). These patients do not have lymphedema, but are often diagnosed as such. They have normal or nearly normal lymphatic flow on lymphoscintigraphy.
3. Venous insufficiency—venous disease is the most common cause of unilateral lower extremity edema, but has a very characteristic physical manifestation of atrophic skin, brawny pigmentation, and dense, hard woody edema that does not resemble lymphedema.
4. Cardiac failure—congestive heart failure often causes bilateral lower extremity edema that may be mistaken for lymphedema. This edema is usually bilaterally symmetric and is accompanied by other signs of cardiac failure, such as presacral edema, exercise intolerance, shortness of breath, and orthopnea.
5. Renal failure—occult or symptomatic renal disease often causes bilateral lower extremity edema. This edema is also bilaterally symmetric and is associated with anemia, oliguria, uremia, and other typical manifestations of renal failure.
6. Hepatic failure—lower extremity edema can occur with hepatic failure due to low plasma protein concentration or due to cysterna chyli obstruction by the liver.
7. Malnutrition—severe protein-calorie malnutrition (kwashiorkor) can cause generalized non-pitting edema due to hypoproteinemia.
8. Reflex sympathetic dystrophy (RSD)—RSD is an uncommon complication of extremity trauma or surgery that is characterized by chronic, severe pain with pitting edema isolated to the affected extremity. The limb is usually hypersensitive to touch and may be associated with trophic changes in the skin.

D. Work-up and Diagnostic Tests

The majority of patients with lymphedema can be diagnosed by history and physical examination alone. Laboratory tests are done for three reasons, however: to make the diagnosis when history and physical exam are equivocal, to rule out other causes of edema, and to determine the cause in cases of unexplained secondary lymphedema. For these reasons, the following laboratory tests may be performed:

1. Lymphangiography—a radiographic study that requires the use of a radiopaque dye to visualize anatomic details of the lymphatic channels. The radiopaque dye can damage the already impaired lymphatics, resulting in worsening of the lymphedema. Because of this concern, lymphangiography is rarely performed today.
2. Lymphoscintigraphy—a nuclear medicine study that uses a radioactive isotope-labeled colloid (gold or technetium attached to sulfur colloid or dextran) that is injected into the dorsal webspaces of the foot or hand. Clearance of the isotope-colloid over time can diagnose impaired lymphatic flow, quantify clearance rates, and determine location of obstructions. This test does not damage lymphatic channels and has become the standard diagnostic test for lymphedema.
3. Computerized tomography—CT scans have been used to diagnose soft tissue masses in patients

with lymphedema (i.e., to rule out the presence of lymphangiosarcoma) and to quantify limb size by cross-sectional area. It is primarily used for research purposes and is not useful for the routine diagnosis or treatment of lymphedema. It is useful as a diagnostic test to look for recurrent cancer in cases with a history of cancer.

4. Magnetic resonance imaging—MRI has become more useful in the diagnosis of lymphedema and in the quantification of edema in the extremities. It is primarily used for research purposes, but may become a good alternative to lymphoscintigraphy for the diagnosis and treatment of lymphedema.
5. Serologic tests—serologic tests for parasites such as *Wucheria bancrofti* can provide evidence of a previous history of filariasis. Eosinophilia and a peripheral blood smear can also be used to diagnose this disease.
6. Laboratory tests—serum albumin, total protein, electrolytes, urea nitrogen, creatinine, and liver function tests should be performed to rule out chronic disease as the cause of bilaterally symmetric lower extremity lymphedema.

IV. TREATMENT OF LYMPHEDEMA

Although the diagnosis of lymphedema is simple, lymphedema treatment is very challenging due to the treatment failures and patient compliance issues that often occur. In general, simpler treatment methods (elevation, compression, and lymph drainage) are recommended for all patients with newly diagnosed lymphedema. More complex treatment methods (medications, pumps, and surgery) are reserved for patients with uncontrolled lymphedema, despite good compliance with simpler therapies. There are many controversies among experts regarding the value of many therapies used to treat lymphedema, however, and great variations exist among Europe, Asia, and the United States in the treatment of this disease. The most commonly prescribed therapies, in order of simplicity, are listed below.

A. Medical Care

Prevention of minor trauma and skin care are very important issues in caring for patients with lymphedema. Elevation of the affected extremity with pillows, foam wedges, or Kodel slings are effective ways of reducing edema at night and during hospitalization. Elevation, combined with antibiotics, is the only method that should be used to treat the edema while the patient has acute cellulitis or lymphangitis. More aggressive therapy may be instituted 24–48 h after antibiotics have been administered and the signs of acute infection have begun to resolve. Elevation alone is not effective in the long-term management of lymphedema, however, and should be combined with the therapies outlined below. The following is a short summary of the medications used to treat lymphedema.

1. Antibiotics—antibiotics are usually only prescribed for episodes of acute cellulitis or lymphangitis. The most common species causing infection in these patients is *Streptococcus*. In patients with recurrent bouts of infection, however, antibiotics may be used to prevent these recurrences. Short courses of antibiotics may be given whenever minor skin trauma occurs (cat scratch, splinter, etc.) in the affected extremity. Long-term antibiotics at low-dose suppression doses may be needed for extreme cases.
2. Benzopyrones—benzopyrones (which include flavonoids and coumarins) are a family of compounds that bind to abnormally accumulated extravascular protein, creating a chemotactic compound 30 times more attractive to macrophages. This promotes phagocytosis and thereby reduces the high protein content that causes the "pitting" in lymphedema. Unfortunately, these compounds are not FDA approved and do have hepatotoxic side effects.

B. Compression

Compression is an effective way to control lymphedema. During the initial phases of lymphedema treatment, when the extremity is large, compression bandaging therapy (CBT) is helpful in reducing limb size. Once the limb volume has been reduced, elastic compression sleeves (upper extremity) or stockings (lower extremity) should be fitted, based on measurements taken by a trained garment fitter. Poorly fitted garments are either ineffective or may cause a tourniquet effect with worsening of the edema. The compression garment should provide at least 20–30 mmHg of graded compression and should extend proximal to the level of edema in the involved extremity. In more severe cases, custom garments may be needed with 30–40 mmHg of graded compression. When elastic compression garments fail to control lower extremity edema, nonelastic Velcro (Circaid) leggings are useful to control edema of the calf and ankle.

C. Lymph Drainage

Manual lymphatic drainage (MLD), first described by Vodder, is a form of lymphedema treatment that has become popular in Europe. Although there is much disagreement among different schools of MLD regarding the massage technique, MLD is a hands-on therapy that attempts to drain edema from the affected extremity into more proximal unaffected areas by manual massage. The unaffected proximal area is treated first, followed by massage from distal to proximal on the affected limb. MLD is usually combined with CBT during the initial treatment phase, followed by elastic compression garment use during the maintenance phase. MLD is best performed by licensed physical therapists with special training in MLD techniques.

D. Compression Pumps

Pneumatic compression pumps (PCP) have been useful in treating more severe forms of lymphedema or lymphedema that has failed the simpler therapy described above. These pumps use air pressure delivered to a sleeve with multiple overlapping air bladders in the sleeve that can be sequentially inflated with air to create a gradient of pressure from distal to proximal. Modern pumps can be adjusted for pressure, gradient, cycle time, and sleeve size. PCP has been condemned by MLD practitioners who claim that the old PCP devices damaged lymphatic channels by the high pressure exerted in the extremity. Modern lymphatic compression pumps no longer use high pressure, however, and are usually adjusted to pressures in the same range as elastic compression stockings. Limb edema will rapidly recur without the concomitant use of elastic compression stockings or Circaid leggings. For this reason, PCP are an adjunct to compression and elevation, not a replacement therapy.

E. Surgery

Surgery for lymphedema is usually reserved for patients who have failed medical management with the therapies listed above. Although numerous surgical procedures have been invented, only a few remain in use at this time. They include the following.

1. Excisional Procedures

The primary purpose of these procedures is to reduce the volume of the extremity by removal of excess subcutaneous tissue and skin, thereby reducing limb size. They include the following:

a. Total subcutaneous excision and skin grafting—this was first described by Charles. The main problems with the Charles procedure are skin graft breakdown, ulceration, poor cosmetic appearance, excessive scar formation, and edema of the foot or hand (distal to the excision).
b. Partial subcutaneous and skin excision—the preserved skin is used as flaps for primary closure of the excision site without skin grafts. The procedure is safest when done as a staged procedure. The main problems with this procedure are the need for multiple staged surgeries and recurrent edema in the preserved soft tissue. Long-term effectiveness in 10- to 15-year follow-up studies has been demonstrated.
c. Liposuction—liposuction has been used for milder cases of lymphedema, but has not gained widespread acceptance due to the high rate of edema recurrence. When combined with MLD and bandaging, however, good results have been shown with 5-year follow-up.

2. Physiologic Procedures

These procedures attempt to restore or improve lymphatic flow by bypassing the level of obstruction with lympholymphatic or lymphovenous shunts. Alternative methods try to establish communication between lymphatic-rich flaps and the edematous limb. They include the following:

a. Buried dermal flaps—this surgery, described by Thompson, attempts to establish new lymphatic connections between the skin's subdermal lymphatics and the deeper lymphatics contained within the muscles, using a deepithelialized skin flap (dermal flap) that is buried into the muscle. Although good results have been published, no study has proven that the buried dermal flap actually transports any lymph fluid. Most surgeons believe that the primary benefit of the procedure is the excision of excess skin and subcutaneous tissue, not the buried dermal flap component. As a consequence, this procedure has largely been abandoned.
b. Lymphovenous shunts—these procedures create a shunt between an obstructed lymph vessel or lymph node in the affected extremity to an unobstructed small vein. This requires tedious microsurgical anastomoses with 10-0 sutures. Blue dye is usually used to help identify the lymphatic channels. The main problem with these procedures is questionable long-term patency.

94

Thoracic and Abdominal Wall Reconstruction

Juliana E. Hansen, M.D.
Oregon Health Sciences University, Portland, Oregon, U.S.A.

Large defects of the thoracic and abdominal wall that result from trauma, tumor ablation, infection, or radiation may significantly impair function of those important structures, may expose vital organs with life-threatening consequences, and may cause gross deformity. Reconstruction of thoracic and abdominal wall defects should aim to restore structure and provide stable soft tissue coverage. Restoring structure will allow for normal respiration, protect viscera and vasculature, and correct or prevent hernias of the abdominal wall. Soft tissue reconstruction should provide stable coverage as well as a cosmetically acceptable result. Judicious use of skin, fascial, and bone grafts, soft tissue flaps, and alloplastic materials for skeletal and fascial support should be used for component restoration of complex defects.

I. CHEST WALL ANATOMY

A. The thoracic skeleton consists of 12 thoracic vertebrae, 12 pairs of ribs with associated costal cartilages, and the sternum. Posteriorly, all ribs articulate with the vertebrae. Anteriorly, the T1–7 costal cartilages articulate with the sternum. The T8–10 costal cartilages articulate with the cartilage above. T11–12 are floating. This structure provides the inherent flexibility of the chest wall necessary to accommodate respiration.

B. Each intercostal space contains three muscular layers and a neurovascular bundle. The external intercostal muscles, the internal intercostal muscles, and the innermost intercostal and transversus thoracis muscles of the chest wall correspond to the anatomy of the abdominal wall musculature. Arterial supply is from the posterior intercostal arteries, branches off the aorta, and the anterior intercostal arteries that are branches of the internal thoracic artery. The intercostal arteries, along with intercostal veins and nerves, run in the costal groove on the underside of each rib.

C. The thoracic skeleton houses both thoracic viscera (heart, great vessels, trachea, esophagus, lungs) and upper abdominal viscera (spleen, stomach, liver, adrenals, and upper poles of the kidneys). These are separated by the diaphragm.

D. Posterior chest wall muscles also include paraspinous muscles, serratus posterior, latissimus dorsi, and trapezius. Levator scapulae, rhomboids, serratus anterior, and pectoralis minor connect the scapulae to the chest wall. Anteriorly, the pectoralis major attaches the chest wall to the proximal humerus.

II. PHYSIOLOGY OF THE CHEST WALL

A. An intact chest wall maintains a negative intrapleural pressure with inspiration. As the diaphragm contracts and moves downward, the lung maintains its contiguity with the chest wall and air flows into the alveoli. With simple expiration, the diaphragm relaxes, the lung returns to its resting state, and the tidal volume is exhaled.

B. When maximal inspiratory effort is made, accessory muscles (primarily the sternocleidomastoids, scalenes, and external intercostals) are used to elevate the ribs and the sternum, allowing for an increased inhaled volume (inspiratory capacity).

C. Forced expiration is aided by contraction of the internal intercostals, the rectus abdominis, external oblique, internal oblique, and transversus abdominis muscles. Maximal expiratory effort causes the additional forced exhalation of the expiratory reserve volume, leaving only the residual volume in the lungs and airways.

D. Resection of a portion of the chest wall may impair the normal pulmonary mechanics. Baseline obstructive or restrictive diseases may significantly contribute to the morbidity of chest wall resection. Generally, a resection diameter of 5 cm is considered functionally significant, requiring rigid fixation to prevent flailing and maintain normal ventilation. In the patient with impaired baseline pulmonary function tests, a much smaller defect may cause functional problems.

III. PREOPERATIVE CONSIDERATIONS AND WORK-UP

A. Patients undergoing large composite resections should undergo preoperative pulmonary function tests and arterial blood gas. A thorough appreciation of any underlying pulmonary dysfunction is critical in planning the reconstruction. Patients with baseline lung disease may not be able to compensate well for a full-thickness defect and may require skeletal reconstruction for even a small (<5 cm) defect. Maintenance of spontaneous ventilation is one of the primary goals of chest wall reconstruction.

B. A thorough physical exam and medical history review should focus on previous incisions that would preclude the use of certain flaps:

- A prior posterolateral thoracotomy eliminates the use of the latissimus dorsi or serratus anterior on that side.
- Subcostal incisions divide the superior epigastric blood supply to the rectus abdominis muscle, thus eliminating the possibility of use of this muscle as a pedicled flap to the chest.
- Prior axillary dissection may also cause damage to the thoracodorsal vessels.
- Prior coronary bypass may have taken one or both of the internal thoracic vessels as bypass grafts, destroying the superior blood supply to the rectus abdominis muscle and the medial blood supply to the pectoralis major, eliminating its use as a pectoralis turnover flap.
- Congenital syndromes such as Poland syndrome may be associated with absence of the latissimus and serratus muscles.
- Prior repair of a pectus excavatum may destroy the medial blood supply to the pectoralis and the superior blood supply to the rectus, depending on the technique.
- The presence of atherosclerotic disease and thrombo-occlusive arterial or venous disease must also be considered when making a flap selection.

C. Adequate debridement is a first critical step toward obtaining a successful reconstruction. Exposed hardware, sternal wires, pacer wires, etc. should be removed whenever possible. Debridement of bone must be performed back to healthy, bleeding margins. A common situation is that of the infected and dehisced median sternotomy wound. In these cases, often the entire sternum and sometimes the costal cartilages require complete debridement to ensure adequate removal of infected or devitalized tissue. In grossly infected cases and in those with mediastinitis, debridement may be done as an initial stage, followed by flap closure when the wound is clean and granulating.

IV. REGIONAL FLAPS AVAILABLE FOR THORACIC RECONSTRUCTION

A. Pectoralis major:

Origin: clavicle, sternum, cartilage of upper 7 ribs

Insertion: humerus

Dominant pedicle: pectoral branch of thoracoacromial artery and venae comitantes

Secondary pedicle: perforating branches off the internal mammary vessels

B. Latissimus dorsi:

Origin: spinous processes of lower 6 thoracic vertebrae, thoracolumbar fascia, and iliac crest

Insertion: humerus

Dominant pedicle: thoracodorsal artery and venae comitantes

Secondary pedicle: perforating branches off posterior intercostal vessels

C. Serratus anterior:

Origin: upper 8 ribs

Insertion: scapula

Dominant pedicle: branches of thoracodorsal artery and lateral thoracic artery and venae comitantes

D. Trapezius:

Origin: external occipital protuberance, superior nuchal line, ligamentum nuchae, and spinous processes of C7–T12 vertebrae

Insertion: clavicle, scapula, and acromion

Dominant pedicle: transverse cervical artery and vein

Secondary pedicle: perforating branches of posterior intercostal vessels

E. Rectus abdominis:

Origin: pubic symphysis and crest

Insertion: costal cartilage of ribs 5–7

Dominant pedicle: superior epigastric artery and vein

Dominant pedicle: inferior epigastric artery and vein

Secondary pedicle: intercostal arteries and venae comitantes

F. Omentum:

Base origin: stomach, duodenum, gastrosplenic ligament

Distal insertion: transverse colon and gastrocolic ligament

Dominant pedicle: right gastroepiploic artery and vein

Dominant pedicle: left gastroepiploic artery and vein

G. Deltopectoral flap:

Dominant pedicle: perforating branches of internal mammary vessels

H. Intercostal flap:

Dominant pedicle: posterior intercostal arteries and venae comitantes

Dominant pedicle: anterior intercostal arteries and venae comitantes

I. Breast flap:

Dominant pedicle: branches off internal mammary vessels

Dominant pedicle: lateral thoracic and thoracoacromial arteries and venae comitantes

Secondary pedicle: perforating branches off intercostal vessels

V. FLAP CHOICE BY ANATOMIC LOCATION

A. Anterior Chest: Pedicled Flaps Available for Use in Reconstruction

1. Pectoralis major: This flap can be used as a muscle or musculocutaneous flap, based on either its main pedicle arising from the thoracoacromial artery or based on its secondary blood supply (perforators from the internal mammary artery). For upper chest wall lesions, the insertion onto the humerus is divided and the entire broad flat muscle is elevated, leaving the thoracoacromial pedicle as the point of rotation. The flap can be advanced medially or rotated superiorly. For midsternal or lower lesions, the flap may be used as a muscle-only turnover flap based on the perforators off the internal mammary artery (Fig. 1).
2. Latissimus dorsi: This is a large, broad, and reliable muscle that can be designed as either a muscle or musculocutaneous flap. Based on its dominant pedicle (thoracodorsal artery), it is released from its origin and can be released from its insertion as well, tunneled through the axilla, and used to cover the anterolateral chest wall.
3. Rectus abdominis: This muscle is very commonly used for both chest wall and breast reconstruction. If a skin paddle is desired, it can be designed either vertically (VRAM flap) or transversely (TRAM flap). The pedicled flap used for the chest wall is based on the superior pedicle (superior epigastric artery, off of the internal mammary artery). When the internal mammary artery has been disrupted, it is possible to raise a pedicled flap based on intercostal, musculophrenic, and costomarginal artery contributions to the superior epigastric artery. Care must be taken, however, to limit the dissection of the upper muscle from the chest wall when raising the flap.

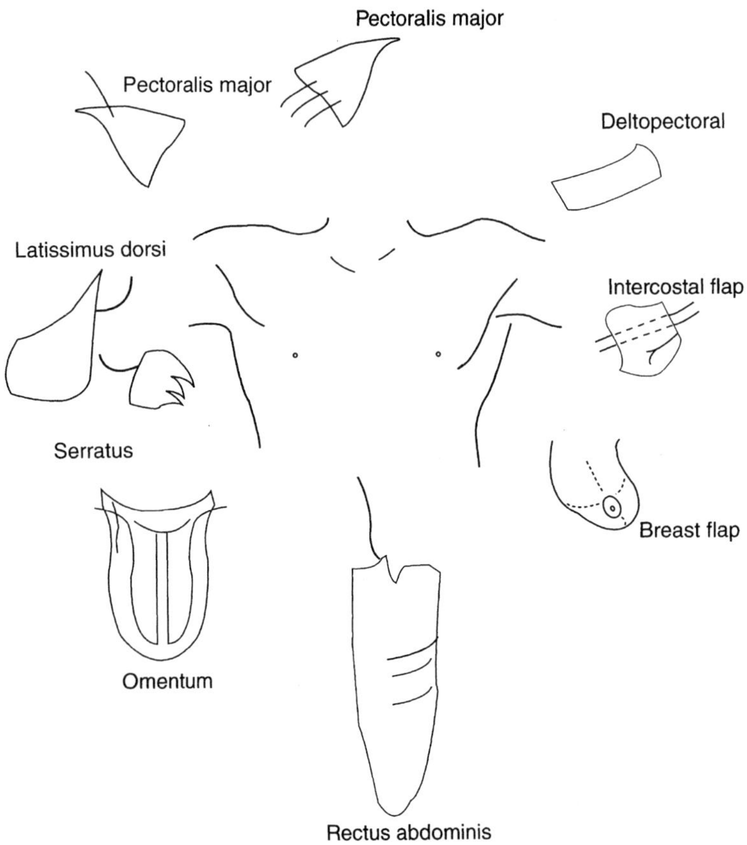

Figure 1 Pedicled flaps available for reconstruction of anterior chest wall.

4. Serratus anterior: This flap can be raised alone or along with the latissimus for coverage of anterolateral chest wall lesions based on a large branch off the thoracodorsal artery. The lateral thoracic artery supplies the upper slips of muscle. Harvest of the upper half of the muscle causes winging of the scapula, however. The small amount of muscle available for use as compared to the latissimus limits the usefulness of this as a pedicled flap when harvested alone.
5. Omentum: Omental flaps can be harvested through a laparotomy or laparoscopically, based on either the right or left gastroepiploic artery. The flap is tunneled into the chest wall defect and skin grafted. This flap is an excellent choice when soft tissue only is needed. It can also be used in full-thickness defects when skeletal reconstruction has been accomplished with alloplastic material. Because it lacks inherent rigidity, it is not a good choice to use alone in full-thickness defects.
6. Deltopectoral flap: This skin flap is based on perforators from the internal mammary artery. It can be deepithelialized and used as a turnover flap or as a rotation flap, or the distal-most portion may be used as a tubed pedicled flap with division of the pedicle and return of the proximal portion back to the donor site at a second stage. The donor site requires grafting and is unsightly.
7. Intercostal flap: Anterolateral chest wall defects requiring both soft tissue and skeletal support may be reconstructed with an intercostal musculocutaneous rib flap. The intercostal vessels of the rib selected for the flap provide the pedicle. The flap can be transferred using either a transpleural intrathoracic approach, maintaining a layer of parietal pleura on the rib segment, or using an extrapleural technique. The 9th or 10th ribs are most commonly used. A musculocutaneous flap alone may also be useful for both intrathoracic and external chest wall defects.

8. Breast flaps: As a last resort, breast flaps may supply ample, well-vascularized tissue for anterior chest wall defects. The donor site has enough laxity to allow primary closure of the donor defect. The donor site defect is quite disfiguring, however. The flap may be designed from a portion of the breast, the entire breast, or as an extended flap including the surrounding chest wall skin.

B. Posterior Chest Wall: Pedicled Flaps Available for Reconstruction

1. Trapezius: Limiting flap elevation to the middle and lower portions of the muscle minimizes the shoulder droop deformity that can develop after loss of trapezius function. The blood supply is from ascending and descending branches of the transverse cervical artery. Muscle-only or musculocutaneous flaps can reach the upper central area of the back (Fig. 2).
2. Latissimus dorsi: For posterior thoracic defects, the latissimus can be used either based on its dominant thoracodorsal pedicle or as a turnover muscle flap based on the medial blood supply (perforator arteries of the intercostal and lumbar vessels). This muscle will provide excellent coverage for scapular defects as well as defects of the lower portions of the posterior thorax.

VI. FREE FLAP COVERAGE

Free flap coverage is an option when no local or regional flaps are suitable for use.

A. Muscle/Musculocutaneous Free Flaps

1. Latissimus dorsi:

   Origin: spinous processes of lower 6 thoracic vertebrae, thoracolumbar fascia, and iliac crest

   Insertion: humerus

   Dominant pedicle: thoracodorsal artery and venae comitantes

2. Serratus anterior:

   Origin: upper 8 ribs

   Insertion: scapula

   Dominant pedicle: branches of thoracodorsal artery and venae comitantes

3. Rectus abdominis:

   Origin: pubic symphysis and crest

   Insertion: costal cartilage of ribs 5–7

   Dominant pedicle: inferior epigastric artery and vein

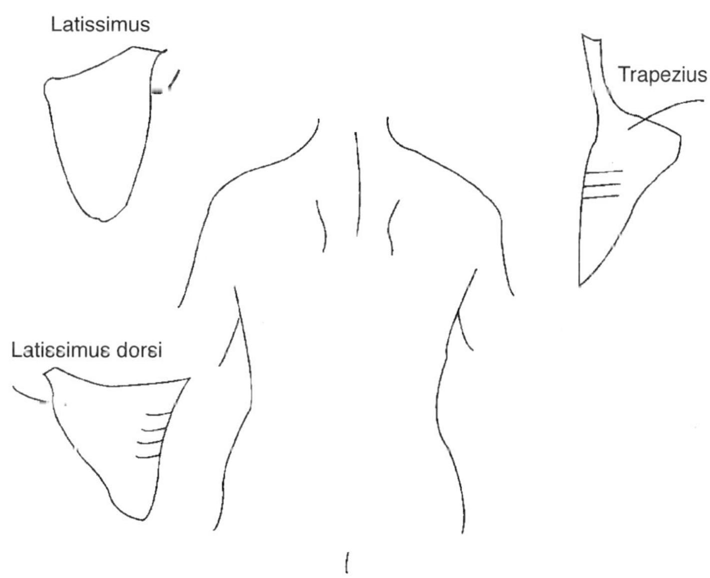

Figure 2 Pedicled flaps available for reconstruction of posterior chest wall.

4. Gracilis:

   Origin: pubic symphysis

   Insertion: tibia

   Dominant pedicle: branch of medial circumflex femoral artery and venae comitantes

B. Flaps for Fasciocutaneous Coverage

1. Radial/ulnar forearm flap:

   Pedicle: radial artery or ulnar artery and venae comitantes

2. Lateral arm flap:

   Pedicle: posterior radial collateral artery and venae comitantes

C. Osteocutaneous Flaps

1. Fibular flap:

   Pedicle: peroneal artery and venae comitantes

2. Scapular flap:

   Pedicle: terminal branches of the circumflex scapular artery and venae comitantes

3. Iliac crest and deep circumflex groin flap:

   Pedicle: deep circumflex iliac artery and venae comitantes

VII. SKELETAL RECONSTRUCTION

A. In small (<5 cm) defects, restoration of structural support may not be necessary. Muscle, musculocutaneous, or fasciocutaneous flaps will generally provide adequate stability.

B. Defects greater than 5 cm generally require skeletal reconstruction to prevent paradoxical motion of the chest wall with respiration and to protect vital organs.

C. The presence of baseline pulmonary dysfunction, the location of the defect, and the rigidity of the flap available for reconstruction will help determine the need for skeletal stabilization.

D. Autogenous tissue:

   - Bone grafts: Segmental or split ribs are most commonly used. Iliac crest may also be used as a source of bone graft. Rigid fixation of grafts with trabecular bone contact between graft and bone at the margin of the defect will provide the best chance for revascularization and minimize resorption. Not more than two ribs should be harvested adjacent to each other to prevent destabilizing the donor site.
   - Bone flaps: Pedicled bone flaps include intercostal rib flaps and scapular osteocutaneous flaps. These vascularized bone flaps have less chance of resorption than grafts. Free composite flaps are also potential sources of skeletal and soft tissue coverage. Free osteocutaneous flaps available include radial forearm, scapula, iliac crest, and fibula flaps.

E. Alloplastic materials:

   - Many different alloplastic materials are available to provide skeletal stabilization. There are meshes (nylon and polypropylene) and sheets of material such as GorTex that can be sewn to periosteum on bone at the wound margins.
   - Alloplastic prostheses are more prone to infection than autogenous reconstructions. If a chronic infection develops with alloplastic material in place, it can be recalcitrant to treatment unless the material is removed.
   - Despite a tight intraoperative repair, flaccidity may develop with time.
   - Methyl methacrylate is a more rigid material that can provide rigidity and that can be custom-molded to provide a desired contour. The plastic may be shaped and allowed to harden, sandwiched between two layers of mesh to facilitate fixation of the implant. Though rigid protection may be desired in such areas as large anterior chest wall defects to protect the heart and great vessels, methyl methacrylate reconstructions can be more problematic than mesh alone, with higher infection and exposure rates.

VIII. ABDOMINAL WALL ANATOMY

A. The abdominal wall is made up of:

   - Paired rectus abdominis muscles centrally
   - Paired pyramidalis muscles inferiorly
   - Three pairs of lateral muscles: the external oblique, the internal oblique, and the transversus abdominis

B. It is the fascial extensions of the lateral musculature that envelop the rectus abdominis and pyramidalis muscles, creating the rectus sheath:

- Above the arcuate (semicircular) line, which runs at the level of the anterior superior iliac spines, there are strong anterior and posterior layers of the rectus sheath. The anterior layer is made up of the external oblique aponeurosis and half of the internal oblique aponeurosis. The posterior sheath consists of half of the internal oblique aponeurosis and the transversus abdominis aponeurosis.
- Inferior to the arcuate line, all of the layers pass anterior to the rectus muscles.

C. Multiple tendinous inscriptions attach the muscle to the anterior fascia. It is these insertions that are responsible for the "six-pack" appearance of the abdominal wall in persons with well-developed musculature.

D. The linea alba is the tendinous raphe that denotes the midline of the abdominal wall, running from the xyphoid process to the symphysis pubis. It is made up of the interlacing aponeurotic fibers of the internal oblique, external oblique, and transversus abdominis muscles. The umbilicus, which crosses through the linea alba, represents the remnants of the umbilical cord, urachus, and yolk stalk. Though these structures close spontaneously a few days after birth, the vestiges remain attached to the deep surface of the umbilicus.

E. The blood supply to the abdominal wall comes from the internal mammary artery, intercostals, the external iliac artery, and the femoral artery.

- In the upper abdomen, the superior epigastric artery is the abdominal extension of the internal mammary artery. It supplies the rectus abdominis muscle and upper abdominal skin.
- Thoracic 8–12th intercostal arteries and segmental lumbar vessels supply the lateral abdominal wall.
- The deep inferior epigastric artery arises from the external iliac artery, supplying the rectus muscles from below and the lower abdominal skin through musculocutaneous perforators.
- There are anastomoses between the superior and the inferior epigastric vessels in the rectus muscle, allowing the muscle and overlying skin to be harvested based on either one of the two blood supplies.
- A deep circumflex iliac artery also branches from the external iliac or the femoral and supplies the iliac crest and surrounding soft tissues.
- The superficial inferior epigastric artery and superficial circumflex iliac arteries are branches off the femoral artery. They run superolaterally to supply the lower lateral abdominal skin and the inguinal ligament area.

IX. PREOPERATIVE PREPARATION BEFORE ABDOMINAL WALL RECONSTRUCTION

A. A thorough understanding of the cause of the defect is critical in planning the reconstruction.

B. Enterocutaneous fistulae must be controlled prior to coverage.

C. A history of radiation is important since all tissues in the radiated field may be severely compromised and unable to support the use of a nonvascularized graft. Pedicled flaps should not be detached when placed into a compromised radiated bed, as they may not be able to reestablish adequate vascularity to survive without the vascular pedicle. Radiation-induced arteritis may obliterate even large vessels, such as the iliac system. As direct line inflow is required for pedicled flaps, the rectus abdominis and all thigh flaps may not be usable after pelvic radiation.

D. A careful examination of pulses should be done and duplex studies and/or arteriogram considered before planning flap reconstruction.

E. Nutritional status may be very poor in patients with chronic open wounds or fistulae. Enteral or parenteral supplementation should be considered and positive nitrogen balance achieved to optimize wound healing.

X. ABDOMINAL WALL CLOSURE WITH EXISTING TISSUES

A. In any location, when all components of the abdominal wall are present, relaxing incisions or component separation can be used to facilitate what would otherwise be a tight or impossible closure.

B. Relaxing incisions can be placed unilaterally or bilaterally in the external oblique fascia, just lateral to the rectus muscles. These incisions are made generously, significantly longer than the area of tight fascial closure. This enables the rectus muscles and surrounding sheath to be transposed medially for several centimeters, closing moderately sized defects.

C. Component separation of the anterior abdominal wall can also be used for tight closures or when there is a unilateral abdominal wall defect. The anterior rectus sheath can be used alone as a medially based turnover flap. Alternatively, by dissecting between the external and internal oblique muscle planes and between the rectus abdominis and the posterior sheath to separate the laminae, the anterior sheath, rectus muscle, internal oblique muscle and transversus abdominis muscle can be transposed medially up to 10 cm in the midabdominal region.

D. Skin grafts directly applied to exposed bowel/omentum are also an option in complex cases with large full-thickness abdominal wall defects. Skin grafts do take well on exposed bowel or intestine, although the patient is left with a hernia that will require secondary reconstruction. Removal of a healed skin graft from intestine is technically difficult and has a high risk of enterotomy.

XI. REGIONAL FLAPS AVAILABLE FOR ABDOMINAL WALL RECONSTRUCTION

A. Rectus abdominis muscle flap; TRAM or VRAM flaps:

Origin: pubic symphysis and crest

Insertion: costal cartilage of ribs 5–7

Dominant pedicle: superior epigastric artery and vein

Dominant pedicle: inferior epigastric artery and vein

Secondary pedicle: intercostal arteries and venae comitantes

B. External oblique flap:

Origin: lower 8 ribs

Insertion: iliac crest and linea semilunaris

Dominant pedicle: lateral cutaneous branches of intercostal vessels

C. Groin flap:

Dominant pedicle: superficial circumflex iliac artery, vein, and venae comitantes

D. Tensor facia lata flap:

Origin: anterior superior iliac spine

Insertion: iliotibial tract

Dominant pedicle: ascending branch of the lateral circumflex femoral artery and venae comitantes

E. Rectus femoris flap:

Origin: ilium and acetabulum

Insertion: patella

Dominant pedicle: descending branch of lateral circumflex femoral artery and venae comitantes

F. Gracilis flap:

Origin: pubic symphysis

Insertion: tibia

Dominant pedicle: branch of medial circumflex femoral artery and venae comitantes

G. Omentum:

Base origin: stomach, duodenum, gastrosplenic ligament

Distal insertion: transverse colon and gastrocolic ligament

Dominant pedicle: right gastroepiploic artery and vein

Dominant pedicle: left gastroepiploic artery and vein

XII. FLAP CHOICE BY LOCATION

A. Epigastrium

1. The omentum is ideal for providing soft tissue coverage in this area. Pedicled on either the right or left gastroepiploic arteries, the intact omentum provides ample well-vascularized tissue that can cover prosthetic mesh and easily accept a skin graft.
2. The rectus abdominis muscle inserts on the costal cartilages of the 5th, 6th, and 7th ribs. The superior blood supply comes from the superior epigastric artery, which enters the muscle at its

posteromedial aspect. Because many epigastric defects involve the superior aspect of the muscle, the rectus abdominis does not tend to be used for closure of wounds in this area. If intact, however, this flap should be considered.

3. The rectus femoris muscle originates from the anterior superior iliac spine and the acetabulum, inserting on the patellar tendon. The blood supply is off the descending branch of the lateral femoral circumflex artery. The arc of rotation centers on this pedicle, about 8 cm below the inguinal ligament. If the flap is designed with either medial or lateral fasciocutaneous extensions, it can reach to the upper abdomen. Donor functional defects include loss of terminal leg extension.

B. Central/Suprapubic Defects

1. The tensor fascia lata originates from the anterior superior iliac spine, inserting on the iliotibial tract of the lateral thigh. Based on the ascending branch of the lateral femoral circumflex artery and venae comitantes, this flap can be mobilized to include a large segment of fascia lata, providing vascularized fascial support for the abdominal wall (Fig. 3).
2. The rectus femoris can be harvested alone or with fasciocutaneous extensions and will reach the middle and lower abdomen easily. There is significant donor site morbidity with loss of terminal leg extension.
3. Omental flaps can be used to provide soft tissue filler for abdominal wall defects extending down into the suprapubic area. In order to gain length, the flap can be pedicled on either the right or left gastroepiploic arteries and backcut as needed.
4. The rectus abdominis can be used as either a superiorly or inferiorly based flap to provide contralateral abdominal wall coverage in these areas.
5. The groin flap can be elevated between the femoral vessels and the posterior iliac spine. Based on the superficial circumflex iliac artery and vein, this flap can provide fasciocutaneous coverage to the lower abdomen. Prior tissue expansion can be used to expand flap dimensions.

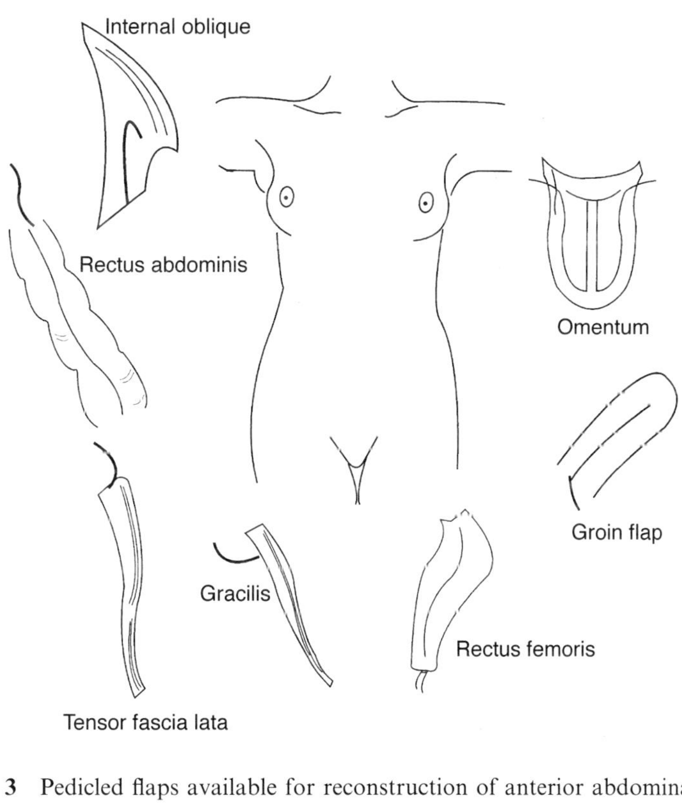

Figure 3 Pedicled flaps available for reconstruction of anterior abdominal wall.

6. The gracilis flap, based on the medial circumflex femoral artery, can provide limited coverage for the lower abdomen and groin. A skin paddle can be harvested with the flap and designed either vertically or horizontally.
7. Based on the ascending branch of the deep circumflex iliac artery, the internal oblique flap can reach the lower abdomen and groin. A segmental (reverse) flap based on the lower thoracic arteries can reach the upper central abdomen.

C. Flank Defects

1. The rectus abdominis flap can be based either superiorly or inferiorly to cover upper and lower lateral abdominal wall defects (Fig. 4).
2. The rectus femoris will reach the flanks and can be designed with a skin island. It may be tunneled subcutaneously as needed.
3. The tensor fascia lata muscle can be harvested with a large strip of fascia lata, providing an excellent source of abdominal wall support. Skin grafts are generally used for coverage, though a skin island can also be designed with this flap.

XIII. FREE FLAP COVERAGE

Free flaps are always an option for coverage of specific problem areas when no regional tissues are available.

A. Latissimus dorsi muscle or musculocutaneous flap:

    Origin: spinous processes of lower 6 thoracic vertebrae, thoracolumbar fascia, and iliac crest

    Insertion: humerus

    Dominant pedicle: thoracodorsal artery and venae comitantes

B. Forearm fasciocutaneous flap:

    Pedicle: radial artery or ulnar artery and venae comitantes

C. Anterior thigh flap:

    Dominant pedicle: descending branch of lateral circumflex femoral artery and venae comitantes

D. Scapula fasciocutaneous flap:

    Pedicle: circumflex scapular artery and venae comitantes

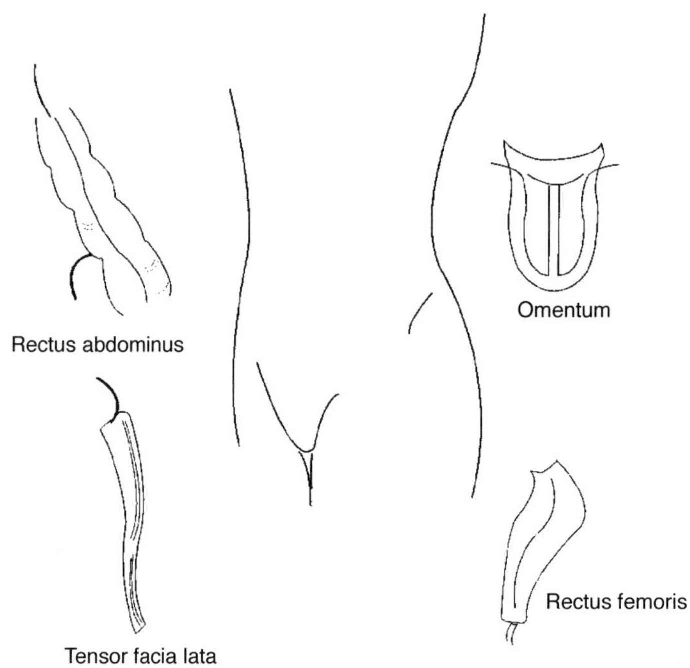

Figure 4 Pedicled flaps available for reconstruction of lateral abdominal chest wall.

XIV. FASCIAL RECONSTRUCTION

Ideally, fascial defects should be reconstructed for structural support. When all abdominal wall components are present in the remaining tissue, relaxing incisions or component separation can be used to close fascial defects. Prosthetic mesh is an alternative.

A. Permanent (polypropylene) mesh is very useful in closing acute fascial defects and repairing large hernias. There is no donor site morbidity. When sewn adequately to innervated muscle fascia, it can provide tight structural support for the abdominal viscera. Mesh can be used in the setting of an open wound when necessary, as granulation tissue will grow through the mesh. Mesh, however, can become infected, cause discomfort, and induce enteric fistula formation.

B. Absorbable mesh (polyglycolic mesh) can be used to prevent evisceration while an open wound is granulating and closing. The advantage is absence of a permanent foreign body in a contaminated area. Though chronic infections are not a problem, the structural support is lost with time and hernia development will occur.

C. Mixed success has been obtained using free fascial grafts to provide structural support. Fascia lata is a readily available source of donor fascia.

XV. TISSUE EXPANSION

Tissue expansion is most appropriately used as a secondary method of reconstruction for improvement of cosmetically unacceptable areas. Expanded local tissues can be used to resurface areas previously skin grafted or areas of severe scarring.

95

Pressure Ulcers

Steven E. Greer, M.D.
New York, New York, U.S.A.

Thomas Mustoe, M.D.
Northwestern University Feinberg School of Medicine, Chicago, Illinois, U.S.A.

Despite the numerous surgical procedures described for treatment of pressure ulcers, surgical flap coverage has not been established as the gold standard of therapy for pressure ulcers. Proper patient education, social support, dedicated wound care, and ulcer prevention are considered more important in achieving complete healing. Unfortunately, these aspects of care can require tremendous healthcare resources and are often not feasible, thereby necessitating a flap. In addition, pressure ulcers involving bone may not heal without surgical closure, and conservative care may take months to achieve healing. In this context, flap closure often becomes an important adjunct to therapy. Flap coverage, however, is plagued by a substantial initial failure rate and an extremely high recurrence rate, with some studies indicating recurrence rates as high as 60–80%. With no consistently effective treatment other than prevention, pressure ulcers represent a considerable morbidity in certain patient populations and a significant economic burden. As a result, the plastic surgeon should have an influential role in the medical community treating this challenging multidisciplinary problem.

I. ETIOLOGY

As the term implies, pressure ulcers (a better term than pressure sores or decubitus ulcers) are an ulceration in the skin (except for stage I ulcers) caused in part by excessive force loads for a duration of time sufficient to cause ischemia and tissue damage. It is believed that the damage often occurs from a deep-to-superficial direction, with muscle being more susceptible to ischemia than connective tissue, and with skin being the most resistant to damage and the last to ulcerate. Although fat is more resistant to ischemia than muscle, the subcutaneous fat is the most susceptible to injury because of its relatively poor blood supply. Large ulcers extending to underlying bone that seem to be the result of egregious neglect may easily develop during a single incident of prolonged immobility. Family members often appreciate this explanation. Controversy still remains as to the precise nature of the destructive force.

A. Pressure

Although definitive evidence is lacking, it has been generally accepted that external pressure greater than the 32 mmHg of capillary pressure is the threshold pressure required to cause ischemia in tissue. Compressed skin is more susceptible to infection and edema, making it more prone to ulceration. When repeated, ischemic events that alone would be subclinical can cause ulceration through an ischemia-reperfusion injury mechanism, in which the initial event leads to polymorphonuclear leukocyte accumulation and endothelial damage. A second ischemic event can then cause an overwhelming tissue insult with resulting necrosis.

B. Sheer Forces

Friction damages skin and makes it more vulnerable to ischemia from pressure. Macerated skin secondary to incontinence is more prone to sheer-force injury.

C. Nonforceful Skin Breakdown

1. Malnutrition
2. Urinary or fecal incontinence

II. DEMOGRAPHICS

A. Prevalence

Accurate data are difficult to collect:

1. Hospitals and nursing homes: 3–11%
2. Spinal cord injury or rehabilitation centers: 20–30%

B. Incidence

Most pressure ulcers originally develop during an acute-care hospitalization. Certain populations are at high risk:

1. All hospital patients: 1–3%
2. Bed-bound hospital patients: 10–15%
3. ICU patients: 33%
4. Hip fracture patients: as high as 66%

III. STAGING

The accepted staging system has four stages: I–IV. Ulcers do not always progress or heal in an orderly stage-by-stage fashion. They may start as a stage IV ulcer.

1. Stage I—nonblanchable erythema of intact skin.
2. Stage II—partial-thickness skin loss presenting clinically as an abrasion or blister.
3. Stage III—full-thickness skin loss extending to but not through underlying fascia. This is the most difficult stage to accurately identify. Based on the common misconception that a stage III is "less severe" than a stage IV, the latter is often underdiagnosed for several reasons. Bony involvement can be more difficult to establish with certainty, and the physician or other caretaker may be reluctant to diagnose the more severe stage, particularly if adequacy of care is being questioned.
4. Stage IV—full-thickness skin loss with involvement of underlying muscle, bone, tendon, ligament, or joint capsule.
5. Unstageable ulcers—closed pressure ulcers with no or small skin openings cannot be staged. Ulcers with non-debrided eschar cannot be staged.

IV. ASSESSMENT AND PREVENTION

A. Risk Factors

One must be aware of and assess for recognized risk factors in order to prevent pressure ulcers. In general, the data indicate that pressure ulcers are a disease of the immobile elderly. The Norton and Braden scales are two popular risk assessment tools. In these scales, points are attached to risk factors, with multiple risk factors dramatically increasing the risk of pressure ulcer formation. Risk factors, in order of strength, are:

1. Mobility limitations, including paraplegia and quadriplegia
2. Incontinence
3. Nutritional factors
4. Altered consciousness
5. Increased age
6. Dry skin
7. Diabetes mellitus

B. Assessing for Signs of Stage I Ulcers

Seemingly insignificant nonblanching erythema can be the early sign heralding a more serious pressure ulcer. Blanching erythema is less serious and reversible within hours. Dark skin is difficult to assess, although warmth and induration are subtle warning signs. Stage I pressure sores are at high risk for progression to more advanced stages if the pressure insults are repeated.

C. Prevention

Since a large proportion of pressure ulcers develops during an acute-care hospitalization (e.g., surgical procedure), surgeons should be aware of preventive measures.

1. Pressure relief:
   - The operating table is a potential source of pressure if the patient is not positioned properly with adequate cushioning. Particularly at risk are the pressure points, including the occiput, heels, elbows, and sacrum.
   - Turning the patient every 2 h in bed.
   - Special pressure-relief devices for the heels.
   - Minimizing elevation of the head of the bed to reduce sacral sheer and pressure.
   - Minimize dragging the patient while repositioning, which causes friction.
2. Special pressure-relief surfaces—consistent with other areas in clinical wound healing research, there are only modest data in the form of prospective randomized trials supporting the effectiveness of specialized air flotation beds in preventing or treating pressure ulcers. Most studies, however, do indicate that some benefit is gained from their use, but the superiority of one type over another has not been conclusively determined. The different types are:
   - Static foam mattress onlays.
   - Low air-loss beds [Flexicair (Hill-Rom), KinAir (KCI)]—these beds can elevate the head and foot of the bed like normal beds and are not heavy or cumbersome. These mattresses are inflated by fan propulsion of air. They are also designed to have a slow air loss through the material, which helps to dry skin moisture. They have achieved widespread use for high-risk patients to prevent ulcerations.
   - Air-fluidized beds [Clinitron (Hill-Rom), FluidAir (KCI)]—these beds are very heavy and filled with silicone beads that become suspended and fluidized by fan propulsion of air. Like low air-loss beds, the air escapes through the fabric by design. Dehydration from increased insensible losses and hypothermia are real concerns, particularly in the spinal cord injury patient without autoregulatory neurologic function. These beds are expensive, costing up to $100 per day. Their efficacy in preventing ulceration or complications from surgery has not been determined in rigorous prospective randomized studies. Nevertheless, they do reduce pressure beneath pressure points to less than 32 mmHg, and they have gained fairly wide acceptance from plastic surgeons who prefer this type of bed for post–flap surgery pressure relief.
3. Skin care—elderly patients tend to have dry skin, which is a risk factor. Moisturizers are likely beneficial.
4. Incontinence:
   - The skin should be cleansed promptly after an episode of incontinence.
   - Urinary incontinence should be treated with a catheter until a more permanent solution is determined.
   - Fecal incontinence is more difficult to treat. Tube feeds frequently cause diarrhea. These can be adjusted to minimize the incontinence. For the patient with no hope of recovering voluntary bowel function, a colostomy can be an appropriate option and may be required to allow a pressure ulcer to heal if the stools are consistently liquid. However, most paraplegics without voluntary bowel function can achieve satisfactory elimination regularly without resorting to a colostomy.
5. Nutrition (see Chapter 7).

V. COMPLICATIONS OF PRESSURE ULCERS

A. Osteomyelitis: Stage IV ulcers with bony involvement are considered to have osteomyelitis until proven otherwise. Swab cultures or bone scans are of little value (Agency for Health Care Policy and Research). The gold standard for diagnosis is bone biopsy and quantitative culture. Physical examination, however, is also very useful. If the ulcer extends to exposed bone on digital exam, then the bone can be considered to be involved. The gold standard for treatment is bone resection (taking no more than necessary in order to avoid future imbalance that may predispose the patient to recurrence), bone culture, and myocutaneous flap coverage with perioperative antibiotic therapy. MRI or nuclear medicine scans can occasionally be useful for ruling out osteomyelitis, and therefore reducing the course of antibiotic therapy, but bone biopsy with culture is more definitive. Refractory ulcers with hip joint involvement may require a girdlestone arthroplasty procedure.

B. Heterotopic bone formation
C. Endocarditis
D. Abdominal and pelvic abscess
E. Bacteremia, sepsis
F. Perineal-urethral fistula
G. Meningitis
H. Maggot infestation
I. Squamous cell carcinoma (Marjolin's ulcers)

VI. TREATMENT

A. Patient Education, Psychiatric Counseling, and Social Support

Perhaps in no other disorder is the bio-psycho-social model of medicine more relevant. Surgical intervention is doomed to fail without proper resources and teaching for the patient and family. The plastic surgeon must form a good partnership with his/her hospital social services.

B. Pressure Relief

Discussed in Sec. IV.C.1.

C. Contractures

Joint contractures can increase pressure over the more prominent flexed joints. Splints should be used as prevention. When contractures exist, they should be surgically released.

D. Spasm Relief

Hip flexion spasm produces tension on most flap closures and must be treated to prevent dehiscence of the suture lines. Dantrolene, baclofen, and diazepam are effective antispasmodic medications. Rhizotomy and nerve blocks are other options.

E. General Wound Care (See Chapter 7)

1. The ulcer needs to be properly debrided of all necrotic tissue, usually in the operating room.
2. Pain and hemorrhage often prevent adequate bedside debridement.
3. In patients who have minimal necrotic debris or who are too debilitated to tolerate surgical debridement, enzymatic debridement can be very useful. Several enzymatic debridement agents are now available clinically.
4. Malnutrition and wound infection also need to be addressed. In general, a serum albumin of less than 2.5 g/dL leads to an unacceptable surgical failure rate. In such patients, definitive flap closure should be delayed until the nutritional status can be improved.
5. A useful clinical sign is the ability of the wound to generate healthy granulation tissue, which is an indication that the patient is capable of healing a surgical wound and that the wound bacterial counts are low enough to allow uncomplicated healing.

F. Wound Care Specific to Pressure Ulcers

1. Stage I—moisturizers to prevent dryness. Promptly clean away incontinence. Avoid skin massages. Careful avoidance of sheering forces, and adequate pressure relief.
2. Stage II—no debridement necessary. Occlusive dressings such as polyurethane film or hydrocolloid are best and can be left in place for several days. To prevent damage to surrounding skin from dressing changes, a border of hydrocolloid or skin sealant is useful. Avoid direct contact of surrounding skin to adhesive tape.
3. Stage III—sharp debridement is essential. Leave the wound covered for 12–24 h after debridement to prevent hemorrhage. Then, saline wet-to-moist gauze dressing changes are preferred. Highly absorptive dressings such as alginates, hydrocolloid beads, foams, or hydrogels can be used for the draining wound. Special adjuvant therapies, such as electrical stimulation or subatmospheric dressings (vacuum assisted) may be helpful, but their role has not been defined by large prospective randomized clinical trials (see Chapter 7).
4. Stage IV—same as stage III. Appropriate bone debridement, as necessary.
5. For all wounds, avoid heat lamps and destructive agents such as Dakin's solution (essentially bleach) or hydrogen peroxide. Dakin's solution can be useful initially in a grossly infected or contaminated wound, but should be omitted as

soon as the wound is cleaner to avoid tissue destruction from the solution itself.

6. Topical antibiotics have a minor role in pressure sores. Adequate absorption of exudate and elimination of all necrotic material are the mainstays of treatment. Silver sulfadiazene (Silvadene) is a broad-spectrum antibiotic that does not generate bacterial resistance; it can be useful in selected cases.

G. Assessment of Healing

1. Wound measurements are difficult to obtain conveniently. At best, any measurement is simply an index of wound progression. The gold standard 2-dimensional method is to trace the wound perimeter on clear sheets and to use digital planimetry techniques to calculate the area. Dental alginate, a liquid that congeals into a rubbery material, is good for measuring the 3-dimensional volume of a wound, but is impractical for other than research purposes. Photography (digital photography) is becoming the documentation of choice for wounds of all types. A useful simple measure is to measure the depth and the diameter at the two longest axes—these can then be followed over time.
2. The wound bed should be beefy red with good granulation tissue if it is healing. Yellow exudate or eschar should be eliminated with dressings and/or debridement.
3. Odor is a sign of possible wound infection or high bacteria counts, both of which will prevent healing.
4. Ulcer margins should be thin with advancing new epithelium. A thickened, rolled-under ulcer edge is termed epiboly. The associated contact inhibition impairs epithelial margin progression.
5. Approximately 50–90% of stage II ulcers will heal by 3 months, while only 20% of Stage III and IV ulcers will heal by 3 months.

H. Surgery

If all of the methods described above fail, surgical flap coverage of pressure ulcers is an option. Ulcers with complications such as osteomyelitis, if left untreated, can lead to progressive amputations of the entire lower half of the body. Therefore, flap coverage is warranted even with the high failure rates mentioned. It is important to appreciate the finite resource of tissue in the "tissue bank account" available to each patient for flaps. Each flap burns bridges for future procedures. For this reason, even partially reducing the size of an ulcer is beneficial by decreasing the required size of the flap.

1. General technique—small ulcers can occasionally be closed by simply excising the bursal sac and primary wound edge advancement. For larger ulcers, the bursal sac is excised, bony prominences are contoured, and a thick myocutaneous flap is inset. Ulcers less than 10 cm in diameter can usually be treated with local tissue flaps. Chronic ulcers that have been present for many years should be biopsied for possible squamous cell carcinoma. Although tissue expanders can be placed at the time of operative debridement to reduce the tension of the flap closure at a later date, tissue expansion in this setting has a very high rate of infection and wound dehiscence. Tissue expansion in generally not recommended in this setting.
2. Sacral ulcers—these ulcers are usually shallow with exposed sacrum. A gluteus maximus fasciocutaneous or myocutaneous flap can be unilaterally rotated (Fig. 1A) or rotated bilaterally for larger defects (Fig. 1B). The lumbosacral flap is another option (Fig. 1C).
3. Ischial ulcers—the ischium should be partially resected and contoured, but radical ischiectomy should be avoided. The gluteus maximus myocutaneous flap can be rotated downward and medially (Fig. 1E). The inferior gluteal myocutaneous flap can also be used. The gracilis flap (Fig. 1F), tensor fascia lata flap (Fig. 1G), and various hamstring-based myocutaneous flaps (biceps femoris, semimembranous, semitendinous) advanced in a V-Y manner (Fig. 1H) are options as well. A posterior thigh fasciocutaneous flap has also been utilized in this setting.
4. Greater trochanter ulcers—the flap of choice is the tensor fascia lata flap (Fig. 1I), with the pivot point 8 cm below the anterior superior iliac spine. Lumbar sensation makes this a sensate flap for lesions below L3 (60% of meningmyelocele patients). Other options include the gluteal, random thigh, and vastus lateralis flaps (Fig. 1F,J,K).
5. Surgery for multiple ulcer—Multiple pressure

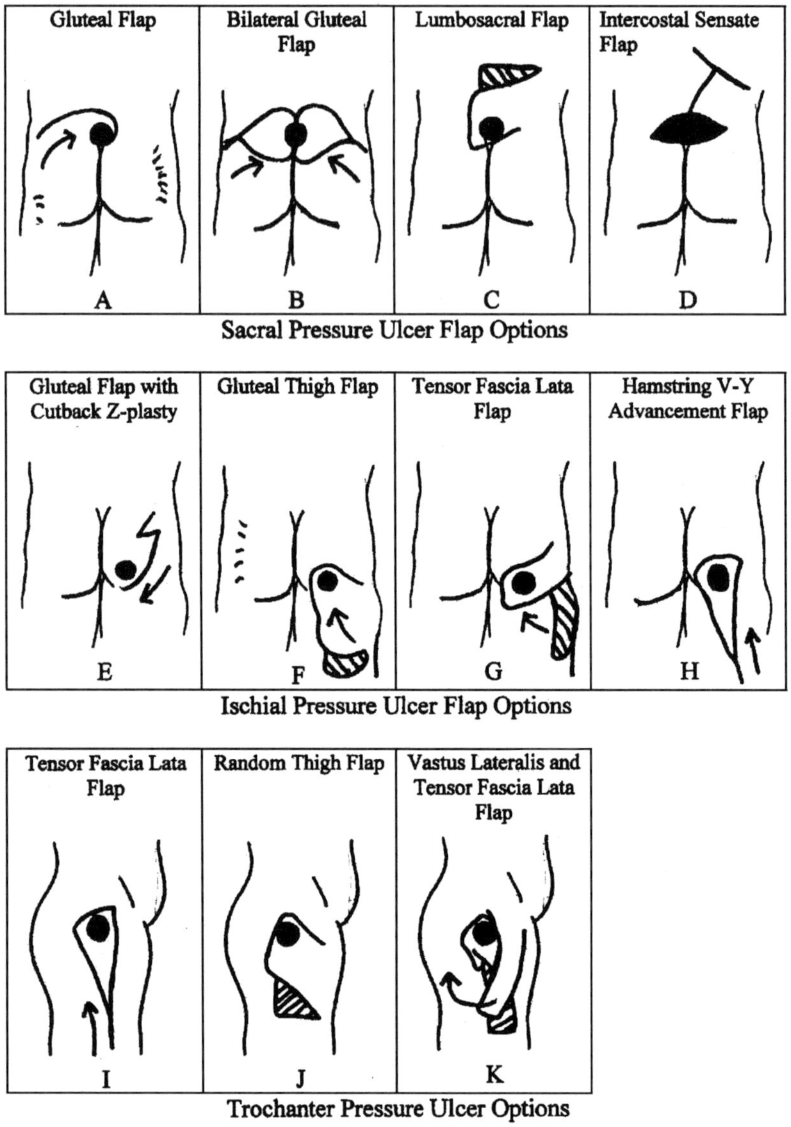

Figure 1 Flap harvesting location. (Artist: Steven Greer, M.D.)

ulcers can be treated in a single-stage procedure more effectively than several staged procedures.

6. Sensate flaps—for spinal cord injury patients, the fundamental cause of their pressure ulcers is the inability to feel discomfort and shift weight. As such, sensate flaps are an intuitive solution. Thoracic island flaps with intact intercostal nerve sensation can be used for pelvic region ulcers (Fig. 1D). Sural nerve grafts can extend the nerve pedicle length. Insensate myocutaneous leg flaps can be neurotized by nerve grafts as well. However, the efficacy of sensory flaps in these patients has not been conclusively demonstrated, and the operations are more complex. The paraplegic with adequate education about his/her condition and with adequate motivation will be able to minimize the risk of recurrences, even with insensate flaps.
7. Salvage flaps—for patients requiring major excision of the hip or pelvis or lower extremity amputation, the nonfunctional soft tissue can be used as flap sources rather than discarded.

8. Procedures to avoid—simple excision of ulcer margins and closure under tension, split-thickness skin grafting of granulating ulcers, or closure with thin flaps using undermined neighboring tissue all have high failure rates.
9. Postoperative management—pressure relief surfaces have traditionally been used for 3 weeks postoperatively. The patient should be completely supine and gradually allowed to use pillows and cushions to elevate the head of the bed. This reduces pressure and sheer forces to the new flap. Adequate nutritional support and incontinence prevention cannot be overemphasized. Measures to minimize postoperative muscle spasms should also be incorporated.
10. The period of pressure relief with expensive beds has been reduced over time, as has the period of hospitalization. In general, it is accepted that a period of 6–8 weeks should pass before the patient resumes normal weight bearing on the operated surface (i.e., sitting for prolonged periods of time).

96

Adult Genital Plastic Surgery

Gary J. Alter, M.D.
David Geffen School of Medicine at UCLA, Los Angeles, California, U.S.A.

I. ANATOMY (SEE CHAPTER 90)

II. GENITAL SKIN LOSS AND RECONSTRUCTION

A. Fournier Gangrene and Other Necrotizing Infections

1. Multiple organisms are commonly cultured from such infections.
2. Patients frequently have other medical problems (i.e., diabetes, chronic indwelling Foley catheter).
3. Infection begins at skin, urinary tract, or rectum. Infection spreads to the penis, scrotum, perineum, abdomen, thighs, and flanks in the dartos fascia, scarpas fascia, and Colles fascia.
4. The corporal bodies, glans, urethra, and testes (including tunica vaginalis) are usually not involved.
5. Treatment:
   - High-dose antibiotics with broad-spectrum coverage
   - Urinary diversion
   - Colostomy if the cause arises from the rectal/perirectal tissues
   - Primary treatment is radical debridement of infected tissue
   - Drains are placed as necessary
   - Serial debridements and dressing changes are performed until all infected and devitalized tissue is adequately debrided

B. Burns

1. Wound care is similar to burn care to other areas, including liberal use of sulfadiazine as a topical antimicrobial medication.
2. Thermal burns:
   - Conservative initial management
   - Excise only necrotic tissue
   - Catheterize bladder or place suprapubic tube if a major genital burn is present
   - Hospitalize if the burn is of significant size and/or depth
3. Electrical burns:
   - Conservative initial management
   - May have deep tissue injury even if cutaneous injury appears small
   - Demarcation may take weeks
   - Excision/debridement may be more significant than the external wound might otherwise predict

4. Chemical burns:
   - Immediately remove clothing to limit amount of contact time of the chemical to the skin
   - Copious irrigation to dilute the chemical concentration

C. Trauma

1. Scrotal and penile avulsion injuries:
   - Tissues separate along the subdartos plane
   - Can track up to the phallus
   - Testicles and spermatic cords are usually intact
2. Penetrating injuries:
   - Immediate repair is indicated
   - Most penetrating injuries are closed primarily
   - Minimize amount of tissue debrided
3. Constrictive injury to the penis:
   - Condom catheters, constrictive rings
   - Minimize amount of tissue debrided

III. RECONSTRUCTION

A. Penile Skin Loss

1. Excise edematous skin, including the distal prepuce up to the coronal sulcus.
2. Skin distal to skin grafts may become chronically lymphedematous.
3. Split-thickness skin graft (STSG):
   - Hairless
   - High rate of success
   - Impotent older patients may be treated as follows:

     Thinner split thickness skin graft (0.015 inch thickness)

     The skin graft may be meshed—higher graft survival; contracts secondarily
   - Potent patients may be treated as follows:

     Thicker split thickness skin grafts (0.020–0.024 inch thickness)

     Do not mesh the skin graft—more elasticity and less contraction. A non-meshed skin graft allows better stretch during an erection than a contracted meshed skin graft

     May take 1 year for graft to slide over areolar tissue on Buck's fascia
4. Full-thickness skin grafts (FTSG):
   - Can be used on potent patients
   - Disadvantages:

     Possible hair growth

     Lower chances of complete take when compared to STSG
5. Management:
   - Use one uniform sheet of skin graft if possible
   - Usually replace all penile skin from base to coronal sulcus
   - Ventral seam suture line should incorporate multiple Z-plasties
   - Sutures of 0000 Vicryl placed on the periphery of the wound are tied over a bolster made of Xeroform gauze and bulky cotton soaked in mineral oil
   - Bed rest for a minimum of 5 days with bolster dressing
   - Foley catheter
   - Penis in vertical position in a bulky splint
   - Antibiotics
   - Mild compression dressings are changed daily for several weeks with Xeroform gauze and Coban to prevent shear and edema

B. Scrotal Reconstruction

1. Partial scrotal skin loss:
   - Usually can close these types of wounds primarily or by rotating local scrotal flaps
   - Meshed split-thickness skin grafts are indicated if primary closure is not possible
2. Total scrotal skin loss (testicle usually within the tunica vaginalis):
   - Initial treatment is with local dressing changes
   - Await clean wound
   - Placement ("burial") of the testicles into thigh pouches is usually unnecessary

- Meshed split-thickness skin grafts are preferred for definitive coverage:
  - Mobilize spermatic cords to the external inguinal rings
  - Suture tunica vaginalis of both testicles and spermatic cords together
  - Meshed split-thickness skin graft is applied (0.018 inch thickness)
  - The meshed skin graft simulates scrotal skin with rugated appearance
  - High success rate
  - Immobilize graft with bolsters for at least 5 days while at bed rest
  - Sutures of 0000 Vicryl placed on the periphery of the wound are tied over Xeroform gauze and cotton soaked in mineral oil. Replace Xeroform daily for several weeks
  - Graft stretches over time to cause a dependent scrotum

3. Thigh pedicle flaps:
   - Rarely necessary; skin grafting easier with excellent cosmetic result
   - Superior and lateral flaps:
     - Preserves branches of the external pudendal, obturator, and medial circumflex arteries
     - Preserves branches of the genitofemoral and ilioinguinal nerves
4. Avulsed skin occasionally regrafted, but results vary.

C. Perineal Defects

Treatment options include:

1. Skin grafts.
2. Local skin flaps.
3. Groin flap.
4. Muscle flaps:
   - Rectus abdominis flap
   - Gracilis flap
   - Rectus femoris flap
5. Fasciocutaneous flaps:
   - Posterior thigh flap
   - Pudendal thigh flap
   - Tensor fascia lata flap

IV. PENIS AND TESTICLE AMPUTATION

A. Penis Amputation

1. Common etiologies include:
   - Circumcision
   - Autoemasculation—usually from acute psychosis
   - Traumatic penile amputation
   - Animal bites
2. Management:
   - Goals:
     - Single-stage replantation or reconstruction
     - Maximize cosmetic appearance
     - Restore sensation
     - Restore ability to achieve adequate erections
     - Maintain an open urethra without significant strictures or fistula formation
   - A multidisciplinary team approach is optimal
   - Management of the amputated part:
     - Irrigate to remove all dirt/foreign debris
     - Wrap in sterile saline-soaked gauze
     - Immerse in saline ice water
     - Avoid excessive cooling that may result in frostbite injury to the amputated segment
   - Reattachment is considered feasible with cold ischemia time of up to 24 h
   - Stabilize patient with respect to hemodynamic status and other possible associated injuries
   - Replantation:
     - Microsurgical approach with operating microscope and microsurgical instruments is preferable
     - Debride wound and opposing surfaces thoroughly
     - Urethra is spatulated and reapproximated: 16 French Foley silicone

catheter serves as a stent for the urethra; suprapubic tube for bladder drainage

Spongiosum is closed as a separate layer

Cavernosal arteries are anastomosed if the injury is proximal

Corpora are reattached with 000 PDS

Dorsal arteries and veins are reanastomosed

Both dorsal nerves are coapted

- Simple corporal reattachment as a composite graft is considered if microsurgery is unavailable:

  High incidence of distal skin and urethral necrosis

  Higher incidence of impotence

- Postoperative care:

  Bed rest for 1 week

  Elevate penis slightly

  Foley catheter removed on postoperative day 14

  Suprapubic tube removed at 3 weeks if no urinary extravasation is noted

  Psychiatric counseling

B. Testicle Amputation

1. Unilateral loss is often not repaired; prosthetic replacement instead.
2. Microsurgical replantation if bilateral testicle amputation is present.

V. PHALLIC RECONSTRUCTION

A. Subtotal Penile Loss

1. Release the penile suspensory ligament.
2. Recess the scrotum and suprapubic skin to increase length of the residual penis segment.
3. Apply skin graft to the remaining penis stump.

B. Total Penile Inadequacy or Loss

1. Causes:
   - Micropenis and other congenital deformities
   - Burns
   - Trauma
   - Ablative cancer surgery
   - Circumcision accidents
   - Female-to-male transsexuals
2. Reconstruction options:
   - Tubed abdominal flap
   - Gracilis myocutaneous flap
   - Groin flap
   - Microvascular free flap
3. Modern phalloplasty options:
   - Advantages of free flap:

     One-stage procedure

     Tactile and erogenous sensation are partially restored

     Better overall cosmetic appearance

     Competent urethra that allows voiding while standing

     Adequate rigidity for intercourse in many patients

   - Radial forearm free flap—multiple variations:

     Radial artery is anastomosed to the inferior epigastric artery

     Venae comitantes of the radial artery are anastomosed to the inferior epigastric vein

     Cephalic vein is anastomosed to the saphenous vein

     Medial and lateral antebrachial cutaneous nerves of the forearm are coapted to the right and left dorsal nerves of the penis or clitoris

     Neourethra is formed from part of the flap and anastomosed to the urethra

     Flap tissue is anastomosed to the residual corporal bodies

   - Ulnar artery free flap
   - Osteocutaneous fibula free flap
   - Lateral arm free flap
   - Penile implants are often inserted as second procedure
4. Transsexual—requires urethral lengthening, vaginectomy, hysterectomy, and oophorectomy.

VI. VAGINAL RECONSTRUCTION

A. Etiology

1. Congenital deformities:
   - Mayer-Rokitansky-Kuster-Hauser syndrome (MRKH)
   - Intersex
2. Extirpative cancer surgery.
3. Male-to-female transsexuals.

B. Procedures

1. Full-thickness skin graft vaginoplasty:
   - Often used for MRKH syndrome
   - Transsexuals—occasionally for primary reconstruction, but useful as a secondary procedure
2. Pudendal thigh flap:
   - Extirpative cancer surgery; sometimes combined with rectus abdominis muscle flap
   - Occasionally used for MRKH—need to depilate
3. Rectosigmoid vaginoplasty:
   - Frequently used for MRKH
   - Occasionally used for transsexuals
4. Less common:
   - Gracilis myocutaneous flaps—extirpative cancer surgery
   - Rectus abdominis myocutaneous flap extirpative cancer surgery

C. Male-to-Female Gender Reassignment

1. Standard technique:
   - Vagina is formed from penile skin inversion
   - Scrotal skin graft can be added to the inverted penile skin if depilated
   - Neoclitoris is formed from a portion of the dorsal glans, retaining the neurovascular pedicle of the dorsal nerves and arteries of the penis
   - Urethra is amputated at the level of the proximal bulb
   - Labia majora are formed from residual scrotum
2. Alternative techniques:
   - Vagina is formed from rectosigmoid colon
   - Vagina is formed from full-thickness skin graft
   - No preservation of the glans for a clitoris

VII. CONCLUSION

1. Challenging.
2. Dependent upon solid knowledge of anatomy.
3. Cosmetic appearance and function should always be considered.

97

Benign Breast Disease

Steven R. Beanes, M.D., and Andrew Da Lio, M.D.
David Geffen School of Medicine at UCLA, Los Angeles, California, U.S.A.

I. ANATOMY

A. Embryology

1. Breast tissue is derived from ectodermal tissue.

B. Layers of Tissue (from Anterior to Posterior)

1. Epidermis.
2. Dermis.
3. Superficial layer of the superficial fascia.
4. Cooper's ligaments.
5. Glandular tissue (ducts and lobules).
6. Deep layer of the superficial fascia.
7. Retromammary space.
8. Deep fascia.
9. Pectoralis major muscle.

C. Lymphatic Drainage

1. Lymphatic vessels do not have valves.
2. 97% of lymphatic flow from the breasts is into the axillae. The remaining 3% is into internal mammary nodes.
3. Rotter nodes are lymph nodes found between pectoralis major and minor.
4. Axillary nodes are found at three levels:
   - Level I—nodes lateral to the lateral border of the pectoralis minor muscle
   - Level II—nodes lying beneath the pectoralis minor muscle
   - Level III—nodes medial to the medial border of the pectoralis minor and extending to the apex of the axilla

D. Histology

1. Breast tissue—consists of lobules and ducts.
2. Alveoli—terminal elongated tubular ducts.
3. Alveolar ducts—consist of low columnar glandular cells with prominent basement membrane.
4. Lobular unit—convergence of 10–100 alveoli.
5. Excretory duct—formation of 20–40 lobular ducts.
6. Excretory ducts—double layer of cuboidal and columnar epithelium.
7. Excretory sinus—formed by the 10–20 excretory ducts. The excretory sinus is located beneath the areola. It is lined with squamous epithelium.

II. EVALUATION ALGORITHM FOR DISCRETE BREAST MASS

A. Younger Than 30 Years

1. Ultrasound:
   - Cyst or fibroadenoma: aspirate and observe; biopsy noncystic masses if suspicious changes develop
   - Other: biopsy

B. Older Than 30 Years, Premenopausal

1. Bilateral mammography.
2. Fine needle aspiration (FNA):
   - Cyst with resolution following aspiration: observe; biopsy if change develops
   - Diagnostic benign cytology: observe; biopsy if change develops
   - Nondiagnostic cytology: surgical biopsy

C. Postmenopausal

1. Bilateral mammography
2. Biopsy

III. BENIGN BREAST DISORDERS—SPECIFIC ENTITIES

A. "Fibrocystic Disease" and Breast Cysts

1. Represents a manifestation of breast tissue response to cyclic hormonal stimulation.
2. Fibrocystic features in a breast biopsy do not confer any increased risk of breast cancer development.
3. Presence of features are dependent upon timing of the biopsy during the patient's menstrual cycle.
4. Mammography is more likely to miss a hidden breast cancer when fibrocystic features are present.
5. 1 in 14 women will develop pure breast cysts (common).
6. Cysts are lined with flattened epithelium.
7. Intracyst carcinoma is very rare (0.1% of all macrocysts).
8. Cysts and cancer risk:
   - No studies demonstrate an increased risk when cysts are small or microscopic
   - The presence of large cysts is controversial: either no increased risk or up to two- to four-fold increase in incidence of cancer

B. Fibroadenoma

1. Benign tumor composed of both stromal and epithelial elements.
2. Most common breast tumor in young women, but also frequently encountered in older women.
3. Multiple fibroadenomas are present in 10–15% of cases.
4. Usually does not change in size with menstrual cycle.
5. Can get larger during pregnancy—suggests response to hormonal stimuli.
6. Mammography plays little role in diagnosis; degenerating lesion can develop calcifications.
7. Pathology—well encapsulated; hallmark is presence of stromal tissue combined with epithelium-lined duct-like structures.
8. Treatment—varies considerably; all include at least FNA, with excision if non-diagnostic or suspicious. Many advocate observation in woman <30 years of age.
9. Not associated with increased risk of breast cancer (as an independent variable).

C. Giant Fibroadenoma

1. Defined as a fibroadenoma larger than 5 cm in diameter.
2. Usually occur just after menarche or just before menopause.
3. Juvenile fibroadenoma is a large adenoma that occurs in young adults and is histologically more cellular than the usual fibroadenoma.

D. Sclerosing Adenosis

1. Histologic subtype of fibrocystic disease.
2. Not associated with increased risk of cancer development.
3. Can be confused radiologically and histologically with cancer.
4. Common presentation includes clustered microcalcifications on routine mammogram.
5. Histology is typified by intralobular fibrosis and proliferation of small ductules.

E. Radial Scar

1. Benign entity; can also be confused with cancer.
2. Mammography—appears as stellate irregular mass.
3. Composed of fibroelastic tissue with entrapped glandular elements.
4. Not associated with increased cancer risk.

F. Fat Necrosis

1. Etiology—traumatic injury to fatty tissue incites inflammatory response, leading to necrosis.
2. Can be confused with cancer; mass is present with skin dimpling and retraction.
3. Histology shows fat-laden macrophages and foreign body giant cells.
4. Not associated with increased cancer risk.
5. No specific therapy is required.

G. Periductal Mastitis (Mammary Duct Ectasia)

1. Uncommon benign disorder.
2. Characterized by presence of dilated mammary ducts with inspissated secretions and marked periductal inflammation.
3. Symptoms include mastodynia, nipple retraction, and nipple discharge.
4. May be the final common pathway that results from obstructed milk ducts.
5. More likely to be infectious in younger women.
6. Treatment usually only requires incision and drainage; antibiotics alone rarely suffice.

H. Breast Abscess

1. Risk factors include lactation and periductal mastitis.
2. Complicates <1% of breast-feeding women, but lactational infections account for 80% of all breast infections.
3. Nonlactational infections are rare; the differential diagnosis should include inflammatory cancer.
4. Most common organism in acute infections is *Staphylococcus*.
5. Organisms that cause chronic infection include *Actinomyces* and *Mycobacteria* (tuberculosis).
6. Treatment:
   - Cellulitis (early)—antibiotics alone are usually successful
   - Abscess (late)—open surgical drainage
   - Recommendation with regard to breast feeding is to continue breast feeding with the contralateral breast and to pump the affected breast

I. Galactocele

1. Breast cyst filled with milk secondary to an obstructed breast duct.
2. Associated with women who are or were recently lactating.
3. Treatment is primarily percutaneous aspiration; repeat if necessary.

J. Mondor Disease

1. Etiology is thrombophlebitis of the superficial veins of the breast.
2. Symptoms include burning breast pain.
3. Can be confused with cancer; mammography can differentiate between cancer and Mondor disease.
4. Is a benign, self-limited process.
5. Treatment is nonspecific, including nonsteroidal anti-inflammatory medications.

K. Intraductal Papilloma

1. Most common cause of bloody nipple discharge.
2. Only 50% of papillomas have bloody discharge; remaining half have serous drainage.
3. Diagnosis is by ductography.
4. Most are located within a few centimeters of the nipple; often have a long stalk.
5. Treatment by subareolar excision of the affected duct is curative.
6. Not associated with increased incidence of breast cancer with solitary lesions.
7. Diffuse papillomatosis is rare:
   - Often bilateral
   - Usually more distant from the nipple
   - Associated with an increased risk of cancer (magnitude unknown, but cancer develops in up to 40% of women with papillomatosis)

98

Breast Neoplasia and Mammography

Andrew Da Lio, M.D., and Steven R. Beanes, M.D.
David Geffen School of Medicine at UCLA, Los Angeles, California, U.S.A.

I. EPIDEMIOLOGY

A. Lifetime risk of a woman developing breast cancer is 10%.

B. Over 50% of women diagnosed with breast cancer are >65 years old.

C. Breast cancer incidence rates have been steadily increasing while the age-adjusted death rate from breast cancer has remained essentially unchanged from 1930 to the present.

D. Breast cancer is the leading cause of death among American women 40–55 years of age.

II. RISK FACTORS

A. Gender

1. The most important risk factor for the development of breast cancer is gender.
2. Female-to-male ratio is 100:1.

B. Age

The risk that breast cancer will develop in a Caucasian American woman in a single year increases from 1:5900 at age 30 to 1:290 at age 80.

C. Family History

1. A positive family history increases a woman's risk of developing breast cancer.
2. The most important increase in risk is associated with the presence of breast cancer in a first-degree relative:
   - The overall risk depends on the number of relatives with cancer, their ages at diagnosis, whether the disease was unilateral or bilateral, and whether the relative was premenopausal or postmenopausal at the time of cancer diagnosis.

D. Prior Breast Cancer

Prior breast cancer will place a woman at risk for developing a second breast cancer with an incidence equal to 0.5–1.0% per year of follow-up.

E. Endogenous Endocrine Factors

1. Age at menarche—women who have regular ovulatory cycles before age 13 have a fourfold increased risk compared with women whose menarche occurred after age 13 and who had a 5-year delay in the development of regular cycles.
2. Duration of menstruation—women who menstruate for more than 30 years are at an increased risk compared with women who menstruate for fewer than 30 years.
3. Age at menopause—the risk of breast cancer for women who experience menopause after age 55 is twice that of women who experience menopause prior to age 44.

4. Age at first full-term pregnancy—the risk of developing breast cancer in a woman who had her first child before age 19 is half that of a nulliparous woman.

F. Exogenous Hormone Use

1. Postmenopausal estrogen replacement:
   - The use of postmenopausal estrogen replacement appears to increase the risk of breast cancer by approximately 40%.
   - When all potential causes of death are taken into account (particularly cardiac and neurologic), estrogen therapy appears to decrease the overall mortality rate among older women.
2. Oral contraceptives:
   - No statistically significant increase in breast cancer risk exists with the use of oral contraceptives.
   - Prolonged use (>10 years) may be associated with an increased risk of breast cancer in women younger than 45 years of age.

G. Atypical Hyperplasia

Patients with atypical hyperplasia and a proliferative histologic pattern are at substantially increased risk of developing breast cancer.

H. Obesity

Obesity is not a significant risk factor for breast cancer.

I. Alcohol Consumption

A positive association exists between alcohol consumption (even at the level of one drink per day) and an increased risk of breast cancer.

J. Genetics of Breast Cancer

1. Approximately 5% of all breast cancers are genetic, but genetic factors may account for 25% of cases in women <30 years of age.
2. BRCA1 gene:
   - Located on the long arm of chromosome 17 (17q21)
   - Inherited as a dominant genetic trait
   - Acts like a tumor suppressor or recessive oncogene, providing negative regulation on cell growth and possibly involved in recognition/repair of genetic damage or spontaneous mutations
   - Large gene, which makes genetic testing technically difficult
   - Accounts for 45% of penetrant hereditary breast cancer
3. BRCA2 gene:
   - Located on chromosome 13
   - Accounts for 30% of familial breast cancer
   - More specific for breast cancer than BRCA1 (ovarian)
   - Large complex gene of unknown function

III. PATHOLOGY OF BREAST CANCER

A. Lobular Carcinoma in Situ (LCIS)

1. Pathologically, proliferation of small round epithelial cells with lumens of multiple breast acini.
2. LCIS never forms a palpable mass by itself nor does it lead to calcification.
3. Usually recognized incidentally after biopsy for another abnormality.
4. LCIS is not a preinvasive condition.
5. Although subsequent breast carcinoma developing in a patient with a previous diagnosis of LCIS has a higher frequency of being invasive lobular carcinoma than in the general population, infiltrating ductal carcinoma remains the most common diagnosis when carcinoma appears after a diagnosis of LCIS.
6. Risk of later invasive breast cancer is equally divided between both breasts.
7. Contralateral LCIS has not been shown to affect risk of cancer development.
8. Approximately 30% likelihood of developing breast cancer in the 20 years after diagnosis.
9. Management is lifetime surveillance in the form of annual mammogram and clinical examination every 6 months.

B. Ductal Carcinoma in Situ (DCIS)

1. More common than LCIS.
2. DCIS is a preinvasive carcinoma.
3. Forms calcifications and thus can be seen on mammography.

4. DCIS is more common late in life.
5. DCIS cells appear cytologically malignant, but the cells do not penetrate deep to the basement membrane.
6. Several subtypes of DCIS are recognized:
   - Solid/comedo type—most common type; more virulent than other types; susceptible to central necrosis
   - Papillary/cribriform type—less likely to form palpable mass. Multiple types can coexist

C. Infiltrating Ductal Carcinoma

1. Most common malignant tumor of the breast (75% of all breast cancers).
2. Lesion is characterized by the absence of special histologic features.
3. Originates from the ductal epithelium.
4. Infiltration distinguishes this lesion from DCIS.
5. May also display an in situ component (DCIS preinvasive).
6. Clinically, usually presents as mass or density lesion with microcalcifications on mammography, and often metastasizes to axillary lymph nodes.
7. Distant metastases are most often found in the bones, lungs, liver, and brain.

D. Invasive Lobular Carcinoma

1. Originates in the breast lobule.
2. Accounts for 3–15% of all invasive breast cancers.
3. Clinically, presents as a mass.
4. No distinguishing mammographic features.
5. Composed of small round cells infiltrating the surrounding stroma. Cells are oriented in a linear array.
6. Multicentricity is more frequently observed than in infiltrating ductal carcinoma.
7. Prognosis is similar to that of infiltrating ductal carcinoma.
8. Known to metastasize to unusual sites, such as meninges and serosal surfaces, more often than other forms of breast cancer.

IV. BREAST CANCER STAGING

Based on the American Joint Committee on Cancer (AJCC), which employs the TNM classification system.

Primary Tumor (T)
Tis = Carcinoma in situ
T1 = Tumor 2 cm or less in greatest dimension
T2 = Tumor >2 cm and <5 cm in greatest dimension
T3 = Tumor 5 cm or larger in greatest dimension
T4 = Tumor of any size with direct extension to chest wall or skin

Regional Lymph Nodes (N)
N0 = No regional lymph node metastasis
N1 = Metastasis to movable ipsilateral axillary LNs
N2 = Metastasis to ipsilateral axillary LNs that are fixed to one another or other structures
N3 = Metastasis to ipsilateral internal mammary LNs

Distant Metastasis (M)
M0 = No distant metastasis
M1 = Distant metastasis (includes metastasis to ipsilateral supraclavicular LNs)

Staging

Stage 0	Tis	N0	M0
Stage I	T1	N0	M0
Stage IIA	T0	N1	M0
	T1	N1	M0
	T2	N0	M0
Stage IIB	T2	N1	M0
	T3	N0	M0
Stage IIIA	T0	N2	M0
	T1	N2	M0
	T2	N2	M0
	T3	N1	M0
	T3	N2	M0
Stage IIIB	T4	Any N	M0
	Any T	N3	M0
Stage IV	Any T	Any N	M1

V. MAMMOGRAPHY

A. General

Mammography is clearly the most sensitive and specific test that can be used to complement the physical examination of the breast.

1. Mammography can be used as either a diagnostic modality (seeking to answer a specific question about the health of the breast) or as a screening test (seeking to find any abnormality within the breast).

2. 10–50% of cancers detected mammographically are not palpable; conversely, palpation recognizes 10–20% of tumors that are not detectable mammographically.
3. The level of radiation exposure during mammography is low and is considered safe in women of screening age.

B. Screening Recommendations

1. Screening studies seek to identify any breast abnormality, maximizing sensitivity and cost-effectiveness.
2. The American Cancer Society Recommendations for Routine Mammographic Screening of Asymptomatic Women advocates routine mammography every 1–2 years for women 40–49 years old, and yearly mammography for women 50 years and older.
3. The National Cancer Institute concluded that randomized trials of women aged 40–49 are consistent in showing no statistically significant benefit in mortality after 10–12 years of follow-up. The National Cancer Institute has confirmed a significant benefit for women aged 50–69, which amounts to a 34% reduction in breast cancer mortality.

C. Mammography Techniques

1. Film screen mammography:
    - Similar to usual radiographic methods
    - Yields black and white radiographs that are viewed on a light box
2. Xeroradiography:
    - Employs an electrostatic detector plate coated with selenium, which distributes electric charge on its surface proportional to the amount of radiation reaching the plate
    - Yields an electrostatic image, which is converted to a blue-on-white photocopy image
3. Both techniques are similar in quality and effectiveness, though film screen imaging involves lower radiation.
4. Regardless of the technique chosen, mammograms should be performed with dedicated instruments and interpreted by radiologists knowledgeable in breast imaging.

D. Nonpalpable Mammographic Abnormalities

Mammographic abnormalities that cannot be detected by physical examination are classified into three broad categories:

1. Lesions consisting of microcalcifications only.
2. Density lesions (asymmetries, architectural distortions, masses).
3. Lesions with both density abnormalities and calcifications.

E. Malignancy

The incidence of malignancy after biopsy depends on the characteristics of the radiographic findings:

1. Overall, incidence of malignancy with mammograms containing abnormalities was 24%.
2. A spiculated density with ill-defined margins is likely to be malignant.
3. In general, lesions with microcalcifications and a mass effect, spiculated masses, and linear branching calcifications carry the highest probability of being malignant. However, even well-defined densities can be malignant.

VI. OTHER IMAGING MODALITIES

A. Ductography

1. Used in the evaluation of nipple discharge.
2. A small volume of contrast dye is injected into the draining duct, with images obtained.
3. Filling defects generally represent intraductal papillomas.
4. Usually requires additional histologic diagnosis.

B. Ultrasonography

1. Uses high-resolution acoustic waves to image the breast.
2. Most useful feature of ultrasound is the ability to distinguish between solid and cystic lesions.
3. Not an effective screening modality for breast cancer. Ultrasound cannot detect microcalcifications or small lesions.

C. PET Scan

1. Produces images reflective of cellular biochemical activities. Provides a functional, as opposed to anatomical, view of thc tissucs.
2. The technique appears to be specific (90% or better positive predictive value).
3. Has been used to image primary breast tumors, as a noninvasive method for staging axillary lymph nodes, and to detect metastatic disease.

D. Magnetic Resonance Imaging

1. Increasing interest in MR imaging of the breast.
2. Excellent sensitivity and adequate specificity have been obtained.
3. Improvements in the method of imaging in addition to a reduction in the cost will be necessary prior to MRI being an acceptable addition to standard imaging of the breast.

99

Primary Treatment of Breast Cancer

Steven R. Beanes, M.D., and O. Joe Hines, M.D.
David Geffen School of Medicine at UCLA, Los Angeles, California, U.S.A.

I. BRIEF SUMMARY OF THE SURGICAL TREATMENT OF BREAST CANCER

Pathology	Treatment
Atypical needle biopsy	1. Open excisional biopsy
Ductal carcinoma in situ	1. Wide local excision 2. Mastectomy
Lobular carcinoma in situ	1. Close observation 2. Bilateral simple mastectomy
Invasive carcinoma	1. Lumpectomy and axillary node biopsy/dissection 2. Modified radical mastectomy
Positive margin or <1 mm margin	1. Reexcision 2. Mastectomy
Tubular carcinoma	1. <6 mm → lumpectomy 2. ≥6 mm → lumpectomy and axillary node biopsy/dissection or modified radical mastectomy
Cystosarcoma phyllodes	1. Benign → wide local excision 2. Malignant → mastectomy

II. SURGICAL PROCEDURES FOR INVASIVE BREAST CANCER

A. Historical Perspective

1. Halsted's patients: 2/3 had locally advanced disease and 60% had clinically evident axillary node metastases.
2. By comparison, in 1980, 85% of patients presented with stage I or II disease and the rate of positive axillary lymph nodes was 40%.

B. Radical Mastectomy (RM)

1. All breast tissue and underlying pectoralis muscles are sacrificed; all regional lymph nodes along the axillary vein to the costo-clavicular ligament are removed.
2. Extended radical mastectomy includes removal of internal mammary nodes; no literature to support improved clinical outcomes.
3. Procedure is of historical value only.

C. Modified Radical Mastectomy (MRM)

1. Combines total mastectomy with removal of axillary lymph nodes in continuity with the mastectomy specimen. Leaves pectoralis major muscle intact.
2. Two forms of MRM:
   - Patey procedure—preserves pectoralis major, but sacrifices pectoralis minor to remove level I, II, and III lymph nodes. Node-negative 10-year survival is 82% with 5% local recurrence; node positive 10-year survival is 48%. The Scanlon modification divides the pectoralis minor, allowing removal of level III nodes, but

sparing the lateral pectoral nerve to the pectoralis major.
 - Auchincloss procedure—does not remove or divide the pectoralis minor muscle; limits the complete removal of high axillary lymph nodes; justified by the fact that only 2% of patients will benefit by removal of the highest lymph nodes.
3. Additional principles:
 - Biopsy site/scar should be included in the specimen.
 - Removal of the nipple in continuity with the major retroareolar ductal complex; nipple is site of unsuspected metastasis in up to 10% of cases.
 - Any skin tethered to the lesion or within 2 cm of the surface should be included in the specimen.
 - >97% of all breast tissue should be removed.

D. RM vs. MRM

1. Directly tested in two large randomized trials in the United States and England (included stages I, II, and operable stage III).
2. At 10 years there was no significant difference in overall survival, but there was a significantly higher rate of local recurrence in the MRM group.

E. Wide Local Excision

1. Referred to by many names: lumpectomy, partial mastectomy, and segmentectomy.
2. Removes the malignancy with a surrounding rim of grossly normal tissue.
3. Removal of the overlying skin if the lesion is within 1 cm of the skin or is tethered to the skin on preoperative examination.
4. Nonpalpable lesions must receive preoperative mammographic needle localization.
5. Contraindications:
 - Multifocal invasive carcinoma
 - Multifocal DCIS or high-risk lesions (atypical hyperplasia)
 - Breasts that are difficult to evaluate by examination
 - Small breast, which will result in poor cosmetic result
6. Must be combined with radiation for local control.
7. Axillary dissection is performed through a separate incision.

III. MANAGEMENT OF EARLY STAGE BREAST CANCER

A. General

1. Includes T1 and T2 primary tumors with N0 to N1 lymph nodes.
2. Accounts for 75% of patients with breast cancer.
3. Three surgical treatment options are available:
 - Wide local excision/axillary lymph node dissection with irradiation
 - Modified radical mastectomy
 - Modified radical mastectomy with reconstruction (immediate vs. delayed)

B. Breast Conservation: Wide Local Excision vs. MRM

Multiple randomized, prospective trials have failed to demonstrate any survival benefit to the more aggressive procedures.

1. NSABP trial B-06: examined women with primary tumors up to 4 cm in diameter with N0 or N1 nodal status.
2. Patients were randomized to one of three groups:
 - MRM
 - Wide local excision with axillary lymph node dissection and radiation therapy
 - Wide local excision with axillary lymph node dissection alone
3. Negative margins were required in the breast-conservation groups.
4. There was no difference in the disease-free survival or overall survival among the three groups.
5. Local recurrence was significantly reduced with the addition of XRT to the breast-conservation group (10% vs. 39% at 8 years).
6. These findings confirm breast-conservation surgery as an acceptable treatment option for early stage breast cancer, but the final decision on the procedure of choice is complex and must be individualized for each patient.

C. Radiotherapy

Postoperative radiation includes at least 4500 cGy to the entire breast with boost to the tumor bed.

D. Axillary Node Dissection

1. A substantial number of women with clinically negative nodes are noted to have nodal disease at the time of surgery.
   - 40% of all patients with clinically negative axillae were found to have positive nodes at the time of resection
   - Rates of 17% histologically positive nodes for clinical T1N0 disease, and as high as 27% for patients with clinical T2N0 disease have been found
2. In addition to contributing to local control, axillary dissection provides important prognostic and staging information.
3. Nodal status remains a major predictor of outcome:
   - Node negative: 10-year survival is >70%
   - One to three positive nodes: 10-year survival is 40%
   - Four to ten positive nodes: 10-year survival is 20%
4. The current recommendation for all patients undergoing mastectomy or wide local excision for T1 or T2 lesions is to undergo axillary lymph node dissection as well:
   - At least 10 lymph nodes should be sampled to allow for adequate prognostic evaluation
   - Dissection should include level I and II nodal tissue
   - Addition of level III nodes is of little benefit to staging and may increase the postoperative complication of lymphedema, especially with XRT

E. Axillary Sentinel Lymph Node Biopsy

1. Sentinel nodes are the one or two initial nodes in the regional nodal drainage basin encountered by the lymphatic drainage from a tumor. These nodes can be identified with an injection of vital dye or radioisotope into the primary tumor site.
2. Examination of sentinel nodes provides a focused histopathologic assessment of tissue most likely to harbor metastases, providing enhanced staging accuracy with a low false-negative rate.
3. Tumor-free sentinel nodes are predictive of a tumor-free axilla, thereby allowing for the possibility of sparing patients the morbidity of a formal axillary lymph node dissection. However, sentinel nodes have been identified in nonaxillary sites, such as the internal mammary nodes.
4. The ultimate role of sentinel lymph node biopsy in breast cancer cannot be defined before the final results of large clinical trials currently in progress.

IV. ADJUVANT THERAPY FOR BREAST CANCER

Menopausal status	Axillary nodes	Tumor characteristics	Recommended treatments
Premenopausal	Positive	Favorable or unfavorable	Combination chemotherapy
Premenopausal	Negative	Favorable	No data to support adjuvant tx
Premenopausal	Negative	Unfavorable	Combination chemotherapy
Postmenopausal	Positive	Favorable	Tamoxifen +/− chemotherapy
Postmenopausal	Positive	Unfavorable	Chemotherapy +/− tamoxifen
Postmenopausal	Negative	Favorable	No data to support adjuvant tx
Postmenopausal	Negative	Unfavorable	No data to support adjuvant tx

V. MANAGEMENT OF NON-INVASIVE (IN SITU) CARCINOMA

A. Lobular Carcinoma in Situ (LCIS)

1. There is no known intervention for or treatment of LCIS.
2. Exists as a risk factor, similar to atypical ductal hyperplasia or family history.
3. LCIS is found in 3.6% of biopsies performed for benign disease.

4. Actuarial probability of developing carcinoma after 35 years is 20%.
5. Subsequent cancer develops equally in the ipsilateral and contralateral breasts.
6. Younger women may opt for mastectomy as treatment option, but would need to be total and bilateral to significantly diminish their risk of developing breast cancer.
7. As mentioned previously, close lifetime surveillance is the current recommendation (yearly mammogram and physical examination every 6 months).

B. Ductal Carcinoma in Situ (DCIS)

1. Excision alone:
   - High likelihood of local control when areas of DCIS are surrounded by 1 cm of normal breast tissue with normal ducts and no DCIS outside the primary focus
   - Average local recurrence rate of 16–20% at 10 years with negative margins and >50% at 10 years with positive margins
   - Local recurrences: 50% are further DCIS and 50% are invasive carcinoma
2. Excision and radiation:
   - Similar approach to that of invasive breast cancer
   - Average local recurrence rate of 7–16% at 10 years with negative margins
3. Mastectomy:
   - Average local recurrence rate of <1% at 10 years
   - Immediate reconstruction is now possible
4. Axillary lymph node dissection (ALND):
   - For pure DCIS, there is no role for ALND
   - For DCIS with microinvasion, the incidence of involved lymph nodes is 0–10%
5. Tamoxifen:
   - Current trials to determine the role of delaying or preventing recurrence or reappearance of DCIS after breast-conserving therapy
   - No role for other systemic therapies currently
6. Determining best treatment option for DCIS:
   - Initially, diagnosis is made through biopsy
   - All patients should receive excision with margins, magnification-view mammography, and detailed pathologic evaluation
   - If the lesion is 1–4 mm in size and has 5–10 mm margins: observe patient
   - If the lesion is 5–20 mm in size and has 5–10 mm margins: radiation
   - If the lesion is >20 mm in size and has at least 10 mm margins: radiation
   - If the lesion is >20 mm in size and has <10 mm margins: reexcision vs. total mastectomy
   - If the lesion is >20 mm: total mastectomy
   - Modifiers to the algorithm include grade of tumor, age of patient, size of tumor, and patient preference
   - Decisions need to be made concerning the patient's overall condition and life expectancy of disease-free survival

VI. INFLAMMATORY BREAST CANCER

A. Accounts for 3% of all breast cancers.

B. Clinical diagnosis is made on the presence of erythema of the breast with rapid progression, associated diffuse edema with dimpling (peau d'orange), warm and tender site, and a discrete palpable mass (present in 70–80% of cases).

C. Axillary lymph node disease in 50–60% of cases.

D. Pathologic hallmark is dermal lymphatic permeation by tumor cells.

E. Since approximately 25% of patients with inflammatory breast cancer have detectable systemic metastasis, full work-up should be performed, including chest x-ray, abdominal and pelvic CT scan, bone scan, and CEA levels.

F. Previously considered uniformly fatal with median survival of 9–12 months.

G. Newer treatment protocols use intensive chemotherapy as the first modality, with 60–80% response rates.

H. If complete or partial response is obtained, local control can frequently be obtained by mastectomy with axillary lymph node dissection:

- Only feasible if primary skin closure can be achieved

- Extensive axillary lymph node dissection is discouraged; prefer to use regional radiation therapy to address residual nodal disease

I. Outcome for these three treatment modalities includes relapse-free survival of 50% at 5 years compared to lesser treatment (7% at 5 years).

J. Current studies evaluating high-dose chemotherapy with bone marrow transplantation.

VII. MALE BREAST CANCER

A. Accounts for 1% of all breast cancers.

B. Average age at diagnosis is 10 years older than for women.

C. Involves the pectoralis major muscle more commonly.

D. Most common type is infiltrating ductal carcinoma.

E. High incidence (84%) of estrogen-receptor positive tumors.

F. Treatment:

- If pectoralis major is involved → radical mastectomy
- If tumor is small and movable → MRM, possible radiation therapy

G. Presence of nodes has same prognostic power as in women.

H. Use of tamoxifen for estrogen-receptor positive cells and use of adjuvant chemotherapy is advocated.

I. 5-year survival of 80% in patients with adjuvant therapy.

VIII. NONEPITHELIAL BREAST TUMORS

A. Cystosarcoma Phylloides

1. Most common nonepithelial tumor of the breast.
2. Occurs exclusively in the female breast.
3. Majority of lesions are considered to be benign.
4. If lesion is benign-appearing, wide local excision is appropriate.
5. If lesion is malignant, total mastectomy is warranted.
6. Axillary involvement in malignant cases is 1%.
7. For metastatic disease, chemotherapy is advocated.

B. Angiosarcoma

1. Malignant tumor characterized by a large and necrotic mass.
2. Hemorrhage can complicate biopsy.
3. Average age of presentation is 10–15 years younger than for ductal breast cancer.
4. Treatment is total mastectomy.
5. Some authors recommend radiation therapy after surgery.

100

Breast Reconstruction After Mastectomy

Chia Soo, M.D., and William W. Shaw, M.D.
David Geffen School of Medicine at UCLA, Los Angeles, California, U.S.A.

I. DEFINITIONS

The boundaries of the breast are from the clavicle superiorly, the sternum medially, the rectus abdominis fascia inferiorly, and the axilla laterally to the anterior border of the latissimus dorsi muscle (Fig. 1).

A. Subcutaneous mastectomy—Removal of all breast tissue with preservation of all skin, including the nipple-areola complex. Subcutaneous mastectomy is associated with a high recurrence rate if used for malignant disease.

B. Simple (total) mastectomy—Removal of all breast tissue, including the nipple-areola complex.

C. Skin-sparing mastectomy—Simple mastectomy with preservation of all skin except the nipple-areolar complex and a 1–2 cm margin around the biopsy site.

D. Modified radical mastectomy—Removal of all breast tissue, nipple-areola complex, pectoralis fascia, as well as level I and II axillary lymph nodes. Level I and II axillary nodes are bounded by the latissimus dorsi laterally, the axillary vein superiorly, and the medial border of the pectoralis minor medially. This may also include dividing or removing the pectoralis minor muscle and level III nodes (medial to the pectoralis minor) and Rotter's nodes (between the pectoralis major and minor).

E. Halsted radical mastectomy—Removal of all breast tissue, nipple-areola complex, pectoralis major and minor muscles, muscular fascia, and all axillary lymph nodes (levels I, II, and III). This procedure does not improve disease control when compared to a modified radical mastectomy and is rarely performed today.

II. OVERVIEW OF RECONSTRUCTION

Breast reconstruction must address both the underlying volume deficit and the overlying skin deficiency for optimal results. Skin-sparing mastectomy techniques with preservation of the inframammary fold and preoperative design of the mastectomy incision with the general surgeon have improved reconstruction results.

A. Goals

The primary goals may vary from simple wound coverage to restoration of breast aesthetics through reconstitution of surface volume and symmetry.

B. Timing: Immediate vs. Delayed

1. Immediate reconstruction does not increase the likelihood or impede the detection of recurrence and is generally preferred over delayed reconstruction.
2. Advantages of immediate reconstruction include: decreased number of surgical procedures, decreased overall cost, improved reconstruction outcomes (decreased mastectomy flap scar formation), and improved self-image.
3. The main contraindications to immediate reconstruction are medical problems that limit surgical

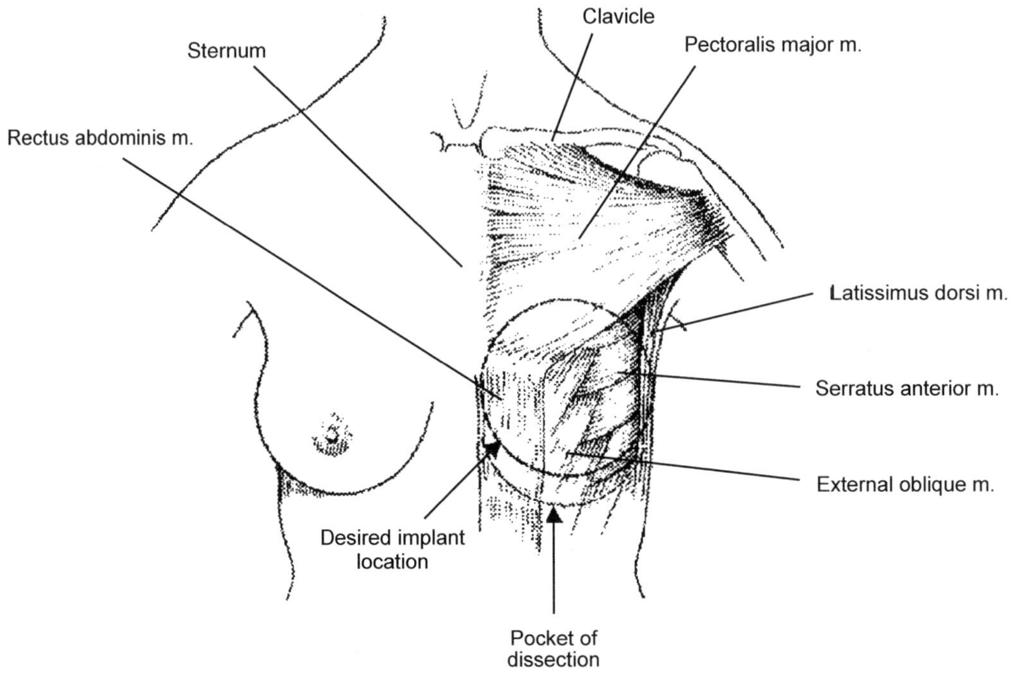

Figure 1 The anatomical boundaries of the breast (see text for full details). The dissection area for prosthesis placement is also depicted. (Modified from Aston SJ, Beasley RW, Thorne C, Grabb WC, eds. *Grabb and Smith's Plastic Surgery*. Philadelphia: Lippincott-Raven, 1997.)

anesthesia time or compromise wound healing (e.g., severe diabetes or peripheral vascular disease). In these instances, the minimal amount of surgery needed for disease control is performed and major reconstruction is delayed.

4. Other relative contraindications to immediate reconstruction include locally advanced breast cancer and the need for postoperative radiation. However, recent studies have shown that immediate autologous tissue reconstruction does not appear to significantly increase postoperative wound complications, even with subsequent chemotherapy and radiation. Implant reconstruction, on the other hand, is associated with increased complications in the setting of immediate postoperative radiation and chemotherapy.

III. IMPLANT AND TISSUE EXPANDER RECONSTRUCTION

A. Indications

1. Medical unsuitability for larger procedure.
2. Patient preference.
3. Disruption of autologous flap blood supply by prior surgeries (e.g., chevron abdominal incision).
4. The ideal patient is thin, with small to medium size breasts.

B. Contraindications

1. Prior or anticipated chest wall irradiation.
2. Obesity (higher incidence of infection/implant or expander extrusion).
3. Thin mastectomy flaps of questionable viability.
4. Excessive skin/suture line tension with wound closure.

C. Advantages

1. No donor site morbidity.
2. Decreased operating time.
3. Decreased recovery time.
4. No additional scar (if mastectomy incision is used for access).

D. Disadvantages

1. Implant or expander rupture/leakage/extrusion.
2. Infection.

3. Flap necrosis.
4. Capsular contracture.
5. Long reconstruction period (expanders).
6. Increased need for reoperation for implant-related problems.

E. Techniques

1. The reconstructive options include immediate implant placement or initial tissue expander placement followed by secondary implant insertion.
2. By necessity, all postmastectomy implant reconstruction should be submuscular because the skin flaps, virtually devoid of breast tissue, are too thin to accommodate subcutaneous implant placement.
3. In general, tissue expansion is more frequently used for breast reconstruction because it minimizes mastectomy flap tension. In addition, gradual stretching of the pectoralis major muscle by tissue expansion also achieves a better breast shape prior to eventual permanent implant placement.
4. The unoperated contralateral breast is used as a guide in marking the inframammary fold on the mastectomy side. For delayed reconstruction, the skin incision may be made at the lateral aspect of the mastectomy scar or through a new incision.
5. After incising the skin and subcutaneous tissue, the muscle-fascial layer is identified and a pectoralis muscle incision made in the lateral thoracic region. Superiorly, the serratus anterior and pectoralis major are elevated as a flap and the inferomedial attachments of the pectoralis major are released. The dissection continues inferiorly beneath the rectus abdominis fascia and external oblique to the inframammary fold (for smooth prostheses, the dissection is extended ~2 cm below the mark of the inframammary fold because of its tendency to migrate upward) (Fig. 1). The anterior axillary fold forms the lateral boundary for dissection. Upward displacement of the prosthesis is avoided by conservative superior dissection.
6. The submuscular implant or expander is inserted and the muscular pocket closed with sutures.
7. For expander reconstruction, only a small amount of saline is placed initially to minimize wound tension.

F. Expander Inflation

1. Generally, expander inflation begins 2 weeks after surgery with injection of 50–100 cc of sterile saline at 1- to 2-week intervals through the injection port. Once 20–30% overinflation is achieved, the expansion is maintained for at least 8 weeks to allow for capsule maturation.
2. Subsequent exchange of the expander with the permanent implant is performed. Nipple-areolar reconstruction and any cosmetic contralateral breast procedures (e.g., mastopexy, reduction mammoplasty) can be performed concomitantly.

G. Complete vs. Incomplete Coverage

Controversy exists as to whether complete submuscular implant or expander coverage in the lower pole is necessary.

1. Proponents of complete coverage argue that it causes less infection, exposure, and extrusion, while opponents believe that complete coverage gives ineffective expansion of the lower pole. Studies have shown no difference in complication rates between complete and incomplete coverage.
2. The decision to use textured or smooth prostheses resides with the individual surgeon. Textured devices are thought to promote more tissue ingrowth with better incorporation of the prosthesis. This allows for more secure positioning of textured prostheses in the chest wall and, possibly, for less pericapsular contraction.

H. Complications

1. The most common include hematoma, infection, flap necrosis, expander malfunction, implant rupture/leakage, infection, and capsular contracture.
2. Overall, prosthetic reconstruction has a higher rate of complications than autologous reconstruction.
3. Implant loss rates have been reported as high as 18%, but should be less with appropriate patient selection.
4. The leakage rate for saline implants is less than 5% over the first 5 years; however, up to 25% of patients undergoing implant reconstruction may need revisional surgery within the first 5 years

for implant displacement, failure, or capsular contracture.

I. Results

Most studies report good to excellent short-term results.

IV. PEDICLED AUTOLOGOUS TISSUE RECONSTRUCTION

A. General Indications

1. Poor quality recipient site tissue (e.g., thin mastectomy flaps).
2. Insufficient recipient site skin or tissue for reconstruction (e.g., after a Halsted radical mastectomy).
3. Problems with previous implant reconstruction.
4. Patient preference.

B. General Contraindications

1. Injury to donor pedicle.
2. Uncontrolled hypertension or diabetes.
3. Obesity.
4. Heavy smoking (nicotine increases platelet adherence and decreases flap perfusion).
5. Severe pulmonary or cardiac disease.
6. Autoimmune disease (e.g., scleroderma, Raynaud's disease).

C. Pedicled Latissimus Dorsi Flap

1. Indications

Patient preference, failure of prior non–latissimus dorsi autologous reconstruction, and prior chest wall radiation.

2. Contraindication

Thoracodorsal artery injury distal to the serratus branch is the only absolute contraindication.

3. Advantages

Reliable source of vacularized muscle and skin; faster recovery and less morbidity relative to transverse rectus abdominis musculocutaneous (TRAM) flap.

4. Disadvantages

Creation of a new donor site scar and generally inadequate autologous tissue for breast mound reconstruction [i.e., may still need implant with all the attendant disadvantages and complications (see above)].

5. Anatomy

a. The latissimus originates from the spinous processes of T6–L5, posterior iliac crest, and ribs 10–12. It inserts into the bicipital (intertubercular) groove of the humerus.
b. It extends, abducts, and medially rotates the arm.
c. It has a type V vascular anatomy with the thoracodorsal artery as the dominant pedicle and secondary segmental pedicles from the posterior intercostal and lumbar artery perforators. The thoracodorsal vein and nerve accompany the thoracodorsal artery.
d. Proximally, the subscapular artery (a branch of the axillary artery) gives off the circumflex scapular artery before terminating as the thoracodorsal artery (Fig. 2).
e. Prior to entering the undersurface of the latissimus dorsi, the thoracodorsal artery also gives off one or two serratus anterior branches. Thus, retrograde flow through the serratus anterior branches can adequately perfuse the latissimus flap if axillary dissection injures the proximal thoracodorsal artery.

6. Flap Design

a. First, determine the recipient site deficiency in terms of underlying volume and overlying skin deficits. Thin irradiated skin or poor quality mastectomy scars will need excision and will increase the total skin deficit.
b. Next, determine the optimal size and position for the flap on the chest. The latissimus skin paddle can be inferolaterally placed and used for inframammary fold definition (Fig. 3A). However, a prominent upper pole mastectomy scar may preclude this approach. In such cases, the mastectomy scar is excised and replaced by the skin paddle.
c. After determining the skin paddle size and position on the chest, the dimensions and location of the actual back skin paddle are configured. With the patient's arms adducted, the tip of the scapula marks the superior margin of the latissimus, while the posterior iliac crest marks the inferior margin (Fig. 3C).

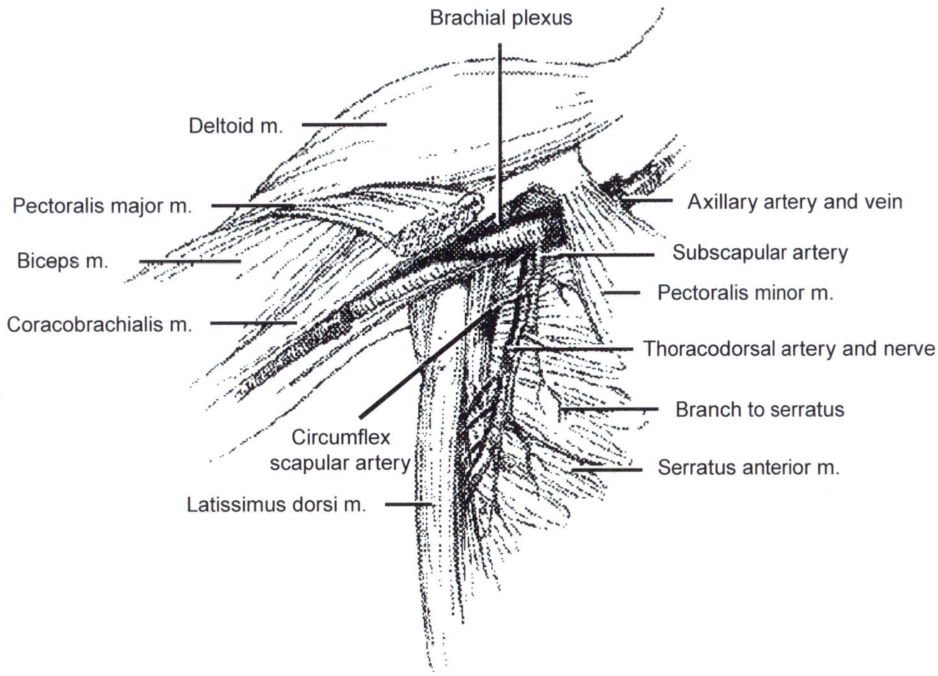

Figure 2 Vascular anatomy of the subscapular system. The subscapular artery arises from the third part of the axillary artery. It gives off a circumflex scapular branch before becoming the thoracodorsal artery. Prior to reaching the latissimus dorsi muscle, the thoracodorsal artery also gives off several serratus anterior branches. (Modified from Riefkohl R, Levin LS, Georgiade GS, eds. *Georgiade Plastic, Maxillofacial, and Reconstructive Surgery*. Baltimore: Williams and Wilkins, 1997.)

d. Removal of the pectoralis major after a radical mastectomy results in an upper chest defect that requires reconstruction with a superiorly placed muscle flap and an inferiorly located skin paddle (Fig. 3B) and thus will require the skin paddle to be located high on the back posteriorly. In contrast, for a modified radical mastectomy reconstruction, there is no superior muscle defect and the skin island can be placed lower in the back. In addition, patient preference for a transverse back scar in a brassiere line or lower oblique scar that allows a lower v-back piece of clothing (Fig. 3C) will sometimes determine placement of the incision.

e. Depending on skin laxity, a flap width of 7–10 cm can usually be obtained.

7. Operation

a. Place patient in the lateral decubitus position.

b. After incision around the skin island, skin flaps are elevated circumferentially. Boundaries for flap dissection include the posterior midline, tip of the scapula, serratus anterior, and 5–7 cm above the posterior iliac spine. Although as much fat as possible is left on the latissimus with the skin island, the surrounding skin flaps should be ~1 cm thick to prevent devascularization after disruption of the latissimus muscle perforators.

c. The thoracodorsal artery is then completely mobilized to avoid kinking of the pedicle. The serratus branch should not be sacrificed unless the thoracodorsal is confirmed to be intact.

d. The thoracodorsal nerve is often transected to prevent involuntary contraction of the transposed latissimus.

e. The tendon of the latissimus can be detached and repositioned to recreate the anterior axillary fold.

f. Except for a tunnel that is made in the apex of the axilla to pass the flap, the intervening skin between the anterior and posterior axillary lines is left undissected to help define the lateral edge of the new breast.

A

B

C

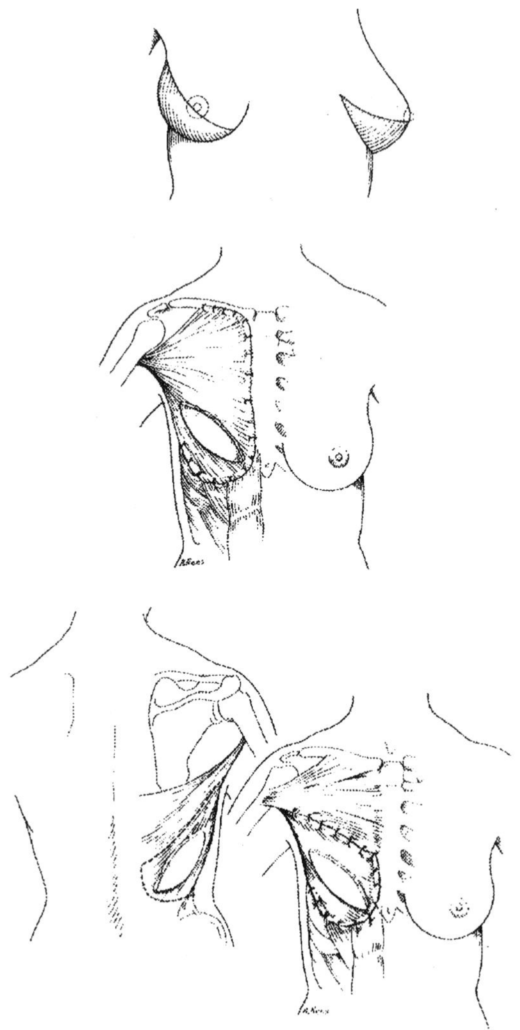

Figure 3 (A) Preferred inferolateral position for the latissimus dorsi skin island. (B) Preferred skin paddle placement for a radical mastectomy reconstruction. Note how the skin island will need to be high on the back posteriorly in order to be located in an inferior position anteriorly. (C) Preferred skin paddle placement for a modified radical mastectomy reconstruction. (Modified from Aston SJ, Beasley RW, Thorne C, Grabb WC, eds. *Grabb and Smith's Plastic Surgery*. Philadelphia: Lippincott-Raven, 1997.)

g. Drains are placed in the back and the posterior incision is closed.

h. The patient is then laid supine and the flap configured. For modified radical reconstruction, the latissimus dorsi is sutured to the inferior edge of the pectoralis major. For radical mastectomy reconstruction, the latissimus muscle is attached to the periosteum of the clavicle. The inframammary fold is determined, and the flap positioned to create the central breast mound. An implant may be used at this point if necessary.

i. The breast reconstruction is then closed and drains placed. The back drains are generally left in position for a longer time than the breast mound drains in order to minimize seroma formation (because of the extensive donor site dissection).

8. Complications

a. Donor site seroma and implant-related problems (if used) are the most common complications, although hematoma, infection, and flap necrosis (rare) can also occur.

b. Flap loss is usually less than 2%.

c. Donor-site morbidity is minimal if the remaining shoulder girdle muscles, including pectoralis major, subscapularis, teres major, and coracobrachialis, are functional.

9. Results

Can be acceptable cosmetically, especially if sufficient back fat is present.

D. Pedicled Transverse Rectus Abdominis Musculocutaneous (TRAM) Flap

1. Indications

Large recipient site defect and patient preference

2. Contraindications

a. Prior abdominal surgeries with injury to the superior epigastric artery or rectus abdominis perforators (e.g., chevron incision, abdominoplasty, abdominal liposuction).

b. Pendulous or inadequate abdominal panniculus.

c. Prior chest wall radiation (may cause radiation fibrosis of the internal mammary vessels).

d. In addition, because the superior epigastric artery is the less dominant vascular pedicle, the TRAM flap is not as reliable as the latissimus dorsi flap. Thus, factors that potentially compromise flap perfusion (see general contraindications above) will have a larger impact on a pedicled TRAM flap than a latissimus dorsi flap.

3. Advantages

   a. Adequate tissue for complete reconstruction (i.e., no need for additional implants).
   b. Reliable perfusion.
   c. Consistently good long-term results.
   d. Better donor site scar.
   e. "Free" abdominoplasty.

4. Disadvantages

   a. Creation of new donor site scar and longer recovery relative to latissimus flap.
   b. With respect to the free TRAM, the pedicle TRAM requires more rectus abdominis muscle sacrifice and has less reliable flap perfusion (higher incidence of fat and partial flap necrosis in the pedicled TRAM).
   c. The reliable flap volume may be unpredictable depending upon the anatomy of the collateral arteries between the superior and inferior epigastric vessels. In some cases, only zone I may be reliable (Fig. 4).

5. Anatomy

   a. The rectus abdominis muscles originate from the 6th, 7th, and 8th rib cartilages and insert into the pubic tubercle and pubic crest.
   b. They function to flex the trunk and stabilize the pelvis.
   c. Each rectus abdominis muscle is encased by an anterior and posterior sheath; however, below the arcuate line the posterior sheath becomes part of the anterior sheath.
   d. The rectus abdominis muscles have a type III vascular anatomy with the superior epigastric and deep inferior epigastric arteries as the two dominant pedicles. The superior epigastric artery travels deep to the rectus muscle but enters it before the first inscription. It is a branch of the internal mammary artery, which itself is a branch of the subclavian artery. The deep inferior epigastric artery is a branch of the external iliac and enters the posterior sheath near the level of the arcuate line.
   e. The deep inferior epigastric artery is the more dominant pedicle, supplying approximately 2/3 of the blood supply to the flap, while the superior epigastric artery only supplies about 1/3.
   f. Perfusion of pedicle TRAM flaps relies on anastomotic choke vessels that connect the superior and deep inferior epigastric arteries with secondary retrograde filling of the deep inferior epigastric artery.
   g. The most important perforators from the superior and deep inferior epigastric arteries to supply the pedicle TRAM are immediately lateral and superior to the umbilicus.
   h. Innervation is from intercostal nerves 8 to 12. They travel between the internal oblique and transversus muscles and enter the lateral third of the rectus muscle posteriorly.

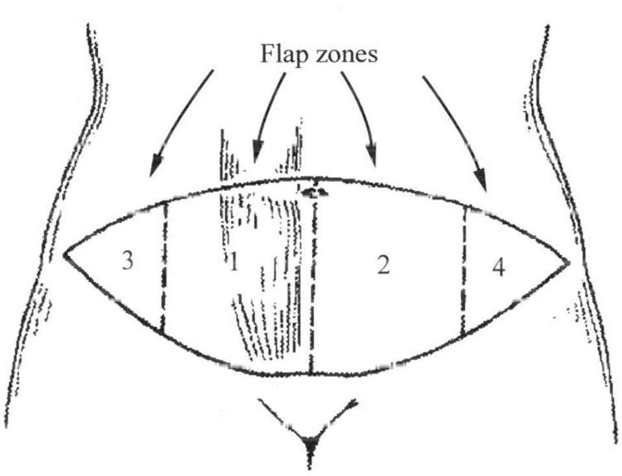

Figure 4 Vascular zones of the TRAM flap. (From Aston SJ, Beasley RW, Thorne C, Grabb WC, eds. *Grabb and Smith's Plastic Surgery*. Philadelphia: Lippincott-Raven, 1997.)

6. Flap Design

   a. In a similar fashion to the latissimus flap, breast tissue and skin deficits, noticeable scars, optimal flap size and position for reconstruction are all determined. For all intents and purposes, the outward appearance of the flap is identical to an abdominoplasty flap.
   b. Because the more dominant perforators are located in the periumbilical area, the superior margin of the flap is always at or above the level of the umbilicus.
   c. The inferior boundary is determined by the degree of upper abdominal skin laxity.
   d. Generally, the contralateral rectus is preferred for breast reconstruction because there is less

twisting/folding of the pedicle, but the ipsilateral rectus can also be used.

e. Four zones of TRAM flap perfusion have been described, with 1 and 3 being ipsilateral to the vascular pedicle and 2 and 4 being contralateral (Fig. 4). Perfusion in zone 1 > 2 > 3 > 4. Zone 4 perfusion in a pedicled TRAM is marginal at best.

7. Operation

a. With the patient supine, the superior portion of the flap is first incised at approximately the level of the umbilicus. More fat is taken on the flap side (i.e., bevel 45° away from the flap) in order to avoid injury to the periumbilical perforators in the flap.

b. Next, the upper abdominal panniculus is dissected off the rectus abdominis fascia to the level of the costal cartilages and xiphoid.

c. The operating table is then flexed and the upper undermined abdominal panniculus pulled down to determine the location of the inferior incision.

d. The inframammary fold location is also confirmed again with the abdomen pulled down.

e. The inferior flap border is incised with less fat taken on the flap side this time (i.e., bevel toward the flap). The lateral aspects of the flap are then dissected. On the side contralateral to the pedicle, the flap is completely elevated past the midline to ~ 1 cm past the medial border of the ipsilateral rectus. The location of perforators on the contralateral side can serve as a guide for the ipsilateral dissection. The flap ipsilateral to the pedicle is then carefully elevated from lateral to medial with care to preserve the perforators.

f. The anterior rectus sheath is then incised longitudinally both medially and laterally to include the perforators (~ 2–3 cm wide strip of sheath). Next, the muscle just lateral to the lateral perforators is incised vertically to expose the posterior sheath. The intercostal vessels and nerves laterally are divided as necessary. The 8th intercostal nerve is divided so that the muscle will atrophy and not create a bulge in the tunnel.

g. The inferior epigastric artery and vein enter the posterior sheath at approximately the levels of the arcuate line and as much length as possible is dissected free in case microvascular anastomosis is needed.

h. Next, the distal rectus muscle is transected near the arcuate line and the deep inferior epigastric artery ligated. In a muscle-sparing approach, the location of the superior epigastric artery is precisely determined by Doppler and carefully preserved as the rectus abdominis is longitudinally divided. This approach preserves the lateral third and a small medial strip of rectus muscle. Alternatively, the entire ipsilateral rectus above the arcuate line may be removed.

i. The umbilical stalk is then completely freed from the flap with enough surrounding tissue to prevent ischemia.

j. At this point, the elevated flap with its pedicle of rectus abdominis and overlying sheath is completely freed.

k. Following this, a tunnel is made over the sternum to allow passage of the flap to the chest. It is important to stay in the midline and not disrupt the inframammary fold. The flap is carefully passed through the tunnel and configured with minimal folding of the pedicle (Fig. 5).

l. If the entire lower abdominal tissue is needed for reconstruction, then a double pedicle or a single pedicle with additional microvascular anastomosis TRAM (“supercharged” TRAM) should be performed.

m. The abdominal wall is reconstructed with the sheath and muscle closed primarily and then oversewn with a second layer of sutures. It is critical to include both the external oblique and internal oblique fascia (tends to retract laterally) in the anterior rectus sheath reconstruction. The costal area of the sheath should be reconstructed without compromising the pedicle. The contralateral fascia may also need plication for symmetry. Mesh may be placed to reinforce the closure.

n. The table is flexed and the abdominal skin closed with a new umbilicus opening. Closed suction drains are placed under the abdominal panniculus.

o. The flap is modified into a breast mound.

p. Lastly, unnecessary skin is removed and the flap sutured with drains in place.

8. Complications

a. Fat necrosis, flap necrosis, abdominal flap skin slough, abdominal weakness/hernia, seroma, infection, and hematoma.

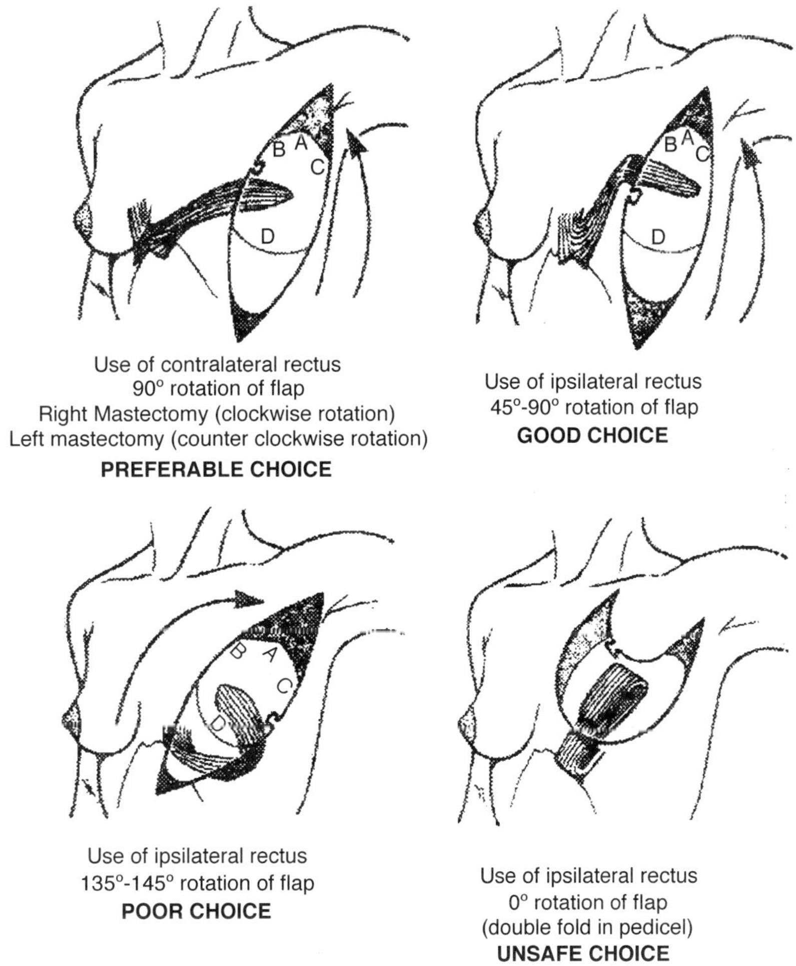

Figure 5 Vascular pedicle options for a left modified mastectomy reconstruction. Shaded areas of flap are possibly unsafe. (Modified from Riefkohl R, Levin LS, Georgiade GS, eds. *Georgiade Plastic, Maxillofacial, and Reconstructive Surgery*. Baltimore: Williams and Wilkins, 1997.)

b. The risk of total flap failure is less than 1%; however, the incidence of fat necrosis reported varies from 5 to 30%, depending on the series.

c. Some authors report lower fat necrosis rates by capturing abdominal perforators above the umbilicus, although this necessitates a higher abdominal scar. Focal areas of fat necrosis result in hard breast tissue nodules that may require subsequent biopsy to rule out malignancy.

d. Abdominal flap skin slough can be decreased by limited fat thinning of the upper abdominal skin flap and cessation of smoking at least a few weeks prior to surgery.

e. The abdominal hernia rate is about 5%, but may be decreased to 1.5% with the routine use of synthetic mesh.

f. Other complications such as deep venous thrombosis from immobilization can be decreased with the routine use of leg compression devices and early ambulation.

9. Results

Results are above average to excellent. One study comparing TRAM, latissimus dorsi, or tissue expander reconstruction found that TRAM flaps gave the best aesthetic results.

V. MICROVASCULAR AUTOLOGOUS TISSUE RECONSTRUCTION

Unconstrained movement of tissue from one part of the body to another is possible as long as suitable donor and recipient vessels are available.

A. General Indications

1. Adequate distant donor site soft tissue and skin.
2. Failure of regional (pedicle) reconstruction.
3. No regional donor sites.
4. Inadequate regional donor site (e.g., not enough tissue).

B. General Contraindications

1. Inadequate distant donor site soft tissue and skin.
2. Injury to recipient vessels or donor vessels and perforators (e.g., abdominal lipectomy).
3. Other contraindications are similar to those for pedicled autologous reconstruction (see above).

C. Free TRAM Flap

1. Indications

Need for a large volume of tissue; pedicled TRAM unfeasible secondary to superior epigastric artery injury.

2. Contraindications

Division of the deep inferior epigastric artery from prior surgery (e.g., inguinal hernia repair, paramedian incision). Other contraindications are similar to those for the pedicle TRAM; however, a free TRAM is preferred over a pedicled TRAM in patients who are at higher risk for flap failure (e.g., obese, heavy smoker) because better perfusion is obtained from the deep inferior epigastric artery.

3. Advantages

Enhanced blood supply (through dominant deep inferior epigastric artery) makes larger flaps possible with less fat and flap necrosis, no pedicle constraints on bulk (more freedom in tissue shaping), less donor site morbidity, and faster recovery (less muscle taken) relative to pedicled TRAMs.

4. Disadvantages

Longer operative times, requirement for microvascular expertise and monitoring, and higher risk of total flap loss relative to pedicled TRAMs.

5. Anatomy

a. In contrast to the pedicled TRAM flap, the free TRAM flap is supplied by the deep inferior epigastric artery and two venae comitantes. This artery arises from the anterior aspect of the external iliac artery just before the inguinal ligament and enters the rectus muscle laterally near the arcuate line.
b. The most common recipient vessels for the free TRAM flap are the thoracodorsal vessels, but they may be unsuitable in an irradiated axilla or may have been injured during axillary dissection.
c. Alternative recipient vessels include the circumflex scapular, internal mammary, thoracoacromial, circumflex humeral, and axillary vessels.

6. Flap Design

Essentially the same as for the pedicled TRAM, but more contralateral tissue (i.e., zone 4) may be utilized because of better perfusion. Also, because the vascular supply will be completely detached and reattached, there is no preference for the contralateral rectus muscle as in the pedicled TRAM.

7. Operation

a. The flap is elevated as for a pedicled TRAM. The side with the largest perforators is selected to be the pedicle side. After selection of the perforators to be retained, the anterior rectus sheath is incised vertically on the pedicle side and the deep inferior epigastric vessels identified. The vessels are then traced to the external iliac and any side branches ligated.
b. The lateral, inferior, and medial portions of the rectus are divided, but the superior portion is left intact until both recipient and donor vessels are completely dissected and deemed appropriate for anastomosis. If not, a pedicle TRAM can still be performed. After division of the superior portion of the rectus muscle, only a free TRAM is possible.
c. The flap is brought to the chest and the microvascular anastomosis performed to the thoracodorsal artery in an end-to-end fashion just proximal to the serratus anterior branch. This preserves retrograde flow though the serratus branch to the latissimus muscle for additional reconstruction, if necessary.
d. Next, the veins are anastomosed with suture or a coupling device.

e. The abdomen is then reconstructed and the flap modified in a similar fashion as the pedicle TRAM.

8. Flap Monitoring

a. Routine monitoring of flap Doppler signal, appearance, and temperature are critical in the first 48 hours.
b. Most complications occur within the first 6–24 hours after vascular anastomosis.
c. Early signs of venous thrombosis include bleeding from flap margins, increased tissue turgor, and a dusky flap color from venous engorgement, as well as loss of Doppler venous augmentation signal. In addition, capillary refill time is decreased to less than 1 second (normal is 1–3 seconds) and the flap surface temperature may fall greater than 3 °C compared with nonflap skin surfaces.
d. Early signs of arterial thrombosis include pale flap appearance, loss of triphasic Doppler signal, increased capillary refill time of greater than 3 seconds, and greater than 3 °C fall in flap temperature.

9. Complications

a. Less than 3% total flap failure, with most series showing less than 1%, making the free TRAM as reliable as the pedicled TRAM.
b. The incidence of fat necrosis or partial flap loss should be less than 5%.
c. The incidence of hernia formation is similar to pedicled TRAMs (~5%), likely because most hernias are inferior and both free and pedicled TRAMs may injure the inferior rectus sheath.
d. Flap failure is most commonly from venous thrombosis, but the flap is generally salvageable if the thrombosis is detected early.

10. Results

Generally better than the pedicled TRAM because of improved flap perfusion (less fat necrosis and partial flap loss), fewer constraints on flap insetting, and no inframammary rectus muscle "bulge."

D. Other Free Flaps for Breast Reconstruction

The TRAM is the most commonly used breast reconstruction flap because other donor sites are technically more difficult with little room for error in skin island design, pedicle dissection, or donor site closure. In addition, these other donor sites generally have shorter vascular pedicles and vessel diameters that are incompatible with the thoracodorsal vessels, necessitating a thorough knowledge of different vascular recipient vessels (e.g., internal mammary, lateral thoracic, circumflex scapular, and thoracoacromial). Table 1 summarizes some of the characteristics of each flap.

1. Gluteus Maximus Flap

a. This flap has a type III vascular anatomy with the superior and inferior gluteal arteries as the two dominant pedicles.
b. It is indicated for patients in whom a TRAM is not feasible because of prior abdominal procedures or in thin patients with inadequate volume

Table 1 Comparison of Flaps for Autologous Breast Reconstruction

	Skin	Bulk	Contour	Donor appearance	Reliability	Technical ease
Free TRAM	++++	+++	+++	+++	+++	+++
Pedicled TRAM	+++	++	++	+++	++	+++
Latissimus	+	+	+	++	++++	++++
Gluteus	+++	++++	++++	+++	++	++
DCIA	+++	+++	+++	+++	++	++
TFL	++	++	++	+	+++	++

+ = poor; ++ = average; +++ = good; ++++ = excellent.
Source: Modified from Riefkohl R, Levin LS, Georgiade GS, eds. *Georgiade Plastic, Maxillofacial, and Reconstructive Surgery*. Baltimore: Williams and Wilkins, 1997.

for TRAM, deep circumflex iliac artery, or tensor fascia lata flaps.

c. If the flap is based on the superior gluteal artery, there is minimal donor site morbidity with the benefit of a thigh "lift" on the donor side.

2. TFL (Tensor Fascia Lata, Lateral Transverse, or Vertical Thigh) Flap

a. This flap has a type I vascular anatomy with the transverse branch of the lateral circumflex femoral artery as the only vascular pedicle.

b. It is not as commonly used for breast reconstruction because of the large lateral thigh scar, thigh asymmetry, potential injury to femoral nerve, and high incidence of seromas.

3. Modified Deep Circumflex Iliac Artery (DCIA, Rubens) Flap

a. There is no muscle involved with this flap.

b. It is based on the DCIA as the only vascular pedicle. The flap encompasses the area overlying the anterior superior iliac spine to posterior axillary line.

c. It is indicated in patients with a large iliac crest fullness and unavailable abdominal donor sites.

d. Disadvantages include injury to the lateral cutaneous nerve of the thigh and increased risk of hernias.

VI. NIPPLE-AREOLA RECONSTRUCTION AND SECONDARY BREAST MOUND REVISION

A. Generally, nipple-areola reconstruction is performed as a secondary procedure after the initial reconstruction.

B. A typical waiting period is 6 weeks to 3 months to allow for sufficient vascularization of the new breast mound.

C. The method of nipple reconstruction is dictated in part by the size and appearance of the contralateral nipple, the type of breast reconstruction, and the surgeon's preference.

D. The nipple and areola are then tattooed after complete healing of the reconstructed nipple.

101

Breast Reduction and Mastopexy

Peter J. Taub, M.D., and Jeffrey D. Hoefflin, M.D.
New York Medical College and Westchester Medical Center, Valhalla, New York, U.S.A.

James Watson, M.D.
David Geffen School of Medicine at UCLA, Los Angeles, California, U.S.A.

I. INTRODUCTION

Breast hypertrophy in women with normal hormonal endocrine function is a common finding in Western societies. Combined with the effects of gravity and involution, the weight of the breasts can cause postural changes. This can result in neck, shoulder, and back pain that is not relieved by exercise, weight loss, or support bras. In patients with and without breast hypertrophy, the effect of gravity also causes drooping of the breasts, eventually resulting in the nipple position falling below the inframammary fold. This is called breast ptosis and is a common indication for surgery.

II. ANATOMY AND PHYSIOLOGY

The breast is glandular tissue that is actually a modified cutaneous gland, an appendage of the skin. This glandular tissue is enclosed between the superficial fascial system and the deep fascia overlying the chest wall muscles.

A. Cooper's Ligaments

The breast parenchyma is attached to the superficial fascia anteriorly and to the deep fascia posteriorly. Sir Astley Cooper first described these anterior "ligaments" as the suspensory system of the breast. These collagenous ligaments stretch with age, resulting in ptosis of the breast.

B. Blood Supply

The breast is supplied by three main arterial branches of the subclavian and axillary arteries:

1. Internal mammary artery—anterior branches of the internal mammary artery perforate through the sternal head of the pectoralis major muscle, providing 60% of the blood supply to the breast. These branches provide blood to the medial flap in a Wise-pattern breast reduction.
2. Lateral thoracic artery—external mammary branches of the lateral thoracic artery, which accompanies the lateral thoracic nerve, provide an additional 30% of the blood supply to the breast. These branches provide blood to the lateral flap in a Wise-pattern breast reduction.
3. Thoracoacromial artery—pectoral branches of the thoracoacromial artery supply the pectoralis major muscle. Myocutaneous branches of this artery provide a minor blood supply to the portion of the breast overlying the pectoralis major muscle. These branches provide blood to the nipple-areola complex in breast reductions with a parenchymal-based pedicle for the nipple.

C. Sensation

Sensory innervation of breast skin is supplied by three sets of nerve branches:

1. Lateral branches of intercostal nerves—lateral branches of intercostal nerves exit the rib cage and enter the breast along the lateral border of the pectoralis major muscle. The lateral 4th intercostal branch provides the major sensory innervation to the nipple.
2. Medial branches of intercostal nerves—perforate the chest wall along with the perforators of the internal mammary artery. These branches of intercostal nerves 2–7 provide sensation to the medial skin of the breast.
3. Cervical plexus—sensory branches of the C3 and C4 nerve roots form the supraclavicular nerve, which provides minor sensation to the superior pole of the breast skin.

D. Physiology of Breast Hypertrophy

The underlying cause of breast hypertrophy is still poorly understood. With few exceptions, hormonal excesses are not usually the cause. The following factors are thought to be the major causes:

1. Body weight—obesity is often associated with breast hypertrophy. Weight loss in obese patients does not always relieve symptoms of neck, shoulder, and back pain, however. Nonetheless, preoperative weight loss should be encouraged.
2. Genetic background—familial tendencies to develop breast hypertrophy have been well documented. The exact genetic transmission of this trait is not yet known, however.
3. End-organ hormonal sensitivity—breast gland sensitivity to ovarian steroid hormones is thought to be a cause of breast hypertrophy. This probably is the major factor in most patients.

E. Breast Measurements and Proportions

Ideal aesthetic proportions of a youthful breast not subject to the effects of pregnancy and gravity have been made with geometric descriptions. These measurements and landmarks are important in surgical planning to determine the proper place to reposition the nipple. The most commonly used landmarks are as follows (Fig. 1):

1. Breast meridian—a line can be drawn vertically down the breast from a point along the mid-clavicle (approximately 5–7 cm lateral to the suprasternal notch). This line can be useful in determining the proper position for the nipple in the horizontal plane.
2. Nipple-suprasternal notch relationship—in the ideal aesthetic breast, an isosceles triangle can be drawn between the two nipples and the suprasternal notch. The distance between each nipple and the suprasternal notch should ideally be the same, usually ranging from 18 to 21 cm. This relationship is a useful one in determining the proper vertical position of the nipple in both breast reduction and mastopexy surgery.
3. Inframammary crease—since the definition of breast ptosis is made by the relationship of the nipple-areola complex to the inframammary fold, the position of the fold is often used as the landmark to determine proper nipple position.
4. Areola—the areola should sit equidistant from all sides of the nipple. Its diameter ranges from 35 to 40 mm.
5. Infra-areolar distance—this distance is approximately 5–8 cm from the inferior aspect of the areola to the inframammary crease.

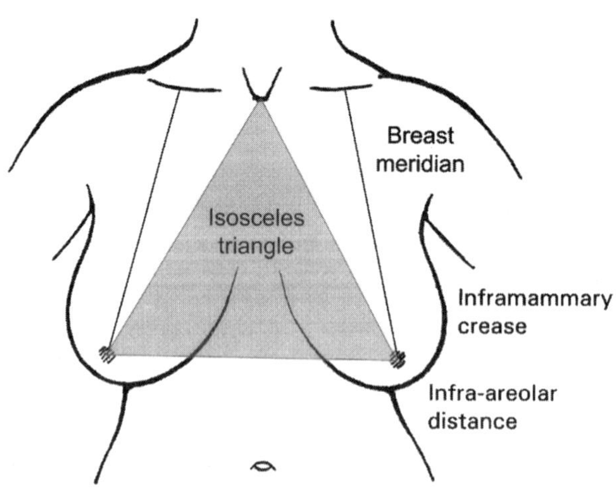

Figure 1 Commonly used landmarks on the breast.

III. REDUCTION MAMMOPLASTY

A. Indications

Most women choose to have breast reduction surgery due to postural problems caused by the weight of the breast. This includes neck and back pain. Bra straps can also cause shoulder pain and create grooves that irritate the skin. Dermatitis within the skin fold at the inframammary crease can also be difficult to control medically, causing maceration and fungal infections. Breast pain due to the weight of the breast can also occur. In most cases, a patient with one or more of these symptoms may be a candidate for breast reduction surgery.

B. Diagnosis and Differential Diagnosis

The diagnosis of breast hypertrophy can easily be made by physical examination. Although large breasts cause neck, shoulder, and back pain, underlying musculoskeletal problems can also cause similar symptoms (e.g., spinal stenosis, arthritis, disc disease, poor posture, trauma, and sports injuries). If the patient's symptoms are due to one of these other causes, reduction mammoplasty may not provide symptomatic relief.

C. Surgical Timing

Breast reduction surgery is ideally performed after breast growth is complete and stable. However, reduction mammoplasty may be appropriately performed before breast maturity in cases where gigantomastia limits the patient's physical activity or normal psychosocial development. Patient counseling should also be provided concerning future plans for pregnancy and breast feeding. Although many patients are able to breast feed following reduction mammoplasty, the surgery may limit their ability to sustain their child on breast milk alone.

D. Preoperative Work-up

A thorough history and physical exam should be performed, documenting the patient's symptoms, as well as personal and family history of malignant and premalignant breast disease.

1. Physical exam—a complete breast and axillary exam should be performed, including documentation of the following:
   - Nipple-to-suprasternal notch measurements.
   - Nipple-to-inframammary fold measurements.
   - Breast asymmetry in terms of size and ptosis.
   - Preoperative sensation of the nipple-areola complex.
   - Breast masses, nipple discharge, skin retraction, and axillary adenopathy must be excluded or evaluated appropriately prior to surgery.
2. Screening mammography—in older patients, preoperative screening mammography should be performed in accordance with current guidelines. Practically speaking, this means that all patients over the age of 35 should have preoperative mammograms. For younger patients, the value of mammography is limited due to the dense nature of the breast parenchyma. In these patients, the need for preoperative mammography is still controversial, especially in patients with normal physical exams.

E. Techniques

A large number of breast reduction techniques have been described historically. Although a complete history and description of each technique is beyond the scope of this chapter, a number of techniques are of historical or current importance. These can be grouped into categories based on the methods of nipple-areola complex movement and perfusion.

1. Breast Amputation and Free Nipple Grafting Techniques

a. Thorek was the first to publish a report of reduction mammoplasty where the nipple was completely removed and then reattached as a free graft. This technique is still used today as a good option for patients with very large breasts with severe ptosis, especially those with a history diabetes mellitus or smoking.

b. In these cases, neovascularization of the nipple graft will be more reliable than perfusion by a long parenchymal or dermal pedicle. For this reason, many surgeons rely on measurements from the inframammary crease (IMC) to the nipple to determine when to use this technique. Although there is no universal agreement on the exact length, many surgeons will consider and consent patients for breast amputation and free nipple grafting if the IMC-to-nipple distance is more than 20 cm.

c. The major disadvantage of this technique is that it results in complete loss of sensation of the nipple-areola complex and inability to breast feed. In patients with very large breasts with severe ptosis, however, preoperative nipple sensation may already be markedly decreased, making this less of an issue.

2. Deepithelialized Dermal Pedicle Techniques

a. Most older techniques of reduction mammoplasty relied on one or more deepithelialized dermal pedicles to provide blood supply to the nipple. These techniques were developed after Schwartzmann described the important role of the subdermal plexus in providing skin perfusion.

b. The techniques described by Strombeck, Skoog, McKissock, and Wise all rely on dermal pedicles to perfuse the nipples. They all utilize inverted T closures for breast reshaping and differ mainly in the way the pedicle for the nipple is designed:

- Strombeck technique—Strombeck described a reduction technique that provided nipple perfusion with bipedicled horizontal dermal blood supply.
- Skoog technique—Skoog modified the Strombeck procedure and based the nipple on a unipedicle dermal pedicle.
- McKissock—McKissock described a reduction technique that provided nipple perfusion with a vertical dermal bipedicle.
- Weiner—Weiner first described a single, superiorly based dermal pedicle for nipple perfusion. This technique had the advantage of eliminating the long inferior pedicle of the McKissock technique and the tethering problems associated with the horizontal pedicle in the Strombeck technique.

3. Dermoglandular Flap Techniques

Rather than relying on the subdermal plexus alone, other surgeons developed breast reduction techniques where the nipple was supplied by both dermal and parenchymal perfusion. These techniques include the following:

a. Regnault B technique—differs from the techniques described above both in the skin closure incisions and the nipple blood supply. In the Regnault B technique, a superiorly based dermoglandular blood supply to the nipple is maintained, with excess skin and breast parenchyma removed laterally. The main advantage of this technique is avoidance of the medial horizontal scar along the inframammary crease.

b. Modified McKissock technique—modification of the original McKissock vertical dermal bipedicle to a vertical dermoglandular bipedicle technique. This technique improved the blood supply and sensation to the nipple-areola complex, compared to the original description.

c. Ribero technique—breast reduction technique based on an inferior dermoglandular pedicle. His technique was later modified by other surgeons into the modern inferior parenchymal flap techniques described below.

4. Parenchymal Flap Techniques

Although the dermal and dermoglandular techniques became popular because of reliable nipple perfusion, they all suffered drawbacks of some loss of nipple sensation. For this reason, several surgeons started experimenting with methods to reduce the breast and yet maintain nipple sensation. They include the following:

a. Central mound technique—Balch first described leaving the nipple-areola complex on a mound of parenchyma directly under the nipple. With this technique, no dermal attachments tether nipple repositioning and nipple sensation can be preserved.

b. Inferior parenchymal pedicle technique—several authors contributed to the development of an inferiorly based parenchymal pedicle for the nipple. They include Courtiss, Goldwyn, Georgiade, and others. These authors are credited for developing the most common technique used today for breast reduction surgery (Fig. 2). It has the advantage of providing both reliable nipple perfusion and nipple sensation. It can be used reliably in all but the largest breast reduction procedures. In these extreme cases, breast am-

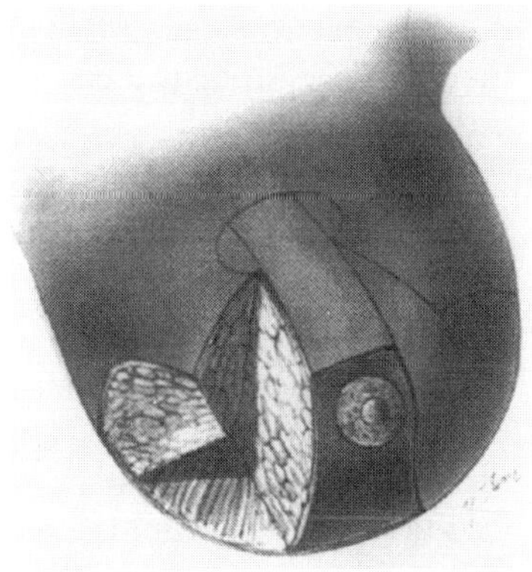

Figure 2 Inferior pedicle technique of breast reduction.

putation with free nipple grafting may still play a role.

c. Central superior pedicle technique—popularized by Lejour, this technique employs a vertical skin and gland resection. Liposuction addresses portions of the medial, lateral, and superior reduction. The gland is sutured to the chest wall superiorly and inferiorly to fix its position and establish contour. The skin retracts in the area of the inframammary fold. Its major advantage is the absence of the horizontal portion of the inverted "T" incision.

IV. MASTOPEXY

A. Indications

Whereas reduction mammoplasty is indicated for correction of physical symptoms as well as aesthetic and psychosocial concerns, mastopexy is largely considered for aesthetic improvement in breast appearance.

B. Diagnosis

Breast ptosis is the term used to describe the descent of the nipple-areola complex and its relative position to the inframammary crease (with the patient standing in the upright position). Determining the degree or grade of breast ptosis is often useful in preoperative decision making with regard to the type of mastopexy that would be appropriate for the patient. The most common classification (Regnault) is as follows (Fig. 3):

1. Pseudoptosis—drooping breast, but nipple still above the inframammary crease.
2. Grade I ptosis—nipple lies at the level of the inframammary crease.
3. Grade II ptosis—nipple lies below the inframammary crease, but above the lowest contour of the breast.
4. Grade III ptosis—nipple lies at or below the lowest contour of the breast.

C. Techniques

Many of the concepts applied to reduction mammoplasty are applicable to mastopexy. The technique chosen is largely dependent upon the amount of breast ptosis.

1. For patients with grade I ptosis, subglandular augmentation mammoplasty may be adequate.

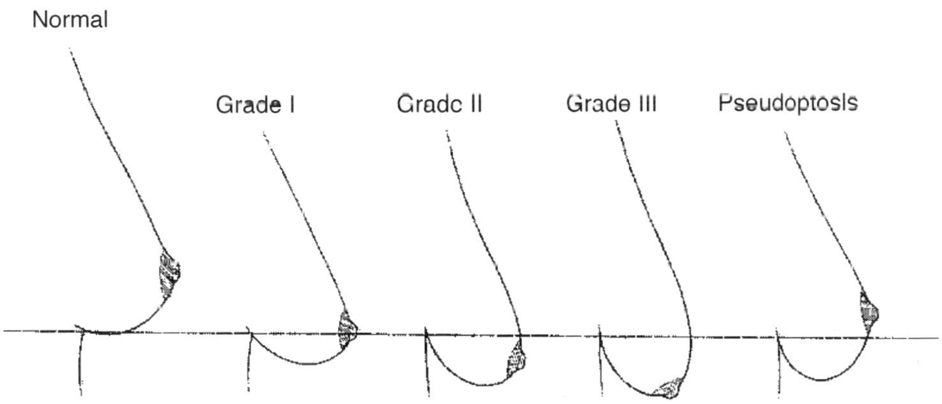

Figure 3 Grading system for breast ptosis.

Another option is crescent excision mastopexy in which a crescent of skin is removed superior to the nipple-areola complex.

2. For patients with grade II ptosis, a circumferential periareolar procedure may be adequate. This technique has limited indications because the results are often poor in the less-than-ideal candidate. The postoperative appearance of the breast is often boxy with enlargement of the areola and scarring around the periphery of the areola. The Benelli, or round-block, excision attempts to avoid these complications. Through a periareolar incision, the technique creates inferomedial and inferolateral dermoglandular flaps that overlap each other in the midline. These flaps are fixed to the chest wall. A nonresorbable, fixed suture encircles the areola.
3. For most patients and especially those with grade III ptosis, mastopexy utilizing the same markings for reduction mammoplasty may be chosen. The breast meridian, inframammary fold, and nipple position are drawn as described above. The areola is positioned around the site of the new nipple and a keyhole pattern is added with inferior, divergent limbs approximately 5 cm in length. The ends of the limbs are joined to the ends of the inframammary fold, often in a lazy "S" to approximate the length of the fold. The area within the pattern is deepithelialized, and the skin is closed with little undermining.
4. Adjunctive augmentation may be used for the ptotic and hypoplastic breast. Subglandular positioning of the implant may lead to future ptosis of the resculpted breast, but avoids the potential double-bubble appearance seen with submuscular placement. *Caution must always be exercised when combining tightening of the skin envelope and augmentation of the breast volume. Undue tension may be created, which may result not only in widening of the scars but also ischemia of the skin and/or nipples.* For this reason, combined augmentation and mastopexy may be best performed in staged procedures.

V. COMPLICATIONS OF REDUCTION MAMMOPLASTY AND MASTOPEXY

A. Diminished nipple sensation and inability to breast feed—reportedly seen in 15–35% of patients, with significantly fewer patients having permanently decreased sensation.

B. Patient dissatisfaction—specific concerns about the postoperative appearance of the breast include the following:

- Improper, or "high" nipple position—largely a function of precise preoperative planning. The ideal position is at or slightly below the inframammary fold with a vertical limb length less than 6 cm from areola to fold. Correction may entail: (1) horizontal excision along the inframammary fold, (2) direct repositioning of the nipple-areola complex, or (3) addition of an implant to improve the projection of the nipple.
- Boxy appearance to the breast—due to inadequate resection of parenchyma at the periphery of the breast.
- Asymmetry—postoperative complaints regarding breast asymmetry may be largely avoided by pointing out to the patient the natural asymmetry in the breasts preoperatively. Significant asymmetry may be improved by limited liposuction of the larger breast.

C. Bleeding or hematoma (~2%)—Although the role of drains remains controversial, postoperative hematoma formation may be ameliorated by judicious use of drains that may be removed early in the postoperative period.

D. Nipple ischemia (1–2%)—More likely to occur with increasing breast size, technical deficiency, tobacco usage, and, most specifically, increased preoperative distance between the areola and inframammary fold. Maintaining an adequate pedicle for the nipple-areola complex is an important component of any technique. The alternative, in exceptionally large breasts, is free nipple grafting. Management of the patient with postoperative nipple ischemia includes removal of sutures, examination of the pedicle, and/or application of nitroglycerin paste.

E. Flap necrosis (1–2%)—due to overly aggressive thinning of the flaps and/or excessive tension in the closure of the breast. This complication is more common in the patient who is actively smoking at the time of surgery, a fact that should be determined prior to performing the procedure. In general, the skin flaps should be approximately 1 cm thick.

F. Cellulitis or abscess formation (<1%).

G. Hypertrophic scar formation.

102

Augmentation Mammaplasty

George H. Rudkin, M.D., and Timothy A. Miller, M.D.
David Geffen School of Medicine at UCLA, Los Angeles, California, U.S.A.

I. HISTORY

A. Attempts at surgical breast augmentation were performed as early as 1895. At first, autogenous tissue was utilized exclusively.

B. Later, paraffin (1942) and silicone (1961) were injected directly into the breast, but these techniques proved to have unacceptable complications.

C. The implantation of Ivalon sponge was reported in 1953, but follow-up again revealed poor results.

D. In 1963, Cronin and Gerow presented a report on the use of silicone gel prostheses for cosmetic breast augmentation, effectively introducing modern breast augmentation.

E. Inflatable prostheses were introduced by Arion in 1965.

F. Early implants were plagued by high rates of capsular contracture, but modifications to the implant shell have decreased the incidence of this complication.

II. THE PREOPERATIVE EVALUATION

Patients and surgeons have a number of options in implant selection and placement. This results in a relatively complex surgical decision-making process, which must be approached in a systematic fashion. An appropriate amount of time must be allocated to the preoperative evaluation to allow a thorough discussion of the options, and the surgeon's rationale for his/her recommendations.

A. Indications

1. A broad range of patients may request breast augmentation.
2. Most commonly, the patient is a young female requesting larger breasts or an older (often postpartum) female requesting restoration of volume that has been lost.
3. Some patients may present with pseudoptosis or Grade I ptosis, which may be appropriately corrected with breast augmentation.
4. More severe forms of ptosis require mastopexy, either with or without augmentation.

B. "Size"

1. Patients may often specify a desired "cup" size, and it is important to note to the patient that the selection of implant size is limited to some extent by the patient's individual anatomy. It is therefore important to engage in frank discussion of the patient's goals and the surgical limitations.
2. Once a size range is selected, having the patient place implants/sizers in her brassiere will allow her to make some assessment of the expected postoperative outcome.

3. Typically, implants of different sizes are brought to the operating room to allow the surgeon a degree of intraoperative flexibility.

III. IMPLANTS

A. Saline vs. Silicone Implants

1. Saline-filled implants are the only option for primary breast augmentation in the majority of women today. These implants have a silicone elastomer shell, and are filled with sterile saline.
2. Prefilled implants are filled to a specific volume by the manufacturer and have the advantages of an optimum fill volume and a factory seal (no valve mechanism/lower leakage rates).
3. Implants may also be inflatable, being filled at the time of surgery through a valve in the implant wall. This offers the advantages of a smaller access incision/scar (as the implant is inserted prior to filling it with saline) and intraoperative volume adjustment for size/symmetry. Care must be taken to keep the volume of saline introduced within the range specified by the manufacturer, as underfilling and overfilling may be associated with an increased rate of rupture and may void the manufacturer's warranty. Underfilling may also be associated with an undesirable degree of visible implant rippling.
4. Silicone implants are filled with liquid silicone gel and may offer a more natural texture and appearance to the augmented breast. In 1992 FDA restricted the use of silicone gel implants due to concerns of a possible link between silicone gel implants and connective tissue diseases, effectively banning their use in primary augmentation mammaplasty. While large-scale clinical trials have failed to substantiate such a link, silicone gel implants currently remain available only for limited reconstructive uses and research studies.
5. Other fill materials have been studied, including soybean oil, hydrogel, and polyethylene glycol (PEG), but their use in the United States is limited at this time.
6. Polyurethane-coated implants are no longer actively being implanted due to concerns regarding carcinogenicity. These implants are of historical and scientific interest because of the extremely low rate of spherical fibrous capsular contracture (SFCC) encountered with their use.

B. Textured vs. Smooth Implants

1. While traditional implants are smooth-walled, the use of textured (rough-surfaced) implants gained popularity in the early 1990s. Texturing lowers the risk of spherical fibrous capsular contracture. The mechanism remains unclear. In theory, texturing may act to "disorganize" the formation of circumferential scarring around the implant.
2. Histologically, synovial-like metaplasia, villous hyperplasia, and foreign body reaction are seen more frequently with textured implants.
3. While texturing reduces the rate of SFCC for implants placed in a subglandular location, the effect is modest for those implants that are placed submuscularly.
4. Smooth implants offer a lower risk of visible implant "rippling" than do textured implants, which tend to adhere to the periprosthetic capsule. This is of particular consideration in patients with little native breast tissue.

C. Round vs. Anatomic Implants

1. Traditional implants are round.
2. "Anatomic" implants were introduced to mitigate the problem of superior-pole fullness sometimes encountered with round implants. These implants are teardrop-shaped and attempt to recreate the shape of the native breast.
3. While anatomic implants may offer theoretical advantages in contour, careful positioning to avoid rotation is mandated. Round implants suffice in most instances of augmentation.

IV. SURGICAL TECHNIQUES

A. Subglandular vs. Submuscular

1. Implants may be placed either in a subglandular position (under the breast gland) or in a submuscular position (beneath the pectoralis major muscle).
2. The principle advantage of submuscular positioning is that it lowers the risk of SFCC, possibly by decreasing potential contamination via breast ducts, or by a "massaging" effect of the muscle itself. As soft tissue coverage of the implant is improved, the risk of visible implant rippling is also diminished.

3. Submuscular positioning may be either subpectoral or total. In contrast to subpectoral placement, in which the implant is placed under the pectoralis major, total submuscular implantation involves implant coverage with the pectoralis major, the serratus anterior, and (if necessary) portions of the anterior rectus fascia. Total submuscular coverage is typically used in breast reconstruction after mastectomy, when soft tissue coverage of the implant is lacking. Subpectoral placement suffices for most cases of breast augmentation.
4. Subglandular augmentation may offer aesthetic advantages in select cases and is significantly less painful in the postoperative period. Subglandular augmentation is preferred in patients who are avid body builders in whom highly developed pectoralis muscles may compromise implant projection/shape.

B. Access Incisions

Implants are generally placed via one of three common approaches:

1. The inframammary approach places an incision at the level of the inframammary fold, immediately lateral to the breast meridian. This approach offers excellent visualization and allows careful modification of the level of the inframammary fold, which is commonly lowered to accommodate the implant. Any future revisions that may become necessary can generally be performed through the same access incision.
2. The periareolar approach places an incision just within the borders of the areola. This approach also offers excellent visualization and allows careful modification of the level of the inframammary fold. Revisions can generally be performed through the same access incision. While some sources cite an increased risk of diminished nipple sensibility and inability to lactate using this approach, careful technique minimizes these risks.
3. The transaxillary approach allows placement of the implant through the axilla. This technique obviates the placement of a scar on the breast, but visualization is poor in the distal (inferior) areas of the dissection, increasing the risk of postoperative inframammary fold asymmetry. Revisions may be difficult, if not impossible to perform via the axilla, necessitating secondary scars on the breast. The use of endoscopic technique improves visualization of the dissection pocket and may alleviate these concerns.
4. The endoscope has also been used to facilitate implant placement via the umbilicus. This technique offers an access scar remote from the breast, but violates the integrity of the inframammary fold, creating a potential for deformity.

C. Anesthesia

Breast augmentation may be performed under local anesthesia with appropriate sedation, or under a general anesthetic, in accordance with the preferences of the surgeon and the patient.

D. Antimicrobials

1. A single preoperative dose of intravenous antibiotic is sufficient; longer courses of therapy offer no additional benefit.
2. Intraoperative breast pocket irrigation with antibacterial solution (dilute povidone-iodine or antibiotic solution) is often recommended and may lower the rate of capsular contracture.
3. Intraluminal Betadine or antibiotic solution may compromise implant longevity, and such use should be avoided.

E. Surgical Protocol

Several principles are involved in augmentation mammaplasty:

1. First, a generous dissection of the implant pocket must be performed.
2. The inframammary fold is usually lowered to a level dictated by implant size, the level of the preexisting fold, and the desire to maintain symmetry.
3. As in any procedure, meticulous hemostasis and attention to sterile technique are important.
4. In the course of surgery, the patient is often placed in a seated position to assess size/symmetry prior to closure.
5. The use of disposable or reusable implant sizers is useful in selecting the appropriate implant size.

F. Drains

1. Drains may be placed in the dissection pocket to facilitate evacuation of blood and serum in the postoperative period.
2. Drain placement does not alter the incidence of postoperative hematoma.

G. Dressings

1. Postoperative dressings may be placed in keeping with the surgeon's preferences.
2. Brassiere/bandeau placement and/or selective taping may assist in implant positioning, but careful intraoperative dissection is of primary importance in achieving the desired result. Early immobilization of the implants with such dressings minimizes patient discomfort.

V. POSTOPERATIVE CARE

1. Most patients may be discharged to home following surgery.
2. Pain is typically well controlled with oral narcotics.
3. Many surgeons advocate the use of implant displacement exercises in the postoperative period. In performing these exercises, the patient is asked to displace the implants manually within the dissection pocket several times daily in an effort to ensure a generous periprosthetic capsule, and possibly alleviate SFCC.

VI. COMPLICATIONS

A. Hematoma

1. Presents as excessive swelling that is typically painful.
2. Prompt drainage/hemostasis under anesthesia in the operating room is the appropriate course of action.
3. If untreated, hematoma may compromise skin viability and increase the rates of SFCC and infection.
4. Small hematomas noted at the first postoperative visit may be treated conservatively, and typically resolve without surgical intervention.

B. Acute Infection

1. Typically due to *Staphylococcus aureus*.
2. Treatment involves removal of the affected implant with drainage and antibiotic therapy.
3. Implant salvage has been described.
4. Subclinical infections may be due to *Staphylococcus epidermidis*, *Propionibacterium acnes*, or other species and may be associated with SFCC.

C. Altered Nipple Sensitivity

1. Occurs secondary to trauma to intercostal nerve branches (T3, T4, T5) during pocket dissection.
2. May occur with any or all approaches described.

D. Implant Rupture

1. Rates quoted in the literature vary significantly and are higher for saline implants.
2. Saline implant rupture presents as deflation, which may be rapid or gradual.
3. Silicone implant rupture may be intracapsular or extracapsular. Extracapsular rupture may present with asymmetry, deformity, or nodularity. Intracapsular rupture is often asymptomatic. If an asymptomatic intracapsular rupture is recognized, many surgeons will recommend implant removal or exchange, though no formal guidelines are established.
4. Mammography, ultrasound, and MRI may be used in the evaluation of implant rupture.

E. Spherical Fibrous Capsular Contracture

1. All patients who undergo breast augmentation undergo some degree of spherical fibrous capsular contracture.
2. SFCC involves scar contracture of the periprosthetic capsule, producing firmness on palpation and/or visible deformity of the breast.
3. Infection, silicone and myofibroblast activity have been suggested to have potential etiologic roles.
4. SFCC is clinically graded using the Baker classification:
   - In Grade I there is no palpable or visible anomaly.

- In Grade II the breast appears normal but is palpably firm.
- In Grade III palpable and visible distortions are present.
- In Grade IV the patient complains of associated breast pain.

5. Variables associated with lower rates of SFCC are saline fill, implant texturing, submuscular placement, and polyurethane coating (no longer available). The use of intraluminal steroids also reduces the rate of SFCC, but results in atrophy of the dependent breast, where the steroid pools by gravitational effect. Implant exposure may result, and the use of intraluminal steroids is therefore not recommended.
6. If treatment becomes necessary for SFCC, options include open capsulotomy or capsulectomy, submuscular placement, and the use of textured implants. Closed capsulotomy, in which the breast implant is vigorously manipulated without surgery, is associated with a high implant rupture rate and is not recommended.

F. Asymmetry

1. Postoperative asymmetry generally results from errors in the surgical dissection of the implant pocket. While improper immobilization may contribute to postoperative implant displacement, a surgical error must be suspected as an etiologic factor.
2. Preexisting asymmetry that remains uncorrected may also lead to patient dissatisfaction. It is therefore important to point out any natural asymmetry preoperatively.
3. The double-bubble deformity may result from improper dissection of the inframammary fold or inadequate release of the pectoralis muscle in submuscular placement. This deformity may also be encountered after augmentation of the tuberous breast.

G. Breast Cancer and Impaired Mammographic Visualization

1. Implants do not increase the risk of breast cancer and do not appear to delay the detection of breast cancer. Interestingly, in one study the incidence of breast cancer in patients with breast implants was significantly diminished vs. controls.
2. While the presence of breast implants does impair mammographic visualization of the breasts, this effect is diminished partly by the use of special "Ecklund" or compression views. However, because of the possibility of impaired breast cancer detection, women with a strong family history of breast cancer should be advised against breast augmentation.
3. All women over the age of 30 should have a preoperative mammogram prior to undergoing augmentation.

H. Human Adjuvant Disease

1. The term "human adjuvant disease" was originally coined in Japan in 1964, after two women developed a connective tissue-like disease subsequent to paraffin injections into the breast for augmentation.
2. An association between silicone gel prostheses and autoimmune disease was first described in 1982, and subsequent reports followed.
3. Due to concerns of a relation between silicone gel implants and human adjuvant disease, FDA placed a ban on the use of silicone gel implants in April 1992. The following exceptions were allowed:

   Women awaiting breast reconstruction with tissue expanders in place.

   Postmastectomy patients in whom silicone gel implants are the only option.

   Women who have silicone implants in place that require replacement.

4. In reviewing the literature, there is no clear scientific evidence of a causal relation between silicone gel implants and connective tissue disorders. Several large studies suggest that the incidence of such diseases is the same in augmented patients and in controls. As such, women who have silicone gel implants in place should be counseled to consider removal only for symptoms or for aesthetic problems.

103

Gynecomastia

Andrew D. Smith, M.D., James L. Watson, M.D., and Marc H. Hedrick, M.D.
David Geffen School of Medicine at UCLA, Los Angeles, California, U.S.A.

Gynecomastia refers to the excessive development of the male breasts associated with an increase in ductal tissue and stroma. Enlargement of the male breast is a common condition. The etiology and natural history of gynecomastia have been clarified in recent years. It is frequently benign, self-limiting, and often reversible. Surgery remains the primary method of correction when the process is longstanding, however.

I. ETIOLOGY

A. Physiological

Gynecomastia occurs at times of hormonal change: infancy, puberty, and old age.

1. Neonatal—palpable enlargement of the breast in neonates is normal and is the result of maternal estrogens. This usually regresses within a few weeks, although it occasionally persists.
2. Adolescence—approximately 75% of pubertal boys have gynecomastia. In most, the gynecomastia disappears within 1–2 years. This is referred to as pubertal gynecomastia. The findings can be asymmetric. Tenderness is common. It is a normal finding and is due to the physiological excess of estradiol relative to testosterone, due to androstenedione production (estrogen precursor). Prepubertal gynecomastia refers to the development of breast tissue in a male before puberty and is pathological. Causes include testicular tumors, adrenocortical carcinoma, tuberous sclerosis, 11β-hydroxylase deficiency, and precocious puberty.
3. Senescence—palpable bilateral breast tissue is present in most older men and is correlated with the amount of body fat. Senescent gynecomastia is thought to be due to the decrease in plasma testosterone and increase in sex hormone binding globulin that occur around age 70.

B. Pathological

1. Hypogonadism—hermaphroditism, cryptorchidism, congenital anorchia, and Klinefelter's syndrome (XXY) are all examples of primary testicular failure. Secondary testicular failure includes orchitis (mumps), castration, trauma, and bacterial infections (leprosy, tuberculosis). All these have decreased testosterone levels and normal estrogen.
2. Endocrine disorders—hyperthyroidism is the most common endocrine disorder associated with gynecomastia. This usually regresses with appropriate therapy. Gynecomastia has also been reported with hypothyroidism (due to increased prolactin levels), hyperparathyroidism, and adrenocortical hyperplasia.
3. Metabolic disorders—cirrhosis is associated with an increase in peripheral conversion of precursors to estrogens and high prolactin levels. Gynecomastia in this scenario usually regresses

with improved liver function. Refeeding after starvation can cause gynecomastia that usually regresses within one year. Renal failure and the institution of hemodialysis are also associated with gynecomastia.

4. Neoplasia—between 2.5 and 6% of testicular tumor patients have gynecomastia. Feminizing adrenal tumors in children can also cause gynecomastia. Bronchogenic carcinoma, hepatoma, neurofibromatosis, lymphoma, stomach carcinoma, renal cell carcinoma, pituitary tumors, colon carcinoma, and prostate carcinoma can all cause gynecomastia.

C. Pharmacological

Exogenous estrogen, testosterone, or anabolic steroids (due to aromatization in testosterone or androgen metabolism) all cause gynecomastia. It has also been reported with spironolactone, cimetidine, digitalis, methadone, drugs (heroin or marijuana), clomiphene, tranquilizers, and chemotherapeutic agents.

D. Miscellaneous

Causes include leprosy, herpes zoster, cystic fibrosis, rheumatoid arthritis, debilitating diseases (severe burns), and idiopathic causes.

II. PATHOLOGY

A. Three types of gynecomastia have been described. They are related to the duration of the condition:

- The florid type has increased ductal tissue in a cellular fibroblastic stroma with markedly increased hypervascularity. The acinar and lobule formation characteristic of female breasts is missing. Florid gynecomastia is associated with symptoms lasting <4 months.
- The fibrous type is characterized by an acellular fibrous stroma with few ducts. Fibrous gynecomastia is associated with symptoms of >12 months duration.
- The indeterminate type is a mixture of the two and is believed to represent a transition between the florid and fibrous types. It is found with symptoms typically present for 4–12 months.

B. Male breast cancer is a rare disease. Klinefelter's patients are the exception, with a 20–60 times greater risk for breast carcinoma than in the normal male. Gynecomastia is not considered to be a premalignant condition.

III. DIAGNOSIS

A. A thorough history and physical exam often helps elucidate the cause of gynecomastia. A history of illegal drug use must be taken. In addition, a review of hepatic, renal, pulmonary, thyroid, prostate, and testicular organ function must be performed.

B. Physical examination is useful in differentiating between carcinoma, pseudogynecomastia, and gynecomastia. Pseudogynecomastia (breast enlargement with obesity due to excess fat) has no palpable subareloar nodule and regresses with weight loss. Carcinoma is typically hard and eccentrically located.

C. Testicular examination for abnormal masses or small size can aid in diagnosis. In addition, examination of the thyroid, liver, lungs, and nutritional status can be helpful.

D. Useful laboratory studies include:

- Liver function studies
- Thyroid function tests
- Renal function tests
- Sex hormone levels
- Urinary markers for 17-ketosteroids, androgens, and gonadotropic hormones
- Karyotyping to exclude Klinefelter's syndrome

E. Mammography is a useful adjunct in making a diagnosis of gynecomastia and excluding carcinoma.

IV. CLASSIFICATION

Gynecomastia can be classified into three categories based on surgical considerations:

A. Grade 1—a localized button of tissue that is concentrated around the areola. The chest is not fatty, and there is no skin excess. These tissue buttons are usually easy to remove.

B. Grade 2—diffuse gynecomastia on a fatty chest where the edges of the tissue are indistinct. This tissue is difficult to taper.

C. Grade 3—diffuse gynecomastia with excessive skin. These patients require external skin incisions or nipple repositioning, or both.

V. MANAGEMENT

A. Recent onset—treatment is determined by the clinical condition. Gynecomastia caused by puberty, hemodialysis, and refeeding regresses spontaneously in most cases. Endocrine causes, such as hyperthyroidism, typically resolve with appropriate treatment of the medical condition. When drugs are the cause, the therapy of choice is to withdraw the agent.

B. Long duration—these cases are unlikely to regress spontaneously. Even if a disorder is identified, it often will not regress at this point. Surgery is the only effective treatment. Medical treatment has been tried, but is largely ineffective. Agents used include antiestrogens and danazol. Radiation therapy has a role in reducing breast pain and tenderness in patients treated with estrogens for prostate carcinoma.

VI. SURGICAL MANAGEMENT

A. Indications

Indications for surgery include symptomatic patients, patients in whom pharmacological therapy has failed, patients who are emotionally distressed by their condition, gynecomastia of long duration, and patients with Klinefelter's syndrome (increased risk of cancer). In addition, adolescent males with gynecomastia of > 2 years duration are candidates for surgery if distressed by this condition.

B. Considerations by Surgical Grade

1. Grade 1—this is usually an uncomplicated surgical procedure. Both traditional suction-assisted lipectomy (liposuction) and ultrasound-assisted lipectomy have been employed in such cases. Traditional liposuction may have difficulty penetrating the relatively fibrous tissue, which may limit its utility. Ultrasound-assisted liposuction has been more successful in this regard. Alternatively, excision of the excess tissue may be performed. The major consideration in all of these techniques is to avoid overexcision of tissue underneath the nipple, which would cause retraction of the nipple.
2. Grade 2—these patients are more complex. Often these breasts have indistinct planes with a subsequent rippled look that can occur postoperatively. Fat necrosis can contribute to this look and can create a depression in contour. The nipple button is also difficult because it is more fatty than fibrous. Tapering the edges of resection is very important and is usually achieved with use of either traditional suction lipectomy or ultrasound-assisted lipectomy.
3. Grade 3—incisions in this case are either circumareolar or mastopexy-type incisions. This dissection is facilitated by the improved exposure. Drains should be brought out through the periareolar incision or through the axilla to prevent additional scarring. A pressure dressing is helpful to prevent fluid accumulation postoperatively.

C. Technique

1. Preoperatively, the patient is marked while in the sitting position. The area to be resected and the peripheral margins are clearly delineated. Anesthesia can be local or general. This depends on the size of the excision and the preferences of the surgeon and patient.
2. A periareolar incision is used and local flaps are created underneath the nipple-areola complex. The excision is then performed to the extent of the surgical markings with tapering at the edges. Traditional suction lipectomy or ultrasound-assisted lipectomy can enhance the appearance by removing adipose tissue and producing a tapered look.

D. Complications of Surgery

1. Hematoma—the most common complication by far.
2. Nipple retraction—it is important to preserve a layer of fat and breast tissue beneath the nipple to allow for the normal projection of the nipple.
3. Rippled look.
4. Dishing at the edges—due to inadequate subcutaneous fat over the pectoral fascia. Ineffective tapering of the edges of resection can also leave a raised look at the edge of resection.
5. Scarring—incisions made outside the areola can produce hypertrophic scarring or keloids. These complications are rare when the incisions are confined to the areola.

104

Sedation for Aesthetic Surgery

Gregory G. Lara, M.D., Kate Huncke, M.D., and Johnathan Pregler, M.D.
David Geffen School of Medicine at UCLA, Los Angeles, California, U.S.A.

I. INTRODUCTION

The demand for sedation has increased as the number of cosmetic procedures performed in ambulatory surgery centers and office-based surgical suites has grown. Sedation offers advantages over general anesthesia in both of these settings. Sedation allows for rapid recovery of patients and discharge within a relatively short period of time compared to a general anesthetic. Recent advances in sedative pharmacology and monitoring have allowed for the administration of safe sedative agents and delivery techniques for aesthetic procedures.

II. PATIENT PREPARATION/ PREOPERATIVE EVALUATION

Patient evaluation plays an important role in outpatient aesthetic surgical procedures. Preoperative evaluation by the anesthesiologist will frequently take place the day of the procedure. In order to avoid unnecessary delays and cancellations, patients, unless they are young and healthy, should be evaluated by their primary care provider prior to the procedure. All necessary lab work, test results, and history and physical should accompany the patient on the day of surgery. The surgeon should be informed of the patient's coexisting disease, since this can affect the decision to proceed with an elective procedure. Outpatient procedures are safe, provided the patient's coexisting medical conditions are optimized, and patients are carefully selected for the outpatient setting.

A. The procedures performed must be matched to the capabilities of the surgical facility.
B. An inpatient hospital or emergency department must be readily available to accept an ambulatory surgery patient when necessary. A protocol for transporting the patient should be clearly established.
C. Patients with preexisting cardiovascular disease, respiratory compromise, neurological disease, and other significant medical problems will benefit from optimization of pre-existing medical conditions. Patients with significant medical problems may not be suitable candidates for ambulatory surgery, even if the procedure is to be performed under light sedation.
D. Preoperative medications should be continued, with the exception of diuretic and hypoglycemic medications, as these may cause fluid and metabolic disturbances that may be difficult to detect or treat intraoperatively.
E. With the exception of prescription medications that can be taken with a sip of water, patients should take nothing by mouth for at least 8 hours prior to surgery.

III. SEDATION TECHNIQUES

The goal of sedation is to provide anxiolysis, amnesia, and analgesia. Sedative agents vary in their ability to provide these goals. In order to achieve the optimal level of sedation, various agents are usually given in combination. The agents selected depend on the procedure and the patient's medical and psychological status. Two primary methods of delivering sedatives include intravenous and oral routes, each having advantages and disadvantages over a general anesthetic.

A. General anesthetics require maintenance of the airway by means of an endotracheal tube or laryngeal mask airway, as well as a means of evacuating anesthetic gases to prevent room contamination and sedation of the operating team.

B. Oral medications are given as a single dose and do not require the use of an intravenous catheter. Oral medications generally have a slower onset and longer duration of action than intravenous agents. These medications are not easily titratable.

C. Intravenous sedation provides a route for continuous delivery of medications, intermittent dosing, as well as the ability to titrate sedation and analgesia both intraoperatively and postoperatively.

D. Benzodiazepines, along with propofol, are the primary medications used for anxiolysis, sedation, and amnesia during aesthetic procedures. Benzodiazepines are the most widely used sedatives for outpatient procedures. All benzodiazepines have hypnotic, sedative, anxiolytic, amnestic, anticonvulsant, and centrally mediated muscle relaxant properties. Benzodiazepines have a mild respiratory depressant effects and cause insignificant cardiovascular depression. Benzodiazepines do not contribute to postoperative nausea and vomiting.

- Midazolam (Versed®) is a water-soluble, short-acting benzodiazepine with a potency two to three times greater than diazepam (Valium®). Midazolam has its most common use as an anxiolytic in the preoperative and intraoperative period:

  Midazolam produces anterograde amnesia lasting 20–30 minutes. Administration is usually intravenous, but it can be given orally or intramuscularly to an extremely anxious patient prior to the insertion of an intravenous cannula. Intravenous midazolam is well tolerated and has a quicker and more predictable onset and duration than oral midazolam.

  Midazolam, in contrast to other benzodiazepines, can cause significant respiratory depression. When it was introduced into clinical practice, several fatalities were attributed to undetected apnea from overdosing. Midazolam should only be used by personnel familiar with its pharmacological effects. Patients should be monitored for hypoxemia and supplemental oxygen, and ventilation equipment should be immediately available.

  Sedative doses cause minimal effect on the cardiovascular system. Usually, midazolam is titrated to effect in 0.5–1.0 mg increments. The oral dose is 0.5–1.0 mg/kg, not to exceed 20 mg total.

- Diazepam (Valium®) can be given orally as an anxiolytic 60–90 minutes prior to the scheduled procedure. Diazepam has an active metabolite, which has an elimination half-life ranging from 20 to 50 hours. The prolonged sedative effect of diazepam, due to its active metabolite, makes midazolam a better choice for the outpatient setting:

  The usual dose is 0.05–0.15 mg/kg P.O. The intravenous dose is 1–3 mg, titrated to effect.

  Diazepam's amnestic properties are less than that of midazolam or lorazepam. Intravenous diazepam causes venous irritation and thrombophlebitis. Intravenous midazolam has replaced diazepam when rapid onset of sedation is required.

- Lorazepam (Ativan®), as a sedative, is approximately four times as potent as diazepam. At equipotent sedative doses, lorazepam provides significantly longer amnestic activity than diazepam despite its shorter elimination half-life:

  The onset and duration of action of an oral dose of lorazepam is greater than that of diazepam. Lorazepam's potent and prolonged amnestic effect may make the drug unsuitable for outpatient surgery.

  If it is utilized for anxiolysis, lorazepam should be given the night before the procedure or several hours prior to the patient's arrival to the surgical facility.

Intravenous lorazepam causes less venous irritation than diazepam. The intravenous dose for an adult is 1–2 mg.

IV. PROPOFOL (DIPRIVAN®)

Propofol has increasingly become the anesthetic of choice for outpatient surgical procedures primarily due to its antiemetic effect and rapid recovery of psychomotor function.

A. The dose and rate of infusion varies widely among patients and is influenced by the patient's age, weight, medical condition, and the intensity of the surgical stimulus.

B. Propofol's short duration of action is due to rapid redistribution. Termination of effect occurs in 5–15 minutes. This allows for rapid recovery and discharge from the outpatient surgical setting.

C. The usual dose of propofol for conscious sedation is 25–100 μg/kg/min. Use of an infusion pump allows for a stable plasma concentration that can be titrated to effect.

D. Pain at the injection site is common and is alleviated or prevented by administration of IV lidocaine, or injection into a large vein.

E. Cardiovascular effects of propofol are a dose-related decrease in myocardial contractility and a decrease in systemic vascular resistance. The patient's preoperative cardiac status should be considered when using propofol. Significant cardiovascular depression is seen primarily at general anesthetic doses.

F. Propofol causes dose-related respiratory depression. Apnea is common and can occur rapidly. Equipment for airway support and positive pressure ventilation and personnel trained in airway management should be readily available. Concurrent use of opioids will increase the likelihood of apnea.

G. Due to the lipid formulation of propofol, it is an ideal microbial culture medium. Therefore, propofol should be used within 6 hours of opening, and sterile technique should be utilized when administering and storing the drug.

V. KETAMINE (KETALAR®)

A. Ketamine, a phencyclidine derivative, produces a unique anesthetic state termed dissociative anesthesia. Patients given ketamine appear to be in a cataleptic state. Unlike the anesthetic state produced by other agents, sedation with ketamine does not resemble normal sleep. Typically, the patient will exhibit a blank stare and nystagmus and will not respond to verbal or physical stimulation.

B. Ketamine has amnestic and sedative effects but, unlike benzopdiazepines and propofol, has intense analgesic properties.

C. Ketamine has a minimal effect on respiration, although apnea has been reported with unusually high doses that are generally not used for sedation techniques.

D. In contrast to other intravenous sedatives, ketamine has a mild sympathomimetic effect that leads to an increase in cardiac output, blood pressure, and heart rate. Due to the sympathomimetic effects of ketamine, local anesthetics containing epinephrine should be used cautiously in patients with cardiovascular disease.

E. Ketamine increases salivation; use of an antisialagogue such as glycopyrrolate preoperatively to limit secretions has been suggested.

F. Unlike propofol, airway reflexes such as gag, cough, and swallowing are usually present with deep sedative doses of ketamine.

G. Emergence and recovery following ketamine administration can be complicated by unpleasant hallucinations causing confusion and fear. This can limit its usefulness in the outpatient setting. The unpleasant psychological side effects of ketamine can be reduced by the administration of a benzodiazepine.

H. Ketamine as a sedative is given intravenously in incremental doses of 0.1–0.15 mg/kg and titrated to effect. A single intramuscular dose of 3–5 mg/kg with glycopyrrolate 0.02 mg/kg can also be given for a short procedure and does not require the insertion of an intravenous catheter.

VI. NARCOTICS

Narcotic medications have long been an effective adjuvant to intravenous anesthesia in the outpatient surgical environment. Although they are primarily used for analgesia, narcotics can potentiate the effects of anxiolytics. Narcotics decrease the sympathetic response to noxious stimuli and decrease intravenous dose requirements for concurrently administered sedative medications. Narcotics can produce nausea, vomiting, respiratory depression, and urinary retention. Narcotics at sedative doses have only minimal cardiovascular effects, causing a mild decrease in peripheral vascular resistance and heart rate. Narcotics also decrease the hormonal stress response to surgery.

A. Fentanyl (Sublimaze®)

1. Fentanyl rapidly crosses into the central nervous system due to its high lipid solubility. Fentanyl is an ideal opioid for pain control in outpatient surgical procedures. Patients who experience excessive amounts of postoperative pain should receive a longer-acting analgesic during recovery.
2. IV fentanyl has an onset of effect in 30 seconds, with peak effect occurring in 5–15 minutes. Duration of action is 30–60 minutes.
3. The dose of fentanyl for an adult patient is 25–50 μg IV (0.7–1 μg/kg), which may be repeated after 5–10 minutes and titrated to effect.
4. Like all narcotics, fentanyl can cause the abrupt onset of apnea when large doses are given.

B. Alfentanil (Alfenta®)

1. Alfentanil has a very rapid onset due to its high lipid solubility at physiologic pH. Its duration of action is also extremely short.
2. IV alfentanil's onset and peak effect occur in 1–2 minutes. Duration of action is 10–15 minutes.
3. Alfentanil can be given as an IV bolus of 100–400 μg just prior to a painful stimulus.
4. Repeated boluses or a continuous infusion of alfentanil have a high incidence of nausea and vomiting that limit its usefulness.

C. Meperidine (Demerol®)

1. Meperidine is a synthetic opioid with an intermediate duration of action. Normeperidine, an active metabolite of meperidine, is a cerebral stimulant. In high concentrations it can lead to seizures. Meperedine also has vagolytic properties, unlike the other opiates. It should not be used with patients taking monoamine oxidase inhibitors due to the severe and potentially fatal cardiovascular and neurologic interactions.
2. IV meperidine has an onset of effect in 1–2 minutes, with peak effect occurring in 5–20 minutes. Duration of action is 2–4 hours.
3. The dose of intravenous meperidine for an adult is 25–50 mg given every 5–10 minutes titrated to effect.
4. Meperidine has an increased incidence of postoperative nausea and vomiting when compared to other narcotics.

D. Morphine

1. Morphine is the prototypic opioid to which other narcotics are compared. It is generally not used in outpatient surgery as a preoperative anxiolytic due to its slow onset. Its long duration of action makes it an excellent choice for postoperative pain control.
2. IV morphine has an onset of effect in 1 minute, with peak effect occurring in 5–20 minutes. Duration of action is 2–7 hours.
3. The intravenous dose of morphine for an adult is 5–10 mg every 10–15 minutes, titrated to analgesic effect. The dose should be reduced in an elderly patient and when used in conjunction with other analgesics or sedatives.
4. Morphine releases histamine and can cause pruritis after systemic administration.

E. Hydromorphone (Dilaudid®)

1. Hydromorphone is a long-acting narcotic with greater potency than morphine.
2. IV hydromorphone has an onset of effect in <1 minute, with peak effect occurring in 5–20 minutes. Duration of action is 2–4 hours.
3. The dose of hydromorphone in adults is 0.2–0.4 mg IV every 10–15 minutes, titrated to effect.

VII. NONSTEROIDAL ANTIINFLAMMATORY DRUGS

Nonsteroidal antiinflammatory drugs (NSAIDs) are essentially devoid of the unwanted side effects that are characteristic of the opioids, such as respiratory depression, nausea, vomiting, urinary retention, addiction, and abuse by healthcare providers. NSAIDs can sometimes be used in place of, or along with, opioids for pain control. Since the side effects of NSAIDs are minimal compared with opioids following administration, recovery and discharge may be quicker.

A. Ketorolac (Toradol®)

1. Ketorolac is the intravenous NSAID used in ambulatory settings. Ketorolac is antiinflam-

matory, antipyretic, and analgesic. The analgesic properties of a 30 mg dose of ketorolac are equivalent to a 9 mg dose of morphine.

2. The onset after an intravenous dosing is less than 1 minute, and the peak effect is seen in 1–3 hours. The duration of action is 3–7 hours.
3. Dosing of ketorolac is 30–60 mg IV or IM (0.5–1 mg/kg), and subsequent doses are given at 6-hour intervals. The maximum dose is 150 mg/day (2–3 mg/kg/day), and use is generally limited to 48 hours. Ketorolac should not be administered to patients with renal insufficiency.
4. There is no significant change in cardiac or hemodynamic parameters seen with ketorolac. There is also not significant respiratory depression with standard dosing.
5. Ketorolac does inhibit platelet aggregation and prolongs bleeding time; thus its use in procedures where the risk of postoperative bleeding or oozing is high is limited.

VIII. REVERSAL AGENTS

Reversal agents can be used to antagonize prolonged or unwanted effects of sedative or analgesic medications. Flumazenil and naloxone are the agents used to temporarily reverse the clinical effects of benzodiazepines and opioids, respectively. The onset of action of flumazenil and naloxone occurs within 1–2 minutes. Patients who have been treated with reversal agents need to be continuously monitored for recurrence of sedative or respiratory effects.

A. Flumazenil (Mazicon®)

1. Flumazenil is a centrally acting reversal agent for benzodiazepines.
2. The dose used in clinical practice range from 0.1 to 0.2 mg every minute, up to a total of 1 mg. This dose may be repeated at 20-minute intervals but should not exceed 3 mg in one hour.
3. Reversal with flumazenil does not precipitate hypertension and tachycardia, even when it is used to treat a benzodiazepine overdose. Chronic benzodiazepine abusers may demonstrate the physiologic effects of withdrawal when given flumazenil.
4. The duration of action is variable and is influenced by the dose of flumazenil and the amount of benzodiazepine being antagonized. Flumazenil lasts 45 minutes to 3 hours, and patients need to be monitored for recurrence of the benzodiazepine effect.

B. Naloxone (Narcan®)

1. Naloxone is an antagonist to all opioids. It can be used to reverse all opioid effects, including analgesia, euphoria, respiratory depression, pruritis, and biliary spasm.
2. Naloxone should be given in incremental doses of 0.5–1.0 μg/kg. Titration of the drug is important, since reversal of the narcotic effect can precipitate severe hypertension and tachycardia.
3. Renarcotization can occur, since the half-life of naloxone is only 30–60 minutes.

IX. MONITORS AND OXYGEN ADMINISTRATION

Monitoring is an essential component of patient safety during intravenous sedation for aesthetic procedures. Cardiovascular and respiratory monitoring must be performed at defined intervals to ensure that the level of anesthesia is appropriate and to detect any adverse response during the procedure. Qualified personnel apart from those performing the surgical procedure should be responsible for the monitoring. The following are the various components that make up guidelines for sedation and patient care during a procedure where an anesthesiologist is not present:

A. In patients receiving intravenous medications for sedation/analgesia, vascular access should be maintained throughout the procedure and until the patient is no longer at risk for cardiorespiratory depression. In patients who have received sedation/analgesia by nonintravenous routes or whose intravenous line has become dislodged or blocked, practitioners should determine the advisability of establishing or reestablishing intravenous access on a case-by-case basis. In all instances, an individual with the skills to establish intravenous access should be immediately available.

B. All patients undergoing sedation shall receive continuous monitoring of heart rate and oxygen saturation.

C. Blood pressure and respiratory rate shall be monitored at least every 5 minutes. For procedures that would be disrupted by a blood pressure measurement at 5-minute intervals, that interval may be prolonged according to procedure-specific protocols approved by the sedation committee.

D. During conscious sedation, the qualified healthcare provider monitoring the patient may perform other brief interruptible tasks to assist the physician.

E. During deep sedation, the qualified healthcare provider monitoring the patient may not perform other tasks, except those related to the administration of sedation; this may require a third qualified healthcare worker to assist the physician, if needed.

F. When an anesthesiologist provides sedation for surgical procedures, the American Society of Anesthesiologists has standard monitoring guidelines, which should be followed.

G. Qualified anesthesia personnel shall be present in the room throughout the conduct of all general anesthetics, regional anesthetics, and monitored anesthesia care.

H. During all anesthetics, the patient's oxygenation, ventilation, circulation, and temperature shall be monitored.

I. Monitors that need to be available include pulse oximetry, EKG, patient temperature, and end-tidal carbon dioxide for any patient who has a laryngeal mask airway or endotracheal tube.

J. Supplemental oxygen should be administered whenever it is suspected that depression in ventilation will occur. Common delivery methods consist of a face mask or nasal cannula. If the operative site dictates that nothing be placed over the face, then oxygen can be delivered through a small suction catheter inserted in the nares. Coating the catheter with lidocaine jelly can minimize nasal irritation.

X. PATIENT DISCHARGE

A. Postoperatively, patients need to be closely evaluated prior to discharge home.

B. Pain control, nausea, vomiting, and sedation must be under reasonable control prior to release from medical care.

C. Prior to discharge, patients who have received any sedation require a responsible adult to accompany the patient to their home.

D. Patients should be informed to refrain from operating machinery or driving, as residual sedation from anesthesia or pain medication may persist for several hours.

E. Taxi rides are not acceptable for the post-operative ride home, as the driver assumes no responsibility for the patient's healthcare status.

F. Patients should be given the names and phone numbers of the physicians involved, since questions and concerns may arise after discharge to home.

105

Chemical Peeling, Dermabrasion, and Injectable Collagen/Fat Implants

Peter Ashjian, M.D., and Marc Hedrick, M.D.
David Geffen School of Medicine at UCLA, Los Angeles, California, U.S.A.

I. HISTOLOGY OF NORMAL SKIN

Despite the variations of skin throughout the human body (thickness, color, presence and degree of hair, glands, etc.), it has a fundamental architecture. The skin has several appendageal structures (hair follicles, sebaceous glands, eccrine glands, and apocrine glands). They are derived from the epidermis embryologically and are essential for reepithelialization.

A. Epidermis—the external surface of skin consisting of a keratinized epithelium. The epidermis has no vascular network. Wounds that only involve the epidermis will usually heal without scarring.

B. Dermis—the cells of the dermis are mainly fibroblasts, but white blood cells, mast cells, and tissue macrophages also reside. Elastin is an important constituent. Dermis is highly vascular and consists of two layers:

- Papillary dermis—the more superficial of the two. Highly vascular, containing the subpapillary arterial, venous, and lymphatic plexuses and papillary vascular loops.
- Reticular dermis—main bulk of the dermis. This layer has coarse interlacing collagen fibers and contains blood vessels connecting the vascular plexuses of the upper dermis to the cutaneous plexuses at the junction of the dermis and hypodermis.

C. Hypodermis—also known as the superficial fascia and contains variable amounts of adipose tissue.

II. CHEMICAL PEELING

A. Indications

1. Elimination of fine facial wrinkles (provided no gross sagging of facial skin).
2. Produces moderate tightening of the skin.
3. Adjunctive procedure to blepharoplasty and/or rhytidectomy for removal of fine wrinkles, especially in the periorbital and perioral region.
4. Telangiectasias.
5. Superficial keratosis.
6. Hyperpigmentation.

B. Patient Selection

1. Ideal candidate is a patient with minimal facial sagging and finely wrinkled skin.
2. Individuals with fair complexions are better candidates. Those with darker complexions are at higher risk for complications. African Americans and other dark-skinned individuals should have a test application.

3. Women are better candidates than men due to their thinner skin.
4. Acne scars respond poorly to this technique.

C. Chemical Agents

1. Phenol—used extensively for deep chemical peeling:
   - Phenol produces immediate keratolysis and coagulation, caused by disruption of sulfur bridges of keratoprotein and aided by denaturation secondary to its acid nature.
   - Common mixture is phenol mixed with distilled water, croton oil, and liquid soap. Croton oil acts as an additional irritant and speeds destruction of the epidermis. Liquid soap acts to retard penetration and absorption of phenol by increasing surface tension.
   - Waterproof tape is used to prolong and deepen phenol's action.
2. Trichloroacetic acid (TCA)—does not burn the skin as deeply as phenol. Highly effective in improving solar-damaged skin, removing superficial keratoses, and irregular pigmentation. Ideal for the thin skin of the hands because the deeper burn induced by stronger agents increases the risk of scar formation:
   - Superficial peel (intraepidermal injury)—TCA concentration 10–25%.
   - Medium peel (papillary dermis injury)—TCA concentration 30–40%.
   - Deep peel (reticular dermis injury)—TCA concentration >40%.
   - TCA can be applied repeatedly at 1- to 3-month intervals. This method decreases the possibility of deep scarring and/or keloid formation.

D. Changes in the Skin

1. An immediate inflammatory reaction after application of acids peaks at 48 hours.
2. Epidermal regeneration begins on the second day and is complete by 2 weeks.
3. The clinical benefits are from the dermal reorganization of collagen from its usual wavy shape to a straight pattern lying parallel to the skin surface.
4. Decrease in the melanin-producing cells in the basal epidermis.
5. Increase in elastic tissue in the dermis.

E. Systemic Reaction

1. Phenol is absorbed into the systemic circulation. After being conjugated and detoxified, phenol is excreted by the kidneys.
2. Phenol can produce cardiotoxicity. A routine baseline electrocardiogram is essential, and continuous EKG monitoring during the procedure is recommended. Only limited areas of the face should be treated at once, with several minute intervals between applications.
3. TCA has no demonstratable blood level, systemic toxicity, or cardiac effects.

F. Precautions

1. Preoperative evaluation:
   - Complete history and physical (special attention to hepatorenal system).
   - History of drug sensitivity or prior chemabrasion warrants skin testing (usually in the preauricular area).
   - History of cold sores (herpes simplex). May require Zovirax prophylaxis.
   - Routine blood analysis.
   - Preoperative photographs (both color and black and white).
2. Chemical peels of the neck have a high potential to form hypertrophic scars.
3. Peeling arms and thorax have been unsuccessful and are problematic.
4. Hands should be peeled with TCA and they should be kept out of water for at least 5–7 days because of possible retarded healing, scarring, and hyperpigmentation.
5. Upper and lower eyelids should not be peeled at the same time because the resulting inflammation can leave the patient temporarily without vision.

G. Procedure

1. The skin is washed on the evening prior to the procedure and on the morning of the procedure.

2. TCA require extensive skin preparation to produce a uniform and effective burn:
   - The skin is first dekeratinized with exfoliants (α-hydroxy, α-keto acids, or retinoic acid). Retinoic acid may require 3–5 weeks of use prior to peeling.
   - Phenol does not require pretreatment of the skin.
3. Although general anesthesia is not necessary, the patient should be premedicated for deeper level peels. The combination of Demerol with titrated amounts of Valium is commonly used.
4. Patient is placed on the operating table with head slightly elevated. Skin oils and residual soap are removed with ether, alcohol, or acetone.
5. The solution is applied with a cotton-tipped applicator stick. Phenol solutions must be frequently stirred to avoid layering and unequal application
6. Tears must be adequately dabbed. They can run down the cheeks, resulting in tracks.
7. Gentle stretching of the skin enables the acid to coat the depths of wrinkles evenly.
8. The peel is extended up into the hairline and down into the eyebrow.
9. The peel must come right to the vermilion border of the lips. If in doubt, include a slight margin of the vermilion border. The lip will blister and be painful, but a band of obvious untreated skin will be avoided.
10. Maintain a 2 mm border on the ciliary margins to avoid corneal or conjunctival burns.
11. Extend the peel to just below the ramus of the mandible.
12. When peeling the entire face, perform individual sections one at a time. Sample sections include:
    - Left cheek (with lower lid, if planned)
    - Right cheek
    - Nose and upper lip
    - Chin and lower lip
    - Forehead (with upper lids, if planned)

H. Postoperative Care

1. Postoperative erythema is normal and may persist for months.
2. Some patients complain of intense itching within first few postoperative days:
   - Trimeprazine (2.5 mg, four times per day)
   - Antihistamines
   - A short course of steroids if the above do not suppress the itching
3. Pulling or picking newly separating skin may result in a scar.
4. An occlusive dressing accomplishes a deeper exfoliation and accelerates healing. It is advised for phenol peels, not TCA peels. There are two methods of occlusive dressings:
   - Occlusive tape dressing:

     Removed in 24–48 hours

     Requires intravenous sedation and/or systemic analgesia

     After removal, gentle surface cleansing with nonallergenic soap
   - Thick layer of petroleum jelly:

     Greater patient comfort

     Ability to evaluate the wound beneath the jelly

     Avoids the unpleasant task of removing the tape dressing
5. Some physicians used hydrocolloid dressings (e.g., Vigilon^{TM}) for the first 2–4 days after a peel. They are extremely hydrophilic polymer dressings.
6. Polysporin ointment or bacitracin are commonly used, but the significant risk of local allergic reaction must be weighed against the benefits.
7. Facial lubrication with standard facial moisturizers is continued for 2–3 months.
8. Sunscreens (SPF >35) and hats are advised to avoid damage to the sensitive skin.
9. Sweating and exercise are contraindicated; they may increase risk of infection.

I. Complications

1. Bleaching of the skin:
   - Most common after a deep peel with phenol.
   - Leads to a line of demarcation between treated and untreated skin.
   - More common in patients with dark skin.

- Fully inform all patients of this potential complication.

2. Hyperpigmentation:
   - More common in patients with darker skin.
   - Patients often have a degree of irregular pigmentation preop.
   - Inform all patients that any such pigmentation may be intensified.
3. Irregular pigmentation:
   - Minimized by thorough cleansing of skin before application of peel.
   - Missed or streaked areas require secondary peeling upon recognition.
4. Hypertrophic scarring or keloids:
   - Rare after chemical peels.
   - Small hypertrophic scars usually disappear after a few weeks. An intralesional injection of triamcinolone may help resorption.
   - Silicone gel sheeting (e.g., Sil-K, EpiDerm) can help prevent keloids after surgery. They are used for at least 12 hours daily for 2 months.
5. Tightness of the face:
   - Frequent complaint.
   - Almost invariably disappears.
   - Treat with reassurance.
6. Ectropion:
   - Usually of the lower eyelids after a full face or eyelid peel.
   - Limited in nature and usually disappears within a few weeks.
7. Milia:
   - Due to temporary blockage of sebaceous glands.
   - Usually resolve spontaneously, but some require opening with needle.
8. Dissemination of herpes simplex infection.

III. DERMABRASION

A. Indications

1. Smoothing of irregularities caused by scar or acne (e.g. acne pits)
2. Used to prepare recipient site for a skin graft

B. Patient Selection

1. Detailed history:
   - Previous episodes of herpes simplex.
   - Prior surgeries to the area.
   - Cold intolerance.
   - Past and present medications, particularly isotretinoin (Accutane). Some patients on Accutane may develop atypical keloid formation after dermabrasion. A yearlong wait after completion of Accutane treatment is currently recommended.

C. Changes in Skin

1. Immediately after procedure, serum forms coagulum across surface.
2. Proliferation of squamous epithelium after 3 days.
3. Thin epidermis regenerated and dermal regeneration evident by 5th day.
4. Pigment formation commences after 3 or 4 weeks.

D. Procedure

1. Although Demerol with Valium is often used, many people still advocate general anesthesia. Nerve blocks can also be employed.
2. Apply ink (Bonny Blue dye) to pinpoint depths of pits.
3. Face is dermabraded in small sections frozen by a refrigerant spray (Frigiderm).
4. To avoid scarring from abrasion to deeper levels, several interrupted procedures are advised with a 3- to 6-month interval.
5. It is extended into the hairline, preauricular region, and under the mandible.
6. Hemostasis:
   - Gauze soaked in lidocaine with 1:50,000 epinephrine
   - Topical thrombin
7. Cover skin with an antibiotic ointment. Dressings are optional.

E. Postoperative Care

1. Patients are discharged on the following day.
2. Daily use of the hair dryer is recommended to maintain eschar.

3. Seventh postop day, begin daily application of vegetable oil to separate the eschar.
4. The use of sunscreens and avoidance of direct sun is essential for at least 6 months after procedure. Failure may result in hyperpigmentation.

F. Complications

1. Hypertrophic scarring.
2. Irregular pigmentation:
   - Usually spontaneously regresses over 3–18 months.
   - If unresolved by this time, secondary chemabrasion may be attempted.

IV. COLLAGEN/FAT INJECTIONS

A. Indications

1. Collagen injections:
   - Facial rejuvenation
   - Elimination of fine to medium wrinkle lines
   - Clinical improvement of soft, untethered scars
2. Fat injections:
   - Autologous wrinkle and lip filler
   - Facial restoration of volume and shape due to aging (e.g., malar eminence, anterior cheeks, infrazygomatic arch, orbital rim, tear trough, etc.)

B. Materials

1. Injectable bovine collagen:
   - Zyderm I—3.5% bovine collagen in normal saline and lidocaine
   - Zyderm II—6.5% bovine collagen in normal saline and lidocaine
   - Zyplast—3.5% bovine collagen cross-linked with glutaraldehyde
2. Autologous fat:
   - Obtained by liposuction

C. Precautions

1. Before use of collagen injections, skin testing for allergic reaction to collagen is mandatory:
   - Initial collagen skin test observed in 48 hours.
   - Second test performed 2 weeks later.
2. Before performing fat injections, it is important to determine if the patient liked his/her young face. With time, the face lengthens and narrows. The goal of facial fat injections is to alter the shape to appear fuller and younger.
3. Faces that were once full but have since lost volume do much better than bony faces that never had much fill.

D. Procedure

1. Collagen injections:
   - Zyderm must be refrigerated until just prior to use.
   - Patient is placed in a sitting position with the back slightly reclined.
   - Skin is thoroughly cleansed with alcohol.
   - Most patients tolerate collagen injections without analgesia or anesthesia.
   - Zyderm I and II are used at a very superficial level in the dermis.
   - Multiple injections are performed with the corrections being immediate.
   - Zyplast is injected deeper into the dermis than Zyderm. It is used primarily to correct contour abnormalities.
   - Zyplast can be overlayed with Zyderm for a finer correction.
   - Zyplast should not be used in the glabellar frown lines due to possible ischemia and necrosis.
2. Fat injections:
   - Most procedures can be performed under local with or without minor oral sedation.
   - After fat is obtained by liposuction, it is centrifuged for about 2 minutes. Fat without supernatant is transferred to 1 mL syringes with a 17-gauge needle.
   - It is essential to deliver fat in fine threads. About 10–20 full-length needle passes per millimeter are made. This increases chance of take and also makes shaping much easier.

- Overinjection is simply treated by aspirating the excess.
- After about 3 months, it is apparent how much fat will last.
- Overcorrection is commonly necessary due to graft attrition.

E. Complications

1. Allergic reaction to collagen:
   - Zyderm test implant—3% develop a reaction
   - 3% with a negative Zyderm skin test develop a treatment reaction
   - Collagen injections do not increase the incidence of autoimmune diseases
2. Abscess or cyst formation after collagen injection:
   - Occurs in approximately 4 of 10,000 injections
   - Treat with incision and drainage or intralesional steroids
3. Complications of fat injection:
   - Irregular distribution and take of injected fat
   - Overly superficial injection
   - Subcutaneous calcifratic
   - Graft Attrition
   - Hyperplasia uncommon

106

Lasers in Aesthetic Surgery

Jenny Kim, M.D., Ph.D., and Gary P. Lask, M.D.
David Geffen School of Medicine at UCLA, Los Angeles, California, U.S.A.

The use of laser (*L*ight *A*mplified by *S*timulated *E*mission of *R*adiation) in medicine and surgery is expanding rapidly. The field of aesthetic surgery has also benefited significantly from its use. Since the development of the first laser by Maiman in 1960, extensive research has provided us with a better understanding of how skin responds to laser treatment. Laser technology has advanced such that it is considered the treatment of choice for a number of conditions.

I. LASER PHYSICS

A. Long before the development of lasers, the concept of stimulated emission was derived by Einstein's quantum theory. When a molecule is in an excited state and returns spontaneously to a stable state, it emits a photon of light. This photon can then stimulate the emission of another photon from a molecule that is in an excited metastate.

B. Inside a laser, photons bounce back and forth in an excited medium between two mirrors, producing an enormous amount of light that is monochromatic, collimated, and coherent.

C. Lasers can emit light in a continuous wave (CW) or by pulses.

D. CW lasers cannot mount the instantaneous power that can be achieved by pulsed lasers. These lasers include CW carbon dioxide (CO_2), neodymium:yttrium-aluminum-garnet (Nd:YAG), argon, krypton, and argon-dye lasers.

E. Copper lasers emit beams with such rapid pulses that they appear to be virtually continuous.

F. High-energy pulsed lasers include pulsed-tunable-dye, Q-switched ruby, and Q-switched Nd:YAG lasers.

G. The Q-switched lasers allow light emission only in short bursts, delivering high energy to tissues.

II. LASER LIGHT AND TISSUE INTERACTIONS

A. When laser light penetrates the skin, two major processes occur: absorption of the light and scattering of the light. With absorption, the energy of the photon is absorbed by the tissue chromophores. With scattering, the direction of the photon traveling is changed and the light moves away from the tissue.

B. The main chromophores in the skin are oxyhemoglobin, hemoglobin, melanin, and carotene.

C. In the epidermis and in the stratum corneum, melanin and other chromophores absorb light of various wavelengths.

D. In the UVC and UVB regions (<320 nm), absorption by proteins and nucleic acid predominates.

E. In the UVA (340–400 nm), visible (400–720 nm), and most of the near-infrared (720–1000 nm) regions, melanin is the dominant epidermal chromophore.

F. In the mid- to far-infrared regions (>1000 nm) water is the most significant chromophore.

G. In the dermis, scattering of the laser light, rather than absorption, occurs. Collagen, which comprises the bulk of the dermis, has a light-scattering property. In the dermis, the only significant light absorption occurs in blood where the absorption peaks of oxyhemoglobin are at wavelengths of 418, 542, and 577 nm.

H. When the high-energy laser light is absorbed by the chromophore, an intense heat is generated and causes destruction of the light-absorbing tissue. This theory of tissue-specific thermal destruction was proposed by Anderson and Parrish in 1983. Since then, more highly selective, pulsed lasers have been developed. With these advanced lasers, specific skin lesions can be targeted and treated with a wavelength corresponding to the absorption peak of the chromophore contained in the lesion. This process of selective photothermolysis is the basis for treating vascular and pigmented lesions, tattoos, and hair. Furthermore, it is the most effective treatment for treating some of these lesions.

III. LASER TREATMENT OF VASCULAR LESIONS

A. Port-wine stain (PWS), also known as nevus flammeus, is a congenital vascular malformation that occurs in 0.3–0.5% of newborns:

- A PWS progressively dilates and persists throughout life.
- Five percent of PWSs have CNS involvement resulting in seizures, mental retardation, and glaucoma.
- Most of the lesions occur in the face and range in color from pink to purple.
- Various treatment modalities including skin grafting, ionization radiation, cryosurgery, tattooing, dermabrasion, and various lasers have been used.
- Lasers presently are the treatment of choice. Hemoglobin absorbs light in the blue, green, and yellow light spectrums. As such, the primary treatment of PWS has utilized a number of lasers including argon, KTP, and pulsed-dye lasers. To date, the pulsed-dye lasers at a 577–595 nm wavelength and a 450 μs to 1.5 ms pulse duration appear to be the most effective lasers and have the least chance of scarring.
- It is generally recommended that treatments take place early, when the lesions are smaller and therefore more likely to respond. Such treatment, when successful, may prevent significant psychosocial trauma.

B. Strawberry/capillary hemangioma is a common vascular lesion of infancy occurring in 2.6% of newborns:

- Lesions occur at birth or soon after and continue to grow rapidly. However, the natural course of the lesion is to spontaneously regress in approximately 50% of patients by 5 years, 70% by 7 years, and over 90% eventually.
- Conservative therapy has been advocated in the past; however, because of reports of scarring after regression of hemangiomas, early laser treatment is now being considered. Furthermore, the treatment of strawberry hemangiomas with lasers can lessen the psychosocial trauma to the patient and family.
- Other indications for laser therapy include ulceration, infection, bleeding, and obstruction of vital organs.
- Treatments including surgery, ionizing radiation, and oral or intravenous steroids have also been used.
- The 585 nm pulsed-dye laser is used to treat macular or enlarging lesions and has been shown to be effective in lightening the lesions and preventing growth.
- The CW Nd:YAG laser has also been used to treat thick hemangiomas but can result in texture changes. It has been used to debulk large hemangiomas prior to excision.

C. Essential telangiectasias and spider angiomas can be treated successfully with pulsed-dye lasers.

D. Phlebectasias (spider veins) on the lower extremities are a common cosmetic problem:

- To date, the most effective method of treating spider veins is sclerotherapy.
- A number of attempts at treating spider veins with lasers have been made, but there

is a high incidence of hyperpigmentation and hypopigmentation. Epidermal cooling devices are now available to decrease the thermal injury to the epidermis.

IV. LASER TREATMENT OF PIGMENTED LESIONS

A. Lentigenes

1. Although a number of lasers can be used for treatment of lentigenes, the Q-switched Nd:YAG at 532 nm, Q-switched ruby (694 nm), and Q-switched alexandrite (755 nm) are the treatments of choice.
2. CW lasers such as KTP, argon, and krypton lasers have been used as well. However, due to the increase in thermal effect, there is also an increase in risk of scarring.

B. Cafe Au Lait Macules (CALMs)

1. Can be seen in association with neurofibromatosis. However, up to 10% of the normal population have sporadic CALMs.
2. These brown macules have increased melanosomes in melanocytes and keratinocytes.
3. Although CALMs appear to be good candidates for laser treatment, Q-switched ruby, Q-switched alexandrite, and Q-switched Nd:YAG lasers have been used with inconsistent results.

C. Postinflammatory Hyperpigmentation

1. In general, laser treatment of postinflammatory hyperpigmentation has not resulted in favorable responses.
2. Laser treatment itself can induce further postinflammatory hyperpigmentation.
3. Some response has been seen with the Q-switched ruby laser on dark infraorbital circles and on drug-induced hyperpigmentation.

D. Melasma

1. Laser treatment, in general, has not been shown to be effective for the treatment of melasma. Lesions can recur. Furthermore, darkening of the lesion after laser treatment has been reported.
2. For this reason, melasma should be treated with topical retinoids, hydroquinone and serial glycolic peels.
3. Sun avoidance and sunscreens are necessary to maintain any improvement of melasma.

E. Tattoos

1. Q-switched lasers are the treatment of choice for tattoo removal. In comparison with previous treatment modalities that include dermabrasion and surgical excision, lasers offer superior results with fewer side effects. With the advent of Q-switched lasers, tattoos can be removed with minimal incidence of scarring.
2. The Q-switched ruby, Q-switched Nd:YAG, and Q-switched alexandrite can all be effective in treating black and blue tattoos. The Q-switched Nd:YAG at 1064 nm causes less hypopigmentation than the Q-switched ruby and the Q-switched alexandrite lasers.
3. On average, amateur tattoos are treated with fewer treatments than professional tattoos.
4. The Q-switched Nd:YAG laser at 532 nm can be used to treat red tattoos.
5. For green tattoos, the Q-switched ruby and alexandrite lasers are used.

F. Nevus of Ota, Ito, and Mongolian Spot

1. These lesions are due to an increase in the dermal melanocytes.
2. Q-switched ruby, Nd:YAG, and alexandrite lasers all have been reported to successfully treat these dermal melanocytoses. The authors have seen more effective results with ruby and alexandrite than the Nd:YAG.

G. Nevomelanocytic Lesions

1. The treatment of nevi, including congenital nevus, has been described using lasers. The Q-switched ruby and the Q-switched Nd:YAG lasers have been used for treatment of nevomelanocytic lesions without significant scarring.
2. Since the development of melanoma in any nevus is a possibility, the authors do not treat nevomelanocytic lesions with lasers. The treatment of choice for nevomelanocytic lesions is surgery.

V. LASER HAIR REMOVAL

1. The concept of laser hair removal is also based on selective photothermolysis, given that the hair

follicle is the only melanin-containing structure in the normal dermis. However, the melanin in the epidermis is a competing chromophore. Selective photothermolysis of hair follicle can be accomplished by using red or near-infrared wavelengths.

2. Currently, permanent hair loss has been achieved by alexandrite lasers, ruby lasers, diode lasers (800 nm), and the xenon flashlamp (700–1200 nm).
3. Theoretically, for a successful outcome, the bulb and the bulge, two components of the hair follicle, must be destroyed. The bulb gives rise to the hair shaft and is responsible for active anagen hair growth. The bulge, thought to be the location where hair stem cells reside, needs to be injured to prevent formation of a new hair follicle. Indeed, studies have demonstrated that laser hair removal consists of immediate destruction of anagen hairs followed by a long-term inhibition of hair growth.
4. The best results are seen in patients with dark hair and fair skin complexion. Patients with light hair do not respond well.
5. Furthermore, all of the lasers mentioned above can result in hyperpigmentation or hypopigmentation, especially in dark-skinned individuals.
6. New technologies, including the use of microwave and longer wavelength lasers such as Nd: Yag laser, are currently used for hair removal in patients with darker skin.

VI. LASER SKIN RESURFACING (LSR)

1. The CO_2 laser (10,600 nm) was originally used to ablate exophytic skin lesions; however, over the past decade, the most common use for the CO_2 laser has been to treat photo-aged skin.
2. Photo-aged skin, including rhytids, dyschromias, solar and senile lentigenes, ephelides, and actinic keratoses, all respond favorably to CO_2 laser skin resurfacing. In particular, periorbital and perioral rhytids respond the best. The deep furrows in the glabellar region, on the other hand, do not respond well to LSR.
3. Acne scars have also been treated with CO_2 lasers with favorable results.
4. The CO_2 laser has a high absorption coefficient for tissue water and allows precise tissue removal with minimal residual thermal damage (RTD).
5. The mechanisms involved in LSR are not certain, but a number of studies have shown that CO_2 resurfacing leads to contraction of collagen I fibers and wound remodeling, which results in reduction of rhytids.
6. The most common side effect is erythema, which is seen in virtually all the patients. The incidence of hyperpigmentation and hypopigmentation is fairly high after CO_2 resurfacing, and other treatment options should be discussed with those patients with Fitzgerald skin type III and higher. However, even patients with skin type I can have significant pigmentation changes.
7. More recently, the 2.94 μm erbium:yttrium-aluminum-garnet (Er:YAG) has been used for resurfacing. The Er:YAG at 2.94 μm wavelength results in strong water absorption and can ablate the epidermis with even more precision than the CO_2 laser and at lower fluences. At fluences between 5–10 J/cm^2, the Er:YAG can ablate to depth of 10–20 μm yet results in only a 10–50 μm RTD. Overall, the Er:YAG LSR is much less painful than CO_2 LSR, and the time of reepithelialization and postoperative erythema is shorter. However, with increasing passes, there is less control of hemostasis due to insufficient heat being generated to seal the vessels.
8. Recently, nonablative LSR has been developed. The 1.32 μm Nd:YAG laser produces selective papillary dermal injury, leading to fibroblast activation and synthesis of new collagen without significant epidermal injury. Although further studies are needed, it appears that the 1.32 μm Nd:YAG laser with a cooling device can achieve improvement in treating facial rhytids while avoiding epidermal injury. This nonablative technique has no recovery time and has a minimal risk of complications relative to the traditional ablative treatments.

Finally, non-laserlight sources such as intense pulse light and radiofrequency are being used as a form of nonablative therapy for facial rejuvenation.

107

The Forehead and Brow

Daniel A. De Ugarte, M.D., and Marc H. Hedrick, M.D.
David Geffen School of Medicine at UCLA, Los Angeles, California, U.S.A.

Rhytidectomy (facelift) corrects lower and midfacial ptosis and aging, but produces little improvement in periorbital and brow ptosis. Furthermore, the action of the superficial muscles of the upper face produces deep furrows or rhytids in some patients. Forehead and brow lifting corrects these problems and rejuvenates the brow and periorbital region.

I. INDICATIONS FOR BROW/FOREHEAD LIFT

A. Ptosis of the brow/forehead.

B. Ptosis of the lateral upper eyelid.

C. Correction of wrinkle lines and creases:

- Transverse forehead lines
- Glabellar creases
- Transverse folds at the root of the nose
- Upper nasal and medial eyelid fullness
- In patients for whom these are the main indications, the goal is not to elevate the brow but to interrupt muscle activity responsible for the lines and creases

D. Upper eye fullness and skin excess *not* correctable by blepharoplasty alone.

II. PATIENT EVALUATION

The patient is examined while seated or standing.

A. Upper and Lower Eyelid Aesthetics

A complete evaluation of both eyelids and globes should be performed. Blepharoplasty surgery may be necessary to improve the appearance of the periorbital area.

B. Brow Position and Ptosis

Manually elevate the brow. The persistence of excess upper lid skin is an indication for concomitant upper eyelid blepharoplasty.

C. Hairline Position

Evaluate the height of the forehead and thickness of the hair to determine the best location for the incision.

D. Ideal Eyebrow Position and Contour (Fig. 1)

1. The brow begins medially at a vertical line drawn perpendicular through the alar base.
2. The brow terminates laterally at an oblique line drawn through the lateral canthus of the eye and the alar base.
3. The medial and lateral ends of the eyebrow lie at approximately the same horizontal level.
4. The apex of the brow lies on a vertical line drawn directly through the lateral limbus of the eye.
5. The brow arches above the supraorbital rim in women and lies approximately at the level of the rim in men.

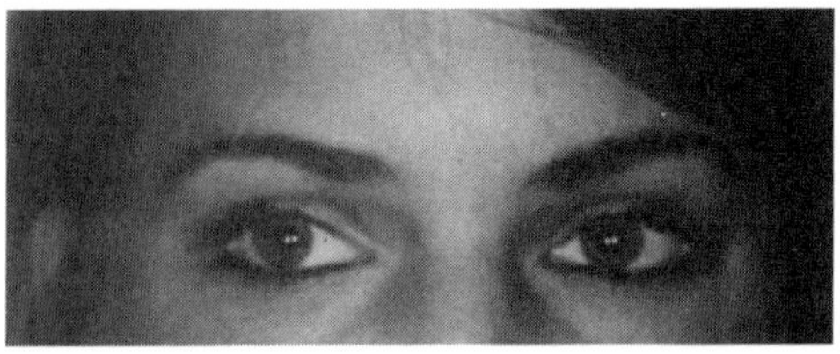

Figure 1 Ideal female brow position. (Courtesy of Putterman AM, ed. *Cosmetic Oculoplastic Surgery: Eyelid, Forehead, and Facial Techniques*. 3rd ed. Philadelphia: W.B. Saunders Co., 1998.)

III. ANATOMY (FIG. 2)

A. Glabella

1. An elevation of the frontal bone between the eyebrows.

B. Frontalis Muscle

1. Part of the occipitofrontalis muscle, the frontalis muscles are scalp muscles that are bilateral extensions of the galea aponeurotica.
2. The frontalis muscles begin at the anterior hairline and insert into the forehead skin.
3. Function—elevate the eyebrows and produce transverse lines in the forehead during frowning.

C. Procerus Muscles

1. Small paired muscles that originate from nasal bones and upper nasal cartilages insert into the skin overlying the glabella.
2. Function—pull the forehead down and elevate the root of the nasal skin to produce transverse lines over the bridge of the nose during frowning.

D. Corrugator Supercilii Muscles

1. Arise from the periosteum along the superomedial orbital rim.
2. Insert into the skin overlying the medial portion of the eyebrow.
3. Function—pull the brow medially and downward to produce vertical glabellar creases.

E. Supraorbital Nerves

1. Are bilateral branches of the frontal nerves which arise from cranial nerve V.
2. Emanate from the supraorbital foramen to provide sensory innervation to the lateral and anterior scalp.

F. Supratrochlear Nerves

1. Are bilateral branches of the frontal nerves which arise from cranial nerve V.
2. Lie in the corrugator supercilii muscles and provide sensory innervation to the middle of the forehead.

IV. BOTOX CHEMODENERVATION

A. Botulinum toxin (Botox®) can be injected subcutaneously or intramuscularly to simulate the surgical results of a brow/forehead lift.

B. Botox acts by paralyzing the glabellar brow muscles medially and the orbicularis oculi muscles laterally.

C. Paralysis of the periorbital muscles can also soften and diminish the depth of many facial wrinkles.

D. Botox can also be used in conjunction with brow/forehead lift procedures.

E. The duration of effect is about 6–9 months.

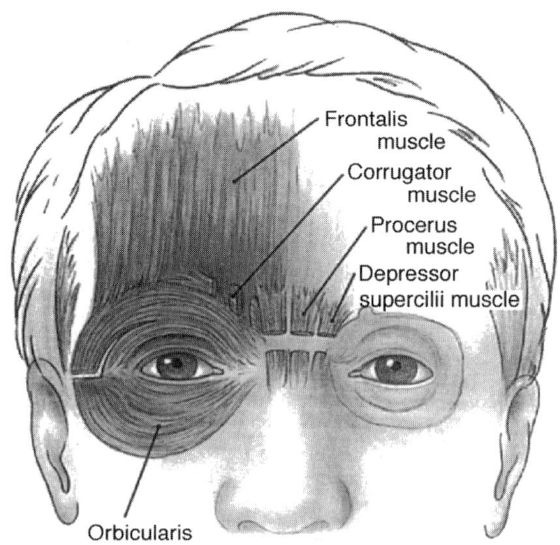

Figure 2 Anatomy. (Courtesy of Putterman AM, ed. *Cosmetic Oculoplastic Surgery: Eyelid, Forehead, and Facial Techniques*. 3rd ed. Philadelphia: W.B. Saunders Co., 1998.)

V. OPEN BROW/FOREHEAD LIFT

A. Types of Incision

Two basic alternative incisions can be used: the standard coronal incision and the modified anterior hairline incision. The modified incision is useful in patients with high hairlines or with excess thinning of the hair.

B. Preoperative Evaluation

1. The vertical glabellar creases and transverse forehead lines should be marked prior to induction of anesthesia or intravenous sedation. The proposed incision should be outlined (Fig. 3).
2. The hair should be parted along the planned incision (shaving is not necessary).
3. Local anesthetic should be administered along the anticipated incision and along the supraorbital rim down to the dorsum of the nose.
4. Corneal protectors should be placed as the eye can be inadvertently injured during the procedure.

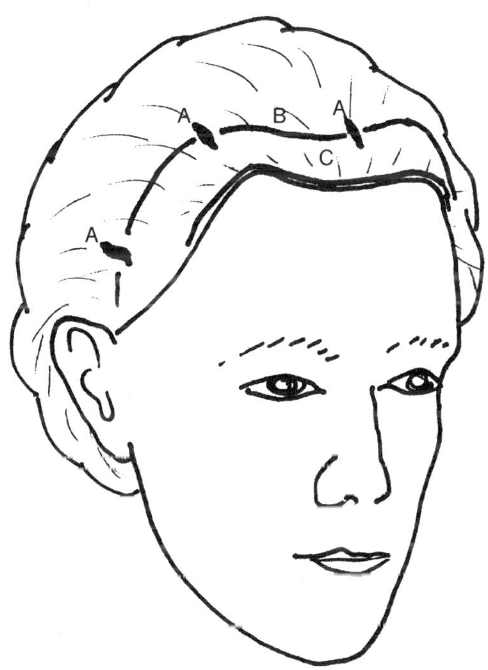

Figure 3 Incisions: (A) endoscopic incisions; (B) coronal incision; (C) hairline incision. (Courtesy of Putterman AM, ed. *Cosmetic Oculoplastic Surgery: Eyelid, Forehead, and Facial Techniques*. 3rd ed. Philadelphia: W.B. Saunders Co., 1998.)

5. During the incision, it is important to bevel the scalpel in the direction of the hair follicles.

C. Creation of Flap

1. A forehead flap is created by dissecting the subgaleal plane.
2. The supraorbital and supratrochlear neurovascular bundles should be carefully identified and preserved.

D. Rhytid Reduction by Muscular Resection and Incision

1. In order to diminish their rhytid-causing actions, the corrugator supercilii muscles should be partially resected and the procerus muscles divided or avulsed.
2. The frontalis muscle elevates the forehead, and its modification, therefore, is controversial.

E. Flap Fixation and Closure

1. The forehead/brow flap is redraped and sutured at specific fixation points in such a manner as to have only light tension on the flap. The remainder of the flap should be trimmed.
2. The galea can be closed with running absorbable suture and the skin closed with staples.
3. Drains are not needed.
4. A light compression dressing can be used.
5. The hair should be combed over the incision and the cut hair removed.

VI. ENDOSCOPIC BROW/FOREHEAD LIFT

1. The endoscopic brow lift has become one of the most common endoscopic plastic surgical procedures.
2. It is associated with a reduced operative time and smaller incisions when compared with the forehead/brow lift. It is also likely to be associated with less frequent, less severe, and more quickly resolving complications of paresthesias, itching, and alopecia.
3. Endoscopic brow lift can be combined with open or endoscopic treatment of the midface and neck regions. It can also be combined with an open rhytidectomy by utilizing the superior ends of the face-lift incisions as lateral entry sites.

4. Generally, three to five incisions are placed to facilitate instrument placement, endoscope access, and fixation of the mobilized brow.

VII. POSTOPERATIVE CARE

A. Mild analgesics are usually adequate. Patients are more likely to experience sensations of pressure and discomfort than pain.

B. Ophthalmic lubricating ointment should be applied liberally to prevent desiccation of the cornea, especially if a concomitant upper eyelid blepharoplasty is performed. The eyelids often do not close completely for the first 24 hours after surgery.

C. Dressings can be removed on the first postoperative day following an isolated forehead/brow procedure or on the second day if done in conjunction with a rhytidectomy.

D. Swelling and periorbital ecchymosis can be anticipated to worsen starting the second or third postoperative day.

E. Staple and fixation or screw removal (in endoscopic procedures) is usually performed 1–2 weeks following the procedure.

VIII. COMPLICATIONS

A. Hematoma is uncommon, but it can lead to flap necrosis or alopecia. Therefore, patients complaining of pain should be carefully evaluated.

B. Frontalis muscle paresis/paralysis can occur if the frontal branches of the facial nerve are injured. Full return of function can occur within 1 year as long as there is some movement postoperatively.

C. Alopecia is rare but can occur in areas of tension (i.e., fixation points) or in areas overlying a hematoma.

D. Paresthesias of the forehead and anterior scalp can result from injury to the supraorbital and supatrochlear nerves. Hypesthesias, dysesthesias, and itching usually resolve within 6 weeks to 6 months.

108

Blepharoplasty and Periorbital Aesthetics

Peter J. Taub, M.D., and Marc H. Hedrick, M.D.
David Geffen School of Medicine at UCLA, Los Angeles, California, U.S.A.

The periorbital area is a complex and dynamic area that changes dramatically with aging. Understanding and performing periorbital aesthetic surgery requires a thorough knowledge of orbital anatomy, physiology, and periorbital aesthetics.

I. ANATOMY OF THE UPPER EYELID

A. The anatomy may be thought of in layers, from anterior to posterior:

- Skin and subcutaneous tissues
- Orbicularis oculi muscle
- Orbital septum—thin layer that covers the periorbital fat compartments
- Periorbital fat compartments:

  The medial fat compartment is bounded by the medial check rein ligament and the superior oblique muscle.

  The central fat compartment is more lateral and is bounded by the same superior oblique muscle and the lacrimal gland.

- Levator muscle superiorly, levator aponeurosis toward the lid margin:

  Expansions from the levator aponeurosis pierce the orbicularis muscle and insert into the dermis of the pretarsal skin. This anchoring produces the characteristic fold in the upper eyelid.

  More superiorly, the preseptal orbicularis glides independently of the skin and dermis because it is separated from the skin by a layer of adipose tissue.

- Müller's muscle superiorly, attached to the tarsal plate inferiorly
- Conjunctiva

B. Whitnall's ligament is the superior transverse ligament.

C. A peripheral arterial arcade is situated at the level of the superior edge of the tarsus posterior to the levator aponeurosis.

II. ANATOMY OF THE LOWER EYELID

As in the lower eyelid, the anatomy may be thought of in layers, from anterior to posterior:

A. Skin and subcutaneous tissues.

B. Orbicularis oculi muscle.

C. Orbital septum.

D. Periorbital fat compartments:

- The medial fat compartment is bounded by the medial check rein ligament and the inferior oblique muscle.
- The central fat compartment is bounded by the inferior oblique muscle and the arcuate band.

- The lateral fat compartment is bounded by the arcuate ligament and the lateral cheek ligament.

E. Horner's muscle is attached superiorly to the tarsal plate toward the lid margin.

F. Conjunctiva.

G. Lockwood's ligament is the inferior transverse ligament that covers the inferior oblique muscle and joins the muscle to the ventral surface of the inferior rectus muscle.

III. TEAR FLOW

A. Tears are produced by basic and reflex secretors.

B. The basic secretors consist of three sets of glands:

- Conjunctival, tarsal and limbal goblet cells produce a mucoprotein layer that lies just above the surface of the cornea.
- Accessory lacrimal glands of Krause and Wolfring are located in the subconjunctival tissues. They produce an intermediate-layer tear film.
- Oil-producing meibomian glands and the palpebral glands of Zeis and Moll. These produce the outer lipid layer of tear film that retards evaporation of the lower layers.

C. The reflex secretors are the lacrimal glands located behind the superolateral orbital rims. Each gland has a larger orbital portion and a smaller palpebral portion separated by the lateral expansion of the levator aponeurosis.

D. Flow is across the cornea from lateral to medial and is aided by opening and closing of the eyelids.

E. Tear fluid drains into the upper and lower puncta just lateral to the medial canthal angle. They join to form a common canaliculus that empties into the lacrimal sac. The sac lies within a fossa on the medial orbital wall. The lacrimal sac is approximately 15 mm long and drains into the nasolacrimal duct that, in turn, opens into the inferior meatus of the nose.

IV. PERIORBITAL AESTHETICS

A. Eyelid

1. Aperture of the eye is almond-shaped.
2. Upper lid covers 2–3 mm of the iris.
3. Intercanthal axis has a gentle upward tilt from medial to lateral.
4. Supratarsal fold is precise and defined in the non-Asian eyelid.
5. Lower eyelid touches the limbus in neutral gaze.
6. Distance from the upper lash line to the lid fold is one third to one quarter of the distance from the lash line to the lower eyebrow.

B. Eyebrow

1. The brow should lie at the level of the supraorbital rim in males and above the rim in females.
2. The medial and lateral ends lie at approximately the same horizontal level.
3. The medial end begins on line with the medial canthus or alar rim. It ends on a line between the alar rim and lateral canthus.
4. The height of the brow is maximal over the lateral limbus.

V. PERIORBITAL PATHOLOGY

A. Dermatochalasis

1. Cosmetic deformity of baggy eyelids.
2. This may be due to redundant skin, malpositioned fat, or a combination of the two.
3. Common in middle age due to loss of elastic tissue.
4. Usually worse in the upper eyelids and often exaggerated by concomitant descent of the brow.

B. Blepharoptosis

1. May be related to either a muscular or a neurologic defect.
2. A myogenic cause is the most common congenital type. It results from dysgenesis of the levator muscle. Striated muscle is replaced with fibrous tissue. May be unilateral or bilateral.
3. A neurogenic cause results from faulty innervation of the upper lid retractors. The superior division of the oculomotor nerve to the levator muscle or the sympathetic innervation to Müller's muscle may be interrupted.
4. Other causes include mechanical or traumatic etiologies.

C. Blepharochalasis

1. Rare, inherited syndrome seen most commonly in young women.
2. Characterized by repetitive episodes of eyelid edema and erythema.
3. Not usually painful.
4. Leads to attenuation and dehiscence of the levator aponeurosis, and possibly the canthal tendons.
5. Late findings include phimosis and ectropion.

D. Blepharophimosis

1. Congenital syndrome of ptosis, telecanthus, and phimosis of the upper eyelids.

E. Orbital Festoons

1. Laxity and malposition of the orbicularis muscle may produce baggy eyelids.
2. True festoons are apparent with contraction of the orbicularis muscle.
3. Treatment involves elevation of the muscle as part of a skin-muscle flap and repositioning.

VI. BLEPHAROPLASTY—PREOPERATIVE EVALUATION

A. History

1. Baseline vision, including use of glasses or contacts.
2. Preexisting ocular pathology, including glaucoma and cataracts.
3. Thyroid disease.

B. Brow Position

1. Must evaluate where the brow rests in relation to the supraorbital rim.
2. Frontalis muscle function.
3. Some describe an abnormal brow position that is less than 30 mm from lower border of the brow to the lash line.

C. Lid Character

1. Must evaluate whether there is excess skin or excess fat.
2. Also must evaluate whether there is malpositioned fat or ptosis.
3. Elasticity of the lower eyelid is tested by grasping the lid and allowing it to "snap back" into position. Poor elasticity may warrant a concomitant suspension procedure during lower eyelid blepharoplasty.

D. Eye Function

Evaluation is performed by the operating surgeon and by a skilled ophthalmologist:

1. Extraocular muscle function.
2. Pupil reactivity.
3. Visual acuity.
4. Fundoscopic examination.
5. Schirmer's test—a 5 mm × 35 mm piece of #41 filter paper is folded 5 mm at one end and placed into the inferior fornix of the eye while the patient maintains a fixed upward gaze for 5 minutes. Normally, the moisture should advance up the paper 10–30 mm. Patients with dry eye syndrome will have decreased moisture advancement on the filter paper. Some authors have failed to point out the validity of the test.

VII. BLEPHAROPLASTY—PREOPERATIVE CONSULTATION

Certain patients should raise concerns about the safety of blepharoplasty. These include:

A. Asymmetry should be pointed out preoperatively.

B. Cheek pads—blepharoplasty will not address this area of bulging.

C. Dry eye syndrome:

- Not seen in contact wearers.
- May require alteration of the surgical technique.

D. Hollow orbits—fat resection should be minimal to prevent worsening of the hollowed appearance.

E. Lower lid hypotonia:

- Tested by pulling the lower lid away from the cornea and observing the quality of the "snap back."
- Poor tone combined with lower blepharoplasty may result in ectropion if a concomitant suspensory procedure is not included.

F. Proptosis:

- Defined by >3 mm forward projection of the cornea.
- 2–3% of these patients have underlying hypothyroidism; 0.3% of patients have hyperthyroidism.
- Skin resection in these patients should be more conservative to prevent postoperative corneal exposure.

VIII. BLEPHAROPLASTY—TECHNIQUE (FIG. 1)

A. Skin incisions:

- Upper blepharoplasty incision is usually placed in the supratarsal crease 7–9 mm above the ciliary margin, approximately at the level of the upper border of the tarsal plate. With the eyes open, the scar should fall within the fold.
- Lower blepharoplasty subciliary incision is placed a 1–2 mm below the lash line. Either a skin only or skin + muscle flap is elevated. A portion of the excess lid skin is resected prior to closure.
- Lower blepharoplasty transconjunctival incision is indicated for removal of herniated fat when there is minimal or no skin laxity. Its major drawbacks are underresection of fat and inability to correct surface rhytids. Many combine this approach with a chemical peel or laser treatment to address the rhytids.

B. Minimal strip resection of the orbicularis muscle. This prevents overlap of the muscle over the pretarsal area and bulging of the tissues with closure.

C. Opening the septum is performed by gently spreading the tissues with a small scissors.

D. Fat resection: Fat is gently teased out of each compartment and the base is cauterized prior to removal. Deep perforators may cause bleeding if disrupted by forcible removal of the fat.

E. Closure:

- Closure of the orbital septum is not necessary.
- Skin closure is performed with a fine absorbable or nonabsorbable suture.

IX. ASIAN BLEPHAROPLASTY

A. The Asian eyelid is characterized by absence of a supratarsal skin crease and the presence of an epicanthal fold medially.

B. In these patients, the levator muscle inserts into the superior edge of the tarsal plate but does not send extensions through the orbicularis. As such, the levator muscle does not insert into the dermis.

C. Treatment traditionally involved anchoring the lower skin-muscle flap to the insertion of the levator aponeurosis at the superior tarsal edge to create a fold. Newer techniques involve one or several transpalpebral sutures without an external incision.

D. The epicanthal fold may be removed by a series of small Z-plasties around the fold, as described by Uchida and others.

X. COMPLICATIONS OF BLEPHAROPLASTY

A. Corneal Abrasion

1. Characterized by the sensation of a foreign body in the eye, pain, and excess tearing.
2. Diagnosed by fluorescein slit-lamp examination.
3. Treated with antibiotic ointment and patching.
4. Most heal within 24 hours.

B. Acute Glaucoma

1. Due to increased intraocular pressure.
2. Characterized by pain in the eye. There may or may not be visual loss.
3. Diagnosed by a Schiotz tonometer, which is designed to measure ocular pressure.
4. Treated with acetazolamide, mannitol (osmotic diuretic), and pilocarpine (pupillary constrictor and vasodilator).

C. Retrobulbar Hematoma

1. Due to bleeding into the posterior orbit.
2. Characterized by pain, proptosis, and limited extraocular movement.
3. Treated with immediate release of all incisions and lateral canthotomy. Additional therapies

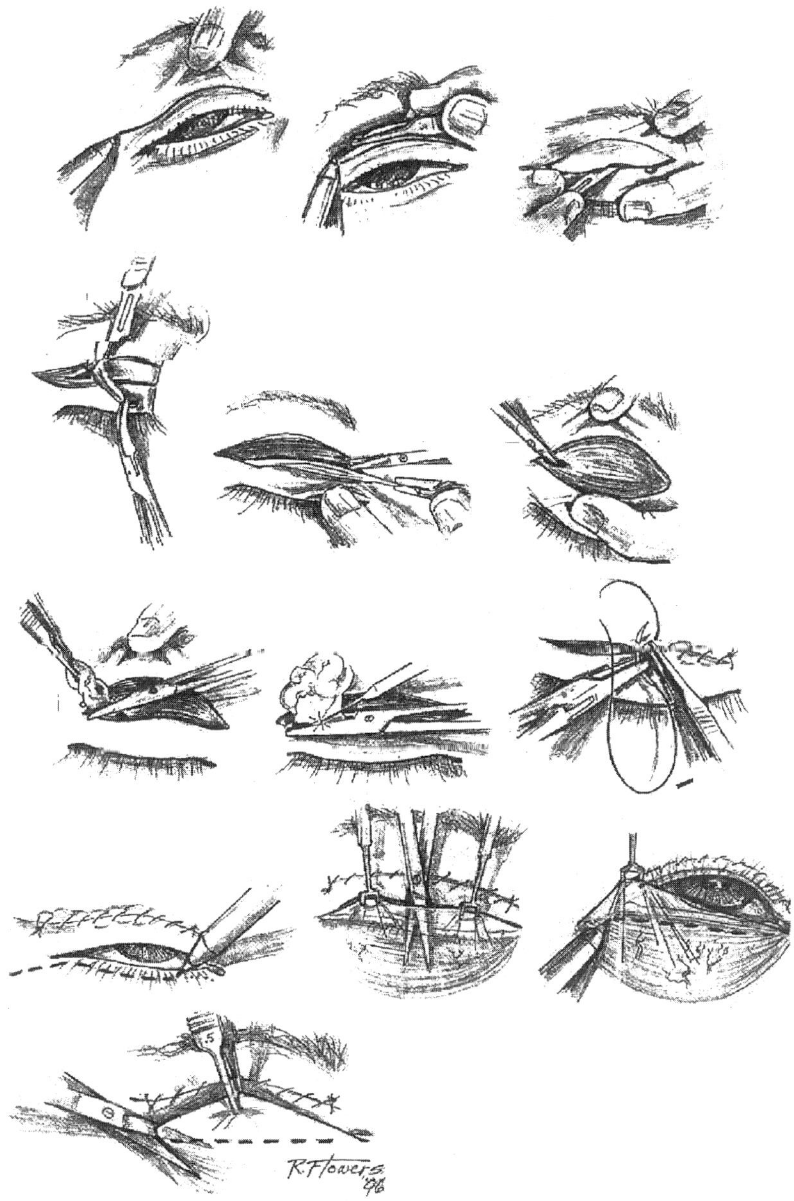

Figure 1 Traditional blepharoplasty technique.

include 20% mannitol (1 g/kg) and acetazolamide (500 mg IV initially, then 250 mg IV q6h).

4. Controversial treatments include an inhalation mixture of 95% oxygen and 5% carbon dioxide and anterior chamber paracentesis.

D. Extraocular Muscle Injury

1. Superior oblique muscle (CN IV) is at risk during upper blepharoplasty. Injury causes difficulty reaching for objects or walking down stairs.
2. Inferior oblique muscle (CN III) is at risk during lower blepharoplasty. Injury causes difficulty with upward gaze.

E. Ectropion

1. Most common complication after lower blepharoplasty (15%).
2. More likely with preoperative hypotonia, as measured by the "snap back" test.

3. Usually due to scarring and septal retraction.
4. Treated with early massage and taping. Failure to improve may warrant skin grafting, resection, and/or lateral suspension.

F. Acute Blindness

1. Seen in approximately 0.05% of cases.
2. Follows a hemorrhagic event involving the optic nerve artery rather than the retinal artery.
3. Characterized by rapid proptosis and ecchymosis.
4. Treated as above for retrobulbar hematoma.

XI. LOWER EYELID LAXITY

A. Hypotonia of the lower lid should be managed at the time of blepharoplasty.

B. Many techniques have been described to address this problem:

- Temporary external support by taping the skin of the lower lid.
- Canthopexy—suturing the lateral canthal tendon to a new position along the periosteum of the lateral orbital rim.
- Canthoplasty—complete detachment and repositioning of the lateral canthal tendon.
- Tarsal suspension to the periosteum of lateral orbital rim.
- Wedge excision of a portion of the lower lid.

XII. BROWLIFT

A. In many patients, hyperactivity of the frontalis muscles has developed to prevent blockage of the line of vision from redundant eyelid skin. This should be identified preoperatively because correction of the eyelids will allow the frontalis to return to a normal level of activity and may unmask a more dramatic descent of the brow. In these patients, concomitant browlift may be indicated.

B. In addition, descent of the brow with aging contributes to the overall periorbital appearance.

C. Correction of brow position maybe addressed in a variety of ways:

- Direct skin excision from the suprabrow area. This may be beneficial in patients (generally male) with preexisting forehead rhytids and a high hairline that might be raised even higher with other procedures.
- Temporal browlift:

  The brow is elevated from incisions placed in the lateral temporal areas of the scalp, which are usually more hair-bearing segments of the scalp.

  Skin excision and closure provides lift solely to the lateral portions of the brows.
- Hairline browlift:

  The incision is placed at the level of the hairline in an attempt to prevent upward displacement of the hairline.

  It is indicated for patients with at least 5 cm between the eyebrow and the hairline

  Leaves the most conspicuous scar.
- Bicoronal browlift:

  Performed behind the level of the hairline to hide the incision.

  Provides the most complete elevation of the forehead, but tends to raise the level of the forehead and anterior hairline margin.
- Endoscopic browlift:

  Performed through separate incisions at the top of the forehead and in the temporal skin.

  The forehead is elevated down to the supraorbital rim. The corrugator and procerus muscles are dissected and transected free of the supraorbital and supratrochlear neurovascular bundles.

109

Rhytidectomy and Cervico-Facial Contouring

R. Michael Koch, M.D., Marc H. Hedrick, M.D., and Timothy A. Miller, M.D.
David Geffen School of Medicine at UCLA, Los Angeles, California, U.S.A.

Rhytidectomy, or facelift, is a primary procedure used to correct the cervico-facial anatomic changes that occur with aging. In addition, adjuvant procedures such as cervico-facial liposuction and injections of "filler" materials may also be used to rejuvenate the face.

I. PATHOGENESIS OF FACIAL AGING

A. General

1. The process of aging involves a combination of wear and tear combined with direct gravitational effects. All facial tissues are susceptible to these forces. These include skin wrinkling and pigmentation changes, structural ptosis producing eyebrow descent, volume loss producing infraorbital hollowing, nasolabial folds, jowling, submental skin redundancy, and overall skin thinning.
2. In addition, sun damage accelerates the aging process and produces characteristic changes such as elastosis, lentigues, and hyperpigmentation (Fig. 1).

B. Morphology of Rhytids

There are three general types of skin rhytids:

1. Animation creases from mimetic muscle insertions.
2. Fine, shallow rhytids caused by disruption of the elastic structural network that develop in sun-protected areas and disappear when the skin is stretched.
3. Coarse, deep, permanent rhytids (solar elastosis) that develop on sun-exposed skin and do not disappear when stretched.

C. Histology

1. Microarchitectural changes of aging include flattening of the dermal-epidermal junction, a decrease in the number of melanocytes and Langerhans cells, decreased gylcosaminoglycans, progressive loss of elastin, and a reduction in dermal collagen.
2. Human rhytids show no histologic or ultrastructural changes that correlate with surface configuration.
3. Theories of elastotic changes and fractured dermal collagen have been proposed. In deeper skin furrows, however, there are apparent fascial insertions of cutaneous muscles that create surface grooves.

II. RARE INHERITED SKIN DISORDERS

A. Ehlers-Danlos Syndrome (Cutis Hyperelastica)

1. This represents a clinically and genetically heterogeneous group of disorders that result in defective collagen cross-linking secondary to reduced lysyl oxidase activity.
2. Features include hyperextensible and extremely fragile skin that is easily traumatized.

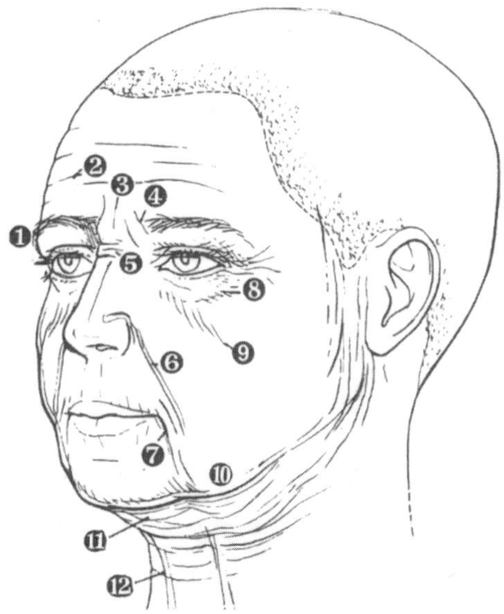

Figure 1 Late signs of brow and cervicofacial aging: 1, medial, arch and lateral brow ptosis; 2, deep transverse forehead lines; 3, marked vertical and 4, oblique glabellar "frown" lines; 5, severe transverse nasion lines; 6, prominent nasolabial crease and fold; 7, multiple labiomental creases and folds; 8, deep malar crescent; 9, severe nasojugal groove; 10, marked jowl; 11, neck obesity or 12, platysmal severe laxity and banding. Significant skin excess and poor skin tone is evident, especially in the neck.

3. Wound healing is impaired and these patients are poor candidates for rhytidectomy.

B. Cutis Laxa

1. In this disorder, there is a decrease in the size and number of dermal elastin fibers with dramatic skin laxity.
2. Affected persons have generalized loose skin in all regions of the body that is inelastic, lacking the springiness of youth.
3. When inherited as a recessive trait, it is often accompanied by pulmonary and cardiac disorders.
4. Rhytidectomy can improve the skin laxity.

C. Pseudoxanthoma Elasticum

1. This occurs in two dominant and two recessive forms.
2. The recessive Type II is characterized by lax and loose-fitting skin infiltrated with degenerated elastic fibers. Rhytidectomy can be of benefit to these patients.

D. Werner's Syndrome (Adult Progeria)

1. This autosomal recessive trait is characterized by scleroderma-like indurated patches of skin that are associated with baldness, skin hyperpigmentation, and atherosclerotic cardiovascular disease.
2. Rhytidectomy is contraindicated because of diabetic-like microangiopathy and subsequent poor wound healing.

III. PREOPERATIVE EVALUATION

A. History and Physical Examination

1. A thorough history and physical examination is required when evaluating a patient for aesthetic surgery.
2. Patients undergoing aesthetic surgery should be healthy without major medical problems. All minor medical problems should be well controlled.
3. Besides rare skin conditions, it is important to note:
   - Factors that may contribute to postoperative bleeding such as renal or hepatic disease, hypertension, and use of medication that causes coagulopathy
   - Smoking history due to the risk of skin ischemia and slough
   - Medical conditions that may increase the risk of anesthesia
   - Steroid use
4. Aesthetic facial surgery is elective and should be postponed if there are any unresolved medical issues.
5. Antiplatelet medications (e.g., aspirin, NSAIDs) and cigarette smoking should be discontinued at least 2–3 weeks prior to rhytidectomy.
6. The cervico-facial examination must be comprehensive and is best conducted in a systematic fashion.
   - First, the skin is inspected for scars, acne, rhytids, or other lesions.
   - Then, it is palpated for thickness, mobility, and elasticity.

- Next, the forehead and brow regions are inspected for furrowing, ptosis, and frontalis hyperactivity.
- The central face, including the nasolabial folds, jaw line, and jowls, are assessed for contour and laxity.
- The face is inspected for submental and submandibular fat deposits, submaxillary gland ptosis, depth of the cervicomental angle, position of the hyoid bone, and platysma muscle anatomy.
- The hairline contour is noted, as are scars from any previous surgery.

B. Preoperative Photographs

1. Preoperative photographs are essential and provide necessary medicolegal documentation.
2. They are also used in preoperative planning, patient discussion, and intraoperative decision making. In addition, they can be used for quality assurance and physician education.

IV. PSYCHOLOGICAL CONSIDERATIONS

A. The psychological assessment is a critical aspect of the preoperative assessment prior to facial rejuvination.

B. Patients should be evaluated for their motivation, expectations for surgery, emotional reactions to the perceived deformities, and overall response to the interview process.

C. It is important for the patient to verbalize his or her appraisal of the problem, and it is essential to determine whether the patient's emotional concern is proportional to the extent of the cosmetic deformity.

D. The ideal surgical candidates are well motivated, with a supportive and stable environment, and are able to develop a strong doctor-patient relationship.

V. ANESTHESIA

A. A rhytidectomy can be performed under either local anesthesia with intravenous sedation or general anesthesia with endotracheal intubation. With both types of anesthesia, lidocaine (0.5%) with epinephrine (1:200,000) can be used at the site of surgery to achieve a local vasoconstrictive effect.

B. Trigeminal and greater auricular nerve blocks may be used for postoperative analgesia.

VI. FACELIFT ANATOMY

A. Layers

There are five anatomic layers of the face that are critical to rhytidectomy (Fig. 2):

1. Skin
2. Subcutaneous fat
3. Superficial musculoaponeurotic system (SMAS)
4. Fascial-muscle layer
5. Facial nerve

B. Layer Arrangement and Characteristics

Though the anatomic arrangement of these layers persists throughout the face, they do exist in varying degrees of thickness and are highly compressed in the region of the zygomatic arch:

1. The SMAS, the most heterogenous layer, lies beneath the skin and subcutaneous fat.
2. Depending on the location, the SMAS may be mostly fibrous, muscular, or fatty.
3. The muscles of facial expression (frontalis, orbicularis oculi, zygomatic major and minor, and platysma) are contained within the SMAS layer.
4. There is some variation in the temporal region, wherein the SMAS layer is represented by the analogous superficial temporal fascia (or temporoparietal fascia).

C. Facial Nerve

1. With few exceptions, facial nerve branches innervate facial muscles on their deep surfaces. As such, dissection superficial to the SMAS layer can be performed safely. If dissection is performed deep to the SMAS layer and superficial to the facial nerve, care must be employed particularly in the temporal scalp, the face anterior to the parotid gland, and neck regions.
2. In contrast to the majority of facial muscles, three muscles are innervated from the superficial aspect:
   - Buccinator muscles
   - Mentalis muscles
   - Levator anguli oris muscles

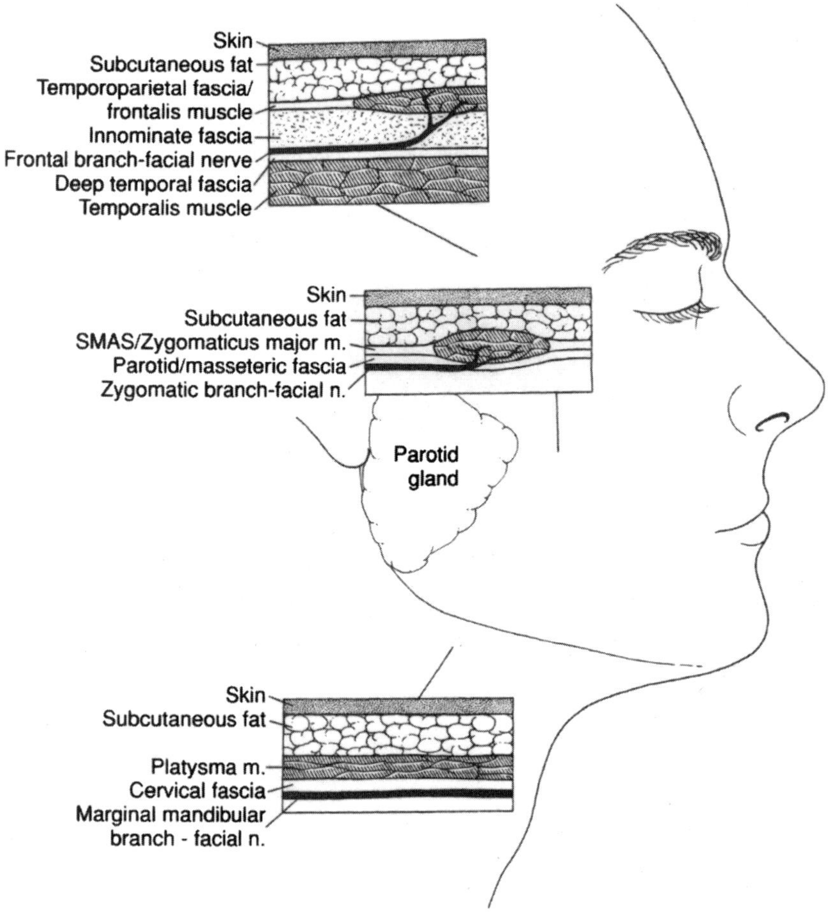

Figure 2 The anatomic layers of the face. Although the names vary, the arrangement persists, regardless of the area of the face. The facial nerve (CN VII) branches innervate their respective muscles of the SMAS layer via the deep surfaces.

3. The facial nerve is comprised of five branches:
   - Temporal
   - Zygomatic
   - Buccinator
   - Mandibular
   - Cervical
4. Crossover communications between the zygomatic and buccinator branches supplying the cheek occur in roughly 70% of patients. However, few communications are observed between the frontal and the marginal mandibular branches. As a result, special care is required in these areas to avoid postoperative paresis.
5. It is important to note that although the facial nerve branches are deep to the SMAS/muscle layer, they will at some point course superficially to innervate the facial muscles. As a result, any continuous dissection in the sub-SMAS plane will eventually denervate some of these facial muscles. In order to avoid this problem during a deep-plane rhytidectomy, the dissection is begun in the sub-SMAS plane laterally and changes to a more superficial plane medially as the zygomaticus major muscle is encountered.

D. Parotid-Masseteric Fascia

1. The parotid-masseteric fascia is a filmy, areolar layer located between the SMAS and the parotid gland and is superficial to the facial nerve.
2. In the temporal region, it lies between the temporoparietal fascia and the deep temporal fascia and extends into the scalp to lie between the analogous galea and pericranium layers.

3. One should consider the galea, frontalis, temporoparietal fascia, SMAS, obicularis oculi, and platysma as structures forming a contiguous superficial layer.
4. The subgaleal fascia, innominate fascia, parotid-masseteric fascia, and cervical fascia can likewise be considered in a similar fashion.

E. Nasolabial Fold

1. The SMAS layer is thin as it courses across the cheek, forming the investing fascia for the muscles of the upper lip. Since the SMAS is anchored by the obicularis oris, lateral traction during a facelift would have little effect on the medial cheek skin.
2. One approach to smoothing the nasolabial fold is a lateral dissection in the sub-SMAS plane with a transition superficially at the zygomaticus major muscle, allowing the transmission of traction to the medial cheek skin.

F. Retaining Ligaments

1. There are two types of ligaments that restrain the facial skin against gravitational pull in the malar region: the zygomatic ligaments (MacGregor's patch) and the mandibular ligaments. These are fibrous bands that run from the periosteum to the dermis and tether the skin to the facial skeleton.
2. There are also the parotid-cutaneous ligaments and masseteric-cutaneous ligaments formed from coalescences between the superficial and deep fascia in certain regions of the face. The laxity of these supporting ligaments is thought to contribute to the deepening of the nasolabial fold and in the formation of jowls.

G. Platysma

1. The platysma is the inferior continuation of the SMAS layer.
2. In the submental region, three distinct configurations are described by the degree of decussation of the two muscles at the midline:
   - In the most common configuration, the two muscles course cephalad as two separate bands and decussate 1–2 cm below the edge of the mandible.
   - In the second type, the platysma decussates all the way from the level of the thyroid to the mandible.
   - The third type shows no decussation. The medial borders of these muscles proceed parallel to each other and insert on the undersurface of the mandible.
3. With aging, the medial borders of the platysma muscles may become redundant and contribute to the appearance of bands in the submental region.
4. The lack of decussation of the platysma muscles also allows pseudo-herniation of submental fat, accentuating the "turkey gobbler" deformity in the anterior neck.

H. Malar Fat Pad

1. The malar fat pad is a subcutaneous structure that overlies the SMAS/muscle layer.
2. Techniques have been described to elevate the malar fat pad and place tension on the nasolabial fold. In the extended SMAS technique, the malar fat pad is elevated in continuity with the SMAS layer.
3. Independent fat pad elevation relative to the SMAS may allow more flexibility in the skin redraping.
4. Finger-assisted malar elevation (FAME) is blunt finger dissection deep to the obicularis oculi muscle (the SMAS layer) and the malar fat pad.

I. Buccal Fat Pad

1. The buccal fat pad is anterior to the masseter muscle and overlies the buccinator muscle. Also anterior to the masseter are the buccal branches of the facial nerve that run superficial to the buccal fat pad.
2. Access to the buccal fat pad can be gained through the facelift incision by a sub-SMAS dissection with spreading of the buccal branches of the facial nerve in the cheek or intraorally via an incision through the buccinator muscle.

J. Facial Sensation

1. A facelift procedure will inevitably result in disruption of sensory nerves to the skin and abnormal sensation may persist for months after surgery.

2. The sensory nerve most frequently at risk in rhytidectomy is the greater auricular nerve (C2, 3). If the patient's head is turned 45 degrees to the contralateral side, this nerve is found crossing the superficial surface of the sternocleidomastoid muscle 6.5 cm below the external auditory canal. The nerve is located just posterior to the external jugular vein beneath the SMAS and proceeds superficially to provide sensibility to the skin of the earlobe. Injury to the nerve may cause dysesthesia, hypesthesia, or neuroma symptoms.

K. Forehead Anatomy

1. The frontalis muscles have vertically oriented fibers that begin at the level of the anterior hairline and insert into the dermis of the forehead.
2. The frontal branch of the facial nerve innervates the frontalis and enters the muscle on its deep surface.
3. The frontalis muscle functions to elevate the eyebrow. Denervation will result in brow ptosis on the affected side.
4. The frontal branch of the facial nerve is typically multiple with 2–5 branches that pass over the zygomatic arch. The most anterior frontal branch of the facial nerve emerges beneath the parotid gland in a line that extends from 0.5 cm below the tragus to 1.5 cm above the lateral brow, passing deep to the SMAS over the zygomatic arch. The point where the frontal branch enters the undersurface of the frontalis muscle is also the point where the circumferential orbicularis oculi muscle intersects the lateral aspect of the frontalis muscle, roughly 1.5 cm above the lateral aspect of the eyebrow.
5. The corrugator muscle originates from the periosteum of the superior orbital rim and inserts into the dermis of the medial eyebrow. Contraction pulls the brow medially and downward, producing a scowling appearance with vertical glabellar creases forming with chronic, repeated contraction.
6. The procerus muscle originates from the surface of the upper lateral cartilages and nasal bones and inserts into the skin of the glabellar region. With contraction, the procerus pulls the forehead down and the root of the nose upward, causing transverse wrinkles.
7. The sensory innervation to the forehead is via the supraorbital nerve, supratrochlear nerve, and the infratrochlear nerve. All of these nerves arise from the first division of the trigeminal nerve (V1).

VII. SURGICAL TECHNIQUES

A. Four General Technical Approaches to Rhytidectomy

1. Skin lifting only.
2. Skin and SMAS/platysma lifting.
3. Skin and SMAS/platysma and mid-face suspension.
4. Deep plane and subperiosteal dissection level, or a combination of the above.

B. Subcutaneous Rhytidectomy

1. This is the original facelift procedure, which consists of subcutaneous undermining (Fig. 3).
2. The planned incisions and the areas to be undermined are marked on the skin before the administration of anesthesia.
3. The incision begins in the temporal scalp approximately 5 cm above the ear and 5 cm

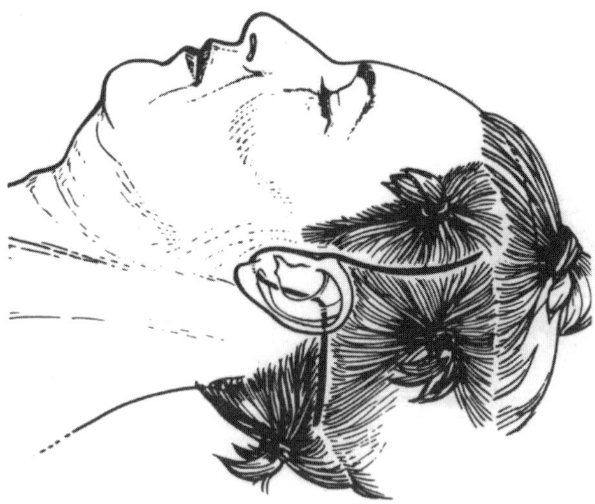

Figure 3 Facelift incision. Alternatively, the incision can be made behind the tragus in an attempt to further hide the preauricular scar. In the retroauricular area, the incision can be made as shown or can run along the hairline for several centimeters before turning posteriorly into the hair-bearing scalp.

behind the hairline, curving toward the superior root of the helix of the ear. At the ear, it curves forward and then downward in the preauricular skin crease, coursing around the ear lobe into the postauricular region.

4. The postauricular skin incision lies 2–3 mm above the retroauricular sulus so that the final scar lies in the concha-mastoid sulcus with the ear covering the resultant scar.
5. The incision is extended onto the mastoid area and to the hairline with a gentle downward curve. The length of this incision is determined by the amount of excess skin. If a large amount of neck skin is to be resected, the incision is extended down to and along the hairline, beveling the incision to preserve hair follicles.
6. The superficial subcutaneous tissue is then progressively undermined, making certain that the dissection extends beyond the areas of redundancy. It commences with elevation of the postauricular skin and the skin that lies over the mastoid region, the sternocleidomastoid muscle (with identification of the great auricular nerve), and continues superficial to the fascia over the muscle and platysma.
7. The cheek is undermined anteriorly through the preauricular incision with dissection extending to within 1 cm of the lateral orbital rim and across the malar area, up to the nasolabial folds to a point 1 cm lateral to the oral commisure, and inferiorly down to the thyroid cartilage in the cervical area (Fig. 4).
8. Release of the zygomatic and mandibular ligaments is also important in order to redrape the skin properly.
9. The mandibular branch of the facial nerve, which lies deep to the platysma, should not be damaged if dissection is confined to the subcutaneous layer and the SMAS is not violated.
10. In the temporal area, the undermining continues along the plane of the temporoparietal fascia, avoiding the frontal branch of the facial nerve.
11. The cervicofacial skin flap is advanced in a cephaloposterior direction, redraped over the underlying base, and fixed at two key points—one in the temporal scalp 1 cm above the ear and the other at the apex of the postauricular incision.

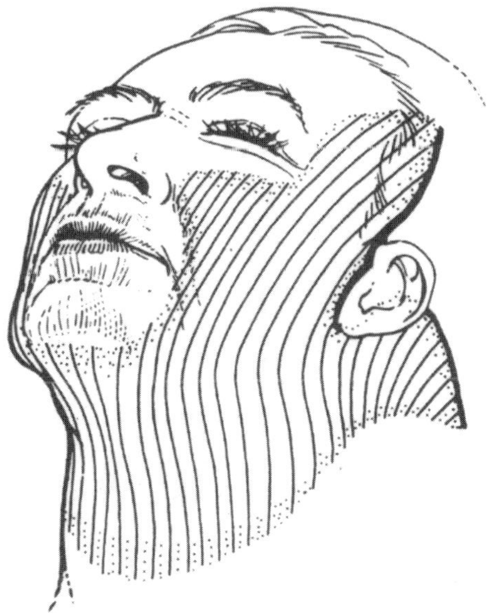

Figure 4 Extent of skin undermining. Maximal skin undermining is shown. In some cases skin undermining may be less extensive, but in general it should be extensive enough to release the zygomatic and mandibular ligaments. (From Furnas D. The retaining ligaments of the cheek. *Plast Reconstr Surg* 1989; 83:11.)

12. It is important to never rotate the sideburn higher than the top of the ear and, if necessary, a triangular skin incision below the sideburn can be made to remove any lax skin.
13. Any overlapping skin in the temporal area is excised and the skin approximated with surgical staples in the hair-bearing areas.
14. The mastoid and postauricular skin incisions are closed with interrupted 3-0 absorbable sutures.
15. The overlapping skin in the prearicular area is excised with conservative trimming of the flap under the earlobe. This ensures tension-free approximation, which is particularly important along the retrotragal suture line and below the earlobe. Incisions are sutured with 5-0 nylon sutures.

C. SMAS/Platysma Facelift

1. The SMAS of the face is continuous with the temporoparietal fascia above and the platysma below and provides the foundation for the overlying skin. The SMAS is connected to the dermis by multiple fibrous septae. Retracting or

pulling the SMAS thus results in a corresponding pull on the overlying skin to which it remains attached medially (Fig. 5).

2. Cervicofacial skin flap dissection is performed as above for the subcutaneous facelift operation. When a submental skin incision is indicated, this incision is made first and the anterior cervical flap is dissected in the subcutaneous plane, with continuity established between the face and neck.
3. The SMAS-platysma unit is then elevated first by identifying the lateral border of the platysma muscle at a point approximately 5 cm below the angle of the mandible. With tension placed by lateral traction, scissor tips are positioned between the anterior border of the sternocleidomastoid muscle and the posterior surface of the platysma muscle.
4. Dissection proceeds inferiorly and anteriorly to pass just superficial to the external jugular vein for a distance of 5–9 cm below the angle of the mandible.
5. Superiorly, the SMAS dissection is begun with a 3–4 cm transverse incision that is placed at a level 1 cm below the inferior border of the zygomatic arch (of note, this cuff of SMAS along the zygomatic arch will later function as a flap anchor and reduce tension on the ear).

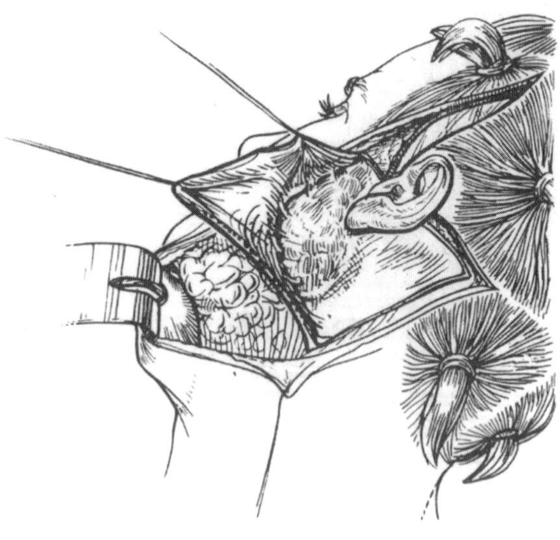

Figure 5 Dissection of SMAS/platysma flap. If a composite rhytidectomy is performed, the same plane of dissection is employed. If SMAS dissection extends to the zygomaticus major muscle, it is termed "extended."

6. A vertical incision through the SMAS is then made approximately 0.5 cm anterior to the auricle. This extends inferiorly from the transverse SMAS incision to continue posterior to the mandibular angle and thus a lateral SMAS flap border is created in continuity with the previously defined lateral margin of the platysma muscle.
7. A scalpel is used to elevate the SMAS from the parotidomasseteric fascia with dissection extending anteriorly beyond the anterior border of the parotid gland, superficial to the deep fascia of the masseter muscle in an areolar plane (where buccal and marginal mandibular nerve branches are frequently seen lying on the masseter). The SMAS flap is elevated until it can freely pull the anterior cheek and jowl without restraint from attachments to the parotid gland, the zygoma, and the fascia of the zygomatic major muscle.
8. The "extended SMAS" dissection also divides the upper masseteric cutaneous ligaments in the subcutaneous level to the level of the oral commissure.
9. With the SMAS and the platysma mobilized as a single continuous flap, they can then be elevated and rotated in a cephaloposterior direction, producing tension on the platysma muscle and lifting the jawline and lower one-third of the face. In addition, the lateral border of the platysma muscle can be advanced and/or partially or fully transected as indicated.
10. To tighten the anterior neck, deepen the cervicomental angle, and contour the jawline, a buried horizontal mattress suture of 3-0 PDS is used to secure the lateral platysma border to the mastoid fascia to create a vector of pull parallel to the mandibular border.
11. Next, a triangle of redundant SMAS is excised at the level of the zygomatic arch and the transverse defect is secured to the previously created cuff of SMAS along the zygomatic arch. Additional vertical-vector fixation of the superior SMAS secures the elevation of the jowls and submental area.
12. The labiomandibular fold is likewise lifted by fixation of the lateral SMAS to the preauricular cuff.

13. Finally, fixation of the platysma to the upper sternocleidomastoid fascia helps define the anterior neck.
14. The edges of the SMAS and platysma are feathered to create a smooth contour with the underlying fascia.
15. The cervicofacial skin flap repositioning, tailoring, and closure are performed as described for the subcutaneous rhytidectomy.

D. Midface Lift

1. This procedure frees the zygomatic ligaments in an effort to correct the malar soft-tissue descent that creates a parenthesis deformity against the nasolabial crease and the so-called nasojugal oblique depression (a parallel hollowing of the anterior malar region, thought to be due to laxity of the zygomatic ligaments) (Fig. 6).
2. By lifting the malar soft tissue fat pad and securing it to the deep temporalis fascia, facial contour is enhanced and a malar prominence in the original anatomic location is created.

E. Subperiosteal Face Lift

1. Craniofacial techniques have been extended to facial rejuvenation procedures in recent years.
2. Through coronal and buccal sulcus incisions, a subperiosteal dissection elevates the midfacial soft tissues off the underlying maxilla and zygoma as far medially as the lateral nasal walls.
3. Deep periosteal tacking sutures are used to plicate and suspend the facial soft tissues.

VIII. COMPLICATIONS

Complications that follow rhytidectomy may be of either minor significance (e.g., a transient loss of hair in the temporal region) or major significance (e.g., skin sloughing).

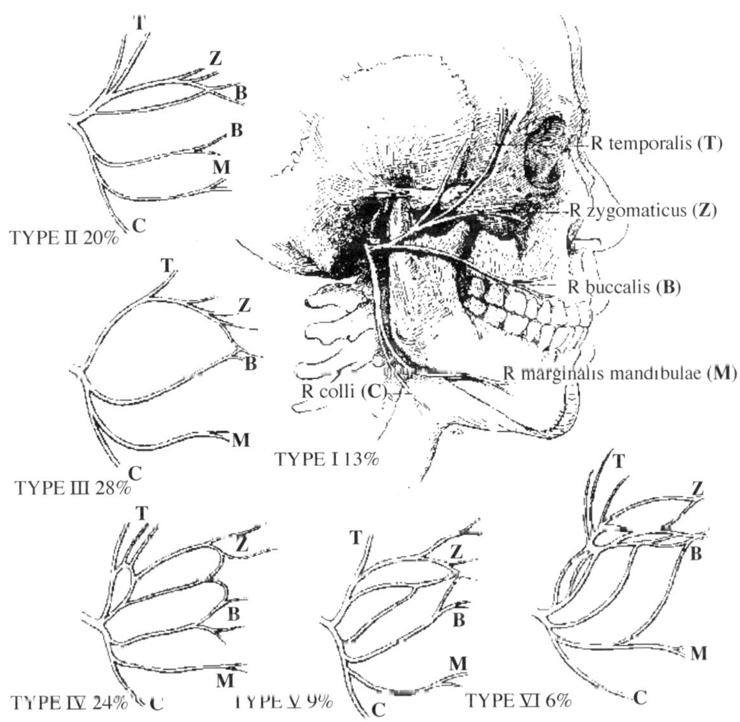

Figure 6 Cross-section of the temporal region showing fascial relationships to the zygomatic arch. The superficial layer of deep temporal fascia inserts along the superficial surface of the arch. The deep layer of the deep temporal fascia inserts along the deep surface of the arch. The superficial temporal fat pad adjoins the superior surface of the arch. The recommended path of dissection to the arch is within the subaponeurotic plane until approximately 2 cm above the arch. The dissection then deepens to penetrate the superficial layer of deep temporal fascia, dissecting within the fat pad inferiorly to the arch periosteum.

A. Hematoma

1. Hematoma after rhytidectomy is the most frequent complication and is twice as common in men.
2. The reported incidence of major hematoma requiring surgical evacuation is about 3.7% and minor hematomas about 15%.
3. Hematomas usually develop during the first 10–12 hours after surgery and can vary from a small collection that is only apparent when facial edema has subsided, to large collections of blood that can threaten skin flap survival.
4. The etiology of hematomas is multifactorial, but correlates most closely with perioperative hypertension, particularly blood pressures above 150/100.
5. Aspirin-containing medications should be discontinued at least 2 weeks before the surgical procedure.
6. The most common presentation of a major hematoma is a restless patient complaining of worsening unilateral facial or cervical pain. Dressings should be removed and the surgical site examined. Evidence of skin flap ischemia is sought, and any sign of respiratory compromise is treated by immediate opening of the incision.
7. Any expanding hematoma should be treated surgically.
8. Sutures are released to relieve tension on the skin flaps and the patient is taken to the operating room. Isolated bleeding vessels may not be found.
9. Minor hematomas usually present as a small area of palpable firmness that can progress to ecchymosis in the overlying skin with or without surface irregularity. Treatment is by either aspiration with an 18-gauge needle or drainage via a small stab incision with a No. 11 scalpel blade. In either case, repeated drainage procedures may be necessary.
10. Occasionally, hemosiderin deposits in the skin result in permanent discoloration.

B. Skin Slough

1. Skin slough is frequently associated with smoking and may be preceded by hematoma or infection. Skin slough occurs most often in the retroauricular region, an area characterized by thin skin with an often-tenuous blood supply.
2. Superficial sloughs of the epidermis usually heal without residual scarring. On the other hand, full-thickness skin sloughs always lead to the development of permanent scarring.
3. The incidence of skin slough after rhytidectomy is 1–3% and is most commonly associated with undiagnosed hematomas, thin skin flaps that may have been damaged during dissection, excessive tension on wound closure, and cigarette smoking (up to 12 times greater risk in smokers than nonsmokers).
4. Treatment is careful observation and meticulous wound care.
5. The final scar is often significantly less than the original defect, but there is generally insufficient skin laxity to allow successful scar excision and closure.

C. Nerve Injury

1. Permanent injury of cranial nerve VII (facial nerve) is a feared complication after rhytidectomy, though permanent injury is rare.
2. Most patients will regain some, if not full, return of motor function.
3. A thorough knowledge of the anatomy and common variations of the facial nerve is essential for any surgeon performing this procedure (Fig. 7).
4. The reported incidence is 0.9%.
5. The buccal branch is injured most often, though injury to either the marginal mandibular or temporal branch is more likely to be noticed and permanent because these branches have very little overlapping innervation.
6. If a facial nerve branch transection is detected during surgery, immediate microsurgical, epineural repair must be performed.
7. Transient numbness of the lower two-thirds of the ear, preauricular area, and the cheeks for the first 3–6 weeks postoperatively occurs as a result of disrupting the small sensory nerves during dissection. This is not preventable, but is usually well tolerated.

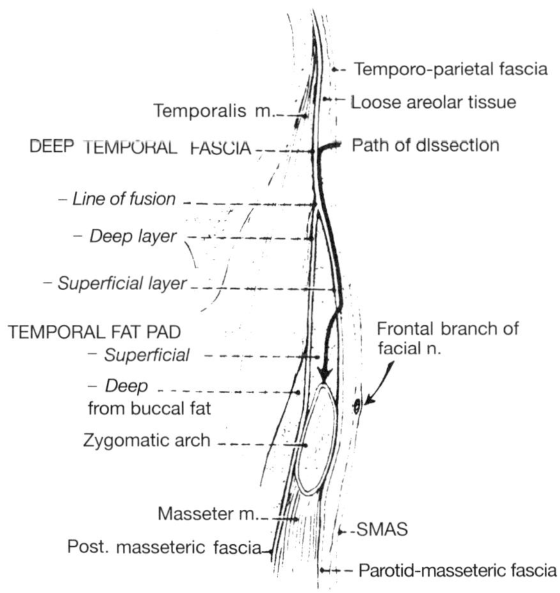

Figure 7 Chief types of branching encountered in 350 cervicofacial halves. Schematically shown, as of the right side of the head. Note that Types III, IV, V, and VI together represent almost 70% of specimens. Type I, absence of anastomosis between the branches of the two divisions (temporofacial and cervicofacial) of the the facial nerve, although, regularly pictured, actually a least common type; Type II, anastomoses within the temporofacial division; Type III, anastomosis between chief divisions; Type IV, two anastomotic loops within the temporofacial part; Type V, two loops from the cervicofacial division, intertwined with branches of the temporofacial; Type VI, extensive intermixture.

8. Injury to the greater auricular nerve is best avoided by maintaining a superficial dissection over the sternocleidomastoid muscle fascia.

D. Alopecia

1. Factors predisposing to hair loss after rhytidectomy include variation in the placement of the temporal incision, extent of undermining, and tension of the closure.
2. The reported incidence ranges from 1 to 3% of patients.

E. Minor Complications

1. Small hematomas (15%).
2. Hypertrophic scars (1–4%).
3. Pigmentation changes (1–3%).
4. Infection (1%).
5. Prolonged edema (rare).
6. Prolonged ecchymosis (rare).
7. Earlobe traction deformity (5%).
8. Chronic pain.
9. Salivary cysts.

IX. FACIAL LIPOPLASTY

A. Facial lipoplasty (suction assisted lipectomy or SAL) can be performed before, during, or after a rhytidectomy or as an isolated procedure to recontour the submental region.

B. SAL poses minimal risk for facial nerve injury.

C. When combined with tumescent local anesthetic infiltration, SAL also carries minimal risk for significant blood loss.

D. Cannula access for facial lipoplasty is gained via hidden sites such as:

- The posterior earlobe (to approach the parotid region, jowl, and submandibular area)
- The submental crease (to approach the submental, submandibular, jowl, and subplatysma regions)
- The lateral nasal vestibule (to approach the nasolabial fold, labiomental fold, jowl, and upper cheek)
- The temporal area above the hairline (to approach the submalar and parotid regions)

E. A suction cannula is introduced through a stab incision and redundant fat is aspirated if possible until a uniform thickness is achieved. In this way, facial fat is sculpted to produce the appearance of a contoured malar eminence and jawline.

F. However, due to the small volume of adipose tissue in the face, lipoplasty in these is frequently ineffective.

G. In the submental region, suction is carried out in a plane between the platysma and overlying skin, often in conjunction with a midline plication of the platysma to complete the cervicoplasty. Skin retraction of the neck is generally good; however, the presence of a low hyoid bone, platysmal bands, and significant skin laxity may limit the success of the lipoplasty. Nonetheless, results in the neck are frequently excellent.

X. FACIAL INJECTIONS

A. The addition of a variety of exogenous materials and implants, along with injection of autogenous fat and collagen, have become increasingly popular over the past several years to augment the common, age-related atrophy of the face.

B. Areas of benefit include those where repeated motion causes deep folds and wrinkle lines. Typical regions include:

- Wrinkle lines around the mouth, such as the nasolabial and labiomental creases (nasolabial folds)
- Forehead (frown lines)
- Sunken cheeks
- Thin lips

C. Autogenous fat grafts have proven to be a safe method with long-term volume enhancement when placed in well-vascularized areas of relative nonmotion, such as the malar and chin regions.

D. During a rhytidectomy, autogenous fat grafting can be performed for volume enhancement in the deep sub-SMAS level as well as in the subcutaneous level in areas outside the field of subcutaneous flap elevation.

E. Autogenous adipose tissue is typically harvested from the thighs, abdomen, or submental area using syringe liposuction. The free lipid is rinsed or centrifuged and then injected through small 1.5 mm incisions pretunneled with a blunt dissector to free up any adhesions or fibrous anchors that could potentially result in a crease or depression.

F. In general, a 20–50% overcorrection is necessary to account for long-term fat resorption. In the facial area, however, this overcorrection may lead to significant edema, prohibiting early return to work and social activities. As such, many patients prefer several sessions to gradually augment over 3–6 months, with potentially longer lasting results.

G. Rigid surface immobilization is obtained by placing steristrips along the skin folds.

H. Bovine collagen has long been available as suture material and as a hemostatic agent. Unlike autogenous fat injections, which can last for years, collagen injections disappear within 3–12 months and can be injected only in relatively small quantities.

- Zyderm I, Zyderm II, and Zyplast are all variants of purified collagen produced by Collagen Biomedical (Collagen Biomedical, Palo Alto, CA) with varying concentrations.
- In addition, however, bovine collagen carries the risk of an allergic reaction.
- All are injected using a fine-gauge needle into the subdermis and deep dermis to correct small contour irregularities and wrinkles and to elevate small depressions.
- Repeated injections at 2- to 4-week intervals are usually required for optimal correction.

110

Primary Rhinoplasty

Nicholas Erik Sieveking, M.D., and Ronald P. Gruber, M.D.
Stanford University, Stanford, California, U.S.A.

Rhinoplasty surgery can be performed using two fundamentally different approaches: the open approach and the closed (or endonasal) approach. The closed approach is the oldest method and leaves the columella skin intact. The open approach incises the columella and retracts the lobule skin cephalically, exposing most of the osteocartilagenous framework. Some surgeons predominantly use the open approach, others predominantly the closed approach, and some will use a combination of approaches depending on the exact patient characteristics.

I. SURGICAL ANATOMY OF THE NOSE

A. The osteocartilagenous framework defines the character of the nose (Fig. 1):

- Cephalic third—comprised of the paired nasal bones. These bones articulate with the frontal process of the maxilla and the frontal bone. The narrowest part of the bony vault at the level of the medial canthus. Anteriorly, the nasal bones broaden to the point where they override the upper lateral cartilages at a junction point called the rhinion.
- Middle third—The upper lateral cartilages define the middle third of the nose, articulating in the midline at the anterior aspect of the cartilagenous septum.
- Caudal third comprised of the lobule. The topography of the lobule is defined by the paired lower lateral (alar) cartilages. The alar cartilages are comprised of 3 crura: lateral, middle, and medial:

  The lateral crura establish the flare of the nostrils and add character to the nasal tip, which is mainly defined by the size and relation of the middle crura.

  The flare of the caudal edge of the middle, and more importantly the medial crura, determines the width of the columella and the lower tip of the lobule.
- Internally:

  The septum (Fig. 1) forms the strut that provides the midline articulation points for the nasal bones, upper lateral cartilages, and alar cartilages. The cephalic third of the septum is the perpendicular plate of the ethmoid bone, articulating at the dorsum with the nasal bones. The caudal two thirds of the septum is cartilage. This quadrangular strut articulates superiorly with the bony septum, posteriorly with the vomer, and inferiorly with the maxilla and anterior nasal spine. This

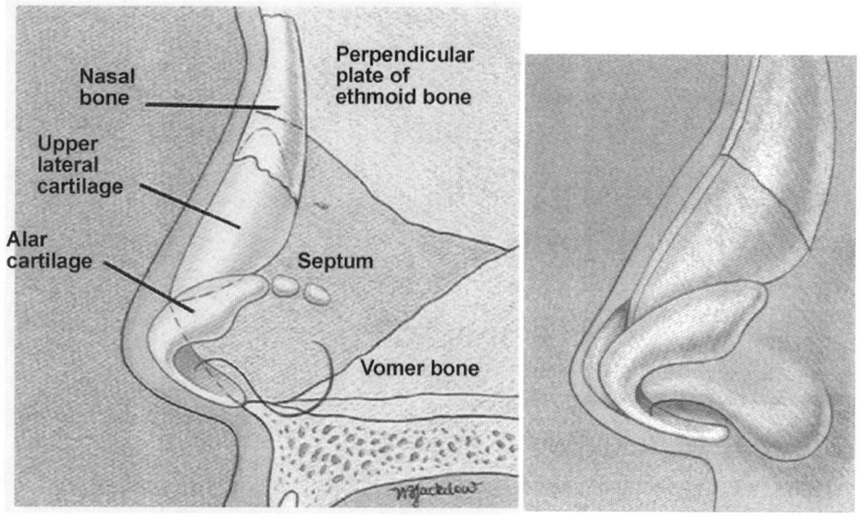

Figure 1 Anatomy of the osteocartilaginous framework of the nose.

cartilagenous septum provides form and support for the nasal dorsum and helps define the nasal tip, caudal septum, and the naso-labial (subnasale) angle.

The external nasal valve is formed by the alar rim, nasal sill, and the columella.

The internal nasal valve is formed by the caudal aspect of the upper lateral cartilages, nasal floor, and the septum.

B. The skin of the external nose varies in thickness from 1.25 to 0.6mm. The skin of the upper half of the nose is thinner and more mobile, while the skin over the tip is thicker and adherent with more oil-producing glands. At the caudal aspect along the alar rim, the skin again thins. Where the skin is thin, irregularities from surgical sculpting errors and cartilage grafts are more prone to be visible upon inspection.

C. The subcutaneous tissue of the nose is divided into four layers: the superficial fatty panniculus, the fibromuscular layer, the deep fatty layer, and the periosteum/perichondrium plane. The main location of the fatty panniculus is directly adherent to the undersurface of the dermis. The fibromuscular layer of the nose is contiguous with the superficial muscular aponeurotic system (SMAS) of the face and frontalis layer of the forehead. The deep fatty layer is found just below the superficial muscular layer and is the location of the neurovascular supply to the nose. Beneath the deep fatty layer is a safe and bloodless surgical dissection plane.

D. Vascular supply:

- External nose—three major blood vessels provide the external blood supply to the nose: the ophthalmic, maxillary, and facial arteries:

  The ophthalmic artery provides the supratrochlear, dorsal nasal, and external anterior ethmoidal branches to supply the upper lateral aspect and dorsum of the external nose.

  The facial artery branches into the angular artery (which feeds the ala and lower lateral nose) and the superior labial artery (which terminates at the columella and caudal tip as the columellar artery).

  The maxillary artery forms collaterals with the branches of the ophthalmic and facial arteries to supply the mid-lateral portion of the external nose. In the open rhinoplasty, knowledge of the blood supply is important. For example, a large alar incision potentially cuts off the blood supply to the tip of the nose during an open approach.

- Internal nose (Fig. 2)—the septum and mucosa of the internal nose also receive their blood supply from the same three major vessels. Kiesselbach's plexus is the vascular network of the anterior septum, the most common site of epistaxis. The lateral nasal cavity and upper septum are supplied by internal branches of the anterior and posterior ethmoidal arteries (ophthalmic artery). The sphenopalatine branches of the maxillary artery supply the posterior lateral wall and posterior septum, while the angular artery and superior labial artery (from facial artery) supply the caudal lateral internal nasal wall and caudal internal septum, respectively.

E. Innervation:

- Sensory nerve supply to the external nose is mediated by the ophthalmic and maxillary divisions of the trigeminal nerve.
- The infratrochlear nerve and the external branch of the anterior ethmoidal nerve from the ophthalmic division innervate lateral and dorsal skin of the nose.

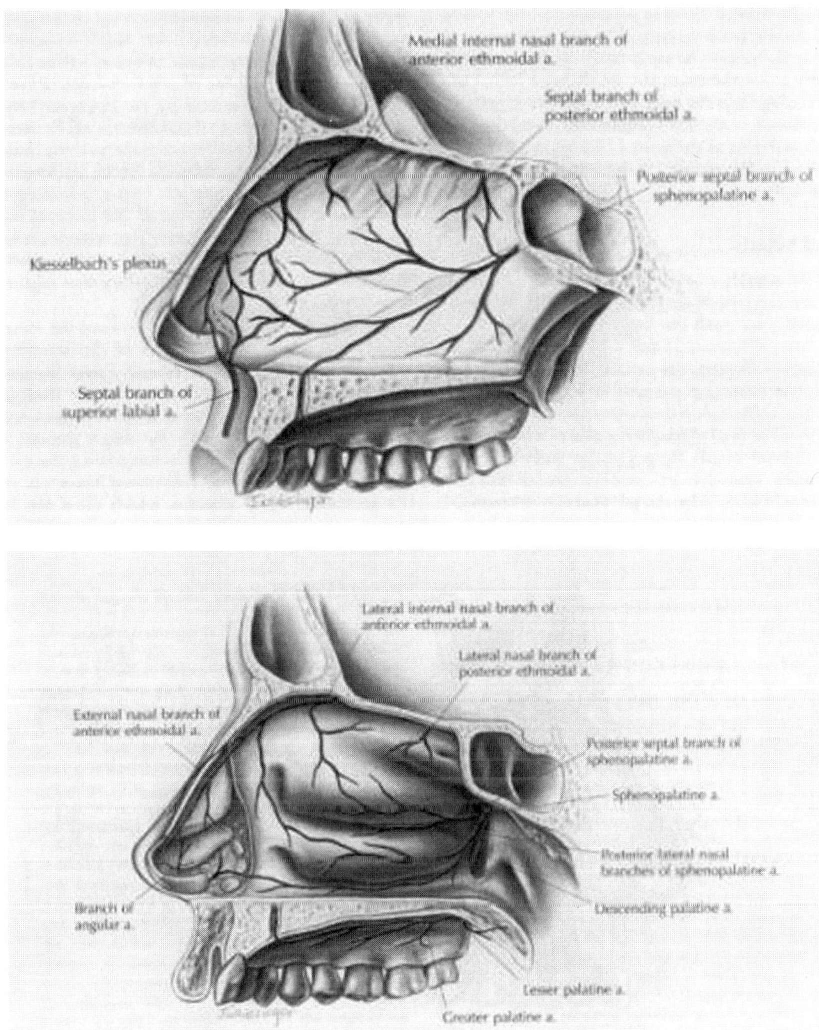

Figure 2 Innervation to the nose.

- The infraorbital nerve (maxillary division) innervates the lower lateral nose, alar rim, and nasal tip.
- The lateral wall of the nasal cavity and the septum receive sensory innervation from the internal branches of the anterior ethmoidal and pterygopalatine nerves.

II. EVALUATION OF THE NOSE

A. Intranasal examination should be performed in any patient seeking aesthetic rhinoplasty. Causes of nasal asymmetry and disharmony can also be responsible for nasal airway obstruction and should be addressed at the time of surgery. Simple speculum examination can reveal nasal valve dysfunction that can be secondary to previous endonasal surgery, trauma, or congenital deformities. Airway obstruction can be caused by collapse of the external valve. Any decrease in the internal valve angle can lead to airway obstruction as well.

B. Other causes of nasal airway obstruction that should be addressed during rhinoplasty include septal deviations and turbinate hypertrophy. Endoscopy is a simple and financially reimbursed procedure that is also routinely performed in addition to the speculum exam. It can diagnose other pathology, such as hypertrophied adenoids or septal bone spurs.

C. While the dimensions of the "ideal" nose are more universally accepted today and trend toward European and western standards, historically ethnic variations of the "ideal" nose have had major cultural implications for patients. In addition, anatomic variations exist among ethnic groups in the soft tissue and skeletal framework, which mandate consideration during rhinoplasty procedures. For example, the African American nose typically has a low radix with and obtuse naso-frontal angle, a wide flat dorsum with short nasal bones, and a thick-skinned and rounded tip with a flattened alar base.

D. With any potential rhinoplasty candidate, whatever the gender or ethnic background, it is essential to establish exactly the patient's ideals for the shape of his or her nose. These ideals should be reaffirmed by repeat office visits prior to any rhinoplasty and by having the candidate display collected pictures of noses they think are suitable for them.

III. THE "NORMALS" OF THE NOSE

A. Naso-facial angle—measures the divergence of the dorsal nasal line from the facial plane, measured from a common point, the nasion. The ideal naso-facial angle is approximately 34 degrees. The naso-facial angle is sometimes referred to as the slope of the dorsum. The slope is steep in boxers who have had their noses broken more than once. The slope is shallow in patients who have an overprojecting tip (Fig. 3).

B. Naso-labial angle—normally ranges from 105 to 108 degrees in females, and 100 to 103 degrees in males. An obtuse naso-labial angle causes people to have too much nostril show and a "piggy nose" (Fig. 3).

C. Concavity of the naso-frontal angle—measured from the glabella (the most anterior point of the soft tissue of the frontal bone) to the nasion (the deepest portion of the naso-frontal groove). The projection of the glabella should be 4–6 mm anterior to the nasion (Fig. 3).

D. Length and height of the nose—measured from the level of the medial canthus to the subnasale. This length should be equal to the distance

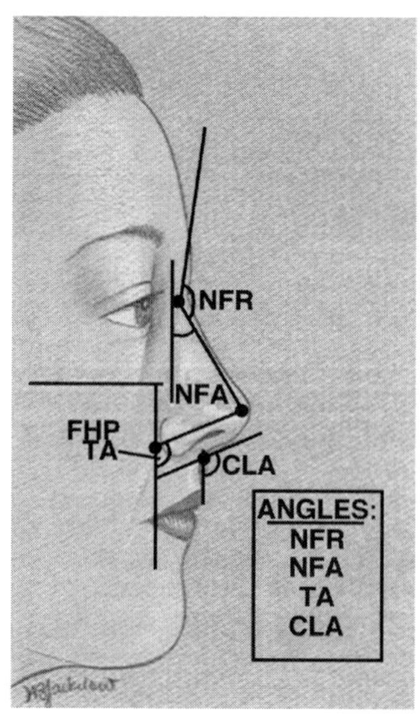

Figure 3 The "normals" of the nose.

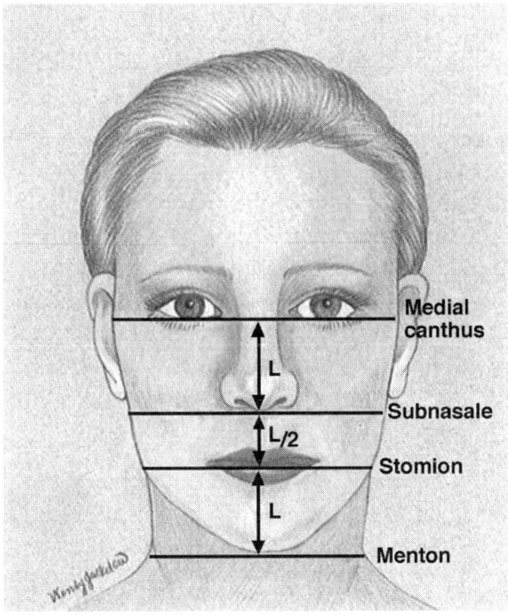

Figure 4 Length and height of the nose.

between the stomion and the menton. The upper lip distance (from the subnasale to the stomian) should be one half of the nasal length (Fig. 4).

E. Alar base—evaluated in the horizontal and the vertical planes. With a normal intercanthal distance, the lateral edge of the alar base should be about 1 mm lateral to the medial edge of the medial canthus, as measured on a vertical line drawn parallel to a vertical facial bipartition line. On profile, the alar base can be evaluated in the vertical plane. A total of 2–3 mm of columellar show below the alar rim on profile are adequate (Fig. 5).

F. Length of upper lip—measured from the subnasale to the stomion, this should be 50% of the nasal length measured from the medial canthal line to the subnasale. More importantly, the length of the upper lip should be approximately the height of the nose or a slightly less (Fig. 4).

G. Angle of rotation of the tip lobule—measures the cephalic angulation of the tip lobule. This angle is measured as the divergence between the line of the tip and the line of the columella. Ideally, the angle of rotation is equal to the angle of divergence (50–60 degrees).

IV. APPROACHES

A. Open rhinoplasty uses a transcolumellar incision combined with a marginal (infracartilage-lower rim of lower lateral cartilage) incision.

B. Closed rhinoplasty has several approaches, depending on the anatomic region to be addressed.

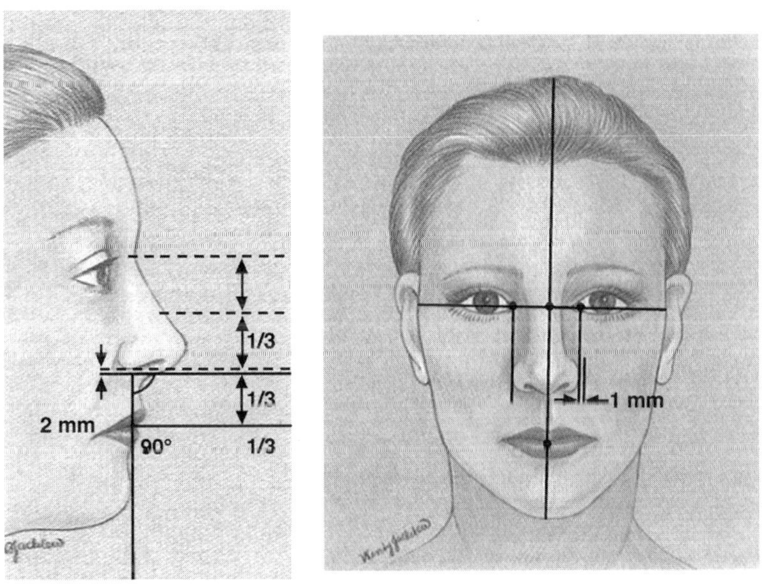

Figure 5 Normal alar base relationships.

Intracartilage (splitting the lateral crura of lower lateral cartilage) and intercartilage (between upper and lower lateral cartilages) incisions are commonly used.

C. A transfixion incision (just below or at the base of the cartilaginous septum) can be included with either open or closed rhinoplasty.

D. The open rhinoplasty approach will be discussed below.

V. COLUMELLA INCISION

Many incisions such as a "V" or a "Chevron" incision may be used to incise the columella. The "stair step" incision is preferred because if any notching occurs from the scar, it will be less visible on profile view (Fig. 6). The incision is usually made through the narrowest part of the columella. Undermining can begin at either the columella or along the rim incision with the use of tenotomy scissors. Dissection proceeds beneath the deep fatty layer and above the perichondrial/periosteal layers. Cephalic exposure even over the nasal bones is important. Defatting the upper and lower lateral cartilages enhances exposure and facilitates repositioning of the cartilaginous framework. One should not defat the flap other than trimming soft tissue that is hanging off because defatting runs the risk of interfering with tip blood supply and causing tip necrosis. Open rhinoplasty allows precision manipulation of the osteocartilagenous framework—the nasal bones, nasal dorsum, and nasal tip.

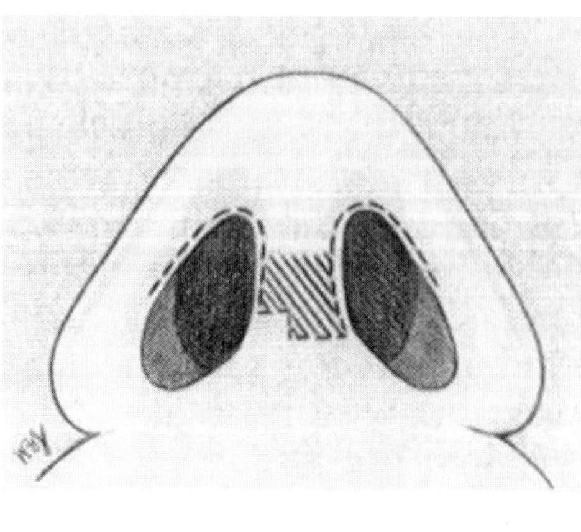

Figure 6 "Stairstep incision."

VI. SURGICAL APPROACH BY NASAL REGION

A. The Septum

Irregularities of the septum can cause nasal airway obstruction, deformities of the dorsum, tip distortions, and columellar abnormalities. Closed or, if necessary, open fracturing and repositioning of the bony septum (vomer and perpendicular plate of the ethmoid) corrects bony septal obstruction. Resection and/or repositioning of the cartilagenous septum at the midline corrects nasal airway obstruction and abnormalities of the nasal dorsum, such as a twisted nose. A vertically oriented mucosal incision at the caudal septum with elevation of the mucosa and perichondrium allows exposure of the septum. The offending segment of cartilage can then be resected, leaving a 1–1.5 cm caudal and dorsal strut to resist septal collapse (Fig. 7). Often, cartilage

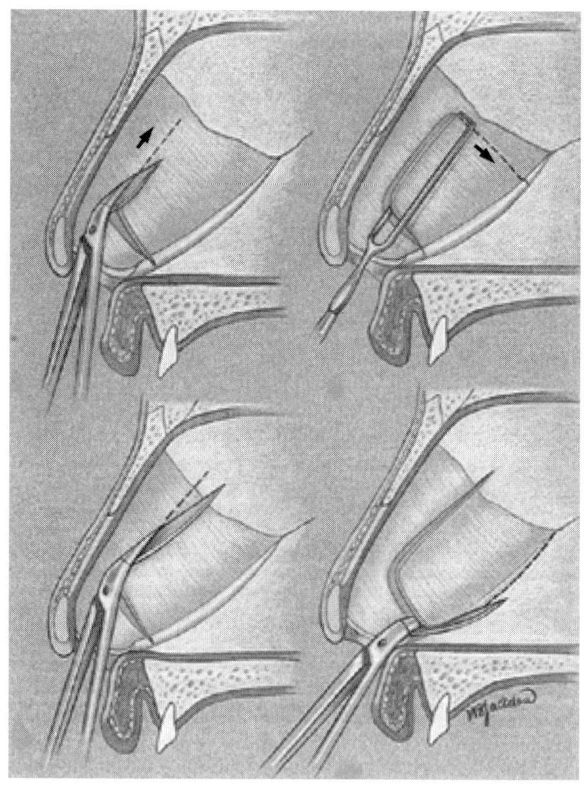

Figure 7 An L-shaped septum is obtained following elevation of the perichondrium bilaterally and resection of the deformed central portion. Note that the septum usually needs only one vertical score in order to bend it into the proper direction.

scoring can correct curvature or angulation of the septum with minimal or no cartilage resection. The resultant L-shaped strut may need to be released from its attachment to the vomerine ridge and set in the midline in order to provide for a straighter nose. Deviation of the caudal septum can cause tip abnormalities, visible columellar deviation, and nasal airway obstruction. Correction of caudal septal deviations includes cartilage resection, scoring, and relocation of the posterior segment in the nasal spine.

B. The Nasal Dorsum

The nasal bones, anterior septum, upper and lower lateral cartilages, and the caudal septum help define the dorsum of the nose.

1. By simply reducing the dorsum of the anterior nasal bones and anterior septal cartilage, the appearance of the nose can be dramatically altered:
   - The dorsal profile of the nose is lowered
   - The width of the nasal bones is decreased
   - The intercanthal distance appears increased
   - The length of the nose appears shortened
   - The nasal tip may appear superiorly rotated
2. Augmentation of the nose produces some opposite results: use of an autograft such as cartilage to augment the nasal dorsum will result in a longer-appearing nose, with a more narrow dorsum, a caudally rotated tip, and a decreased intercanthal distance. Augmentation should be considered before reduction to avoid the risk of over-reduction and supratip deformity (Fig. 8).

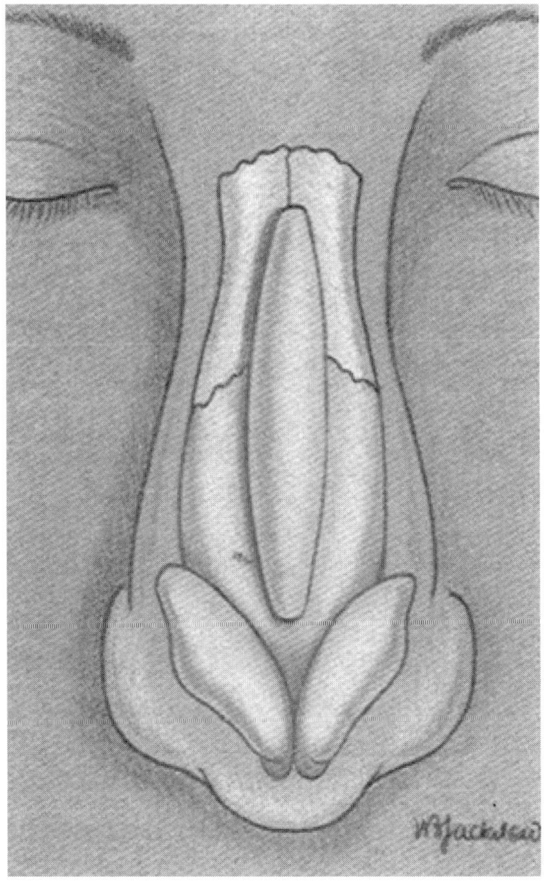

Figure 8 Dorsal augmentation.

C. The Tip (and Lip)

The nasal tip is defined by a dynamic interplay of the soft tissues, septum, lower lateral cartilages, and nasal spine. Alterations in these elements can elicit changes in tip width and symmetry, projection, height, and nasolabial angle.

1. Tip width reduction is achieved by transdomal and/or interdomal sutures, tip grafting with a narrow graft, or conservative resection of the cephalic part of the lower lateral cartilages. The simplest maneuver is transdomal (also known as dome sutures) and interdomal (also known as intercrural) suturing. Transdomal sutures can narrow a widened domal segment and create improved symmetry. Once the domal arches are symmetrical and desirable, interdomal sutures can be used to converge the domes and narrow the tip. Narrowing of the tip can increase tip projection.
2. Increasing nasal tip projection can be achieved by tip grafting, transdomal suturing, fixation of the medial crura to a more anterior location on the caudal septum (with sutures), and the use of a columellar strut. Onlay grafts, shield grafts, or anatomic tip grafts can be used for moderate augmentation of the nasal tip. The anatomic tip graft uses the concepts of the Peck and Sheen grafts while maintaining the surface morphology of an aesthetic nasal tip (Fig. 9). The graft achieves a well-projected and contoured nasal tip by emphasizing the high point (pronasale), the

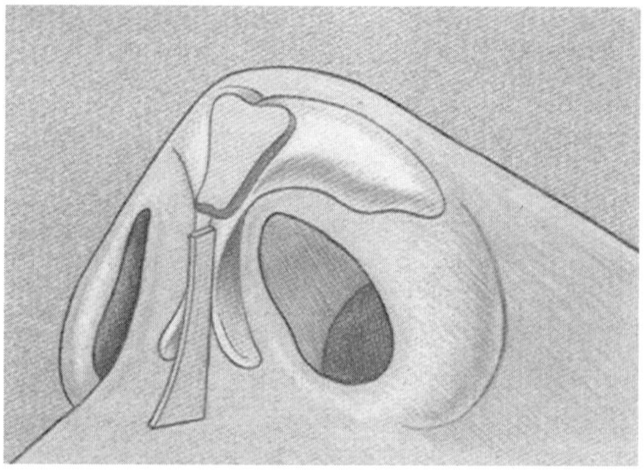

Figure 9 The "anatomic tip graft."

full length of the domes, and the normal relationship between the domes and the middle crura. A columellar strut is a predictable and reliable means to increase tip projection without increasing the size of the infratip lobule. Transdomal suturing can provide tip augmentation as it narrows the overall tip width. Anterior transposition of the medial crura along the caudal septum is difficult, unpredictable, and creates a rigid lower nose as the tip and columella now move as unit. However, it can be a useful maneuver on certain occasions.

3. Reduction of tip projection can be achieved by:
   - A deep transfixion incision
   - Shortening the lower lateral cartilages (by transecting the lateral-most aspect of the lower lateral cartilages)
   - Transecting the middle crus (and allowing the elements to overlap)
4. A less common method to reduce tip projection is actual resection and repositioning of the domal segments. The surgeon must note that reduction of tip projection makes the alar base appear wider and causes anterior projection of the dorsum on profile. Furthermore, laxity of the external nasal valve and bowing of the columella may result.

D. Infracturing the Nasal Bones

A wide cephalic nasal dorsum or nasal bridge can be corrected by inward fracturing of the nasal bones.

1. A small osteotome (~4 mm) is introduced in the nasal cavity at the level of the pyriform ridge. The mucosa is punctured and the caudal borders of the nasal bones are contacted with the osteotome.
2. Osteotomies are performed along the base of the nasal bone in a posterior-superior direction to the level of the medial canthus. At that point, osteotomies are directed more superiorly to the midline near the nasal-frontal junction (Fig. 10).
3. Prior to infracturing the bones, medial osteotomies (with a saw) may be needed if there is no open roof (as is sometimes observed following hump removal).
4. After bilateral osteotomies are completed, gentle external pressure completes the infracturing, thus narrowing the nasal bones and creating a narrower dorsum.
5. Rasping is often required after completion of the infracturing to smooth any rough edges. Alternatively, small external stab wounds can be used to introduce the osteotomes along the skin at the pyriform ridge with minimal scarring.
6. Lastly, an alternative method of lateral osteotomies to approach the bone is via a buccal sulcus approach. Advantages include postoperative bleeding that tends to exit the mouth instead of the nostrils and avoidance of an external scar. Infracturing may narrow the internal nasal valve and can cause airway obstruction.

VII. HOW TO EFFECT SPECIFIC CHANGES IN THE NOSE

A. How to Modify Nasal Length

1. Using a transfixion incision and an intercartilaginous incision, the lower lateral cartilages are retracted to expose the caudal septum. The

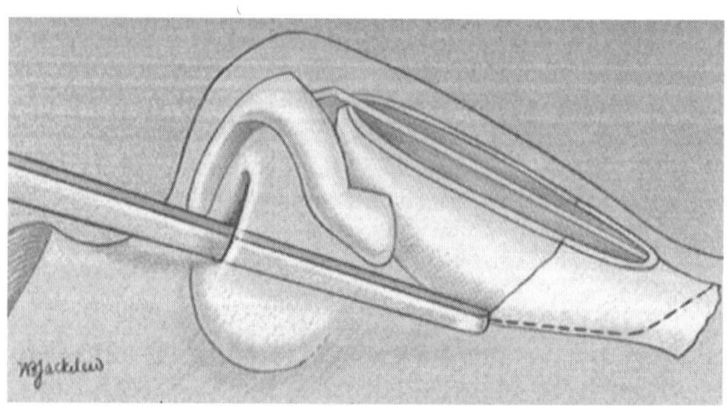

Figure 10 Infracture of nasal bones.

caudal edge of the septum can then be reduced to the desired length.

2. The loss of tip support as a result of these incisions should be stabilized by suture repair prior to completion of rhinoplasty. Some degree of tip modification likely will be necessary when shortening the caudal septum.
3. Occasionally, the anterior nasal spine has to be removed with an osteotome to shorten the posterior aspect of the caudal nose.

B. How to Narrow a Broad Tip

1. Large lower lateral cartilages and wide domes create a broad or bulbous nasal tip.
2. After delivery of the lower lateral cartilages through the open incision, the dome is inspected to see how weak it is. If it is soft, no scoring is required. If it is moderately firm, mild scraping with a scalpel will weaken it.
3. Only in unusual circumstances is it required to put two superficial scoring incisions about 1 mm apart at each dome. These maneuvers will decrease the spring tension of the domal cartilage.
4. By placing a 4-0 PDS dome or transdomal suture at the posterior aspect of each dome, the narrowness of the tip can be maintained.
5. Further narrowing can be obtained with an intercrural (interdomal) suture. This is done by suturing the posterior aspect of the middle crura together just below the domes with a 4-0 PDS. The intercrural suture provides tip symmetry and tip projection (Fig. 11).

C. How to Decrease Lateral Convexity of the Lower Lateral Cartilages

1. Prominent lateral crura of the lower lateral cartilages can cause excessive lateral convexity of the lower nose. Trimming of the lateral crura is required to address this deformity. Although minor lateral crura resections can be achieved through a closed approach, an open approach is often recommended.
2. The amount of lateral crus to be resected on each side is based on intraoperative assessment, but as a general rule, leaving a 4–6 mm caudal rim of the lateral crus is suggested.
3. Following cephalic resection of the lateral crus, the dome is usually 4–6 mm wide.

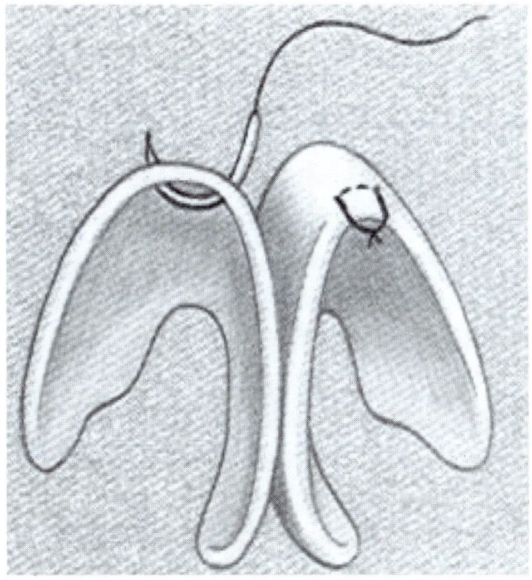

Figure 11 The intercrural ("interdomal") suture.

D. How to Elevate and Rotate a Drooping Tip

1. A drooping tip can be caused by a combination of an excessively long nose with a caudal rotation of the lower lateral cartilages. Both problems can be corrected by a cephalic rotation of the tip cartilages and fixation to the caudal septum.
2. An open approach with transfixion and intercartilaginous incisions allows adequate visualization of the caudal septum and alar cartilages. After mobilization of the tip cartilages, a 4-0 PDS suture is used to fix the medial crura to the caudal septum, rotating the tip superiorly. This may have the effect of shortening the length of the nose and obliterating some of the membranous septum. Care must be taken not to overtighten this "crural-septal" suture for this could cause a retracted columella.
3. The tip can also be held in place with a spanning suture of Tebbetts, a horizontal suture that brings the cephalic aspect of the lower lateral cartilages together. The suture rests on the dorsal septum, which helps prevent the tip from falling (Fig. 12).

E. How to Increase Dorsal Width

1. Occasionally, the dorsal width needs to be increased. This is especially true in the nose that

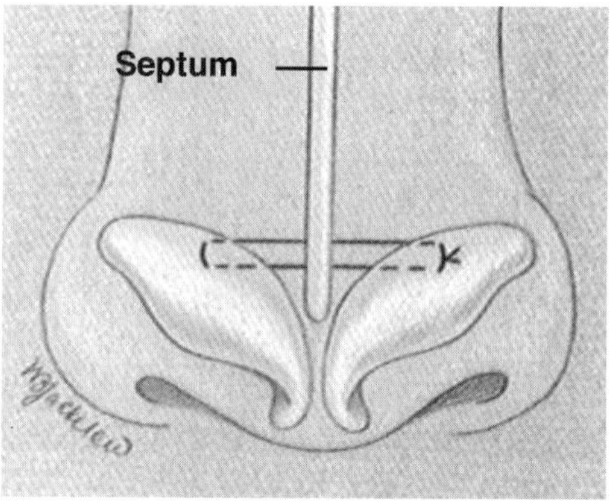

Figure 12 The spanning suture developed by Tebbetts narrows the nasal tip but also helps prevent the tip from falling.

has had overresection of the dorsum with a resulting collapse of the middle vault and an "inverted V" deformity. In such cases, the internal nasal valve has been destroyed.

2. The treatment involves replacing the missing cartilage with spreader grafts. A small single-layer graft is placed on either side of the dorsal septum to not only increase the width of the dorsum, but also to open up the angle of the internal nasal valve (Fig. 13).

F. How to Decrease Dorsal Width

1. Decreasing the width of the bony dorsum is a formidable task. It involves medial osteotomies

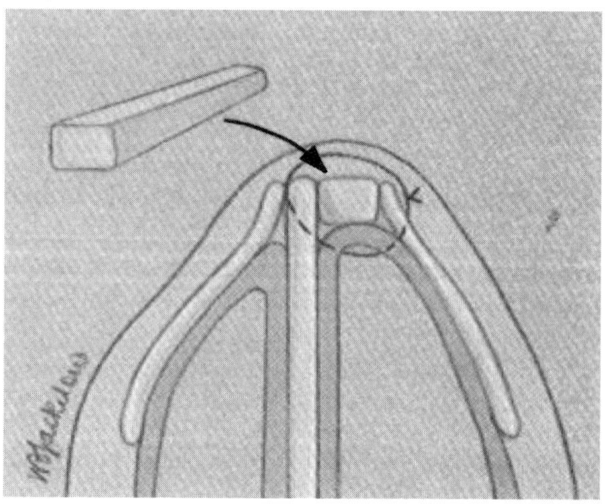

Figure 13 Spreader grafts to increase dorsal width and to open the internal nasal valve.

with a saw as well as lateral osteotomies followed by gentle infracturing.

2. Very broad noses may also need resection of the dorsal aspect of the upper lateral cartilages at a point where they approach the dorsal septum.

G. How to Lengthen a Short Nose

1. To lengthen the short nose is a difficult task in aesthetic rhinoplasty (Fig. 14). Using an open approach, the mucoperichondrium is released bilaterally from the dorsal aspect of the septum. Bilateral releasing incisions in the dorsal perichondrium may also be needed. If the releasing incisions are staggered, the septal cartilage will reepithelialize. The soft tissue attachments between the upper and lower lateral cartilages are also released. A "batten" graft is attached to the caudal septum, pushing the tip cartilages caudally to provide additional length to the nose. Occasionally a batten graft or composite graft will be necessary to fill the defect left after

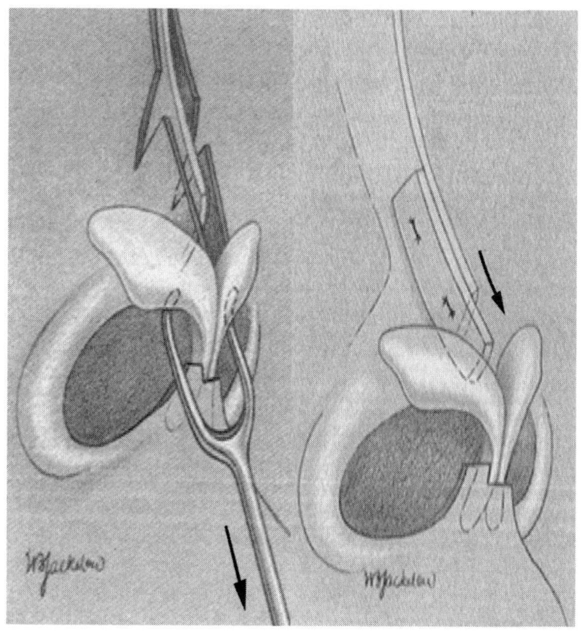

Figure 14 Lengthening the short nose requires (1) bilateral elevation of the mucoperichondrium, (2) occasional releasing incisions of the mucoperichondrium, and (3) releasing incision between the upper and lower lateral cartilages and a batten graft to project the tip cartilages caudally.

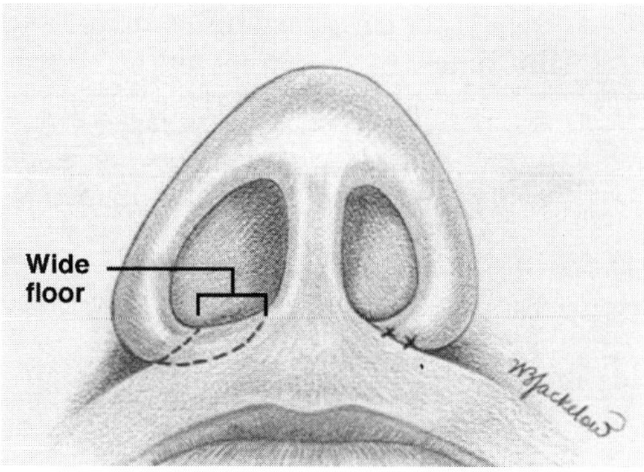

Figure 15 Reduction of the alar base.

releasing the soft tissue between the upper and lower lateral cartilages. Smaller degrees of nasal lengthening can be obtained by a closed approach using the batten graft, but this is much more difficult than in the open approach.

2. Often, the nose is apparently shortened without actually being absolutely shortened. This is because of an obtuse columellar-labial angle and excessive tip projection. This can be corrected by a "derotation" of the tip, allowing the tip to drop while decreasing the naso-labial angle and providing minimal nasal lengthening. A complete through-and-through transfixion incision is connected to an intercartilaginous incision to allow de-rotation of the tip.
3. Placement of a dorsal graft can provide small degrees of nasal lengthening by raising the nasion (if needed) and pushing the tip cartilages and tip-defining point in a caudal direction.

H. How to Decrease Nasal Base Width

1. The nasal base includes the alar base, the nostril sill, and the columellar base (Fig. 15).
2. Maneuvers to reduce the base depend upon which component is causing the abnormal width. It is usually the alar base. A wide alar base can be narrowed by a wedge excision with medial rotation of the ala. The incision should be designed to follow the anatomic contours of the alar groove, allowing the final scar to be in the alar-facial groove. The size of the wedge excision is determined by preoperative analysis of the excess of alar base width. Usually, the amount to resect is equivalent to the width of a Brown-Adson forceps. Resection of excessive tissue not only leads to aesthetic deformities that are difficult to correct, but can also cause severe nostril stenosis with airway obstruction. Usually less than 3 mm of rim are excised. The ala is advanced medially and sutured with 4-0 nylon.
3. Sometimes the sill itself is excised (as may be required in ethnic noses).
4. Sometimes the entire nasal base, including the columellar base, needs reduction. By turning from one alar incision to the other, a heavy, permanent suture is placed across the base to literally squeeze the nasal base together.

I. How to Reduce a Dorsal Hump (Fig. 16)

1. Through an intercartilaginous incision, dissection scissors are introduced along the nasal dorsum below the deep fatty plane. Blunt dissection with the scissors then separates the soft tissue envelope along the dorsum from the osteocartilagenous framework.

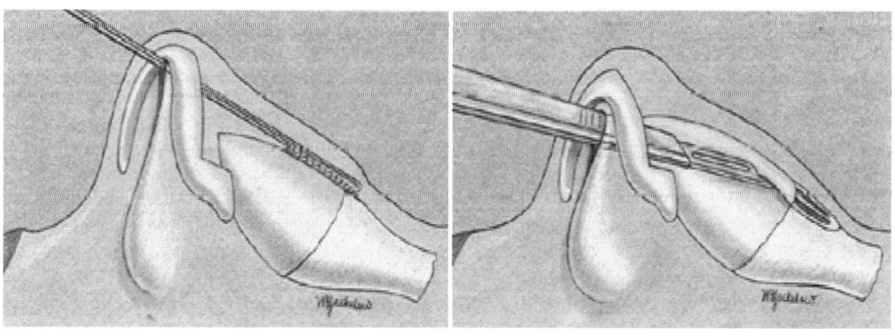

Figure 16 Dorsal hump reduction.

2. Various methods can be used to reduce the hump. The senior author prefers the following method:
   - Elevate the mucoperichondrium from the undersurface of the upper lateral cartilages.
   - Release the upper lateral cartilages from the dorsal septum.
   - Resect the cartilagenous hump followed immediately by osteotomy of the bony hump.
   - Score and fold over the dorsal aspect of the upper lateral cartilages to act as a spreader graft. Technically, the last maneuver is a "spreader flap".
   - Primary open reduction rhinoplasty.

111

Nasal and Sinus Pathology

Edward J. Damrose, M.D., and Nina L. Shapiro, M.D.
David Geffen School of Medicine at UCLA, Los Angeles, California, U.S.A.

I. NASAL ANATOMY

A. External Anatomy

1. Arterial supply: facial artery branches.
2. Venous drainage: angular vein. Infection may spread from angular vein to ophthalmic vein and then to cavernous sinus, resulting in cavernous sinus thrombosis.

B. Nasal Cavity

1. Lined by respiratory and olfactory epithelium.
2. Internal nasal valve: junction of upper lateral cartilages with the septum.
3. External nasal valve: junction of lower lateral cartilages, septum, and inferior turbinates.

C. Septum

1. The most anterior segment of the septum contains Kiesselbach's plexus, a series of arterial anastomoses that are the origin of 90% of cases of epistaxis.

D. Turbinates

1. Paired inferior, middle, and superior turbinates.
2. They function to humidify and filter air.

E. Sinus Ostia

1. Maxillary, frontal, and anterior ethmoid sinuses drain just inferior to the middle turbinate at the hiatus semilunaris.
2. Posterior ethmoids drain lateral to the superior turbinate.
3. Nasolacrimal duct drains lateral to the inferior turbinate.

II. SINUS ANATOMY AND EMBRYOLOGY (FIGS. 1 AND 2)

A. Maxillary Sinus

1. Rudimentary until seventh year of life, after which the maxillary sinus enlarges to a volume of 15 cc.
2. Orbital blowout fractures result in herniation of orbital contents into the maxillary sinus.
3. Spread of infection from upper (maxillary) teeth results in acute maxillary sinusitis.

B. Frontal Sinus

1. Absent in 5% of the population.
2. Develops after birth, fully formed in the second decade.
3. Posterior wall abuts the anterior cranial fossa.

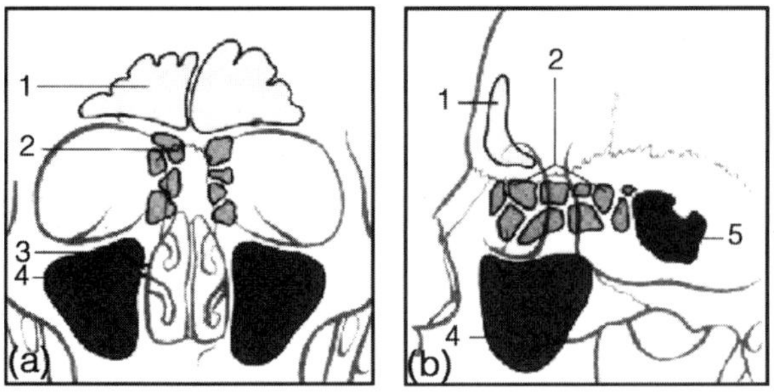

Figure 1 Paranasal sinuses. (a) Frontal section. (b) Sagittal section. 1, frontal sinus; 2, ethmoid sinus; 3, maxillary ostium; 4, maxillary antrum; 5, sphenoid sinus.

4. Frontal sinus infection may spread to the meninges and brain through the posterior wall of the frontal sinus.

C. Ethmoid Sinus

1. Fully formed at birth.
2. Infection may spread through the roof of the ethmoid sinus (fovea ethmoidalis) to involve the anterior cranial fossa or laterally through the lamina papyracea to involve the orbit.

D. Sphenoid Sinus

1. Absent in 3–5% of the population.
2. Develops after the sixth year of life.
3. Infection may spread intracranially from the sphenoid sinus or may result in thrombosis of the cavernous sinus.

III. SYMPTOMS AND SIGNS OF SINONASAL DISEASE (TABLE 1)

IV. RADIOLOGICAL EVALUATION OF SINONASAL DISORDERS

1. Computed tomography (CT) of paranasal sinuses with axial and coronal views provides excellent bony detail of the nose and sinuses.
2. Magnetic resonance imaging (MRI) can delineate the extent of soft tissue masses of the nose and paranasal sinuses.

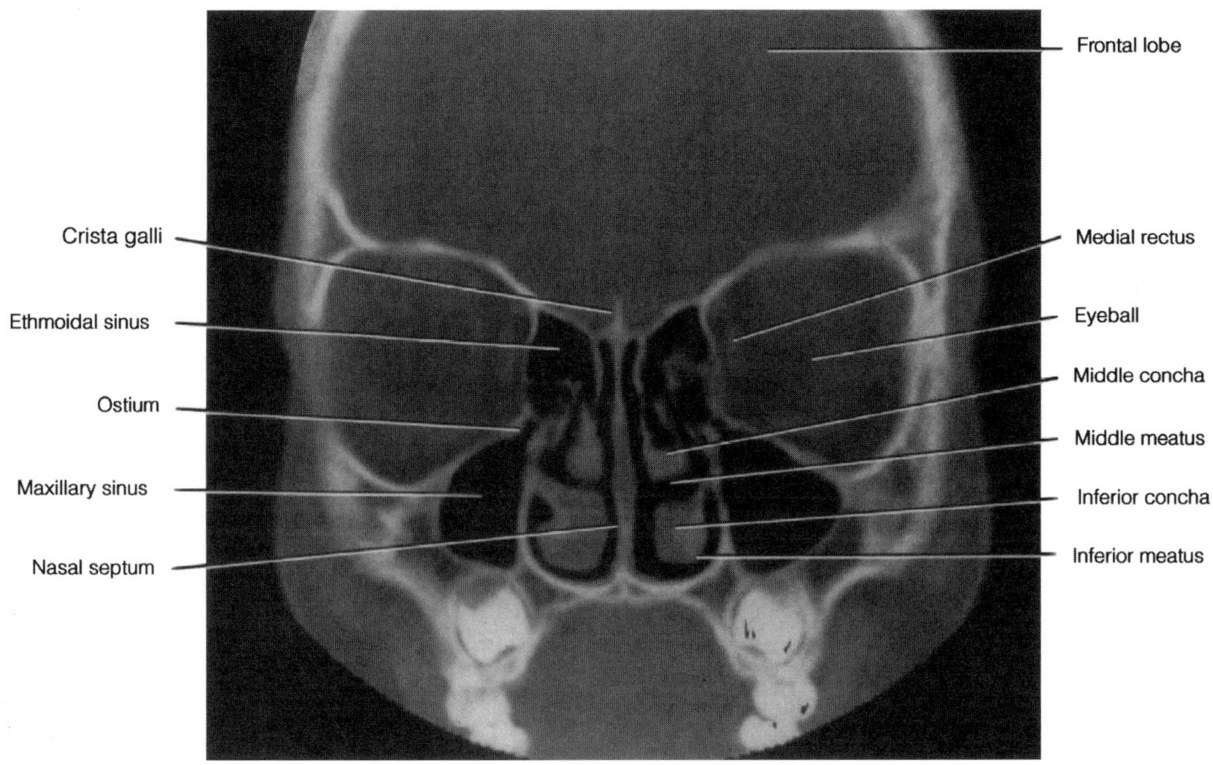

Figure 2 CT scan of normal sinuses, coronal view.

Table 1 Symptoms and Signs of Sinonasal Disease

Nasal airway obstruction	Foul odor
Facial fullness	Hyponasal speech
Headache	Hyposmia/anosmia
Rhinorrhea (clear, mucoid, purulent)	Facial deformity
	Soft tissue destruction
Pain	Cranial nerve deficits
Epistaxis	Epiphora
Ophthalmologic complaints (diplopia, decreased visual acuity, proptosis)	

Source: Adapted from Gluckman JL. The clinical approach to nasal obstruction. *J Respir Dis* 1983; 4:13–29.

3. Plain sinus radiographs provide little information and are not routinely obtained.

V. NASAL DISORDERS

A. Rhinitis

1. Acute rhinitis:
   - Common cold
   - Secondary to *Rhinovirus*
   - Disease is usually self-limited
   - Treatment: supportive
2. Allergic rhinitis:
   - Hay fever
   - Secondary to inhaled allergens (pollen, dust, houseplants, foods, and mites)
   - Symptoms include sneezing, nasal congestion, watery rhinorrhea, and facial fullness
   - Treatment: desensitization and avoidance; antihistamines; steroid sprays; decongestant sprays (e.g., oxymetozalone)
3. Vasomotor rhinitis:
   - Paroxysmal attacks of nasal congestion and profuse clear rhinorrhea secondary to nonspecific reflex hyperactivity of the nasal mucosa parasympathetic nerves
   - Symptoms resolve within hours
4. Rhinitis of pregnancy:
   - Nasal obstruction and rhinorrhea occurring in second and third trimesters
   - Resolves after delivery
5. Rhinitis medicamentosa:
   - Rebound mucosal edema and nasal congestion from prolonged abuse of over-the-counter nasal sprays (e.g., oxymetazoline, phenylephrine)
   - Treatment: stop offending spray; intranasal or systemic steroids

B. Foreign Body

1. Unilateral nasal obstruction and purulent rhinorrhea.
2. Common in children.
3. Treatment: removal of object.

C. Epistaxis

1. 90% of nosebleeds originate in Kiesselbach's plexus from the anterior nasal septum. Digital trauma is the most common etiology. Most cases resolve with local pressure.
2. Treatment: cautery; nasal packing; ligation of anterior ethmoid or internal maxillary artery; angiographic embolization.

VI. NASAL SEPTAL DISORDERS

A. Septal Deviation

1. Congenital or traumatic, producing unilateral nasal obstruction on the deviated side.
2. Treatment: septoplasty.

B. Septal Hematoma

1. Secondary to trauma.
2. Pressure of accumulated blood under mucoperichondrium can destroy cartilage.
3. Exam shows ballotable mass at the nasal septum.
4. Treatment: immediate incision of the septal mucosa and evacuation of the underlying hematoma.

C. Septal Abscess

1. Secondarily infected septal hematoma.
2. Causes septal destruction, meningoencephalitis, and cavernous sinus thrombosis.
3. Treatment: immediate incision and drainage of the abscess with concomitant intravenous antibiotics.

D. Septal Perforation

1. Secondary to trauma, surgery, or cocaine abuse
2. Symptoms include nasal crusting, whistling noise on inspiration, and epistaxis.
3. Treatment: surgical closure of the perforation.

VII. SINUSITIS

A. Acute Sinusitis

1. Secondary to bacterial infection (*Streptococcus pneumoniae*, *Moraxella catarrhalis*, *Haemophilus influenzae*) within a poorly aerated sinus.
2. Symptoms include pain and facial pressure over the affected sinus, nasal obstruction, purulent rhinorrhea, and fever.
3. CT scan reveals opacification or an air/fluid level within the sinuses.
4. Treatment: antibiotics, oral and nasal decongestants. Persistent sinusitis may require surgical drainage.

B. Chronic Sinusitis

1. Symptoms include persistent nasal congestion, postnasal drainage, headache, facial pressure, and hyposmia/anosmia.
2. Exam may reveal obstruction of the sinus ostia by polyps.
3. CT scan reveals mucoperiosteal thickening of the involved sinuses and opacification of ethmoid air cells.
4. Treatment: endoscopic removal of polyps and ethmoid air cells; surgical enlargement of sinus ostia; nasal steroid spray.

C. Fungal Sinusitis

1. Noninvasive
   - Allergic reaction to fungus (e.g., *Aspergillus*).
   - Primarily involves maxillary and ethmoid sinuses.
   - CT scan demonstrates opacification of the affected sinus with central calcifications.
   - Grossly appears as a firm, rubbery, translucent mass (mycetoma).
   - Treatment: surgical evacuation of the involved sinus. Antifungal therapy is recommended only when histologic soft tissue invasion by fungi is seen.
2. Invasive
   - Primarily aspergillosis and mucormycosis.
   - Primarily affects immunocompromised patients.
   - Extensive soft tissue and bone destruction with rapid invasion of the cranium and orbit from paranasal sinuses.
   - Treatment: emergent radical debridement and systemic antifungal therapy (e.g., amphotericin B).

Table 2 Complications of Acute Sinusitis

Facial cellulitis	Epidural/subdural abscess
Periorbital cellulitis	Intracranial abscess
Orbital cellulitis	Meningoencephalitis
Cavernous sinus thrombosis	Osteomyelitis of facial skeleton

D. Complications (Table 2)

VIII. MUCOCELE

A. Cystic lesion lined by respiratory epithelium and filled with mucus.
B. Secondary to obstruction of the sinus ostium.
C. Commonly involves frontal and ethmoid sinuses.
D. Slowly enlarge and compress adjacent sinus walls.
E. May become secondarily infected.
F. CT scan shows bony thinning, sclerosis, and erosion. The tissues appear hyperintense on T2-weighted MRI images.
G. Treatment: complete surgical excision.

IX. TUMORS (TABLE 3)

A. Benign

1. Prolonged nasal obstruction, facial fullness, headache, rhinorrhea, hyposmia/anosmia, and sinusitis.
2. Lesions enlarge slowly over time.

B. Malignant

1. 60% arise from the maxillary sinus, 20% from the nasal cavity, 15% from the ethmoid sinuses, and 1% from the frontal and sphenoid sinuses.

Table 3 Neoplasms of the Nose and Paranasal Sinuses

Benign	Malignant
Schneiderian papillomas	Squamous cell carcinoma
Capillary hemangioma	Adenocarcinoma
Benign fibrous histiocytoma	Mucosal melanoma
Fibromatosis	Lethal midline granuloma
Leiomyoma	Neuroblastoma
Ossifying fibroma	Malignant fibrous histiocytoma
Osteoma	Fibrosarcoma
Myxoma/fibromyxoma	Leiomyosarcoma
Ameloblastoma	Angiosarcoma
	Osteosarcoma
	Teratocarcinosarcoma

2. Symptoms and signs are similar to those of benign tumors, but evolve more rapidly and include: epistaxis, pain, facial numbness, unilateral nasal airway obstruction, unilateral rhinorrhea, cranial nerve palsy, diplopia, loose teeth, epiphora, and regional adenopathy.

C. Diagnosis

1. Tissue biopsy.
2. CT scan (bony remodeling or postobstructive sinusitis with benign tumors, bony destruction with malignant tumors).
3. MRI to delineate soft tissue extension of tumors and to differentiate tumor from postobstructive fluid.

D. Management

1. Surgical excision.
2. Radiation therapy and/or chemotherapy in cases of malignancy.

112

Aesthetic Otoplasty

Cheryl T. Huang, M.D.
Kaiser Medical Center, San Rafael, California, U.S.A.
H. Peter Lorenz, M.D.
Stanford University Medical Center, Stanford, California, U.S.A.

I. GENERAL CONSIDERATIONS

Abnormalities of the external ear can cause great distress to the child, who becomes the easy target of schoolyard teasing. Successful treatment relies on knowledge of normal ear anatomy, accurate diagnosis of the deformity, and application of one or more sculpting techniques.

II. SURFACE ANATOMY

Key topographical landmarks include (Fig. 1):

A. Helix
B. Antihelix
C. Scapha
D. Superior and inferior crus
E. Fossa triangularis
F. Tragus
G. Antitragus
H. Concha (cymba and cavum)
I. Lobule

III. BLOOD SUPPLY

A. Arterial

1. Superficial temporal artery (from external carotid artery)
2. Posterior auricular artery (from external carotid artery)

B. Venous

1. Superficial temporal vein
2. Posterior auricular vein

IV. NERVE SUPPLY

A. Greater auricular nerve (C2–3) to helix, antihelical fold, concha, lobule, and postauricular skin
B. Auriculotemporal nerve (V3) to crus of helix and tragus
C. Lesser occipital nerve to posterior concha
D. Auricular branch of Vagus (X): Arnold's nerve to external auditory meatus

V. EMBRYOLOGY

The ear develops from six auricular hillocks or swellings during the 6th week of gestation:

A. The first branchial arch (mandibular arch) gives rise to the 1st, 2nd, and 3rd hillocks. These evolve into the tragus (1st) and the helical root (2nd and 3rd).

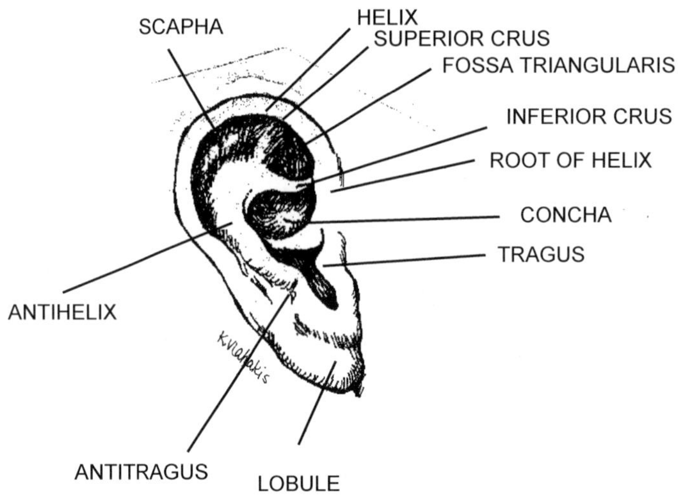

Figure 1 Surface anatomy.

B. The second branchial arch (hyoid arch) gives rise to the 4th, 5th, and 6th hillocks. These evolve into the helix, antihelix, scapha, antitragus, concha, and lobule.

VI. AESTHETIC CONSIDERATIONS

Awareness of the following general observations of normal ears is important in determining the presence of a deformity:

A. The long axis of the ear normally lies 20 degrees posterior from the vertical (coronal) plane.

B. The long axis of the ear normally lies 15 degrees more upright than the dorsum of the nose. It is not parallel to the nose as had been described in the past.

C. The normal distance from helix to mastoid skin is as follows:

- 10–12 mm at the superior ear
- 16–18 mm at the middle ear
- 20–22 mm at the lower ear

D. The ear projects 23 degrees away from the temporal scalp.

E. The top of the ear is at the level of the brow. The bottom of the ear is at the level of the base of the nasal columella.

F. The ear sits at a distance of one ear's length posterior to the lateral orbital rim.

VII. ANATOMY OF THE PROMINENT EAR DEFORMITY

The prominent or protruding ear is a common type of external ear abnormality. The three anatomic characteristics are:

A. Underdeveloped antihelical fold: There is effacement with poor definition of the antihelical fold, such that the conchal concavity is in continuity with the fossa of the helix.

B. Overdeveloped concha: There is excessive height of the conchal wall. The concha is deeply cupped.

C. Increased conchoscaphal angle: The angle is greater than 90 degrees.

VIII. TREATMENT

By age 4, the ear has reached 85% of its adult size. Surgery is usually performed before the child starts elementary school. The choice of techniques is tailored according to the specific deformity present.

A. Overdeveloped Concha

1. Suture technique (Furnas): An elliptical excision of postauricular skin is resected to assist setback of the ear. Excessive skin excision will lead to obliteration of the posterior sulcus and should be avoided. Care must also be taken to avoid distorting the external auditory canal. Next, the

perichondrium is stripped from the posterior conchal cartilage. An ellipse of posterior auricular muscles and ligaments may need to be resected. Care must be taken to avoid the branches of the greater auricular nerve. Horizontal mattress sutures are placed full-thickness between the concha and the mastoid fascia/periosteum. Usually three or four nonabsorbable, clear monofilament sutures are required.

2. Direct excision (Morestin): Similar to the Furnas technique, but a full-thickness ellipse of cartilage is also excised from the base of the excessive conchal bowl to decrease its excessive height.

B. Underdeveloped Antihelical Fold

1. Mustarde technique: The location of the proposed antihelical fold is determined. Paired ink marks are made with a 25-gauge needle 1 cm away from the fold. These marks precisely guide suture placement. A posterior ellipse of skin is excised. The posterior skin is undermined and all soft tissue is stripped off the cartilage. Three or four full-thickness horizontal mattress sutures are placed between the scaphal and the conchal cartilage according to the marks. These sutures incorporate the anterior perichondrium to decrease the chance of sutures pulling through and subsequent relapse. The sutures are tied simultaneously to create an antihelical fold.
2. Scoring technique (Stenstrom): From a posterior incision, a rasp is passed to the anterior cartilage surface in the area of the antihelix and crura. Rasping these areas weakens them. The endpoint is weakening of the cartilage spring and a folding back of the antihelix. An accurate amount of posterior skin must be excised, as this dictates the degree of folding. Scoring techniques are based on original observations made by Gibson and Davis (1963) on rib cartilage. They noticed that cartilage bends in a direction opposite the scored surface due to a "release of interlocking stresses."
3. Incision technique (Luckett): A full-thickness crescent of posterior skin and cartilage is excised along the antihelical fold. Contact between the cut surfaces of cartilage is reestablished with Lembert sutures. An unnaturally sharp edge may result.
4. Molding of cartilage: This may be possible within the first few days of life, due to circulation of maternal estrogens that make cartilage moldable. A variety of tapes or dental compounds may be used to achieve the desired molding effect. This window of opportunity lasts only a few days, after which the maternal estrogens have decreased and the cartilage hardens.

C. Complications

1. Hematoma: This usually presents as sudden pain. Prompt evacuation is necessary to prevent cartilage necrosis and permanent deformity. A bolster dressing or head dressing may be applied to decrease recurrence.
2. Infection: This needs to be treated with IV antibiotics and sulfamylon if cartilage is exposed in order to prevent chondritis and late deformity.
3. Inadequate setback and asymmetry: These can be minimized with careful intraoperative assessment.
4. Relapse: This may occur as intrinsic cartilage forces emerge due to insufficient scoring, sutures pulling through, or ear growth. Revision may be needed. To avoid this complication, full-thickness suture placement should always be used. Sutures should not be too close to the peak of the fold and should not be tied too tightly.
5. Poor result:
   - Sharp antihelical fold: This is encountered more often with cartilage excision and repair techniques (Luckett) but may also be the result of overly vigorous scoring. Treatment options include recontouring and camoflauge techniques with a dermal graft.
   - Telephone deformity: This is the result of inadequate setback of superior and inferior thirds of the ear or overcorrection of the middle pole. The ear resembles a telephone receiver.
   - Protruding earlobe: This can be corrected by extending the posterior ear incision down to remove posterior lobular skin, excising a fishtail pattern of posterior skin, or scoring the anterior surface of the helical tail.
   - Hidden helix: This is due to overcorrection. The helix is abnormally recessed behind the antihelix.

- Obliteration of the posterior sulcus: This can be the result of excessive post-auricular skin excision or overly aggressive setback.
- Contour irregularities: Kinks may occur if too few sutures are used or sutures are spaced too far apart.
- Suture sinus tracts: This is a result of using permanent sutures. Sutures may need to be removed.

IX. SPECIFIC DEFORMITIES

A. Constricted ear: This is also known as "lop ear," "lidded ear," "cup ear," and "canoe ear." The rim of the ear appears as if a pursestring tightens it. Some features of protruding ear may be present. A range of treatment options exists, which depend on the degree of deformity. If minimal deformity exists, the overhanging segment may be excised. In the most severe forms, total ear reconstruction may be necessary.

B. Stahl's ear: Also known as Spock's ear, this deformity is characterized by the presence of a third crus, flat antihelical fold, and a malformed scapha. Treatment options include molding in infancy, Z-plasty, cartilage reversal, wedge excision, and third crus advancement.

C. Cryptotia: Other names include "hidden ear" and "pocket ear." This rare deformity occurs when the upper pole of the ear is buried under the temporal skin. There is absence of the superior sulcus. Treatment consists of molding in infancy or later surgical division of intrinsic auricular muscles and skin graft placement in the retroauricular area.

113

Aesthetic Osteotomies and Genioplasty

Gordon K. Lee, M.D.
David Geffen School of Medicine at UCLA, Los Angeles, California, U.S.A.
H. Peter Lorenz, M.D.
Stanford University, Stanford, California, U.S.A.

I. BASIC DEFINITIONS

A. Osteotomy—the cutting of a bone

B. Genioplasty—altering the size and/or shape of the mandibular symphysis (i.e., chin)

C. Retrogenia—condition in which the chin is positioned more posteriorly than is aesthetically desirable

II. PREOPERATIVE EVALUATION

A. History and physical examination

- Address specific concerns of the patient.
- Inquire about previous orthognathic surgery, which could affect further surgical interventions.
- Careful physical examination with attention to projection of cheek and chin, and upper/lower lip relation. Should also include intraoral examination with evaluation of dentition and temporomandibular joint examination.

B. Cephalometric analysis

- Plain radiographs of head with anterior, posterior, and lateral views.
- Used to determine dentofacial skeletal relationships.

C. Panorex radiograph

- Assess temporomandibular joint, mandible, and dentition.
- Can identify bone, or dental pathology, that could be a contraindication to genioplasty.
- Allows for check of the distance between the incisor roots and the inferior border of the mandible to ensure enough room for internal fixation in genioplasty.

III. ZYGOMATIC ARCH

A. Augmentation may be performed with alloplastic implants, or by osteotomy and repositioning. Osteotomy is preferred by many surgeons due to potential complications of infection, migration, and underlying bone resorption associated with implants.

B. Augmenting facial width:

- Exposure is achieved through an intraoral incision.
- An osteotomy is made at the junction of the zygoma and the maxilla. A greenstick fracture is made in the zygomatic arch, and a bone graft or hydroxyapatite block is placed in the osteotomy site.

- Can be combined with buccal fat pad removal for greater emphasis of malar projection (Fig. 1A).

C. Augmenting anterior zygomatic projection:

- Through a maxillary vestibular and lower eyelid approach, the zygomatic arch, inferior orbital rim, zygomatic body, and anterior maxilla can be exposed. An osteotomy is made in the zygoma posterior and lateral to the infraorbital foramen.

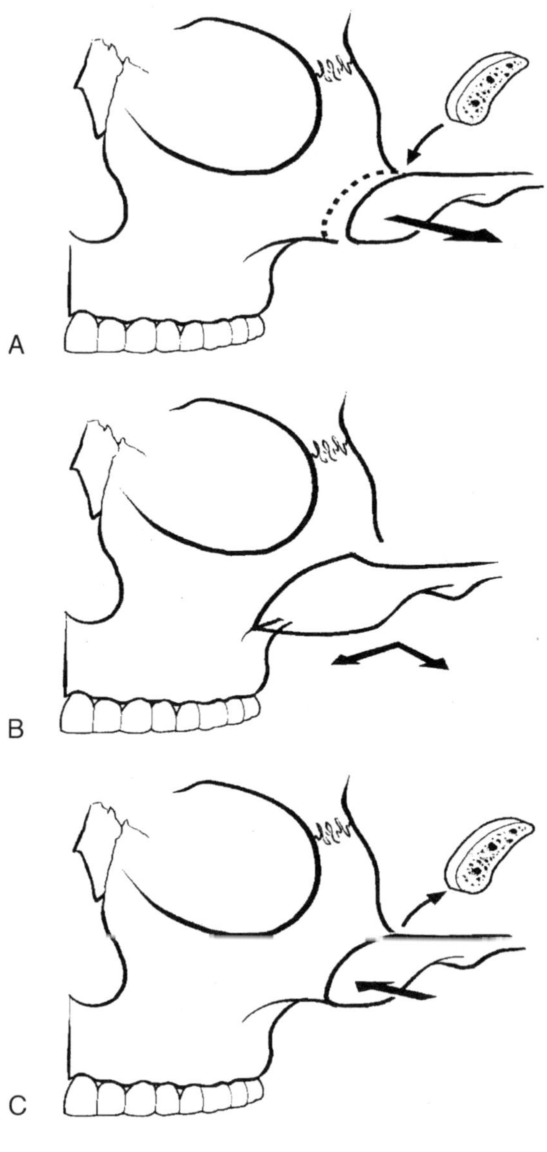

Figure 1 Zygomatic arch: (A) Augmenting facial width; (B) augmenting anterior-zygomatic projection; (C) reduction of the zygoma.

- A bone graft or hydroxyapatite block can then be wedged into the osteotomy site, usually without the need for fixation devices since recoil forces of the zygoma will usually fix the graft well (Fig. 1B).

D. Reduction of the zygoma:

- Can be achieved by simple burring down of the zygoma.
- For larger reductions, parallel osteotomies at the junction between the maxilla and the zygoma, with removal of a zygoma wedge, are necessary. The entire zygoma can then be repositioned more medially and held in position with either wire or plate fixation. Midface suspension is required after reduction due to the compromise in skeletal support of the overlying soft tissue. The deep temporal fascia is suspended to the periosteum overlying the zygomatic complex (Fig. 1C).

IV. MANDIBULAR BODY AND ANGLE

A. Reduction

- Usually for treatment of benign masseteric muscle hypertrophy, which produces a broad lower face.
- Exposure of the mandibular angle, proximal body, and ramus is via an intraoral approach. The muscle is resected off from the mandibular angle and body. The bone is then burred or cut with a reciprocating saw. Care must be taken not to injure the inferior alveolar neurovascular bundles (Fig. 2A).

B. Augmentation

- Although various osteotomies and bone grafts have been described, inconsistent aesthetic results have limited their use. Therefore, implant augmentation has proven to be more reliable, and technically easier to perform.
- Through an intraoral approach, a subperiosteal pocket along the body and angle is created for direct placement of the implant (Fig. 2B).

V. GENIOPLASTY

A. Altering the shape or size of the chin can be achieved with alloplastic material or through autogenous bone grafts, depending upon the type and extent of deficiency.

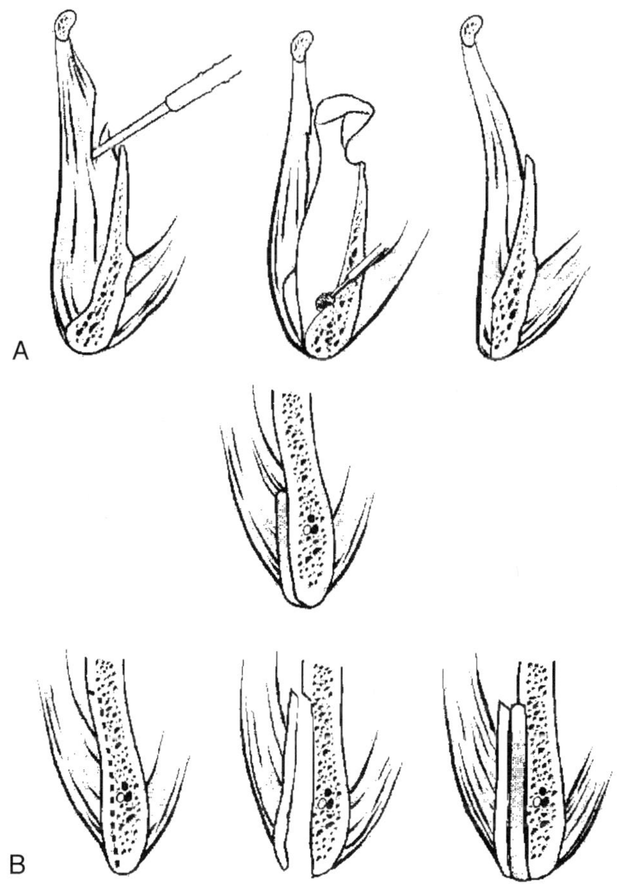

Figure 2 Mandibular body and angle: (A) Reduction; (B) augmentation.

B. Alloplastic genioplasty (Fig. 3A)

- Employs prosthetic material to augment the chin; usually silastic implants
- Is simpler to perform than osseous genioplasty
- Can often be performed under local anesthesia
- Is limited in correcting vertical excess of the anterior mandible
- Is more suitable for patients with mild to moderate anterior projection
- Is associated with complications of bony erosion, infection, and implant migration

C. Osseous genioplasty (Fig. 3B)

- Surgical method:

    Intraoral incision, from canine tooth to canine tooth in the mandibular buccal sulcus

    Subperiosteal exposure of the mandibular symphysis to the inferior border of the anterior mandible

    Horizontal osteotomy of the anterior mandible 2–3 mm below the mental foramina in order to protect the mental nerves

    Osteotomy extends posteriorly to the vicinity of the molar teeth

    The bony segment is then repositioned, depending upon the deficiency that is to be corrected (i.e., anteriorly for greater chin projection, laterally to correct chin asymmetries, or with interposition bone grafting or hydroxyapatite to increase chin vertical height)

    The bone is fixed with wires, screws, or rigid plates

- Key points:

    Technically more demanding than im plant genioplasty

    Not performed in children under the age of 12 years, because their incisor

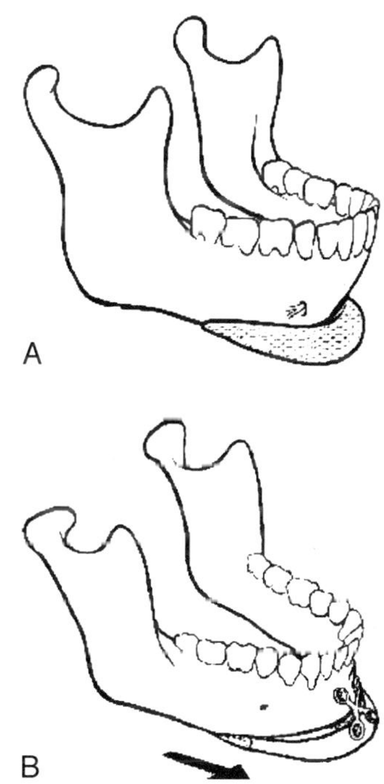

Figure 3 Genioplasty: (A) Alloplastic genioplasty; (B) osseous genioplasty.

roots extend deeper into the mandible than in adults

Can be used in patients with Treacher-Collins syndrome

Osteotomy creates a symphyseal segment that is essentially a pedicled flap, which is attached posteriorly by attachments to the geniohyoid, genioglossus, and anterior belly of digastric muscles

The angle of the osteotomy will affect vertical height of the chin (e.g., a steeper osteotomy angle will allow for augmentation of chin projection as well as reduction in vertical height)

Parallel osteotomies may be made to allow for removal of a wedge of mandibular bone, in order to reduce vertical length of the chin

Labiomental folds will be deepened with vertical shortening, and slightly effaced with vertical lengthening

D. Complications of genioplasty

- Lower lip paresthesias secondary to injury to the distal inferior alveolar nerve (mental nerve)
- Lower lip ptosis
- Mentalis muscle dysfunction
- Avascular necrosis of symphyseal segment
- Infection
- Bone resorption
- Unsatisfactory aesthetic outcome.

114

Alloplastic Facial and Body Implants

Edward O. Terino, M.D.
Plastic Surgery Institute of Southern California, Thousand Oaks, California, U.S.A.

This chapter describes the concepts and techniques for using alloplastic implants to restructure facial and body form in three dimensions. Alloplastic implant contouring through the use of alloplastic materials is a fundamental and new addition to the specialty of plastic surgery (Fig. 1). Contour changes are created that imitate soft tissues, as well as bone.

I. TERMINOLOGY

The basic terminology used in this chapter includes the following:

A. Alloplastic: Materials of synthetic origin (other than metal) or human tissue.
B. Implant: A material or object inserted into the human body for therapeutic or cosmetic purposes.
C. Contouring: Shaping or molding an object to create a desired outline or form.
D. Three-dimensional: Having the dimensions of length, width, and depth, thereby comprising volume and mass.
E. Sculpturing: The art of making or forming a three-dimensional representation.

II. SIGNIFICANCE OF AESTHETIC CONTOURING IN PLASTIC SURGERY

A. Three-dimensional sculpturing procedures using alloplastic materials are a recent innovation in plastic surgery. Operations that attempt to create three-dimensional structural changes by using only soft-tissue manipulations suffer from lack of permanent results. In contrast, alloplastic implant augmentation produces permanent, effective, three-dimensional contour alterations. Moreover, the risks and morbidity are minimal.
B. Another advantage of alloplastic techniques over the use of natural tissue is the ease of exchange and the reversibility of contour that accompanies the use of implants of non-human material. When human tissue is transferred or transplanted, it always reabsorbs to a significant and unpredictable degree, regardless of its source. This does not happen with alloplastic implants. Use of alloplastic implants also eliminates morbidity associated with autogenous tissue donor sites.
C. Perhaps the most valuable function of alloplastic implants is in facial contouring, especially when they are used in conjunction with traditional two-dimensional tightening procedure or with the newer midface repositioning methods for restoring and rejuvenating facial changes of aging. The aging process causes tissues to atrophy. They become inelastic, and their biological composition is weakened. When they are placed under tension during traditional tightening techniques, the results often dissipate, sometimes within the first months or first few years following the surgery. Because the volume and

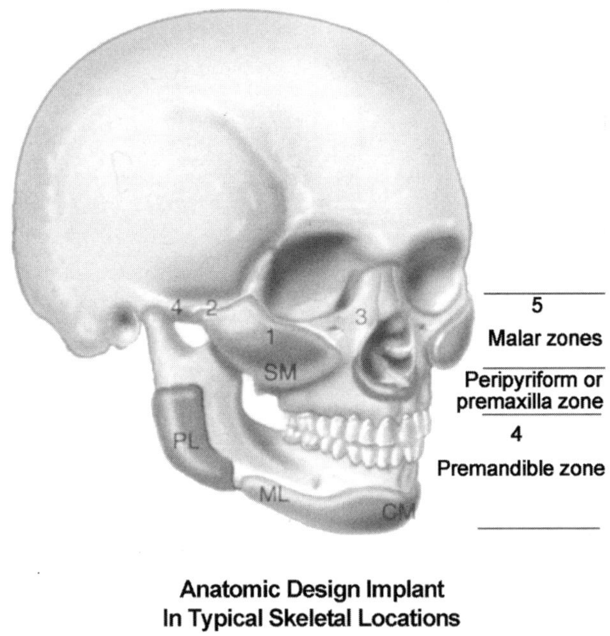

Figure 1 The most commonly needed implants and their anatomic locations. All of these implants are commercially available.

mass properties of alloplastic implants do not change over time, they are an ideal complement to soft-tissue surgeries.

III. OPTIMUM QUALITIES FOR IMPLANTS

A. An ideal alloplastic implant should possess the following characteristics:

- Easy to place
- Nonpalpable
- Readily exchangeable
- Malleable and conformable
- Biocompatible
- Easily modifiable by the surgeon
- Resistant to infection

B. Ideal implants should be malleale and compressible enough to allow insertion through small incisions. Limiting the entrance site minimizes possibilities for extrusion. Soft silicone rubber implants make it possible for the surgeon to introduce them with ease and minimal morbidity.

IV. ALLOPLASTIC BODY IMPLANTS

A. Alloplastic implants for contouring parts of the body other than the face are used at the present time, mostly in the form of mammary prostheses for aesthetic and reconstructive breast surgery. To date, there are very few successful or commonly requested alloplastic implant operations for any other parts of the body.

B. Custom-shaped silastic rubber implants are used to augment the muscle contours of the upper chest in males. The implants are inserted through a transaxillary approach into the retropectoral region to augment upper chest contours. Additionally, calf implants with a special "torpedo" or spindle shape have been designed for placement between the medial and lateral heads of the gastrocnemius muscle for calf augmentation. Other specialized implants have been occasionally used to augment the contour of the male forearm.

C. Smooth silicone rubber implants become rapidly and circumferentially immobilized in the body by a thin and smooth biologic capsule consisting of collagen. By simply incising the capsule, the implant can be easily exchanged or removed, when necessary. Implants made from porous materials permit ingrowth of natural tissue into the implant. Examples are Proplast, Porex, hydroxyapatite, and Gore-Tex. Implants made from porous materials or implants with fenestrations are considerably more difficult to remove and exchange.

D. These implant techniques into unusual body sites have been performed in limited numbers and mainly in patients in whom correcting hereditary deficiencies or improving aesthetic contours in the areas described above are of great emotional significance. While implants in the pectoral and calf region are successful, their predisposition to malposition, palpability, and mobility is greater than that for implants placed on the bony skeleton of the face.

V. ALLOPLASTIC FACIAL IMPLANTS

A. The surgeon who seeks to use alloplastic implants successfully in operations designed to alter aesthetic form must first become thoroughly familiar with certain basic principles of facial aesthetics.

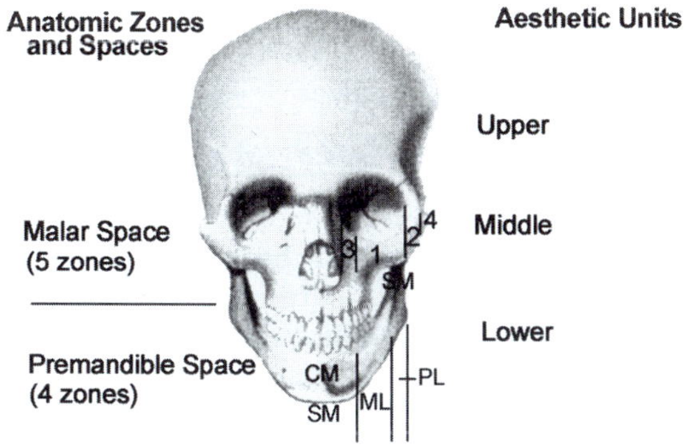

Figure 2 The three aesthetic segments of the face and the anatomic zones of the malar-midface and the chin-jawline.

B. The human face is divided into three major aesthetic units: upper, middle, and lower (Fig. 2):

- The upper facial aesthetic segment extends from the hairline to the lateral canthi of the eyes. It contains the eyebrows, as well as the glabella, frontal, and supraorbital brow components of facial contour.
- The middle-third aesthetic facial segment extends from the lateral canthi to the lateral oral commissures. It contains two of the three major architectural promontories of facial form: the nose and the malar-submalar midface-cheek complex.
- The lower facial aesthetic segment includes the lower lip, mandible, and jawline. It is frequently of smaller dimensions, including vertical height.
- The shape of the midface-cheek is a primary determinant of facial aesthetic beauty. This region of the face contains the eyes and nose, which are the main focal points that attract the attention of the viewer. There are also a variety of contour configurations to the central midface and nasolabial elements (Fig. 3).

VI. VOLUME-MASS RELATIONSHIPS

A. In addition to perceiving a face in terms of aesthetic units, there also must be an understanding of the several areas of significant volume and mass that constitute the three-dimensional characteristics of the face. These include the following important promontories:

- Malar-midface prominence
- Nasal size and projection
- The entire lower third jawline and mandible segment
- The supraorbital brow ridges (of lesser significance)

B. Altering any one of the three facial volume-mass units directly and inversely affects the aesthetic importance of the others. When any one structure is significantly larger, the other two appear relatively diminished. For example, when the size of the nose is reduced, the volume and projection relationships of the midface-cheek and mandible jawline assume more importance.

C. Furthermore, when two areas are enlarged (as by facial implant augmentation), the size significance of the others is deemphasized. Therefore, by accentuating the malar/submalar-midface

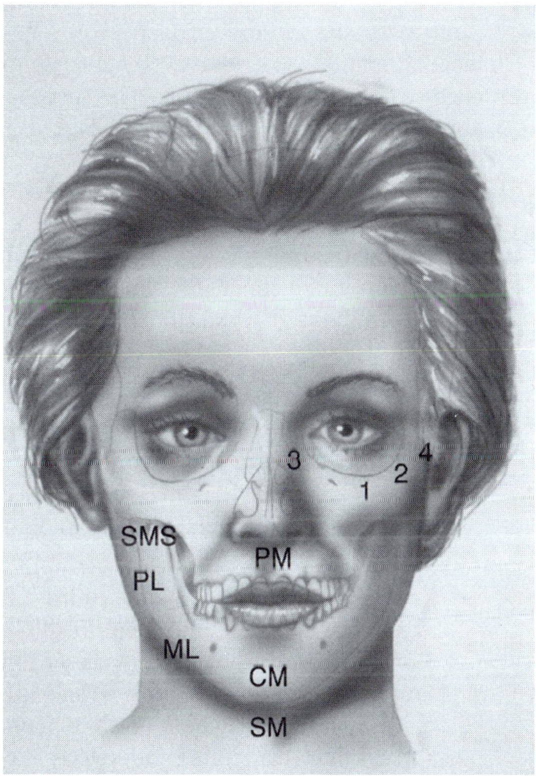

Figure 3 The relationship of the skeletal zones to the overlying facial features and soft tissue anatomy.

component, and at the same time augmenting the chin-jawline, the apparent size of a prominent nose is significantly diminished.

VII. FACIAL BALANCE

A. The interrelationships of volume and mass are what determine a relative balance called aesthetic beauty.

- For example, an extremely prominent nasal characteristic accompanied by an extremely small receding chin is considered unattractive.
- Lean-faced individuals who have long, narrow facial contours and an inadequate malar/midface and/or central chin development, can appear "ugly."
- Patients with round, full, fleshy facial contours that contain an abundance of subcutaneous fat are rarely considered beautiful by contemporary standards. These types of faces are aesthetically imbalanced.

B. In order to assist the surgeon in selecting the right size, shape, and proper positioning of facial implants, several types of facial imbalances will be described below. The surgeon can apply the syste of facial analysis by zonal principles, as well as an understanding of six basic types of aesthetic midfacial deficiencies to achieve planned predictable results. It is useful to think of the malar/midface aesthetic unit as divided into five distinct anatomic zones (Figs. 2 and 3). Analysis by zonal principles:

- Zone 1 includes the major portion of the malar bone and the anterior third of the zygomatic arch. Augmentation of Zone 1 maximizes anterior/posterior projection of the malar eminence and produces a high, sharp, prominent facial skeletal and cheekbone contour.
- Zone 2 overlies the middle third of the zygomatic arch. Enhancement of this zone, along with Zone 1, gives a broader dimension or width to the upper third of the face. Excessive augmentation of Zones 1 and 2 will give an unnatural, overly skeletal appearance.
- Zone 3 is the paranasal area lying between the infraorbital foramen and the pyriform aperture. Augmentation in Zone 3 produces medial fullness, especially in the upper medial nasolabial area, and can produce an unattractive effect. Zone 3 is the location of the medial suborbital "tear trough" or nasojugal soft-tissue sulcus. This area can be improved either by using a specialized implant that surrounds the infraorbital nerve or by releasing bony origins of the orbicularis musculature, with placement of autogenous tissue (e.g., fat or dermis) beneath this medial area.
- Zone 4 overlies the posterior third of the zygomatic arch. Augmentation in this area is never needed and would produce an unnatural appearance.
- Zone 5 is perhaps the most important midfacial region. It is bounded posteriorly by the masseter muscle, superiorly by the malar bone, and medially by the nasolabial fold. This "submalar triangle" is the region that, with aging, develops soft-tissue atrophy and a medial descent of these tissues to create a nasolabial fold. This results in a tired, haggard appearance. It can occur even in people in the age range of 30s to 40s. Alloplastic augmentation within the submalar zone mimics soft-tissue restoration and produces a fuller, rounder, and more youthful contour.

VIII. TYPES OF MIDFACIAL AESTHETIC DEFICIENCIES

There are six basic types of aesthetic deficiencies in the midface area.

A. Patients with Type I deficiency have insufficient malar and suborbital skeletal development, but have good midface soft-tissue fullness. The basic deficiency is in Zones 1, 2, and possibly 3. Malar shell implants or possibly tear-trough implants, when used medially, significantly correct the aesthetic deficiency of a Type 1 face. This is especially true when used in conjunction with midface suspension procedures.

B. Type II facial aesthetic deficiency consists of adequate bony and soft tissue volume in the upper Zone 1 and Zone 2 areas, but inadequate volume of midfacial soft tissue in the submalar zone location. This can be corrected by placing alloplastic malar shell implants of various sizes and thicknesses on the masseter tendon, extending 1–3 cm below the lower border of the malar bone. In this location, these implants provide fullness and projection for a flat face, as well as for atrophic changes of the aging face. Alloplastic implantation into this submalar Zone 5 is the most frequently required and most desirable placement for improving facial contour. Implants in this location mimic midfacial soft tissue fullness.

C. Type III facial pattern is a more extreme version of Type II and is rare. It consists of dramatically prominent malar bones accompanied by a severe soft-tissue deficiency in the submalar region. An abrupt transition from the strong Zone 1, 2 malar bone area to an area of extreme submalar deficiency and hollowness makes the patient appear gaunt and emaciated. Traditional rhytidectomy techniques often accentuate this unattractive skeletal appearance. Newer midface suspension techniques can improve a Type III face. When accompanied by submalar implant placement, the restoration can be corrected to an even greater degree.

D. Type IV aesthetic deficiency is also rare. It is a combination of the severe malar-suborbital skeletal hypogenesis and a deficiency of the midfacial soft tissues. It appears more commonly in men. Since this type of midface is totally deficient in volume, it requires augmentation of both the malar and submalar zones (Zones 1 and 5). A large shell or a "combined" implant can augment both the malar eminence and the submalar triangle soft-tissue hollowness.

E. Type V aesthetic deficiency exists where there is significant suborbital bony recession, as well as descent of the malar soft tissues. This is accompanied by a visible, unattractive infraorbital sulcus or valley that is frequently accentuated medially in the Zone 3 tear-trough region. Whether the origin is from hereditary skeletal deficiency or an aging descent of the entire soft-tissue envelope of the midface, the correction can be either autologous, alloplastic, or both. Optimum repair requires subperiosteal midface suspension in conjunction with alloplastic augmentation.

F. Type VI face has a retrusive central premaxillary appearance. This aesthetic facial deficiency is a lesser variant of a cleft lip deformity. It exhibits a malformed central premaxillary hypoplasia. A peri-pyriform premaxillary augmentation with specialized alloplastic implants can successfully improve the appearance of such patients.

G. A thorough understanding of the zones of facial anatomy, their interrelationships, and the six facial types described above enables the surgeon to create facial contours that can correct a variety of aesthetic deficiencies and can thereby accommodate the needs of a broader number of patients. The three most crucial parameters the surgeon must control are:

- Appropriate choice of implant shape
- Correct implant size
- Precise zonal placement

IX. ZONAL ANATOMY OF THE LOWER FACE

A. Alloplastic facial implants can alter the entire chin/jawline contour. Anatomic-shaped implants can be inserted that extend laterally beneath the mental nerve, thereby creating a widening of the lower third of the face (Fig. 2). The traditional smaller, centrally placed implants that were positioned between the mental foramina often produce an abnormal central protuberance.

B. The mandibular anatomy consists of four zones:

- Zone 1 (CM) consists of the central mentum between the mental nerves.
- Zone 2, the midlateral zone (ML), extends to the middle of the mandibular body.
- Zone 3, a posterior-lateral zone (PL), overlies the posterior aspect of the mandibular body, including the angle of the mandible and the lower third of the ascending ramus. Augmentation of this posterior lateral zone widens the face at the posterior jawline and gives prominent sculptured definition to the mandibular angle.
- Zone 4 exits beneath the inferior border of the mandible. This can be referred to as the submandibular zone. Traditional implants do not create extension of the mandibular segment in a vertical direction. New implant designs, however, are available that wrap

around the inferior bony margin of the chin. These can increase the vertical height of the face from the lower lip to the inferior border of the chin.

X. GENERAL GUIDELINES FOR IMPLANT SELECTION

A. The author has found in his experience that 4 mm of augmentation in the malar/midfacial zones will almost always be optimal. A malar shell implant of 3 mm size will produce a subtle effect, and a 5–6 mm implant will produce a bold, dramatic result.

- In the central mentum region of the chin, 5–7 mm of projection are suitable for the majority of patients. When severe microgenia is present, an implant providing 8–10 mm of augmentation is necessary.
- In cases where an extreme degree of mandibular projection is needed, patients may be better served by mandibular osteotomy bone advancement techniques.
- The posterior mandibular angle (PL) can be adequately contoured by an implant with 8 mm of lateral thickness. For strong accentuation in a male patient, 10 or 12 mm (2–2.4 cm total widening) may often be indicated.

B. Technical considerations include:

- Four basic routes can be used for introducing malar-midface implants: 1) intraoral, 2) subciliary—blepharoplasty, 3) preauricular—face lift, and 4) coronal. Each of these approaches has its own advantages and may be performed successfully according to the experience of the individual surgeon.
- Implant placement through the lower eyelid should be accompanied by malar/midface suspension and canthopexy techniques to minimize the chance of lower lid retraction.
- Chin/jawline implants are introduced by three routes: 1) intraoral anterior, 2) intraoral posterior, and 3) submental. The intraoral posterior incision is 2 cm in length, curvilinear in shape, and placed 1 cm anterior to the gingival-buccal attachment. The intraoral incision is 1.5 cm transversely and 1 cm from the gingival attachment.
- A vertical separation of the mentalis muscle pillars is used in order to minimize laxity or weakness of the central chin mound. The intraoral approach is used for chin implant placement when the implant size is moderate. A submental approach is necessary whenever other procedures are used to access the fat and platysma musculature of the neck region. This approach is most commonly associated with rhytidectomy operations. This type of incision is also used for accurate placement of submandibular vertical-extension implants.

XI. TECHNIQUE OF OPERATION

Some of the basic principles that should be observed when performing implant surgeries are the following:

A. Elevate soft tissues from the bone at the subperiosteal level. Implants placed directly on bone become firmly encapsulated and immobilized. Capsular contraction has not been observed when implants are placed on the bony plane.

B. Avoid trauma to the soft tissues and do not dissect into the area of the mental or infraorbital nerves.

C. Create an adequate pocket to accommodate the implant. Do not make the pocket too large.

D. Minimize bleeding by staying on the bone and by using a copious injection of a solution containing epinephrine.

E. Irrigate frequently with antibiotic solution (e.g., Ancef, 2 g/L normal saline).

F. Once the anatomic space has been created, the implant can be inserted. With a posterior angle implant or a midfacial implant, place a straight, serrated clamp transversely across the long axis of the implant to facilitate insertion through the small incisional aperture. This maneuver facilitates placement into the malar Zones 1 and 2, zygomatic tunnel, and the angle of the mandible space. In the midface, two percutaneous Ethibond arthroscopic sutures are placed, first through the tail of the implant and then transcutaneously posterior to the temple hairline. Traction on these sutures stabilizes the tail of the implant and ensures proper positioning. The sutures are tied over a large tonsil sponge for 3 days, until they are easily removed.

G. Fiberoptic Aufricht retractors or a headlight are used to illuminate the operative space, reveal the internal anatomy, and confirm the correct positioning of the implant.

H. Creation of the submalar zonal space entails removing the soft tissues from the shiny, white, fibrous masseter muscle tendon in an inferior and lateral direction.

I. Through the use of adequate local and general anesthesia, the surgeon can obtain excellent visualization of the skeletal anatomy and musculature. This is critically necessary to facilitate precise placement of the implant and to minimize bleeding. Excessive bleeding can lead to hematoma, seroma, and infection.

J. The intraoral approach for midfacial implant placement involves a 1.5–2 cm incision made obliquely above the canine tooth and extending upward over the buttress of the maxilla. The surgeon avoids the facial musculature and nerves by entering inferior to them and elevating the periosteum from the bone over the malar prominence at the origin of the masseter muscle. The dissection then continues onto the anterior surface of the malar bone in Zone 1.

XII. COMPLICATIONS

In the author's 25 years of experience with over 3000 facial implants, the following complications have occurred. They are listed in order of importance and frequency:

Complication	Rate
Patient and/or doctor dissatisfaction	10%
Minor asymmetries	5%
Malposition requiring correction	2%
Hematoma, seroma	1%
Infection and removal	0.25%
Transient infraorbital nerve dysfunction (intraoral route)	1%
Transient zygomaticus lip elevation dysfunction (intraoral route)	1.5%
Lower eyelid ectropion (subcilial route)	1.5%

A. With mandibular implant placements, asymmetries and malposition occurred in a slightly higher incidence (5–10%), but the deformities that resulted were often so minimal that the patients overlooked them. They were easily corrected by secondary repositioning of the implants under local anesthesia.

B. Despite the fact that complication rates are relatively low when using alloplastic implants, the surgeon must nevertheless remain aware of the inherent risks in utilizing foreign materials in the body. The surgeon must be prepared to remove implants promptly if infections do not immediately respond to treatment. Otherwise, severe undesirable consequences can occur.

XIII. CONCLUSION

A. Through the insertion of volume-mass implants, surgeons are now able to make permanent changes in the facial and body contours of human beings.

B. Implants in the body are used mostly in male patients mainly for the purpose of augmenting the pectoral upper chest region and the calves.

C. Alloplastic facial implants help to create facial balance and improve aesthetics, especially when accompanied by the newer midfacial and upper subperiosteal suspension techniques (Fig. 4).

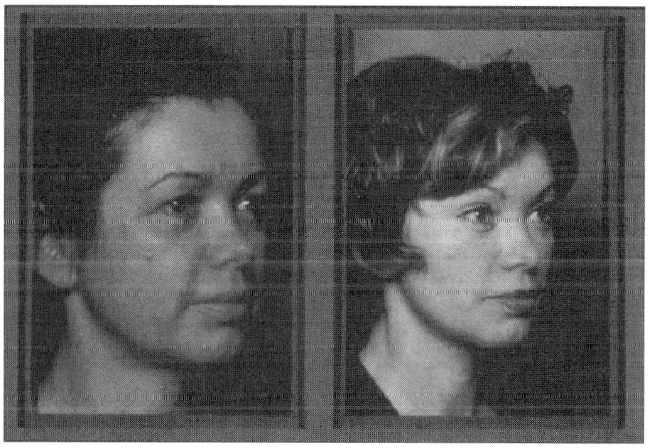

Figure 4 48-year-old patient demonstrating the use of malar and chin implants in conjuction with mid-facial and upper suspension surgery and lower rhytidectomy to enhance facial balance and create aesthetic beauty.

Facial implants are, by definition, three-dimensional in nature. They alter facial form by manipulating volume and mass in certain prescribed zones of facial anatomy. They are used to correct various types of aesthetic facial deficiencies and thereby achieve a balance of facial form called facial beauty.

D. Autogenous tissue implants have generally been considered preferable. On the other hand, because of their impermanence in relation to shape and size retention, they have become a less desirable alternative than the current methods of contouring the face through the use of alloplastic implant techniques.

115

Endoscopic Facial Rejuvenation and Remodeling

Nicanor G. Isse, M.D.
Burbank, California, U.S.A.

I. INDICATIONS

A. Endoscopic facial rejuvenation is indicated for those cases where tissue repositioning is desired, in the presence of minimal to moderate dermatochalasia. These procedures complement dermal-planing techniques such as chemical peeling, dermabrasion, and laser resurfacing.

B. In severe dermatochalasia, an open approach might be indicated (bicoronal forehead lift, direct brow-pexy, or bi-planar technique).

II. PRINCIPLES OF ENDOSCOPIC PLASTIC SURGERY

A. The goal of the endoscopic technique is to develop a plane of dissection between the superficial and deep facial fascia. These two fascias have multiple areas of fusion (ligaments); therefore, it is necessary to detach those ligaments and develop a plane of dissection to allow gliding and repositioning of the superficial plane over the deep plane. All of the facial structures contained in the superficial layer will be elevated to a more harmonic position by suture fixation.

III. ANATOMIC CONSIDERATIONS

A. Superficial Plane Structures

These include skin, subcutaneous adipose tissue, and the following structures:

1. Forehead area:
   - Superficial plane (fascia):

     Fronto-galea aponeurotica

     Periosteum
   - Muscles:

     Frontalis (Fig. 1.4)

     Orbicularis oculi (Fig. 1.3)

     Depressor supercilii (Fig. 1.2)

     Procerus (Fig. 1.1)

     Corrugator muscle, partially elevated (not shown), covered by other muscles
   - Fat pad—retro-orbicularis fat pad lies underneath the orbicularis oculi muscle (not shown)
   - Facial nerve:

     Terminal branches of the frontal nerve

     Terminal branches of the corrugator nerve

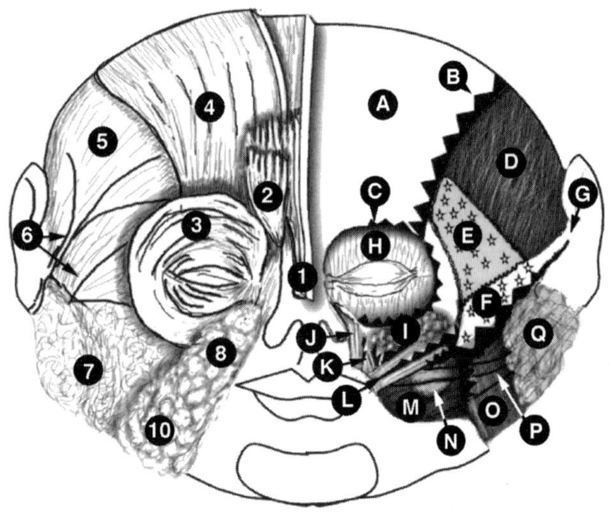

Figure 1 The plane of dissection: Left side shows the superficial layer of dissection; right side shows the deep layer of the dissection. The dark-shaded areas represent different points of fusion between the two planes of dissections.

Terminal branches of the superior zygomatic nerve

2. Temporal area:
   - Superficial fascia:

     Temporo-parietal fascia (TPF) (Fig. 1.5)
   - Muscles:

     Temporo-parietal muscles (not shown) lie underneath the TPF

     Orbicularis muscle (Fig. 1.3)

     Fat pad—subcutaneous fat (not shown)
   - Facial nerve:

     Temporal branches of the facial nerve (Fig. 1.6)

     Superior zygomatic branches of the facial nerve (Fig. 1.6)
3. Mid-face area:
   - Superficial fascia—investing fascia of the orbicularis oculi muscle
   - Muscles—orbicularis oculi muscle (Fig. 1.3)
   - Fat pad:

     Malar fat pad (Fig. 1.8)

     Subcutaneous fibrous fat pad (Fig. 1.7)
   - Facial nerve:

     Middle branch of the zygomatic facial nerve (not shown)

     Underneath subcutaneous tissue and SMAS
4. Lower face area:
   - Superficial fascia—superficial musculo-aponeurotic system (SMAS) (Fig. 1.7)
   - Muscle—risorius (not shown) underneath subcutaneous tissue
   - Fat pad—subcutaneous fat (Fig. 1.7)
   - Facial nerve—not present at this level

B. Deep Plane Structures

1. Forehead area:
   - Deep fascia (plane)

     Frontal bone (Fig. 1A)
   - Muscles, fat pad, and facial nerve are not present in this layer
2. Temporal area:
   - Deep fascia—deep temporal fascia (superficial and deep layer) (Fig. 1D).
   - Muscles—temporalis muscle (Fig. 1D)
   - Fat pad—superficial temporal fat pad (Fig. 1E)
   - Facial nerve—not present in this layer
3. Mid-face:
   - Deep fascia—not present
   - Muscles:

     Zygomaticus major and minor muscle origins (Fig. 1L)

     Levator labii superioris (Fig. 1J)

     Levator angularis oris (Fig. 1K)

     Levator alaqui nasi (not shown)
   - Fat pad—SOOF (sub-orbicularis oculi fat) (Fig. 1I)
   - Facial nerve—not present on the deep plane at this level
4. Lower face:
   - Deep fascia:

     Deep facial fascia, masticatory fascia—covering masticatory muscles

Muscles—buccinator (Fig. 1M) and masseter (Fig. 1O)

- Muscles:

  Zygomaticus major and minor muscles (Fig. 1L)

  Buccinator (Fig. 1M)

  Masseter (Fig. 1O)

- Fat pad—Bichat's fat pad (Fig. 1N)
- Facial nerve:

  Inferior zygomatic branch (Fig. 1P)

  Buccal branches (Fig. 1P)

C. The Interface Structures (Fusion Lines, Areas, Ligaments)

1. Forehead area—temporal crest ligament (Fig. 1B)
2. Temporal area—orbicularis-temporal ligament (temporal fusion line or area) (Fig. 1E)
3. Mid-face:
   - Zygomatic arch fusion line or area (Fig. 1F)
   - Zygomatic ligament—black structures lateral to zygomaticus major (Fig. 1)
   - Malar ligament—black structures between zygomaticus major and minor (Fig. 1)
   - Maxillary ligament—black structures around levator labii muscles (Fig. 1)
4. Lower face:
   - Superior parotid-masseteric ligament, black structures on top of masseter muscle (Fig. 1)
   - Inferior parotid-masseteric ligament, black structures on top of masseter muscle (Fig. 1)
   - Parotid-cutaneous ligaments (not shown)

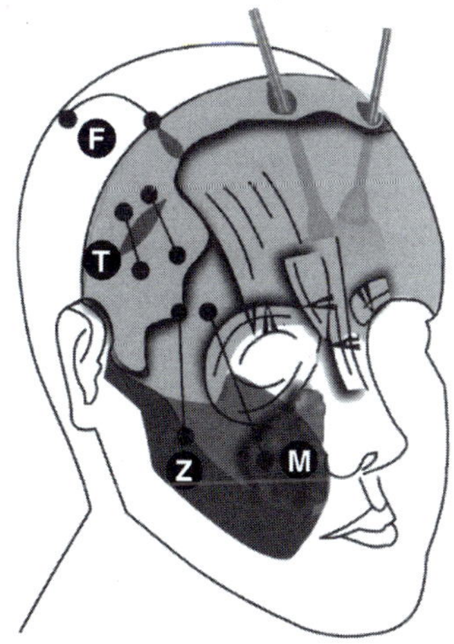

Figure 2 Basic technique. Dissections: endoforehead (lighter-shaded area); endo mid-face (medium-shaded area); endoface (darker-shaded area). Myotomies: dark arrows over the orbicularis, procerus, depressor supercilii, and corrugator muscle. Fixations: fronto-paramedial (F), temporal (T), malar (M) and zygomatic (Z).

IV. CLASSIFICATION

A. Endoforehead—Endoforeheadplasty is a procedure designed to improve brow ptosis, pseudoptosis of the upper eyelid, and peri orbital wrinkles around the lateral orbit, forehead, and glabella area. The whole forehead and temporal areas are dissected (Fig. 2, light-shaded area).

B. Endo-midface—Endoscopic mid-face lifting and peri-orbitoplasty are indicated for the improvement of the lower eyelid area and mid-face area, correction of the palpebral-malar depression, correction of the vertical length of the lower eyelid, improvement of ptosis of the malar fat pad, and improvement of the naso-labial fold. The dissection is performed medially to the naso-labial fold, laterally to the origin of the zygomatic major muscle, and inferiorly to the level of the corner of the mouth (Fig. 2, medium-shaded area).

C. Endo-face—Endoscopic lower facelifting is done in conjunction with the endoforehead or endo-midface procedures. It is also indicated for the improvement of the mandibular fat pad (jowl) and tightening of the soft tissue of the mandibular area. The dissection is carried out inferior to the corner of the mouth and lateral to the origin of the zygomaticus major muscle, detaching the zygomatic and superior masseteric ligaments (Fig. 2, darker-shaded area).

V. INSTRUMENTATION AND ORGANIZATION

A. Surgical Instruments

1. A series of periosteal elevators and soft tissue dissectors.

2. Electrosuction and suction fulguration devices.
3. An irrigation system to keep the lens clean from blood, fog, and debris.

B. Video Instruments

1. A 4 mm telescope (arthroscope) with 30-degree angle.
2. A telescope protection sheath.
3. Irrigation.
4. An endo-retractor and endo-dissector, to create and maintain an optical cavity.
5. A video monitor.
6. A video camera to connect the telescope and to transfer the image to the video monitor.
7. A VCR to tape record a procedure and to help review the same to improve your skill.
8. The setup of the monitor is usually next to the "foot" of the table, either to the right or left of the patient, depending on the surgeon's needs.

VI. BASIC TECHNIQUE

A. Incisions

Generally, five incisions are used: one medial incision, two para-medial incisions (5 cm apart from the medial incision), and two temporal incisions slightly parallel to the hairline and located 2 cm behind the hairline.

B. Dissection

1. The dissection on the forehead may be either sub-galeal or sub-periosteal.
2. The dissection in the temporal area is between the superficial temporal fascia (TPF) and the superficial layer of the deep temporal fascia.
3. The dissection on the mid-face is under the orbicularis muscle and under the SMAS (superficial musculo-aponeurotic system).
4. The dissection on the lower face is under the SMAS.

C. Tissue Modifications

1. Tissue modifications are performed mostly in the forehead area, where the aging signs are mainly due to muscle hyperactivity.
2. Tissue modifications are also performed on the periosteum and galea to allow the tissues to expand vertically as well as horizontally, improving the wrinkles on the glabella and supra-orbital rim areas.
3. The myotomies of the orbital portion of the orbicularis oculi muscle prevents further ptosis of the brow, and decreases the wrinkles of the glabella area (frown lines) and the crow's feet wrinkles above the lateral canthal raphe. Myotomies of the procerus muscle improve the horizontal wrinkles of the radix of the nose.
4. Myotomies of the depressor supercilii muscle improve the frown lines. Myotomies of the corrugator muscle further elevate the head of the brow and increase the interbrow distance.
5. Myotomies of any muscle performed in the glabella area will elevate the head of the brow.

D. Fixation

After undermining, tissue modification, and ligament detachment, the forehead and facial tissues are repositioned to a more superior location. Suture fixation is used to maintain the position of the tissue and to prevent recurrent ptosis. There are several potential methods of fixation.

1. Forehead area: para-medial fixation (Fig. 2F) from the fronto-galea aponeurotica to the underlying bone (cortical tunnel or screw fixation), or to the posterior galea aponeurotica by means of subperiosteal suture fixation.
2. Temporal area: temporal fixation (Fig. 2T). The superficial temporal fascia is fixed about 1 cm caudal to the temporal incision and sutured to the deep temporal fascia.
3. Mid-face: malar fixation (Fig. 2M). A suture is placed 3 cm lateral to the alae of the nose in the undersurface of malar fat pad and is suspended to the superficial layer of the deep temporal fascia.
4. Lower-face: zygomatic fixation (Fig. 2Z). A suspension suture from the undersurface of the SMAS at the level of the origin of the zygomaticus major muscle to the superficial layer of the deep temporal fascia is applied. The author prefers a 3-0 or 4-0 nylon, Gore-Tex, or PDS suture. Drains are applied to prevent fluid collection and to speed recovery.

VII. PITFALLS AND PROBLEMS

A. The most common pitfall is the combination of overresection or modification of the glabellar muscles, with undertreatment or poor elevation of the tail of the brow. Generally speaking, the brow should be higher laterally than medially.

B. Lack of dissection of the deep galea at the supraorbital rim. This problem will lead to poor elevation of the body of the brow and early recurrence of brow ptosis.

C. Excess belief in tissue fixation over complete tissue undermining and modification.

D. Note: emphasis should be placed on fixation at level of the lateral brow (temporal fixation) at all times.

116

Hair Restoration

James P. Watson, M.D.
David Geffen School of Medicine at UCLA, Los Angeles, California, U.S.A.

Androgenic alopecia, or male pattern baldness, is a common progressive disorder that is characterized by a premature decrease in scalp hair density in the bitemporal and vertex areas of the scalp. Because a full head of hair is associated with youth and vitality, hair is an important part of self-image for both men and women. Recent advances in hair restoration techniques have been able to create a much more natural result than in the past. As a consequence, an increasing number of patients are seeking hair restoration today.

I. HAIR ANATOMY AND PHYSIOLOGY

Hair is a complex organ that is made up of the pilosebaceous unit and undergoes three distinct phases of growth.

A. Types of Hair

1. Lanugo hair—prenatal.
2. Vellus hair—fine hair in "hairless areas"—hair at birth.
3. Terminal hair—coarse hair, pubertal hair.

B. Pilosebaceous Unit

The pilosebaceous unit is made of three components:

1. Hair follicle—made up of epithelial and dermal components:
   - Epithelial components—hair follicle matrix + outer root sheath
   - Dermal components—dermal papilla + connective tissue sheath
2. Sebaceous gland—this produces sebum, which is comprised of triglycerides, wax esters, squalene, and cholesterol.
3. Arrector pili muscle—smooth muscle that inserts into the hair follicle.

C. Hair Growth

New hair is made when the hair follicle matrix divides. This process is controlled by the dermal papilla. Three distinct phases in the hair growth cycle occur:

1. Anagen—growth phase.
2. Catagen—transition, or regression, phase.
3. Telogen—resting phase (no hair visible).

D. Natural History of Hair

Scalp hair is constantly going through a phase of the life cycle, which ranges from 2 to 5 years in length. The hair is divided up into the following phases:

1. Telogen phase—10% of total hair is in this phase. It lasts for 3 months.
2. Anagen phase—90% is in this phase (growing hair).
3. Catagen phase—approximately 50–100 hairs are lost per day (<1% of total).

II. CAUSES OF HAIR LOSS

Many different etiologic agents can cause hair loss (alopecia). For this reason, it is important to do a thorough history and physical examination of any patient seeking hair restoration. The following are the most common causes of hair loss.

A. Senile Alopecia

Senile balding occurs during the seventh and eight decades of life in both men and women, where universal scalp hair thinning occurs. This thinning is a uniform decrease in hair density, whereas male pattern baldness is a nonuniform thinning of hair.

B. Androgenic Alopecia

Male pattern baldness is the thinning of scalp hair that occurs first in the temporal area and then spreads to the vertex of the scalp. This hair loss is not readily apparent for the following reasons:

1. 50% of the hair density of a region (frontal or vertex) may be lost before most people may notice thinning.
2. 20% of hair density can be lost without being detectable by even the trained clinician.

C. Cicatricial Alopecia

1. Balding due to scarring can occur following many types of trauma.
2. The common denominator is permanent hair follicle destruction, which cannot be reversed with medical treatment (minoxidil, finasteride, etc.)
3. The only effective treatment is to bring in new hair follicles with transplantation, tissue expansion, or excisional techniques.
4. A variety of causes have been reported, including chemical burns, thermal burns, surgery, severe infections, scleroderma, and radiation.

D. Telogen Effluvium

1. Telogen effluvium is a temporary form of hair loss that is defined as a transient increase in the number of hairs in the telogen (resting) phase of the growth cycle. Instead of the 50–100 hairs normally lost per day, hair loss often exceeds 150 hairs per day. Patients rarely become completely bald, however, and the hair loss is reversible.
2. These patients do not need hair restoration.
3. Although the etiology is still unclear, many authors believe this phenomenon is related to iron deficiency. A variety of triggering events have been reported, including normal gestational delivery, "crash dieting," high fever, surgery, shock, malnutrition, and oral contraceptives.

E. Alopecia Areata

1. Alopecia areata is the loss of hair in salmon-colored patches without evidence of scarring. These patches are smooth and often have small hairs in the lesions that measure only 2–3 mm in length ("exclamation hairs").
2. Although the exact cause is unknown, it is believed to be an autoimmune phenomenon and is usually treated with medications such as intralesional steroids or other topical drugs.
3. These patients are not good candidates for hair transplantation.

F. Drug-Induced Alopecia

1. Although the most common drugs causing alopecia are chemotherapeutic agents, many other drugs can also cause hair loss. The hair loss caused by drugs is almost always reversible and needs no treatment other than to stop the drug when possible.
2. The common drugs associated with drug-induced alopecia include thallium, excess vitamin A, retinoids, anticoagulants, antithyroid drugs, oral contraceptives, allopurinol, propranolol, indomethacin, and amphetamines.

III. MALE PATTERN BALDNESS: MATHEMATICS AND CLASSIFICATION

Since androgenic alopecia is partly a hair density problem, it is helpful to look at the mathematics of male pattern baldness. Although these numbers are only approximations, they still are helpful in surgical planning and patient decision making. Since androgenic alopecia is also partly a hair location problem, a classification system makes it easier to describe the extent of frontal and vertex hair loss.

A. Mathematics of Balding

The average person with a full head of hair has approximately 100,000 hairs. Since an individual often does not perceive the hair loss until there is a 50% reduction in density, a typical patient with early stages of androgenic alopecia may present with only 50,000 follicular units on his scalp. Because as few as 25% of these hairs may be genetically stable, this leaves the hair transplant surgeon with only 12,500 follicular units to cover both the donor and recipient sites. Understanding the mathematics of hair density and available donor follicles is helpful in planning restoration surgery.

1. Hair density—normal hair density is approximately 2 hairs/mm^2 or 1 follicular group/mm^2. Since $\leq$50% loss in hair density will not be clinically noticeable, the surgeon only needs to restore a hair density of 1 follicular unit/2 mm^2 along the frontal edge to create a natural hairline. In areas behind the hairline, areas less than 50% of the original density can be hidden with hair styling.
2. Hair number—based on the observed natural history of male pattern balding, a patient presenting with 50,000 follicular units may be at risk of losing an additional 37,500 units (75%). This means that the remaining 12,500 follicular units must be used to cover both the donor and recipient sites. In most cases, half of the genetically stable available follicles can be used for grafting, since the other half must remain in the donor site to avoid donor site deformities. As such, only 6,500 follicular units are available to cover an area previously covered by 37,500 hairs. In other words, hair restoration surgery can only replace one-sixth of what the patient had to begin with. This clearly illustrates the point that increasing graft density is not the answer to the treatment of male pattern balding. Rather, by separating the grafts into smaller and smaller "units," more total grafts can be obtained, thus "spreading" the grafts out over a larger area.

B. Norwood Classification System

Although many classifications have been developed, the Norwood system has become the most widely used. It breaks down androgenic alopecia into seven stages and helps determine if the patient is a good candidate for hair restoration.

Norwood class	Balding areas: Temporal	Balding areas: Vertex	Candidate for surgery
Type I	Mild	None	Good
Type I_{Vertex}	(Same)	Minimal	Good
Type II	Moderate	None	Good
Type III	Extensive	None	Good
Type IV	Extensive	Mild	Good
Type V	Nearly complete	Moderate	Good
Type VI	Complete	Severe	Poor
Type VII	Complete	Complete	Poor

IV. INCIDENCE AND ETIOLOGY OF MALE PATTERN BALDNESS

Although as many as 95% of males may develop some mild forms of androgenic alopecia, it is usually not severe enough for most men to seek treatment. The following factors appear to be associated with severe androgenic alopecia:

1. Family history—a strong positive family history is the best predictor of the development of androgenic alopecia. A negative family history does not exclude the diagnosis, however. The genetic inheritance pattern is consistent with an autosomal dominant transmission with variable penetrance, but no linkage with a specific gene or set of genes has been made to date.
2. Race—the highest incidence of androgenic alopecia is in Caucasian, with a 50% incidence in men and women after age 40. Asian, Native American, and African American men have a much lower incidence. The severity is also usually much less (lower Norwood type).
3. Androgens—testosterone (or its metabolites) must be present to induce androgenic alopecia, but testosterone levels do not correlate with the severity of balding. On the other hand, castration prevents male pattern baldness, but does not reverse it once it has developed. Administration of subphysiologic exogenous testosterone will cause male pattern baldness in these castrated men.
4. Androgen metabolites—dihydrotestosterone (DHT) is the major metabolite produced by the enzyme 5α-reductase. DHT has been shown to be five times more potent than testosterone in producing benign prostatic hypertrophy, prostate cancer, hirsutism, acne vulgaris, and androgenic alopecia. In women, weak andro-

gens are converted by three enzymes in the skin to more potent androgens, such as testosterone or DHT.

5. 5α-Reductase—the enzyme required for converting testosterone to DHT. Patients with 5α-reductase deficiency do not develop androgenic alopecia, despite normal or slightly elevated levels of testosterone. This has proved that DHT, rather than testosterone, is the cause of androgenic alopecia. 5α-reductase exists as two isoenzymes, type I and type II. Type I 5α-reductase is predominant in the liver and the sebaceous glands of the skin. It is responsible for one-third of the circulating DHT. Type II 5α-reductase is primarily found in the prostate, seminal vesicles, epididymis, and hair follicles (as well as the liver). It is responsible for two-thirds of the circulating DHT. The expression of these two isoenzymes in normal males and subjects with 5α-reductase deficiency in different tissues has led to the following conclusions:
   - Androgens are not required for normal expression of scalp hair, but they are required for the nonscalp body hair.
   - DHT is required for full expression of beard, chest, and suprapubic hair, whereas testosterone is sufficient for the production of pubic and axillary hair.
   - DHT is required for the development of androgenic alopecia in men.
6. Androgen receptors—androgens are capable of producing seemingly paradoxical effects on hair follicles, inhibiting growth of scalp hair while stimulating the growth of facial hair in the same individual.

V. MEDICAL TREATMENT OF MALE PATTERN BALDNESS

The understanding of androgen metabolism, the role of DHT, and the enzyme 5α-reductase have helped in the development of several methods of treating androgenic alopecia medically. Although these drugs may halt or even reverse some of the hair loss, the main disadvantage is the need to continue the use of the drug indefinitely. The hair loss will recur or continue with discontinuation of the drug. The current methods for medically treating hair loss include:

1. Finasteride (Propecia, Proscar) is a competitive and specific inhibitor of the type II isoenzyme of 5α-reductase, which converts testosterone into DHT. Oral finasteride is effective in treating male pattern baldness and benign prostatic hypertrophy. In double-blind, placebo-controlled studies, finasteride has caused hair regrowth in anterior midscalp areas in patients with Norwood types II and III androgenic alopecia. In these same studies, hair regrowth was demonstrated in scalp vertex areas in patients with Norwood types II, III, IV, and V. Because finasteride has no affinity for the testosterone receptor, it does not have any androgenic or antiandrogenic effects. It also does not have any estrogen or progesterone effects.
2. Minoxidil (Rogaine, Apo-Gain, Gen-Minoxidil, Minoxigaine) is a potassium channel opener that can help slow or stop hair loss when used topically on the scalp. The mechanism whereby it affects androgenic alopecia is unclear, but research has shown that it stimulates follicular cell proliferation and activates prostaglandin synthesis. Others believe that minoxidil increases blood flow to the scalp skin, which in turn increases hair growth and preservation. Although hair regrowth with topical minoxidil does occur in some patients, it does not routinely occur in all patients. When hair regrowth occurs, it may be finer and thinner than the normal hair texture. Stronger topical solutions (5% vs. 2%) recently made available show increased efficacy. The product must be topically applied to the scalp twice a day, and it often takes months before any effect is noticeable.
3. Unproven hair loss products—hundreds of hair loss prevention remedies have been marketed with little or no evidence to prove their efficacy. These products generally fall into one of the following categories:
   - Scalp cleansers—these products "cleanse the scalp" of shampoos, conditioners, and hair spray that have "sullied" the scalp.
   - Nutritional products—these products claim that hair loss is due to poor nutrition and that nutritional supplements can correct this problem.
   - Scalp vibrators and massagers—these devices claim that scalp stimulation will result in follicle stimulation and hair growth.

VI. SURGICAL OPTIONS FOR MALE PATTERN BALDNESS

Although most of these procedures are no longer advocated, there are many options for the surgical treatment of androgenic alopecia. This section presents a short summary of the most widely used methods of the past and present. Many of these techniques have been used in combination to improve results.

A. Alopecia Reduction (Scalp Reduction)

Alopecia reduction is defined as the excision of an area of alopecia or prospective alopecia. Except for mild cases of isolated vertex alopecia, these procedures will not completely remove all of the balding scalp. For this reason, it is usually combined with other techniques, such as scalp expansion, scalp flaps, or hair grafts. The larger the area that can be removed, the less of an area will be left to cover with these other techniques. For this reason, the main role for alopecia reduction today is as an adjunct for the treatment of severe cases of male pattern baldness (Norwood types V, VI, and VII). The size of the area that can be excised is dependent on two factors:

1. Natural scalp laxity—this tends to be greater in older patients.
2. Surgical maneuvers to increase scalp laxity, such as undermining.

B. Scalp Extension

Scalp extension, or scalp stretching, is the technique of gradually stretching out the scalp with an elastic sheet (silicone) attached to a series of hooks (MXM Laboratories & Applied Biomaterials Technologies). The sheet is placed in the subgaleal space under the bald area, and stretched out to twice its original length. With the sheet under tension, the hooks are attached to the galea, and the device is left in place for 1 month. After this period of scalp stretching, the bald area is excised and the process repeated. The main advantage of this technique is that it avoids the disfigurement associated with tissue expansion, which is unacceptable to many patients. The main disadvantage is the unidirectional extension of the scalp (from lateral to medial). Multidirectional extenders that will bring the hairline forward have not been widely accepted yet.

C. Scalp Flaps

Scalp flaps were first developed as stand-alone methods to treat male pattern baldness. The most popular, described by Juri, was the parietal-occipital flap. These flap techniques would often require multiple stages, including flap delay, flap rotation, dog ear excision, and scar revisions. The one problem with these techniques that could not be improved with subsequent revisions was incorrect hair orientation. With the Juri flap, the hair orientation would be in the wrong direction, creating a very unnatural hairline. Without tissue expansion, tension at the flap donor site often produced unacceptable scars with significant donor-site alopecia. Recipient-site scars along the hairline were also difficult to hide. As a consequence, flap reconstruction without the use of tissue expansion has largely been abandoned.

D. Scalp Expansion with Flap Advancement or Rotation

Tissue expansion consists of subgaleal placement of a tissue expander under hair-bearing scalp. The expander is placed 6–12 weeks before expansion begins, after which weekly expansion is performed with saline infusion until the skin is overexpanded. After 6–12 weeks, the expander is removed and the hair-bearing scalp is advanced over the balding areas as a rotation or advancement flap. The balding areas are then excised, being replaced with expanded hair-bearing scalp. Many technical designs have been described for expander shape, positioning, and number of expanders used. Two of the most common techniques include:

1. Bilateral advancement transposition (BAT) flaps—this technique utilizes tissue expanders placed in a crescent-shaped formation under the genetically stable occipital and parietal hair follicles. The expanders are placed through an incision along the fringe of the receding hairline. The expanded occipital scalp is advanced toward the scalp vertex, and the expanded parietal scalp is rotated toward the forehead.
2. Triple advancement transposition (TAT) flaps—this technique utilizes a similar expansion strategy, but differs in that a posterior occipital random flap is raised and transposed, rather than just advanced (as in the BAT flap technique).

E. Strip Grafts

Strip grafts are useful for eyebrow reconstruction when harvested from the parietal area with correct orientation of the hair follicles (i.e., where the hair shafts are running laterally and obliquely). This technique has not been useful for treating male pattern baldness, however, becaue the donor hair is not spread out to a wider recipient area. There may be a significantly high rate of hair follicle loss as well due to delayed follicle neovascularization of the composite graft.

F. Graft Harvesting with Open Treatment of Donor Sites (Punch Graft Technique)

Trochars as large as 6–12 mm in diameter were used in the "rediscovery" of hair transplantation in the 1950s. These large punches had an unacceptably high rate of follicular loss in the center of the punches. This led to progressively smaller punch sizes. For technical reasons, 4 mm was accepted as the standard punch size. Problems included donor-site alopecia and scarring, as well as incorrect orientation of hair "plugs," giving the patient a very unnatural hairline. These large punches were inefficient and limited the number of grafts that could be harvested. As a consequence, only 20–50 grafts were usually harvested at a time. The donor site wounds would heal by secondary intention, which required a prolonged period of time between grafting sessions.

G. Graft Harvesting with Closure of Donor Sites (Mini- and Micrografting Techniques)

With time, punch graft techniques were abandoned in favor of strip-graft harvesting and primary closure of the hair donor site with sutures. This greatly reduced the donor site deformity and allowed the surgeon to section the strips into smaller "units" that could be spread over a larger recipient area. Initially, single-blade scalpels were used to harvest the strips, but it was difficult to create separate parallel incisions without injuring or destroying many hair follicles. Then, multi-blade scalpels were developed that allowed the surgeon to make simultaneous parallel incisions, thereby harvesting multiple thin strips that were easier to section. Grafts were then categorized by the number of hair follicles per "unit." The common "units" were categorized as follows:

1. Minigrafts—small "follicular units" consisting of 2–4 terminal follicles, 1 (or rarely 2) vellus follicle, associated sebaceous lobules, insertions of arrector pili muscles, perifollicular vascular plexus, neural net, and fine adventitial collagen. These "follicular units" have high follicular survival rates (>90%) with minimal donor-site scarring. Their only disadvantage is that the "clumps" of hairs are noticeable at the hairline.
2. Micrografting—in an effort to create a perfectly natural hairline with no apparent signs of surgical hair "reorganization," smaller "units" consisting of 1–2 terminal follicles have become increasingly more popular not just for hairline reconstruction, but for entire areas. The main disadvantage of micrografting techniques is the increased time for graft sectioning and graft transplantation, since the same amount of donor scalp can produce many more grafts. Without taking appropriate technical precautions to avoid follicular trauma, there is a potentially higher chance of damaging the follicles when sectioning them into micrografts when compared to minigrafts.

H. Technical Refinements in Follicular Unit Grafting

With the growing popularity of "follicular unit" grafting, many refinements have been developed to reduce follicular trauma and decrease graft loss. The following technical advancements have been developed and advocated, although they have not all been universally adopted by hair restoration surgeons.

1. Single-strip harvesting—although simultaneous multistrip harvesting was developed as a time-saving method, many authors now believe that 3- and 4-bladed scalpels often transect many follicles even before they can be sectioned into follicular units. As a consequence, most authors believe that harvesting one thin strip at a time with either a single blade or two closely spaced parallel blades will result in the lowest follicle transection rate during graft harvest.
2. Microscope-assisted strip sectioning—follicular dissection consists of dividing the donor strip into smaller strips, then dividing the smaller strips into follicular units. The dissecting microscope provides much better visualization by magnifying the strip by 5–6 times, compared to 2–3.5 times surgical loupe magnification. Microscopes usually provide better illumination than overhead lights or headlights, as well. Studies have demonstrated both an increase in the number of hairs successfully sectioned and an increase in graft survival when microscopic

dissection was used versus loupe magnification. Most studies now conclude that microscope dissection yields a 5–10% increase in graft yield (graft number and graft survival).

3. Illumination — good lighting is vital for both the harvest and graft preparation, whether or not a microscope is used.
4. Automated implanters—although follicular unit grafting provides more grafts and more natural hairlines, more units must be implanted, which is more time consuming. The smaller grafts also require more skill to implant and are more susceptible to trauma. The Rapid Fire Hair Implanter (Carousel) has been developed to address these problems. The device creates a recipient site with a knife, then "drags" the graft into the site as the knife is withdrawn. The "dragging technique" reduces hand motion and avoids compression or bending of the follicle. As a consequence, the speed is increased and graft trauma is decreased.

VII. CURRENTLY USED TECHNIQUES FOR THE SURGICAL TREATMENT OF MALE PATTERN BALDNESS

Current trends in hair restoration have been driven by the patient's desire for more natural-looking hair. Invisible scars, uniform hair density in transplanted and untransplanted areas, and hair shafts oriented in a normal orientation have now become the standard that patients expect and demand. As a result, fewer and fewer patients will accept the scars associated with flaps and punch graft donor sites, the temporary disfigurement associated with tissue expanders, or the irregular density or contour ("corn rows," "cobblestoning") associated with punch graft recipient sites. For this reason, almost all hair restoration surgeons use "follicular units" of 1–4 terminal hairs per graft as the first line of therapy. Although much can be said for the continued usefulness of alopecia reduction, scalp extension, and scalp expansion with advancement/rotation flaps (BAT, TAT), these techniques are still often combined with "follicular unit" transplantation.

117

Liposuction and Body Contouring

Lloyd M. Krieger, M.D., Marc H. Hedrick, M.D., and Peter B. Fodor, M.D., F.A.C.S.
David Geffen School of Medicine at UCLA, Los Angeles, California, U.S.A.

Liposuction is the most commonly performed cosmetic surgery procedure in the United States. The market for liposuction has been growing at a rate of 35% per year since 1992, according to data from the American Society of Plastic Surgeons. While it may seem among the simplest of the procedures performed by plastic surgeons, there is the potential for unfavorable cosmetic results and high morbidity. This chapter will describe the anatomic and surgical principles of liposuction and endermologie.

I. LIPOSUCTION

A. Anatomy

1. Gender differences in fat distribution are pronounced. Women tend to accumulate fat in the hips, lower trunk, upper thighs, and buttocks. Men tend to accumulate fat evenly around the entire trunk.
2. Surgical fat layers determine the safest planes to perform liposuction. These layers are best defined in the torso and thighs:
   - The deep layer is composed of loose fatty tissue with few septae.
   - The superficial layer is composed of denser fat within firm fibrous septae.
   - The deep layer is quite "forgiving" when subjected to liposuction. The superficial layer must be approached with caution as it is prone to surface irregularities as a result of treatment.
3. Five "zones of adherence" display close adherence between the skin and underlying fat. Liposuction is contraindicated in these areas as it is likely to result in contour irregularities. These areas include the following:
   - Inferolateral iliotibial tract
   - Gluteal crease
   - Lateral gluteal depression
   - Middle medial thigh
   - Distal posterior thigh

B. Technique

1. Wetting solution, or subcutaneous infiltration, is an essential part of liposuction:
   - Rationale for subcutaneous infiltration is that it promotes ease of fat aspiration, helps to achieve even contour, aids in hemostasis, and minimizes patient discomfort.
   - Components of the subcutaneous infiltrate include a base fluid of normal saline or lactated Ringer's solution. Epinephrine is generally added to this solution. Lidocaine and/or bupivicaine for analgesia may also

be used. Some add gentamicin for infection prophylaxis and hyaluronidase to potentially aid in lipolysis.

- Lidocaine toxicity must be avoided. Traditionally, the maximum allowed dose of plain lidocaine is said to be 5 mg/kg; it rises to 7 mg/kg when combined with epinephrine. The accepted maximum safe dose when used in conjunction with liposuction is 35 mg/kg. In liposuction, this higher dose is accepted because the lidocaine is injected into the fat layer of subcutaneous tissues with epinephrine, which delays systemic absorption, and much of the lidocaine is immediately removed as part of the liposuction aspirate.
- The sequence of infiltration is such that infusion is generally done sequentially for each body area treated (to minimize overall fluid and pharmacologic load) and with a 10- to 20-minute latency period prior to aspiration (to allow for epinephrine to have a maximal vasoconstrictive effect).
- The typical volume of infusion has evolved over the last 10–15 years. Table 1 shows the various techniques, including the overall volume infused as well as the resulting amount of blood in the aspirate. The "tumescent" technique was originally developed so that liposuction could be performed in the office setting, with minimal additional anesthesia. Most plastic surgeons now use the "superwet" technique in conjunction with some form of sedation or anesthesia.

2. Cannulas have also evolved over the last 10–15 years. Originally, large-bore sharp cannulas with a single suction hole were the mainstay of treatment. Now, smaller-bore cannulas (2–3 mm) are often used to minimize contour irregularities. Cannulas with a single aspiration hole now represent just one type of cannula in the armamentarium of suction devices. Variations in cannula design may include a hole at the tip of the cannula, on one side of the end of the cannula, or the "Mercedes" tip that includes three holes at the tip of the cannula. Blunt tips are now standard, as they serve to minimize overly aggressive dissection with the cannula tip and resulting contour defects.
3. Pretunneling serves to establish an even plane for later suctioning. This is performed in one of two ways. Some surgeons use the suction cannula for pretunneling but keep the suction inactive. Others do it at the same time they inject subcutaneously with specialized injection cannulas.
4. Overlapping cannula movement helps to determine the cosmetic result. This "cross-hatching" motion serves to create an even contour. The technique uses multiple access incisions for each area treated so that they are approached with radially overlapping passes with the cannula. Different anatomic areas are approached through different directions. Examples are shown in Figures 1–3.
5. Feathering of edges helps to eliminate step-offs between suctioned areas and surrounding non-treated areas. It is achieved through minimal suctioning around those areas that have been subjected to the greatest amount of liposuction treatment.
6. Superficial suctioning, though once considered unsafe under all circumstances, is slowly gaining growing acceptance as part of liposuction procedures. It must be done with extreme caution, however, because of the increased risk of complications. Important steps to assure safety include the use of small-bore cannulas, careful pretunneling, and keeping cannula holes pointed away from the dermis.

Table 1 Subcutaneous Infiltration Volumes

Technique	Infiltrate	Hematocrit of aspirate (%)
Dry	No infiltrate	20–40
Wet	200–300 cc/treated area	4–10
Superwet	1 cc infiltrate:1 cc estimated aspirate	1
Tumescent	2–3 cc infiltrate:1 cc estimated aspirate	1

C. Complications

1. Perforations of the underlying fascia, peritoneum, and abdominal structures have been reported during liposuction, but these events are quite rare. They can be minimized with careful pretunneling to establish an even layer for later (more aggressive) suctioning, and constant attention to the location of the cannula tip.

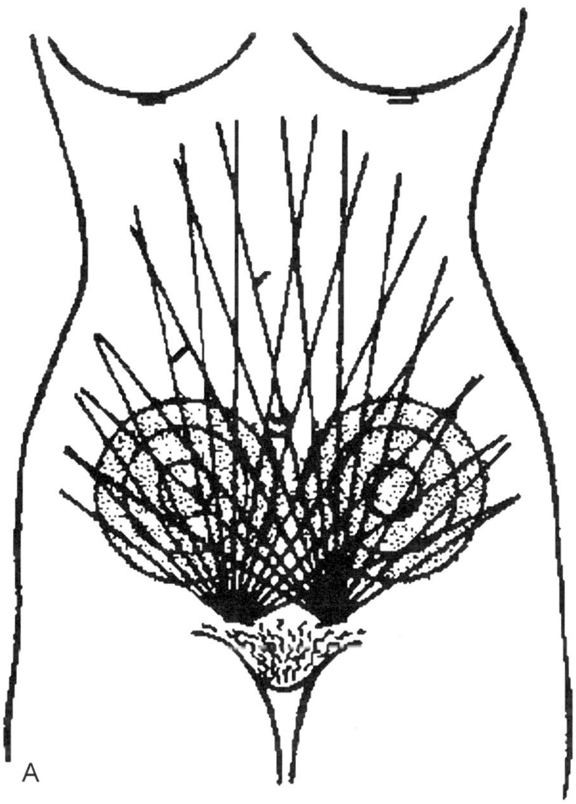

Figure 1 Direction of cannula passage for liposuction of abdomen.

2. Fluid balance must be closely monitored. This is especially true in cases of "large-volume" liposuction, which is generally defined as greater than 4 liters of aspirate. These procedures should be performed with the patient's urine output monitored intraoperatively and postoperatively with a Foley catheter. Liposuction results in physiologic fluid shifts similar to patients who suffer burn injury. For this reason, patients who have more than 1500–2500 cc of aspirate removed generally need postoperative intravenous fluids. With larger volume of subcutaneous infiltration, particularly using the tumescent technique, patients must also be monitored for fluid overload. Indeed, if volume status is not closely monitored in cases of large volume liposuction, patients may suffer severe fluid overload, pulmonary edema, or hypovolemia.
3. Blood loss used to be a major concern with liposuction, with many authorities quoting various formulas for recommended transfusions according to the volumes of aspirate. Recent advances in wetting solutions have radically decreased the need for transfusions, but there is always the risk of bleeding during and after the procedure. Attention to blood loss is crucial. The "rule of 150" predicts that the patient's hematocrit will fall 1% for each 150 cc of fat aspirated. A 3-liter suctioning will thus lead to a 20% decline in the patient's hematocrit. This rule was generated based on using 15–30 cc of wetting solution per 100 cm^2 of area treated. New, higher-volume approaches to wetting solution will decrease blood loss from the rule's predicted values.
4. Contour irregularities can negatively impact the cosmetic results of liposuction. These manifest as dents or waves in areas subjected to treatment. They can be minimized by confining suction to the deep layer of fat or treating the superficial layer of fat with extreme caution, pretunneling, avoidance of the "zones of adherence," and the

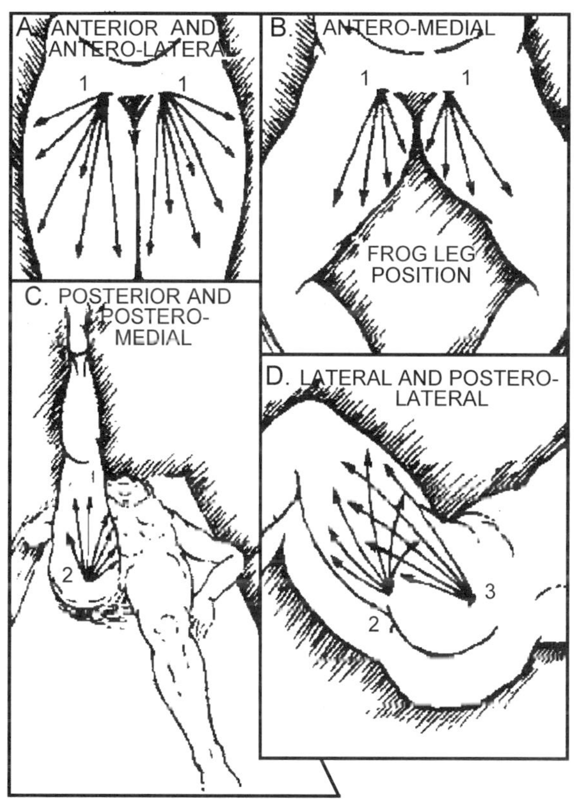

Figure 2 Incisions and cannula passage for liposuction of inner and outer thighs.

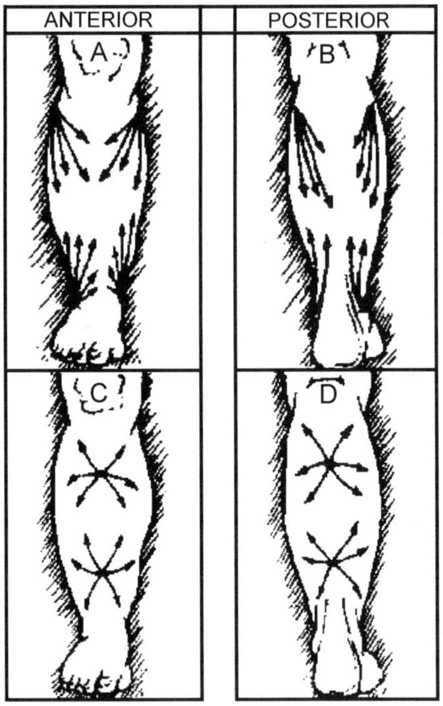

Figure 3 Incisions and cannula passage for liposuction of calves and ankles.

use of wetting solution. When they do occur, contour defects are difficult to treat. Possible remedies include repeat suction to attempt to even out the superficial fat layer, fat transplants to the deepened areas, and direct excision of particularly glaring contour defects.

5. Seromas and ecchymoses may occur with liposuction and can be minimized with the use of pressure garments postoperatively. Many surgeons treat their patients for 6 weeks postoperatively with the garments. Some add further padding to these garments in the form of Reston® foam or bulky surgical dressings in order to apply additional pressure to treated areas.
6. Hypesthesia is a common, though typically transient, problem that occurs in essentially all treated areas. Normal sensation generally returns within 6 months.
7. Deep vein thrombosis and fat embolism have been reported following liposuction. Pneumatic pressure devices are recommended for medium- and large-volume procedures.

D. Ultrasonic-Assisted Liposuction (UAL)

1. The physiology behind UAL differs from that of traditional liposuction. In the traditional technique, fat tissue is avulsed, broken apart, and then evacuated under suction. UAL treats subcutaneous tissue with ultrasonic energy. This results in cavitation, which serves to "liquefy" the fat by means of cellular emulsification. The cellular contents accumulate in the interstitial space. This material is then aspirated using a hollow cannula.
2. The results of UAL, despite an initial burst of enthusiasm on the part of surgeons and the public, have not been clearly shown to be superior to those of traditional liposuction. UAL may offer added benefits in fibrous areas, such as in the gynecomastic breast, in the buttock, and with secondary liposuction procedures. Since it supplies its own source of energy to break up fatty tissue, rather than relying on mechanical effort to avulse it, UAL is said to be less tiresome for the surgeon in difficult or long procedures.
3. The current recommended technique for UAL combines UAL with traditional liposuction. Wetting solution is essential for the ultrasonic energy to travel in the subcutaneous space. After infusion, UAL is used first, and then traditional aspiration techniques are applied to evacuate the treated contents. This helps to speed the procedure (UAL is slower than the traditional method because of the time required for cavitation) and minimize the risk of seroma.
4. Complications of UAL are the same as those of traditional liposuction, along with those related to the use of ultrasonic energy within the subcutaneous space. This energy can generate heat (particularly at the cannula tip), and care must be taken to keep the cannula moving so that thermal burns do not occur. Care must also be taken to protect access incisions from repeated bursts of ultrasonic energy. UAL also serves to liquefy a great deal of fatty tissue within the subcutaneous space, leading to an increased incidence of seroma. At the conclusion of the procedure, all liquefied tissue must be thoroughly evacuated.

II. ENDERMOLOGIE

A. Cellulite is a term that describes the dimpling of skin often seen in the thighs and buttocks. It most commonly affects women. The physiology of cellulite is thought to involve the anatomy of the superficial layer of fat in these areas. The adipose tissue is separated into pockets by fibrous septae that are firmly attached to the overlying skin. When there is hypertrophy of the fatty tissue, the fat pockets expand. The septae remain anchored to the skin. The result is bulging of these fat pockets between the intact septae.

B. Endermologie gained prominence in France in the early 1990s. The process consists of 12–14 treatments with a device that vacuums and then massages the skin of areas affected by cellulite. Although some surgeons note positive results in terms of both cosmetic improvement and patient satisfaction, no large well-controlled studies have documented these results as of yet.

118

Abdominoplasty

Alan Matarasso, M.D.
New York, New York, U.S.A.

Victor Schingo, M.D.
Schenectady, New York, U.S.A.

I. INTRODUCTION

Despite different cultures and fashions, the appearance of an ideal abdominal contour has remained relatively constant over the ages. The appearance of a narrow waistline with full hips in a female is rooted in the mating aspects of evolutionary psychology. Diet, exercise, and lifestyle modifications are considered appropriate means, often in conjunction with surgery by which one can rejuvenate the waistline and abdominal region. However, acquired abdominal disfigurement (e.g., from pregnancy, aging, or massive weight change) may be more suitable to surgical intervention, particularly if nonsurgical methods fail to improve the appearance of the abdomen. The purpose of this chapter is to provide guidelines for the diagnosis, evaluation, and treatment of patients seeking abdominal contour improvement.

II. DIAGNOSIS AND PATIENT EVALUATION

The etiology of acquired abdominal contour deformities stems from weight fluctuations, pregnancy, prior abdominal surgery, genetics, hormones, medications, and age-related changes. During the examination of patients considering abdominal contour surgery, the focus is on the treatable soft-tissue layers of the abdomen, which include skin, subcutaneous adipose tissue, and the musculofascial layer. In addition, the nontreatable causes of abdominal disfigurement, such as intraperitoneal fat (intra-abdominal or apple fat) position or size of pelvic organs, and lumbar lordosis, should be noted and brought to the patient's attention.

A. Skin—the quality, tone, laxity, presence of striae gravidarum, and location of previous surgical scars should be noted during the evaluation of the skin.

B. Adipose layer:

- This layer is examined for excess fat as it is distributed among the aesthetic units of the abdomen.
- In addition, the width, height, and thickness of the mons pubis are also noted. The mons often needs treatment during abdominal contour surgery to bring the entire abdomen into aesthetic balance. Liposuction and wedge reduction (both vertical and horizontal) are the most common techniques used to treat the mons.

C. Musculofascial layer—this layer is carefully examined for the presence of abdominal wall hernias (i.e., umbilical or ventral), generalized weakness, or diastasis of the rectus abdominis muscle.

D. After the examination is complete, patients are classified according to the abdominolipoplasty

Table 1 Abdominolipoplasty Classification System. It is based on an evaluation of the skin, fat, and musculofascial systems

Category	Skin	Fat	Musculofascial system	Treatment
Type I	Minimal laxity	Variable	Minimal flaccidity	SAL alone
Type II	Mild laxity	Variable	Mild lower abdominal laxity	Mini abdominoplasty
Type III	Moderate laxity	Variable	Moderate lower or upper abdominal flaccidity	Modified abdominoplasty
Type IV	Severe laxity	Variable	Significant lower or upper abdominal flaccidity	Standard abdominoplasty with or without SAL

Source: Reprinted with permission from Clin Plast Surg, April 1989.

system of diagnosis and treatment (Table 1). This classification system stratifies patients into four categories (Types I–IV) based on skin, adipose, and musculofascial pathology. It incorporates liposuction as a primary treatment modality (Type I) as well as an adjunct to more excisional procedures (Types II–IV).

III. ANATOMY

Before discussing specific surgical options available to treat abdominal contour deformities, an understanding of the pertinent anatomy of the abdominal wall is necessary. The anatomy of the abdominal wall can be divided into topographic, vascular, musculofascial, and nervous systems.

A. Topography

1. The abdomen is divided into six aesthetic units in men and seven in women, based on areas of fat accumulation that are of concern to patients.
2. For men, the units include the epigastrium, periumbilical region, lower abdomen, mons pubis, flanks, and sacrum.
3. The dorsal back roll is the seventh aesthetic region, which is seen in women when examining the posterior trunk.
4. These units are particularly helpful in preoperative planning for suction-assisted lipectomy when used either as a primary modality or as an adjunctive procedure.

B. Vascular

1. The arterial supply of the abdomen has been previously described by Huger and can be divided into three anatomic zones (Fig. 1).
2. In the unoperated abdomen, the primary blood supply is from the deep superior and inferior epigastric arcades (Huger zone I). When the blood supply is interrupted, such as during the elevation of the abdominoplasty flap, secondary vascular arcades become the dominant supply.
3. The secondary arcades include the subcostal, intercostal, and lumbar perforators (Huger zone III), as well as a minor contribution via retrograde flow into the superficial circumflex iliac system from the deep circumflex iliac system (Huger zone II).
4. When combining flap undermining during abdominoplasty with suction-assisted lipectomy (especially in the scarred abdomen), the surgeon attempts to preserve the integrity of these secondary vascular arcades in order to avoid flap ischemia and necrosis. The region of the flap most susceptible to ischemia is known as the "terrible abdominoplasty triangle" that is located between the "neo-umbilicus" and the mons pubis.

C. Musculofascial System

1. The muscular anatomy of the abdominal wall can essentially be viewed in two layers.
2. The superficial or vertical layer is composed of the paired rectus abdominis and external oblique muscles, which primarily act to flex the torso.
3. The deeper or horizontal layer is composed of the internal oblique and the transversus abdominis muscles. In addition, the aponeurosis of both the internal oblique and transversus abdominis muscles pass anterior to the rectus abdominis below the arcuate line of Douglas, creating an inherent anatomic weakness in this region due to the lack of the posterior rectus sheath.

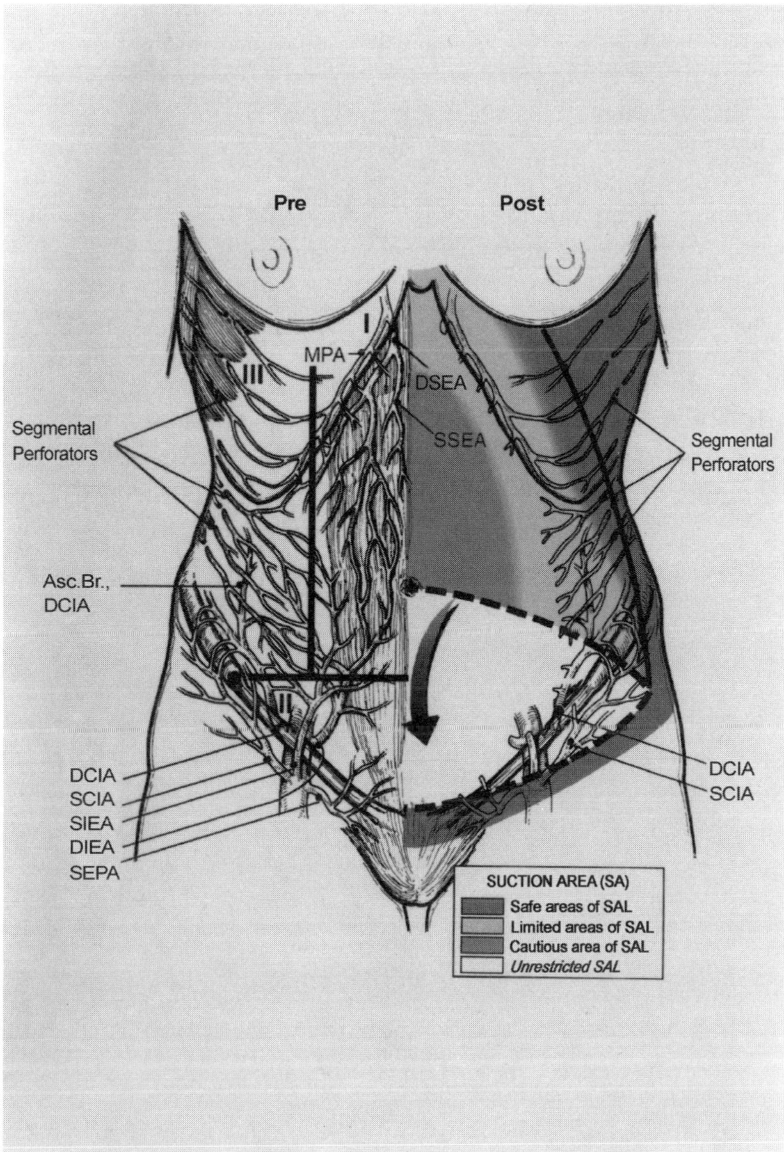

Figure 1 (Left) Pre: The blood supply to the anterior abdominal wall. Note Huger zones I to III. (Right) Post: Vascular anatomy in the postabdominoplasty patient and its relationship to potential areas of suction lipectomy. DSEA = deep superior epigastric artery; SSEA = superficial superior epigastric artery; MPA = marginal phrenic artery; DIEA = deep inferior epigastric artery; DCIA = deep circumflex iliac artery; SCIA = superficial circumflex iliac artery; SIEA = superficial inferior epigastric artery; SEPA = superficial external pudendal artery; segmental perforators (zone III) = intercostal, subcostal, lumbar arteries. (Reprinted with permission from *Plast. Reconstr. Surg.*, April 1995.)

4. In women who have previously had children, there is an even greater tendency for lower abdominal musculofascial laxity and diastasis of the rectus muscle.
5. Additionally, the effects of pregnancy on the appearance of the abdomen include both transient (e.g., linea nigra) and permanent (e.g., striae) cutaneous alterations. Moreover, intra-abdominal and skeletal changes occur in pregnancy.

D. Innervation

1. In general, the innervation of the abdominal wall is segmentally supplied by the lateral cutaneous branches of the intercostal nerves.

2. The lateral femoral cutaneous nerve is of particular surgical significance because of the risk of entrapment during deep wound closure for up to 6 cm within the region of the anterior superior iliac spine.
3. The ilioinguinal and iliohypogastric nerves are also susceptible to injury during wound closure and rectus muscle plication, leading to recognizable deficits.
4. Entrapment of any these nerves can lead to persistent postoperative pain and dysesthesjas.

IV. SURGICAL TECHNIQUES

When choosing a particular surgical technique to treat abdominal contour deformities, the abdominolipoplasty system of diagnosis and treatment is a useful initial guide that is then reconciled with the patient's tolerance for the morbidity associated with each procedure (Fig. 2).

A. Type I: Suction-Assisted Lipectomy

1. Patients who are candidates for suction alone have minimal cutaneous and musculofascial laxity with a variable amount of adipose tissue. The primary aim is fat removal to restore a more youthful and contoured appearance to the abdomen.
2. Preoperatively, areas of excess adipose tissue are marked with the patient standing.

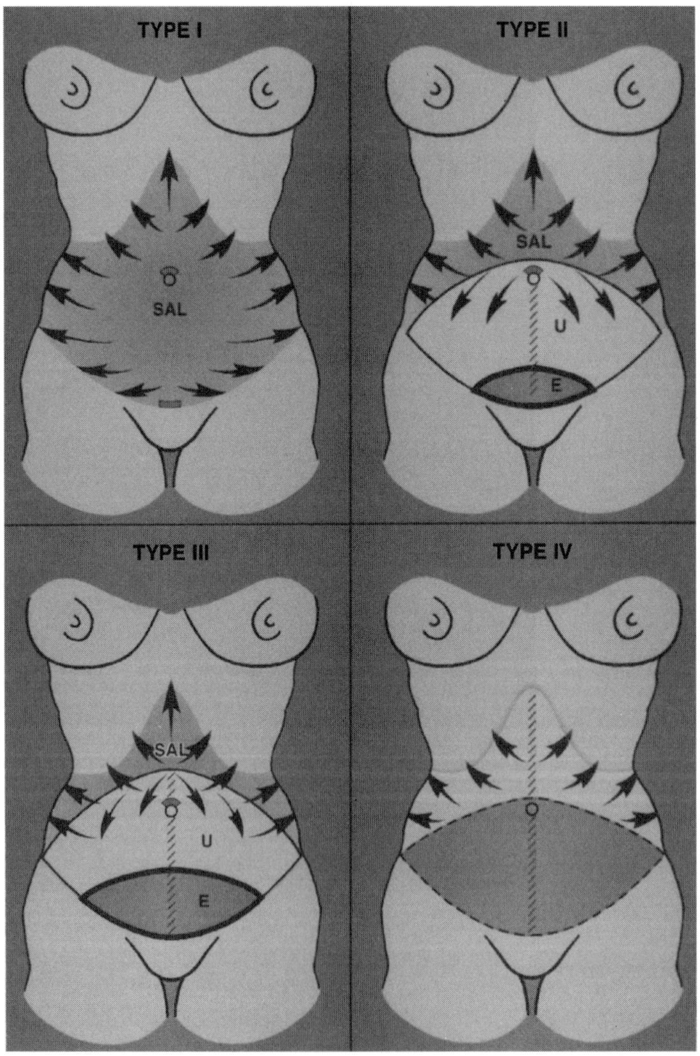

Figure 2 Abdominolipoplasty Types I–IV surgical techniques. (Reprinted with permission from *Clin. Plast. Surg.*, April 1989.)

3. Superwet fluid (1 liter of Ringer's lactate, 20 cc of 1% lidocaine, and 1 cc of 1:1000 epinephrine) is evenly infiltrated into the subcutaneous space in the areas to be treated.
4. Liposuction is then performed with small-caliber mercedes cannulas through inconspicuous pubic and umbilical access incisions.
5. The ultimate success of any liposuction procedure is dependent on the capability of the skin to contract after suctioning. Therefore, in patients with significantly damaged skin (e.g., flaccid skin or pregnancy-induced striae), its ability to shrink after treatment is limited. In these patients, an excisional procedure may be the best treatment option. Nevertheless, liposuction remains the most commonly performed and requested surgical procedure for abdominal contour deformities.

B. Type II: Mini-Abdominoplasty

1. The ideal candidate for this procedure has mild skin laxity and musculofascial flaccidity primarily limited to the infraumbilical region.
2. The procedure begins with liposuction as indicated. An incision approximately 6–10 cm in length is placed at the level of the pubic hairline and the upper flap is elevated in the suprafascial plane to the level of the umbilicus. The musculofascial diastasis is plicated in the midline from the umbilicus to the pubic region. A small ellipse of skin is excised, and the wound is closed in layers over suction drains.
3. Occasionally, patients may undergo a panniculectomy of the lower abdomen without any flap undermining.

C. Type III: Modified Abdominoplasty

1. Patients suitable for modified abdominoplasty have moderate skin excess and musculofascial laxity that is not necessarily confined to the lower abdomen. In addition, these patients may have previous upper abdominal scars (i.e., subcostal scar) that may limit the extent of safe flap undermining routinely performed in full abdominoplasties.
2. As with Type II patients, the procedure is begun with liposuction as needed. In order to excise more skin, a larger curvilinear incision is made at the level of the pubic hairline and is usually confined to the area between the anterior superior iliac spines. The abdominal flap is elevated to a level above the umbilicus and any musculofascial laxity is plicated in the midline from the umbilicus to the pubis. If needed, additional plication sutures can be placed above the level of the umbilicus by retracting the intact umbilical stalk. The table is flexed minimally, excess skin is excised, and the wound is closed as described previously for Type II patients.
3. In certain situations, such as in long-waisted individuals or when the umbilicus is tethering the abdominal flap during wound closure, the umbilical stalk can be transected at its base and translocated (floated) inferiorly with the upper abdominal flap. If this is done, the fascial defect at the site of transection should be repaired, and the umbilicus is sutured to the fascia at its new location. In order to preserve proper aesthetic proportions, the new umbilicus should not be relocated to greater than 2–3 cm below its previous position (approximately 10 cm superior to the top of the pubic hairline).

D. Type IV: Full Abdominoplasty

1. A full abdominoplasty is reserved for patients who have more significant skin laxity and musculofascial flaccidity in both the upper and lower abdomen.
2. The procedure begins with liposuction as indicated. In these patients, suction-assisted lipectomy is useful to treat residual "dog-ear," flank fullness, or to reduce the thickness of the upper abdominal flap. However, when performing liposuction in the region from the inframammary fold to the inguinal crease in combination with full abdominoplasty, the surgeon should be aware that the contribution from the dominant blood supply to the undermined flap stems from this region (Huger zone III). This is also referred to as suction area one (SA-1), which is the lateral-most zone depicted in Figure 1. Therefore, every effort should be made to preserve the blood supply by performing limited liposuction, parallel to the vessels in one or two sites only, and for a limited distance (15–20 cm). Additionally, caution should be used when suctioning the central upper abdominal flap (SA-3), since it has a random blood supply. This area corresponds to suction areas 2 and 3 as one moves laterally to medially on the abdominal wall, as shown in Figure 1. Therefore, flap thickness should be

maintained by preserving the fat between Scarpa's fascia and the dermis.

3. Following liposuction, the umbilicus is circumscribed and freed from the surrounding skin. The upper abdominal skin incision is made in a vest-over-pants fashion. The upper flap is undermined superolaterally to the level of the xyphoid and costal margins in an inverted "V" type fashion in order to maintain the lateral intercostal blood supply from Huger zone III. Rectus musculofascial diastasis is repaired vertically with a "0" nylon loop suture and 2-0 neurolon sutures.
4. The wound is closed in layers over drains with absorbable sutures and staples.
5. The umbilicus is palpated through the abdominal wound, a full-thickness 2.5 cm curvilinear incision is made, and the umbilicus is exteriorized. The skin flaps are defatted and the umbilicus sutured in place and then packed with preform gauze.

V. MINIMAL ACCESS VARIATIONS IN ABDOMINOPLASTY

The abdominolipoplasty system can subdivide most abdominal contour patients into four pathological groups. However, there are additional smaller subsets of patients who benefit from an additional subgroup classification system known as the minimal access variations in abdominoplasty (Types 1a–3a). These represent offshoots from the standard Type I–IV categories.

A. Type 1a: Extended Liposuction

1. Extended liposuction in this context is defined by the treated layers (superficial and deep fat), extent (multiple areas), and volume (up to 2000 cc total lipoaspirate).
2. Patients who are candidates for this procedure have an abundance of adipose tissue but do not require skin or muscle treatment.
3. The success of this procedure depends on skin that has good tone and a reasonable potential to contract after the removal of a substantial volume of adipose tissue or pseudoptotic skin that is not irreversibly damaged.

B. Type 2a: "Open" Mini-Abdominoplasty

1. Patients who fall into this subgroup have a previous vertical lower midline scar and lower abdominal laxity.
2. Liposuction is performed as indicated.
3. The old vertical scar is excised and muscle tightening is performed through this incision. Consequently, no additional incisions are necessary.

C. Type 3a: Endoscopically Assisted Abdominoplasty (Muscle Access Abdominoplasty)

1. These patients have abdominal wall pathology characterized by minimal skin excess and upper/lower rectus abdominis muscular flaccidity.
2. Liposuction access sites are made and standard liposuction is performed as needed. The diastasis of the rectus abdominis muscles can be visualized and treated utilizing a fiberoptic scope.
3. A rare group of patients with minimal skin laxity and extensive diastasis extending to the xyphoid require endoscopic-assisted muscular closure.

VI. ADDITIONAL CONCEPTS IN MINIMAL-ACCESS ABDOMINAL CONTOURING

A. Downstaging

1. This term refers to the downward deviation from a more extensive to a less invasive surgical procedure. The decision to perform the less extensive procedure is based on the patient's preferences and on an analysis of risk factors that may mandate a less invasive procedure. Often patients who are downstaged from an open procedure to a closed (liposuction) procedure can still achieve good results.
2. Smaller incisions are ultimately needed.

B. Access Abdominoplasty

1. This also refers to a conceptual approach in abdominal contour surgery where the large abdominoplasty incision is used as an "access" site to perform additional procedures. For example, breast augmentation, liposuction, and lateral thigh lifting can be performed through this incision.
2. Ultimately, fewer incisions are needed to perform these additional procedures.

VII. SPECIAL CONSIDERATIONS

A. Male Abdominal Contour Surgery

1. In general male skin tone is better than females; consequently males most often undergo liposuction

of the abdomen or a full abdominoplasty. The limited abdominoplasties are infrequently indicated.

2. Intra-abdominal adiposity will not be improved with any form of abdominal contour surgery that is seen increasingly in males as they age and in perimenopausal females. In these circumtances rectus muscle plication will enlarge the waist line.

B. Secondary Abdominal Contour Surgery

1. Reoperative surgery occurs either early (<18 months) or late (>18 months) versus a revision or complete redo surgery.
2. The most common indication for repeating abdominal contour surgery is for additional liposuction or wound margin revisions.

VIII. COMPLICATIONS

Complications associated with abdominal contour surgery can be discussed by individual category of treatment (i.e., SAL); time in which they occur (early vs. late); and whether they are local or systemic in nature.

A. Types I and 1a

1. Contour deformities, errors in patient classification and diagnosis, and fluid balance are the most commonly encountered problems.
2. Patient satisfaction hinges on proper patient selection and their education and understanding of the limits and benefits of the procedure.

B. Limited Abdominoplasties (Types II, 2a, III, and 3a)

1. Fluid collections and pseudobursa formation (from persistent fluid collections) are seen.
2. Errors in diagnosis and classification can occur when performing these procedures on patients with excess skin that requires more extensive skin resection (e.g., Type IV) for adequate correction.

C. Full Abdominoplasties (Type IV)

1. Local complications such as wound dehiscence, fluid collections, skin ischemia, unsightly scarring, and nerve entrapment syndromes can be seen.
2. Systemic complications are potentially more common in this group of patients and include but are not limited to pulmonary complications such as atelectasis, pulmonary embolus/deep vein thrombosis, pulmonary fat embolism syndrome, anesthesia complications, blood transfusions, and death.

IX. CONCLUSION

The introduction of suction-assisted lipectomy has permanently altered body contour surgery. Utilizing the abdominolipoplasty system of classification and treatment, liposuction has become a primary treatment modality as well as an adjunct to more traditional excisional techniques. Now there are a variety of procedures available to successfully treat patients with a wider range of deformities.

119

Body Contouring with Excisional Surgery

Timothy D. Santoro, M.D., and Marc H. Hedrick, M.D.
David Geffen School of Medicine at UCLA, Los Angeles, California, U.S.A.

I. GENERAL PRINCIPLES

A. Patients with body contour deformities, primarily due to poor skin and soft-tissue tone, frequently do not benefit from liposuction alone. Severe degrees of skin excess may occur secondary to massive weight loss, senile skin laxity, and contour abnormalities following liposuction. These patients are good candidates for body contour surgery. Although liposuction and body contour surgery are easily combined, liposuction of significant localized fat deposits 3–4 months prior to the latter is recommended.

B. Lockwood has described the repair of the superficial fascial system (SFS) in relation to excisional body contour surgery. Repair of the SFS with permanent sutures provides a more secure wound closure with a decreased risk of hypertrophic scarring or scar widening.

C. Patient selection is important in obtaining optimal results. Liposuction may be preferable for younger patients with good skin tone, and weight loss is indicated in obese patients. Those patients using nicotine in any form should not undergo excisional body contour surgery.

II. BRACHIOPLASTY

A. Pathophysiology and Indications

1. Posteromedial arm soft tissues are suspended by a tough, dynamic fascial system sling that ultimately derives its strength from the clavicular periosteum, clavipectoral fascia, and axillary fascia. Loosening of the arm SFS from these structural support results in skin and soft tissue laxity.
2. Liposuction is generally reported to have poor results in these areas, and most authors report superior results with direct excision.
3. Patients undergoing surgical brachioplasty must be willing to accept a longitudinal scar along the inner aspect of the arm that extends from the axilla to the elbow.
4. Abnormal scars, disproportionate resection, and other wound complications are potential problems following brachioplasty.
5. Partly because of the resulting scar, the popularity of this procedure remains low. Brachioplasty accounted for only 0.16 % of all cosmetic procedures performed in the United States in 1994.

B. Markings

1. The shoulder is abducted and the elbow flexed.
2. For the Lockwood brachioplasty (Fig. 1a), a vertical ellipse of redundant axillary tissue is marked initially within the axillary fold. The lateral line of the ellipse is angular at two points; these facilitate closure of the axillary wound. The inferior angle position is determined by digitally forcing the lax arm tissues into the axillary dome.

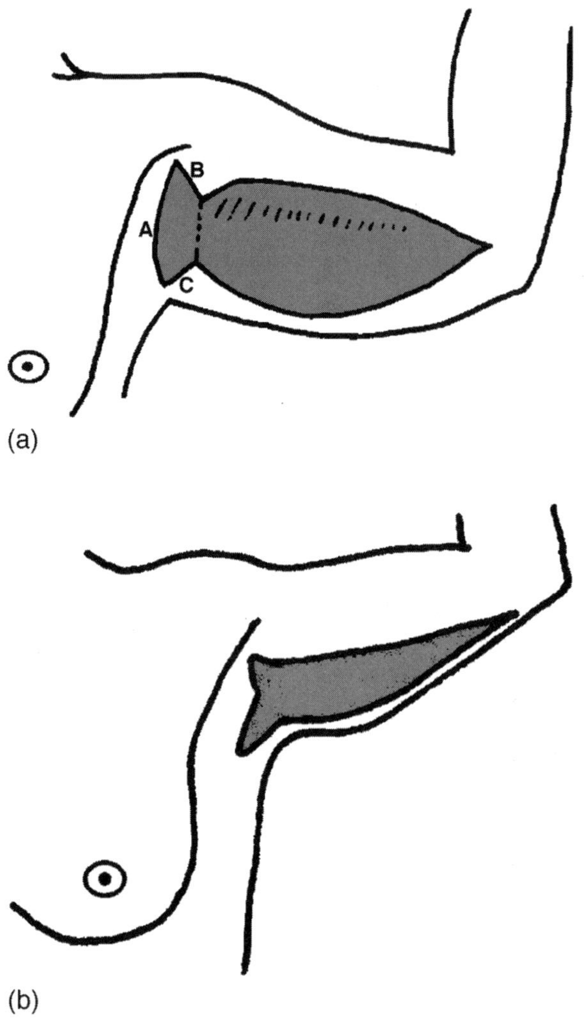

Figure 1 (a) The Lockwood brachioplasty. The lengths of lines A and B should equal the length of line C. Excised area is shaded. (b) Brachioplasty markings with axillary "fishtail." Excised area is shaded. This technique may prevent axillary retraction.

The point that produces the best correction of arm ptosis is used. A longitudinal ellipse, marked along the inner arm, spans the lateral line of the axillary ellipse and the medial epicondyle. The superior line of the ellipse is drawn 4 cm above and parallel to the medial bicipital sulcus. The inferior line is estimated based on the vertical length of redundant skin and fat.

3. A variety of other brachioplasty incisions have been successfully used. Regnault employs a "fishtail" incision in the axilla (Fig. 1b), in order to prevent axillary retraction that may result from a T-type incision.
4. Regardless of the incision used, it should not be visible posteriorly and should not cross the elbow joint.

C. Operation

1. The axillary ellipse of skin and fat are excised to the level of the axillary fascia. The incision is then temporarily closed with towel clips, and the superior incision along the arm is made. A flap is elevated inferiorly in a plane just above the brachial aponeurosis to the resection estimate, and the redundant tissue is resected.
2. Permanent sutures are used to anchor the SFS along the lateral line of the axillary ellipse to the axillary fascia.
3. The wound is then repaired in layers over a drain in the axilla. The SFS and remaining layers of the arm incision are repaired similarly.
4. Liposuction can be performed at this time if necessary.
5. One of the most common problems associated with the procedure is that the incisional scars are prone to widening.

III. MEDIAL THIGH LIFT

A. Indications

1. Those patients with contour deformities due to skin and soft-tissue laxity affecting the upper, inner thigh region can benefit from this procedure. If the skin in this area is relatively flaccid and excessive, liposuction alone is relatively contraindicated.
2. The medial thigh lift removes an elliptical strip of skin and fat from the superior medial thigh. The resulting scar is confined to the groin and thigh-perineal crease and is designed to be concealed by a bathing suit.
3. The amount of vertical redundancy is usually 8–12 cm.

B. Markings

1. The patient is marked in the standing position (Fig. 2).

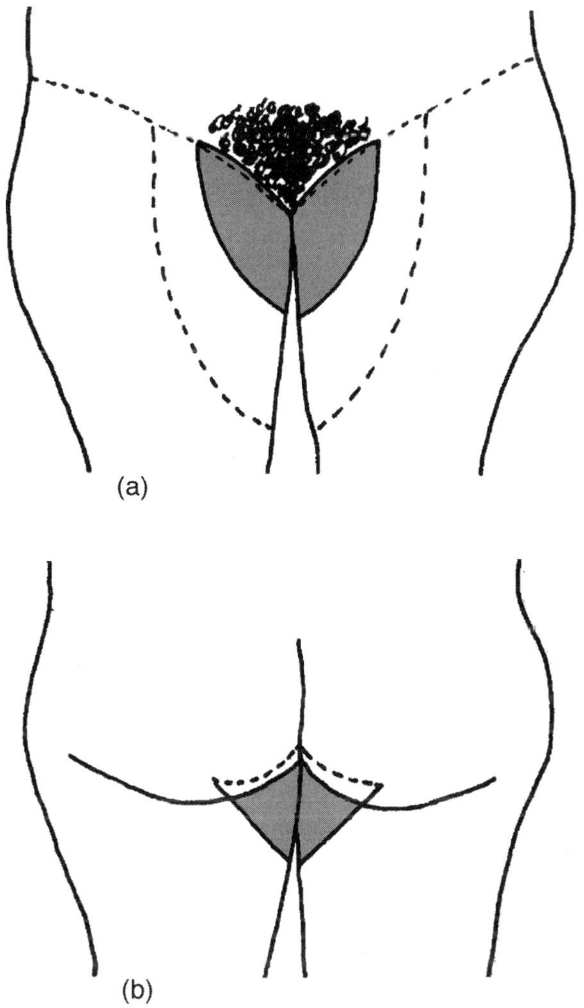

Figure 2 The medial thigh lift corrects contour deformities along the superior and medial thighs. Dotted lines, along the inner thighs and gluteal regions, border the contour deformities. The shaded area is excised.

2. The superior incision is marked in the perineal-thigh crease.
3. The anterior extent should stop medial to the femoral triangle in order to avoid damage to lymphatic channels.
4. Posteriorly, the incision continues to the medial buttock crease.

C. Operation

1. The patient is placed in supine position with the thighs abducted and hips flexed. The medial thigh is liposuctioned (possibly combined with trochanteric liposuction). Redundant tissue is resected and Colles' fascia is identified medially, deep to the thigh-perineal crease.
2. No undermining or drains are necessary.
3. Deep sutures placed to approximate the SFS to Colles' fascia prevent lateral traction on the vulva. The remainder of the wound is closed in layers.
4. Complications include wide scars, distortion of the vulva, and recurrence. Anchoring the undermined thigh flaps to the perineal or Colles' fascia has helped to minimize these complications.

IV. TRANSVERSE FLANK-THIGH-BUTTOCK LIFT

A. Pathophysiology and Indications

1. The transverse flank-thigh-buttock lift allows for an improved contour of the lateral thighs, hips, and buttocks.
2. The technique involves transverse resection of redundant inferior trunk and thigh skin and fat, with scars designed to be covered by a bathing suit. Resected tissue is within the watershed area between the major vascular territories of the inferior trunk and gluteal regions. Oblique incisions across the buttocks, used by Pitanguy, transect the dominant (superior gluteal) vascular territory and are avoided.
3. Indications include trunk and thigh laxity, buttock ptosis, and trochanteric contour deformities.
4. This procedure can be combined with an abdominoplasty in selected patients.

B. Markings

1. Bathing suit lines are marked while the patient stands with the feet 12 inches apart (Fig. 3).
2. The reference line (line of final closure) is marked 2 cm below the superior bathing suit line.
3. The resectional ellipse extends from or near the posterior midline to the inguinal or pubic areas anteriorly.

C. Operation

1. The patient is placed in lateral decubitus position with foam wedges between the thighs to keep the

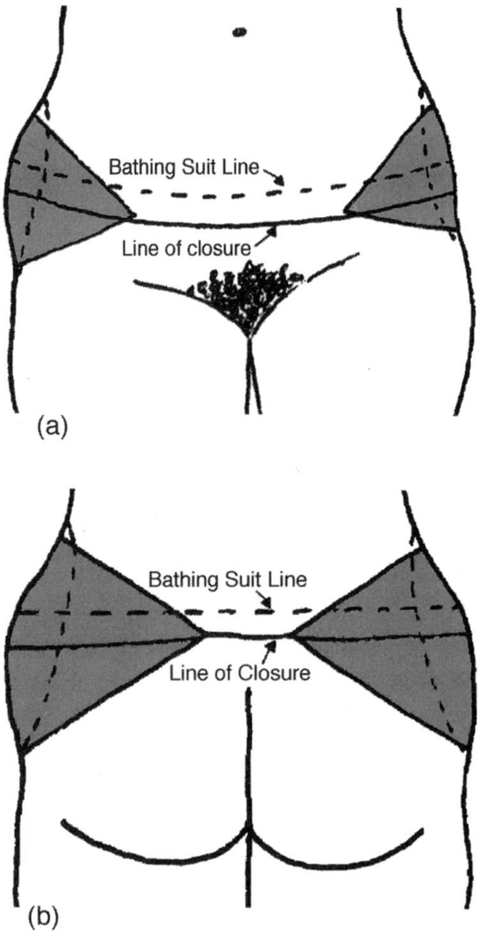

Figure 3 The transverse flank-thigh-buttock lift provides contour improvement in those patients with thigh and trunk laxity, buttock ptosis, and trochanteric deformities. The reference (line of closure) and superior bathing suit lines are depicted. Vertical dotted lines along the hips border the contour abnormalities. The shaded area is excised. The position of the line of closure is within the area covered by a high-cut bathing suit.

knees 10–12 inches apart. Liposuction is performed if needed.

2. Incision along the reference line is made, followed by elevation of the superior flap in the plane deep to the SFS. Undermining the inferior flap is performed to the greater trochanter level.
3. In the inguinal region, undermining should include the area parallel and inferior to the inguinal ligament for improved lifting of the anterior thigh.
4. Redundant tissue is removed from the superior and inferior flaps, and the wound is repaired in a moderately overcorrected position.
5. The wound is closed in layers, including SFS. The SFS is sutured to underlying fascia anterior to anterior superior iliac spine. Liposuction can be used to equalize the thickness of the flaps.
6. Superiorly or inferiorly based deepithelialized flaps may be useful to correct supratrochanteric depressions, producing a more youthful and rounded contour.
7. Sitting is not allowed for 4 weeks in order to reduce tension on the suture line.

V. LOWER BODY LIFT

A. Pathophysiology and Indications

1. This procedure combines the medial thigh and transverse flank-thigh-buttock lifts.
2. It is indicated for patients with laxity of the entire lower trunk and thighs, and corrects mild epigastric and hypogastric laxity without direct surgical undermining or umbilical transposition. For severe abdominal wall laxity, a standard abdominoplasty can be performed 3–4 months prior to a lower body lift. Patients of relatively normal weight with significant soft-tissue laxity and a positive hip pinch test are ideal candidates.
3. Incisions are placed within bathing suit lines, between the major vascular territories of the abdomen and thighs.

B. Markings

1. The planned line of closure begins in the thigh-perineal crease, coursing vertically along the lateral mons pubis and curving laterally to lie 2–3 cm below the top of the bathing suit outline (Fig. 4a).
2. Posteriorly, the incision curves gently downward toward the superior aspect of the gluteal crease (Fig. 4b).
3. The amount of soft-tissue redundancy superior to the line of closure is estimated with the knees 6 inches apart (usually 4–5 cm).
4. Anteriorly, soft-tissue redundancy is estimated by pulling from either side.

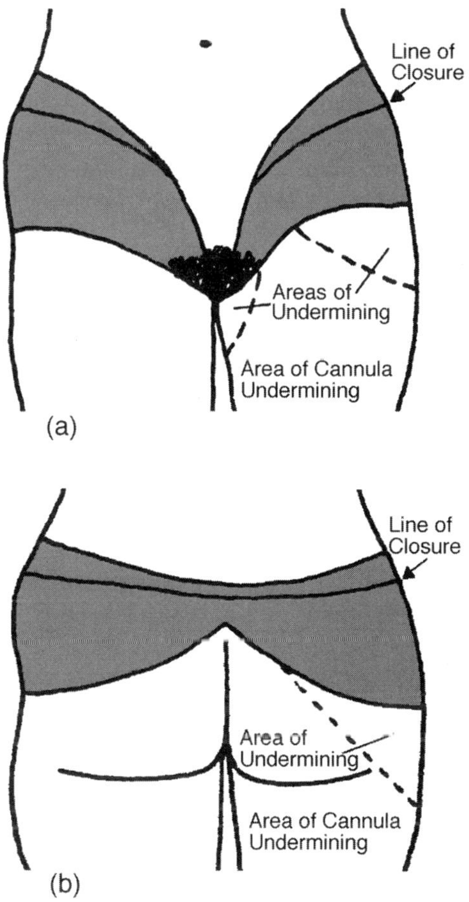

Figure 4 The lower body lift combines the medial and transverse flank-thigh-buttock lifts for resections in patients with skin and soft tissue redundancy of the entire lower trunk and thighs. The lines of closure are depicted, and shaded areas are resected. Areas of direct surgical undermining and cannula undermining (with no suction) are shown.

5. Redundant tissue inferior to the line of closure is estimated (usually 10–15 cm vertically along the lateral contour).
6. Finally, tissue excess in the inguinal and medial thigh areas is marked. The incision should end in the thigh-perineal crease rather than extending to the buttocks fold.

C. Operation

1. The patient is placed in a lateral decubitus position, with the knees held 12–15 inches apart with foam blocks.
2. Liposuction is performed if needed.
3. The incision is started anteromedially, superficial to the deep fascia, staying lateral to the femoral triangle. As the incision proceeds laterally and posteriorly, the plane of dissection is more superficial in order to preserve the superior gluteal vessels. Excess fat excision in this area is by liposuction following wound closure. The SFS is directly undermined in trochanteric and inguinal regions. A straight suction liposuction cannula (without suction) can be used to undermine the SFS circumferentially to the knee level. Following excision of redundant tissue, the wound is repaired in layers over drains.
4. The patient is then repositioned, and the contralateral resection is performed.
5. To complete the procedure, the patient is placed in the supine semi-frog leg position. Lateral mons and thigh-perineal incisions are made, preserving the femoral lymphatics as described above. Undermining and resection proceeds as in medial thigh lift.

VI. COMPLICATIONS

A. Seroma
B. Hematoma
C. Wound infection
D. Superficial wound dehiscence
E. Scar hypertrophy
F. Migration of scar
G. Contour abnormalities

Appendix A: Important People and Events in Plastic Surgery

Steven E. Greer, M.D.
New York, New York, U.S.A.
Prosper Benhaim, M.D.
David Geffen School of Medicine at UCLA, Los Angeles, California, U.S.A.
William Newmeyer, M.D.
University of California at San Francisco

Any list like this will inevitably leave out deserving people. Please excuse us in advance.

I. PLASTIC SURGERY

700 B.C.—**Sushruta**: India, described forehead flaps for nasal reconstruction

25 B.C. to 50 A.D.—**Celsus, Aurelis**: used advancement flaps

Renaissance period—the anatomical text of Vesalius "Fabrica" was published in 1543

1597—**Tagliacozzi**: Bologna, popularized the use of the upper arm pedicle flap to reconstruct the nose

625–690 A.D.—Arabian and Indian surgical practices became incorporated in Western thinking in the Roman Empire

1791—**Sommering**: observed that calvarial growth occurs along suture lines

1814—**Carpue**: London surgeon who used a technique originally performed in India to reconstruct a nose with a forehead flap in less than one hour using crude anesthesia and hemostasis

1817—**Cooper**: first to report a successful human skin graft

1818—**Von Graefe**: used the term "plastic" for the first time in association with plastic surgery in his publication *Rhinoplastik*, which described various nasal reconstruction techniques

1800s—**von Langenbeck, Bernard**: pioneer in cleft palate and jaw surgery

1827—**Mattauer**: performed the first cleft palate operation in the Western world using homemade instruments

1844—**Mirault, G.**: France, described the repair of unilateral cleft lip by using lateral lip flap

1851—**Virchow**: observed compensatory growth of the skull to allow for the growth of the brain

1861–1865—introduction of anesthesia and antiseptic techniques during the American Civil War allowed surgery to flourish

1886—**Thiersch, Carl**: innovator of skin graft harvesting techniques

1887—**Roe, John**: described the first intranasal rhinoplasty before Joseph, and later described the first endonasal approach for hump removal

1898—**Joseph, Jacque**: published *Surgical Correction of the Nose* and is considered a founder of modern aesthetic surgery

1900—**von Mangold**: described the use of rib cartilage for the correction of a saddle nose deformity

1907—**Handley**: described excisional techniques for melanoma treatment

1907—**Miller**: Chicago, published *Cosmetic Surgery: The Correction of Featural Imperfections*

1912—**Blair, Vilray P**: wrote *Surgery and Diseases of the Mouth and Jaws*

1914–1918—**World War I**: modern plastic surgery, including aesthetic surgery, takes root

WWI era—**Morestin** (general surgeon): France, used wide subcutaneous undermining and Z-plasty techniques for contractures

WWI era—**Gillies, Sir Harold**: (otolaryngologist, pupil of Morestin) Britain, "father of modern plastic surgery," established a plastic surgery medical center for the war effort to treat facial wounds and other injuries; became a founder of modern plastic surgery and innovator of numerous techniques including the tubed pedicle flap (along with Filatov)

WWI era—**Ivy, Robert** (pupil of Gillies and Blair): headed the plastic surgery team at Walter Reed Hospital for the U.S. Army

WWI era—**Kazanjian, Varaztad H.**: (D.D.S. dental surgeon and M.D.) became the first Professor of Plastic Surgery at Harvard and applied his dental knowledge to the treatment of facial injuries; completed his MD in Boston at age 42 and became a plastic surgery pioneer

WWI era, 1917—**Blair, Vilray P** (general surgeon, collaborator with Gillies): headed the plastic surgery team at Jefferson Barracks for the army; set the stage for multidisciplinary approaches to complex facial problems, described the delay phenomenon in flap design, and later set up the premier U.S. plastic surgery training center in St. Louis; founder of the American Board of Plastic Surgery

Post-WWI peacetime era—**Gillies, Harold**: renowned as a reconstructive surgeon, also performed breast reductions and other cosmetic procedures

Post-WWI peacetime era, 1930–1935—**Safian and Aufricht**: learned from Jacque Joseph and brought rhinoplasty techniques to the United States

1919—**Davis, John Staige**: published the first American textbook in plastic surgery, *Plastic Surgery—Its Principles and Practice*, one of the first to specialize completely in plastic surgery

1921—**American Association of Oral and Plastic Surgeons** is formed, including only members that had both dental and medical degrees. This organization later became the American Association of Plastic Surgeons

Post-WWI peacetime era—"aesthetic" and "cosmetic" surgery further develops as a branch of plastic surgery

1928—**Smith, Ferris**: the landmark text *Reconstructive Surgery* was published in the United States

1929—**Blair and Brown**: published an important work on split-thickness skin grafting

1930s, 1940s—**Bunnell, Sterling**: pioneered reconstructive hand surgery

1930—**Aufricht, Gustave**: organized unofficial dinner meetings of plastic surgeons as a precursor to the official formation of the American Society of Plastic and Reconstructive Surgeons (ASPRS)

1932—**Maliniac, Jacques**: convened the first official meeting of the American Society of Plastic and Reconstructive Surgeons; Gustave Aufricht, Lyndon Peer, and Clarence Straatsma were also integral to the early success of the ASPRS

1936—**European Society of Reconstructive Surgery** is formed

1937—**Padgett** (pupil of Blair) **and Hood** (engineer): developed the Padgett-Hood dermatome for skin grafting, presented in 1939

1937—**Blair, Vilray P**: spearheaded the formation of the American Board of Plastic Surgery; The American Board of Medical Specialties officially recognized plastic surgery

1939—**Fomon**: (not a plastic surgeon) published *Surgery of Injury and Plastic Repair*, which became a popular textbook among surgeons

1939–1945—**World War II**: subspecialization takes root; elective and cosmetic surgery became more common

1940—**Brown, James Barrett** (pupil of Blair): performed extensive research on skin homotransplantations, setting the stage from modern-day transplant surgery

1941—The name of the American Association of Oral & Plastic Surgeons formed in 1921 was changed to the American Association of Plastic Surgeons

1942—**Converse, John Marquis**: developed the scalping flap for nasal reconstruction from WWII experiences; became the Chief of Plastic Surgery at The Institute of Reconstructive Plastic Surgery of NYU and the first president of the International Transplant Society

1942—**Cannon, Bradford**: treated victims of the famous Coconut Grove fire, making large advancements in burn management

1942—**Hofer, Alex**: described cadaver work with the genioplasty osteotomy

1943—**Medawar and Gibson**: laid the foundation for immunology and transplantation; Medawar won the Nobel Prize in 1960

1944—**Brown, James Barrett**: Head of Plastic Surgery for the U.S. Army in Europe and headed the plastic surgery effort at Valley Forge Hospital to care for the injured during and after World War II

1946—**Aufricht, Gustave**: formed the journal entitled *Plastic and Reconstructive Surgery* (first issue published July 1946); Warren Davis was the first editor; Maliniac was intentionally left out

1948—The *British Journal of Plastic Surgery* was published

1949—**Converse and Kazanjian**: publish the landmark *Surgical Treatment of Facial Injuries*

1940s–1980s—**Converse, John Marquis** (pupil of Kazanjian): received his M.D. in France and trained at Massachusetts General Hospital and at the Massachusetts Eye and Ear Infirmary; wrote the 7-volume text *Reconstructive Plastic Surgery* (with McCarthy and Littler), now referred to as "the bible of plastic surgery"; founded the prestigious Institute for Reconstructive Plastic Surgery at New York University Medical Center

1949—**Maliniac, Jacques**: initiated the ASPRS and later created the Educational Foundation of the ASPRS, now known as the Plastic Surgery Educational Foundation

1954—**Murray, Joseph E.**: as a plastic surgeon, he performed the first human kidney transplantation between identical twins; later developed the first immunosuppressant, azathioprine, and won the Nobel Prize in Medicine in 1990

1955—**Millard Jr., Ralph D.** (pupil of Gillies and Brown): Received M.D. from Harvard and began in pediatric surgery until WWII interrupted his training; described his rotation advancement lip flap repair of the unilateral cleft lip and wrote the classic *Cleft Craft*

1955—**The International Confederation of Plastic and Reconstructive Surgery** was founded in Stockholm

1960—**Brown, Adolph**: first plastic surgeon to describe the phenol deep peel formula from the Miami estheticians

1961—**Baker and Gordon**: popularized a deep chemical peel using phenol formulas from Miami aestheticians

1963—**Cronin, Thomas and Gerow, Frank**: introduce successful prototype for the silicone breast implant

1964—**Converse and Wood-Smith**: popularized the osseous genioplasty

1967—**The American Society for Aesthetic Plastic Surgery** was founded

1967—**Pitanguy, Ivo**: further described the modern abdominoplasty

1967—**Tessier, Paul L**: described surgical principles for hypertelorism repair and later became the pioneer of modern craniofacial surgery; used the multidisciplinary craniofacial team approach

1967—**Converse, John Marquis**: elected president of the International Transplantation Society for his work on immunology

1970s—**McCarthy, Joseph** (pupil of Converse and Tessier) **and Marchac** (pupil of Tessier): developed techniques promoting infant craniofacial surgery

1970s—**Tessier, Paul L**: Introduced the term and concept of the SMAS layer

1970s to present—**Buncke, Harry J.**: Canadian-born and now in California, he pioneered microsurgery; also a pioneer in hand surgery (see below)

1972—**Buncke and McClean**: performed the first free flap (omentum)

1973—**Taylor and Daniel**: Australia, perform free flaps of the groin; Taylor was later instrumental in mapping the angiosomes of the body

1973—**Snyder, Charles**: described distraction osteogenesis of the mandible in a canine model

1974—**Skoog, Tord**: described the importance of the platysma in the facelift as a precursor to the formal description of the SMAS

1975–1976—**Sheen, Jack**: introduced the concept of supratip deformity; later formally introduced the concept of augmentation correction, rather than further reduction, for supratip deformity in secondary rhinoplasties

1976—**Tessier, Paul L**: France, described facial clefting classification

1979—**Mathes, Stephen and Nahai, Foad**: published *Clinical Atlas of Muscle and Musculocutaneous Flaps*, a landmark text that described detailed anatomy and vascular supply of the major muscle flaps now in common use

1982—**Hartrampf, Carl**: described the TRAM flap

1983—**International Society of Craniomaxillofacial Surgery** was founded

1984–1987—**Sheen, Jack**: described the importance of adequate nasal bone structure and spreader grafts to maintain nasal valve function after rhinoplasty surgery

1990s—**McCarthy, Joseph** (pupil of Converse): pioneered craniofacial distraction osteogenesis by clinically applying the principles in humans, thereby creating an alternative to conventional osteotomies and autogenous bone grafting; co-author and later editor of the "bible" of plastic surgery (see Converse above)

1989–1990—**Jurkiewicz, Maurice**: served as President of the American College of Surgeons; started the plastic surgery program at Emory; his pupils include Vasconez, McGraw, Nahai, and Mathes

1990—**Murray, Joseph**: work in transplant immunology led to the first successful renal transplant in 1954; was awarded the 1990 Nobel Prize for medicine (shared with Edward Thomas)

1997—**Ganske, Greg** (pupil of Murray): first plastic surgeon elected as a United States Congressman (Iowa)

II. HAND SURGERY

1834—**Dupuytren, Guillaume**: described operation for palmar fibromatosis and classified burns according to depth

1834—**Bell**: published treatise on the hand

1867—**Duchenne, Guillaume**: wrote *The Physiology of Motion* that described the neuroanatomy and physiology of the arm and hand

1881—**von Volkman, Richard**: published his first article on ischemic contracture of the hand

1868–1940—**deQuervain, Fritz**: described deQuervain's tenosynovitis of the 1st dorsal extensor tendon compartment

1871–1953—**Kienbock, Robert**: described Kienbock's disease (avascular necrosis of the lunate)

1879–1942—**Kirschner, Martin**: developed Kirschner wires

1879–1952—**Tinel, Jules**: described Tinel's sign in cases of compression neuropathy and nerve regeneration following nerve injury

1882–1957—**Bunnell, Sterling** (general surgeon): the most prominent pioneer of reconstructive hand surgery; wrote the first definitive textbook on hand surgery, *Surgery of the Hand*, that guided surgeons in WWII and for the next 30 years; in 1944, asked by Surgeon General of the U.S. Army to set up regional hand centers in the United States to treat patients whose hands had been mangled in the course of military duty in World War II (see below) (9 such centers widely spread throughout the country were organized under Bunnell's direction)

1891—**Nicoladini**: Italy, pioneered thumb reconstruction

1912—**Kanavel, Alan** (general surgeon): described the synovial sheaths of the hand and numerous infectious conditions in his *Infections of the Hand*; started the "Chicago school" succession of influential hand surgeons from Northwestern University; a president of the American College of Surgeons; he and Bunnell became two of the pioneers of hand surgery

1913—**Lexer, Erich**: Germany, performed a toe-to-hand transplantation

1914–1918—World War I

1920—**Wood-Jones**: Britain, published his book on the anatomy of the hand

WWI to 1940s—**Koch, Sumner**: second of the "Chicago school," established the Hand Clinic at Cook County Hospital, studied wound healing of tendons and the hand

WWI to 1950s—**Mason, Michael**: followed Koch in the "Chicago school" lineage, wrote the *Rate of Healing of Tendons*

1930s—**Steindler, Arthur and Mayer, Leo**: made important contributions to the field of tendon transfers in the late 1930s with seminal papers on the topic

1930s—**Brand, Paul**: worked in India and Carville, Louisiana, for many years with leprosy patients; studied tendon transfers scientifically and made major contributions over many years

1939–1945—**World War II**: more hand injuries seen than in WWI; birth of modern hand surgery

WWII era—**Allen, Harvey**: followed Mason in Chicago, began the practice of early burn excision and used the principles learned in WWII

1940s–1960s—**McIndoe, Archibald** (pupil of Gillies): New Zealand, applied plastic surgery techniques to hand burn reconstruction

1940s—**Littler, J. William** instrumental in bringing hand surgery into the specialty of plastic surgery

1944—**Bunnell**: sets up regional hand centers

1946—**Boyes, Joseph**: American Society for Surgery of the Hand (ASSH) was founded in Chicago at the suggestion of Dr. Bunnell, under the organizational skills of Joseph H. Boyes, M.D.; there were 35 founding members; Dr. Bunnell was the first president of the organization

1947—**Shaw and Payne**: developed the abdominal flap for hand coverage

1953—**Littler, J. William**: presented his work on digital transfer based on a neurovascular pedicle

1960s—**Dieter Buck-Gramcko**: expanded on the work by Littler on digital transfers when he treated a large number of children with thalidomide-induced absent thumbs by index finger pollicization

1962—**Malt**: performed first successful arm replantation

1960s—**Phalen, George**: reported treatment of a large series of carpal tunnel syndrome cases in the middle 1960s and gave us the Phalen test, one of the standard diagnostic maneuvers used in the physical examination for this problem

Late 1960s—**Swanson, Alfred B.**: introduced the silastic implant used as a flexible prosthetic spacer to substitute for joints damaged by rheumatoid arthritis and other joint-destroying problems; despite problems with some of these implants (the carpal bones), his PIP and MCP implants have withstood the test of time, and the derivatives of these first implants are still the most commonly used ones today

1967—**Kleinert, Harold and Kutz, Joseph**: primary flexor tendon repairs were performed rarely until these two reported a large series of such repairs with very good results at the ASSH meeting in 1967; old-school hand surgeons challenged the work, but the results were indisputable and this has become the standard of treating acute flexor tendon injuries

1972—**Hanno, Millesi**: building on the work of Sir Herbert Seddon and Sir Sydney Sunderland, Millesi and coworkers gave us the idea of using carefully placed nerve grafts to achieve a tension-free method to overcome median and ulnar nerve deficits

Late 1960s and early 1970s—**McFarlane, Robert**: Canadian hand surgeon and former ASSH president; detailed and delineated the anatomy of the pathological fascia in Dupuytren's disease; promulgated the proper surgical concept of treating Dupuytren's disease

Late 1960s—**The Swiss ASIF/AO group**: standardized the introduction of reliable, solid internal fixation, which allowed the active mobilization of soft tissues during bone healing; ASIF (Association for the Study of Internal Fixation)/AO (Arbeitsgemeinschaft für Osteosynthesefragen

1960s to current—**Buncke, Harry**: extensive experimental and clinical work in microsurgery and digital replantation from the 1960s to the present time

1960s to current—**Linscheid, Ronald and Dobyns, James**: both Mayo Clinic surgeons who have done extensive work about the wrist for many years and coined the well-known terms DISI (dorsal intercalary segmental instability) and VISI (volar intercalary segmental instability); other major contributions in this field made by Julio Taleisnik and David Lichtman

1982—**Green, David**: the first edition of *Operative Hand Surgery*, conceived and edited by David P. Green, published; now in its fourth edition and several assistant editors have been added; the major textbook in hand surgery today

1998—**Dubernard, Jean-Michel**: attempted the first hand transplantation; patient refused to adhere to the immunosuppression regimen and the transplanted hand was subsequently amputated

1999—**Breidenbach, Warren**: performed the first U.S. hand transplant in Louisville, Kentucky

Appendix B: The Cardiac History and Physical and Electrocardiography (ECG) Interpretation

Charles A. Bush, M.D.
The Ohio State University College of Medicine, Columbus, Ohio, U.S.A.

I. CARDIOVASCULAR HISTORY

A. Symptoms

- Chest pain: discomfort, tightness, unusual awareness or similar symptoms likely to occur with exertion or emotional stress; most frequently located substernal, epigastric, shoulder, neck, jaw or either arm. Indigestion may be an ischemic symptom.
- Dyspnea: subjective awareness of shortness of breath may be related to pulmonary congestion, low cardiac output or active ischemia.
- Fatigue: lack of energy may indicate chronic low output state
- Palpitations: awareness of heartbeat may indicate rhythm disturbance
- Syncope: loss of consciousness; dizziness, light-headedness suggest cardiac rhythm disturbance or intermittent hypotension.

B. Past medical history and risk factors

- History of myocardial infarction, bypass surgery or angioplasty
- Known congenital or acquired heart murmur
- Risk factors of current or remote smoking, diabetes, hyperlipidemia, hypertension, or family history of any cardiac events

II. CARDIOVASCULAR PHYSICAL EXAMINATION

A. Vital signs: The most significant marker of an unstable cardiovascular system

- Blood pressure: alert levels, systolic under 100 or over 170 and diastolic pressure over 86.
- Heart rate: alert levels below 60 or above 100, be aware of any irregularity
- Respiratory rate: alert levels below 8 or over 14, be aware of depth of respiration.

B. Pulses: Characterize bilateral carotid, brachial, radial, femoral, posterior tibial and dorsalis pedal pulses on a 0 to 4+ scale.

C. Venous pressure: Venous pressure identified in the neck is abnormal if the patient is sitting a 45 degree angle or greater.

D. Apex impulse: Location should be within the mid-clavicular line and the size no greater than one fingertip.

E. Heart sounds: Identify S-1 and S-2. Sounds difficult to hear may be related to low cardiac output or pulmonary disease. Listen for third or fourth heart sounds that could be gallop sounds or valve opening sounds.

F. Murmurs: Systolic murmurs may or may not be indicative of pathology. A 'holosystolic' murmur is heard through the second heart sound. Any diastolic murmur is pathologic.

- Apex murmurs:

  late systolic-mitral valve prolapse (MVP) frequently with one or more mid-systolic clicks

  holosystolic-ventricular septal defect, mitral regurgitation

  diastolic-mitral stenosis

- Right and/or left sternal border murmurs:

  systolic-aortic stenosis (transmitted to neck, decrescendo)

  diastolic-aortic valve insufficiency, pulmonic valve insufficiency

H. Pulmonary exam: Dullness at bases may indicate pleural effusion. Rales or crackles may indicate pulmonary congestion.

III. ELECTROCARDIOGRAPHY (ECG) INTERPRETATION

The first assessment is a brief overall evaluation of the rate, rhythm, and vectors. Abnormalities are noted and evaluated in detail on the second assessment. All electrocardiograms are recorded in standard fashion with the horizontal axis measuring time. Each millimeter of paper (1 little box) represents 0.04 seconds. The vertical axis measures voltage with each millimeter representing 1 millivolt.

A. Determine rate: If rhythm is regular, it is determined by the formula: 60 divided by the time between R-R waves in seconds (multiply the number of little boxes between beats by 0.04) equals heart rate. Estimation method: 1 big block between beats is 300 bpm, 2 big blocks is 150 bpm, then 100, 75, 60, 50 bpm.

B. Determine rhythm: A single P wave must precede every QRS complex by a constant interval for the rhythm to be a sinus mechanism. Any other rhythm requires an in-depth evaluation during the second assessment to determine the exact rhythm.

- Abnormal rhythms

  Atrial fibrillation: no identifiable P waves, irregular RR intervals, inconsistent fluctuation of the baseline. Ventricular response rate is likely to be rapid (140–160)

  Atrial flutter: no identifiable P waves. The baseline has a 'sawtooth' appearance with flutter waves at rate of 200 or greater. QRS complexes are variably conducted usually in a repeating pattern.

  Ventricular tachycardia: Wide complex (QRS duration 0.12 seconds or greater) tachycardia. Ventricular rate usually greater than 80. P waves not defined or bear no relationship to QRS complex.

  Ventricular fibrillation: No definable P waves or QRS complexes. Inconsistent but continuous electrical activity identified.

C. Measure intervals:

- P-R interval is measured from the onset of the P wave to the onset of the QRS complex. Normal range is 0.16 to 0.22 seconds.
- QRS duration is measured from the initial deflection from baseline to the final return to baseline. Normal range is 0.06 to 0.09 seconds.
- QT interval is measured from the onset to the QRS complex to the end of the T wave and must be corrected for heart rate. Usually the QT interval should be about 0.4 seconds with heart rates between 60 and 80. A general rule is that the QT interval should always be less than half of the RR interval. The corrected QT interval normal range is 0.35 to 0.45 seconds.

D. Determine vectors:

- Frontal plane axis determination requires knowledge of the hexagonal reference system where Lead 1 'points' to the left side and is the 0 degree point, AVF 'points' to the foot and is the 90 degree point.
- QRS vector: (frontal plane axis) is normally between −30 and +100 degrees. It is easily determined by identifying if the QRS complex in leads 1 and AVF are both net positive deflections (the distance in little blocks above the isoelectric line is greater than the distance below it). If so, then the

QRS vector must be between 0 and 90 degrees and normal. Any axis less than −30 is left axis deviation or greater than + 100 is right axis deviation.

- Horizontal plane axis QRS vector: (determined by R wave progression in precordial leads. The 'transition zone' from a net negative to a net positive QRS complex usually occurs between leads V3 and V4. The QRS vector will be either more anterior or more posterior depending on shift of that transition zone.
- T wave vector: should be within 45 degrees of the QRS vector in both planes indicating that depolarization and repolarization vectors are similar.
- Ventricular Hypertrophy:

  Left ventricular hypertrophy: Increased precordial voltage, left axis deviation (QRS vector −30 degrees or less), T waves inverted, ST segment depression with downsloping ST segment. Single criterion is voltage in AVL exceeds 11 millivolts.

  Right ventricular hypertrophy: QRS vector towards the right (right axis deviation + 100 degrees or more), prominent anterior forces in V leads (prominent R waves in V1, V2).

E. Identify Q waves:

- The duration of the Q wave is more significant than its depth. An initial negative deflection of 0.04 seconds or greater is highly significant. Q wave location correlates highly with location of infarction. Q waves indicative of infarction should be 'grouped' to reflect infarction of a myocardial wall. An isolated Q wave to a single lead is likely not significant. Short duration Q waves (less than 0.02 seconds) may not indicate infarction. The only lead where a Q wave is normal is AVR.
- Abnormal conduction

  1st degree heart block: prolonged PR interval

  2nd degree heart block:

  Mobitz 1: progressively longer PR intervals with eventual non-conducted sinus beat (dropped QRS)

  Mobitz 2: repetitive non-conducted sinus beat with 2:1, 3:1 or similar conduction

  3rd degree heart block: (complete heart block) no sinus beats are conducted. QRS complex originates in the junctional tissue (narrow complex) or the ventricle (wide complex)

  Left bundle branch block: (LBBB) prolonged QRS duration of 0.12 seconds or greater. Delayed left ventricular depolarization results in otherwise normal QRS pattern. The ST segment may be depressed and the T wave vector is opposite the QRS vector (inverted T waves).

  Right bundle branch block: (RBBB) The QRS duration is 0.12 seconds or greater. The right ventricle depolarization is delayed with no delay of the left. Thus the initial portion of the QRS complex is unchanged with the prolongation of the QRS occurring exlusively because of the delayed right side conduction. Thus a prominent R' wave in V1 and AVR with the RSR' pattern.

F. Identify ST segment:

- Determine if the ST segment is exactly isoelectric with the PR segment
- ST segments that originate below the baseline and are upsloping are not specific for cardiac ischemia or injury.
- ST segments that originate below the baseline and are downsloping may indicate hypertrophy.
- ST segments originating above the baseline may represent injury, pericarditis or repolarization variant.

G. Identify T wave:

- Determine if the T wave vector is within 45 degrees of the QRS vector (calculate the QRS vector and compare it to the calculated T wave vector in either the frontal or horizontal plane). If not, the T waves are likely 'inverted' or 'flipped' indicative of an abnormality of repolarization.

- Determine the morphology of the T wave. Tall or peaked T waves are indicative of hyperkalemia or myocardial injury. Flat or absent T waves may indicate hypokalemia or other electrolyte or metabolic disturbance.

IV. ISCHEMIA, INJURY, AND INFARCTION

A. Ischemia

- T wave changes with localized T wave inversion.
- ST segment depression in a horizontal fashion is indicative of myocardial ischemia.
- ST segment that originates below the baseline and is upsloping is not specific for cardiac ischemia.

B. Injury

- ST segment elevation in a horizontal fashion is indicative of myocardial injury
- ST segment that originates below the baseline and is upsloping is not specific for cardiac injury
- ST segment originating above the baseline may represent injury, pericarditis or repolarization variant.

C. Infarction

Region	Anatomy	Coronary artery	ECG changes
Anterior	Left ventricle (LV) septum	LAD	ST changes and Q waves in V2, V3, V4, V5
Lateral	LV	LAD diagonal circumflex marginal	ST changes and Q waves in leads I, AVL
Septal	Septum	LAD	Q waves in leads V1,V2
Inferior	RV, LV, or both	RCA	Q waves in leads 2,3 and AVF
Posterior	LV	RCA circumflex	R wave of prominence in leads V1 and V2 ("posterior wall Q waves")

D. Considerations in the Management of Myocardial Infarction

Discontinuation of aspirin or anticoagulants prior to surgery may make some patients more prone to the development of acute infarction. If MI is suspected, emergency cardiology consultation or emergency monitored transport to a hospital is mandatory. The treatment objective is to reduce or eliminate myocardial necrosis resulting from infarction. Treatment includes beta-blockers, nitrates, ACE inhibitors and aspirin. In addition either primary coronary angioplasty and/or aggressive thrombolytic and anti-platelet aggregation therapy is frequently indicated. Managment must be closely coordinated between surgeon and cardiologist to maximize therapeutic benefit and minimize hemorrhagic complications.

Index